Pediatric Epilepsy Surgery

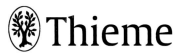

Pediatric Epilepsy Surgery

Preoperative Assessment and Surgical Treatment

Oğuz Çataltepe, MD
Associate Professor
Departments of Surgery and Pediatrics
University of Massachusetts Medical School
Chief
Pediatric Neurosurgery
Co-Director
Epilepsy Surgery
Division of Neurosurgery
UMass Memorial Medical Center
Worcester, Massachusetts

George I. Jallo, MD
Associate Professor
Departments of Neurosurgery, Pediatrics, and Oncology
Director
Neurosurgery Residency Program
The Johns Hopkins University
Clinical Director
Division of Pediatric Neurosurgery
The Johns Hopkins Hospital
Baltimore, Maryland

Thieme
New York • Stuttgart

Thieme Medical Publishers, Inc.
333 Seventh Ave.
New York, NY 10001

Editorial Director: Michael Wachinger
Executive Editor: Kay Conerly
Editorial Assistant: Lauren Henry
International Production Director: Andreas Schabert
Production Editor: Print Matters, Inc.
Vice President, International Sales and Marketing: Cornelia Schulze
Chief Financial Officer: James W. Mitos
President: Brian D. Scanlan
Compositor: Manila Typesetting Company
Printer: Everbest Printing Company Ltd.

Library of Congress Cataloging-in-Publication Data

Pediatric epilepsy surgery : preoperative assessment and surgical intervention / [edited by] Oğuz Çataltepe, George I. Jallo.
      p. ; cm.
   Includes bibliographical references and index.
   ISBN 978-1-60406-254-0 (alk. paper)
   1. Epilepsy in children—Surgery. I. Çataltepe, Oğuz. II. Jallo, George I.
   [DNLM: 1. Child. 2. Epilepsy—surgery. 3. Neurosurgical Procedures—methods. 4. Postoperative Care—methods. 5. Preoperative
      Care—methods. WL 385 P3705 2010]
   RJ496.E6P435 2010
   618.92'853059—dc22
                  2009026104

Important note: Medical knowledge is ever-changing. As new research and clinical experience broaden our knowledge, changes in treatment and drug therapy may be required. The authors and editors of the material herein have consulted sources believed to be reliable in their efforts to provide information that is complete and in accord with the standards accepted at the time of publication. However, in view of the possibility of human error by the authors, editors, or publisher of the work herein or changes in medical knowledge, neither the authors, editors, nor publisher, nor any other party who has been involved in the preparation of this work, warrants that the information contained herein is in every respect accurate or complete, and they are not responsible for any errors or omissions or for the results obtained from use of such information. Readers are encouraged to confirm the information contained herein with other sources. For example, readers are advised to check the product information sheet included in the package of each drug they plan to administer to be certain that the information contained in this publication is accurate and that changes have not been made in the recommended dose or in the contraindications for administration. This recommendation is of particular importance in connection with new or infrequently used drugs.

Some of the product names, patents, and registered designs referred to in this book are in fact registered trademarks or proprietary names even though specific reference to this fact is not always made in the text. Therefore, the appearance of a name without designation as proprietary is not to be construed as a representation by the publisher that it is in the public domain.

Printed in China

5 4 3 2 1

ISBN 978-1-60406-254-0

To the memory of
Fred
Our dear teacher, mentor, and friend

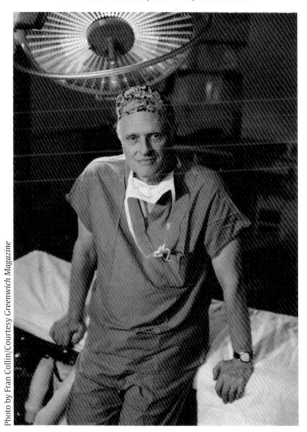

Fred Epstein
July 28, 1937–July 9, 2006

To my wife, Sule, whose love and boundless energy has made it all possible, and to my daughter, Deniz, and my son, Arda, who remind me every day how unique and precious all children are and how big the responsibility of a pediatric neurosurgeon is

To my mother and my sister for their limitless love, trust, and support

Oğuz Çataltepe

To my best friend and wife, MZ, without whose encouragement and support I would not be able to be the person I am

To my family for their support and to all the residents who taught and continue to teach me about pediatric neurosurgery

George I. Jallo

Contents

Foreword

Drs. Cataltepe and Jallo have assembled a book on surgery for epilepsy in children that is impressive in its completeness and in its list of authors. It does honor to the person to whom it is dedicated, Dr. Fred Epstein, and I am sure that he would be extremely proud of his two former fellows. The book is organized to be useful not only to the student desiring an overview of the subject but also to the clinician needing information about a certain aspect of managing a child with epilepsy.

As the editors correctly emphasize, surgery on the nervous system of children has distinctive demands and is not simply an extension of surgeries performed on adults. Children have unique conditions that result in epilepsy and the surgical management of these conditions requires unique approaches, much as does their medical management. The book extensively covers preoperative assessment and surgical techniques in pediatric epilepsy and includes numerous chapters that discuss the wide range of surgeries that can be used to treat a child with refractory epilepsy. The chapters are organized in a thoughtful manner allowing easy access to information needed by the reader and an impressive list of very experienced clinicians and surgeons has been called upon to write these chapters. This lends a considerable weight of authority to this book. Consequently, this text is a welcomed addition to the literature of pediatric neurosurgery and childhood epilepsy.

It is an honor to be asked to write the foreword to what should be a book destined to be owned and read by many. I congratulate the editors and authors for assembling and contributing to such a work.

Rick Abbott, MD
Attending Physician
Department of Neurosurgery
The Children's Hospital at Montefiore
Professor
Department of Neurosurgery
Albert Einstein College of Medicine

Preface

Epilepsy is one of the most common neurological disorders in children. The burden of epilepsy in children is not limited to seizures but also involves cognitive and psychosocial damage as well as developmental stagnation—even decline. Despite many new antiepileptic medications, approximately 20% of the children with epilepsy continue to suffer from medically intractable seizures. Surgical management of epilepsy stays as a single remaining treatment option for most of these children.

Surgical management of epilepsy in childhood is challenging in many ways and requires the special expertise of a multidisciplinary team. Although epilepsy has many common features in both adults and children, pediatric epilepsy disorders and their surgical management have many significant differences and peculiar characteristics. Cause and nature of the seizures in children are much more diverse, including perinatal injuries, stroke, and certain pediatric epilepsy syndromes such as infantile spasms. Hemispheric pathologies such as Rasmussen encephalitis and Sturge-Weber syndrome constitute a significant group among pediatric epilepsy patients, and some epileptic syndromes are seen exclusively in children but rarely or never occur in adults. Each one of these disorders has its own unique challenges as an epilepsy syndrome and requires a great deal of expertise and experience during the presurgical assessment stage, selection of surgical candidates, and surgical strategy.

Although patient age is almost never significant in adult epilepsy, it dominates the discussion in many areas in pediatric epilepsy surgery, including feasibility and reliability of certain diagnostic techniques during preoperative assessment, surgical indications, timing of the surgery, surgical approaches, and even outcome measures. Catastrophic epilepsy syndromes seen in very young ages are another significant and challenging topic relevant only in pediatric epilepsy surgery. Therefore, awareness of age-related characteristics, special paradigms, and controversies have the utmost importance in pediatric epilepsy surgery. Finally, the types and frequency of commonly performed surgical procedures in pediatric epilepsy also differ from adult epilepsy surgery. Some surgical procedures, such as hemispheric or multilobar resections, disconnections, and multistage resections are performed almost exclusively in pediatric epilepsy patients as opposed to adults. Considering that an intracranial operation in an infant is a challenge by itself, the significance of expertise and experience in performing a challenging and complex procedure such as hemispherectomy or hemispherotomy in an infant can be easily appreciated. Therefore, we believe that pediatric epilepsy surgery should not be seen as a simple extension of adult epilepsy surgery. Pediatric epilepsy surgery requires surgical expertise and experience extending to both specialties: pediatric neurosurgery and epilepsy surgery. Therefore, having experience in both surgical areas is equally significant in the management of this unique group of patients.

Over the past two decades, surgical treatment of epilepsy in children has become more widely available. Many specialized pediatric epilepsy surgery centers around the world have been established, and the number of neurosurgeons with expertise and experience in both areas has increased significantly. We have witnessed tremendous advances in diagnostic studies and significant refinement and sophistication in surgical techniques during this period. As a result, epilepsy surgery in children has become a widely acceptable, established treatment option. Therefore, we believe that more focused efforts on pediatric epilepsy surgery, including the publication of epilepsy surgery textbooks devoted to pediatric epilepsy, are needed to further support the development of this field.

We conceived this book as an attempt to integrate the many facets of the epilepsy surgeon's and the pediatric neurosurgeon's focus. Although there are several excellent and comprehensive books on epilepsy surgery, there is no pediatric epilepsy surgery book in print. Therefore, an up-to-date book devoted to pediatric epilepsy surgery that is accessible to epilepsy surgeons, pediatric neurosurgeons, general neurosurgeons, and neurosurgeons-in-training with an interest in this topic, as well as pediatric neurologists and epileptologists managing children with epilepsy, is a long-delayed effort. This book focuses on pediatric epilepsy surgery by presenting the current state of the art, highlighting the controversial issues by mainly focusing on surgical strategies and diagnostic techniques, and describing details of the widely used surgical techniques in pediatric epilepsy surgery.

We have attempted to choose all the relevant topics in pediatric epilepsy surgery and have recruited well-known experts to provide an up-to-date review of these topics. This book starts with an overview of pediatric epilepsy surgery followed by chapters describing the selection of surgical candidates, including young patients with congenital or early lesions. The first part of the book deals with preoperative assessment techniques with sections on electrophysiological, neuroimaging, and neuropsychological assessment. The second part constitutes the backbone of the book: surgical approaches and techniques. This part includes all relevant surgical epilepsy techniques. The resective surgical techniques for temporal and extratemporal lobes have been covered under separate sections with chapters devoted to different surgical approaches. The section that follows extensively covers hemispherectomy and hemispherotomy techniques with comprehensive reviews of each technique in separate chapters that are written by well-known experts on each technique. The next several sections define the surgical techniques currently used for disconnection procedures, neuromodulation procedures, and radiosurgery. The third part of the book is concerned with postoperative outcomes, and the book ends with a fourth section on advances by providing a brief overview of promising diagnostic and management techniques in three separate chapters.

Overall, we believe this book offers some unique features to the reader. Unlike other epilepsy surgery books, it was prepared by organizing related surgical approaches under separate sections, such as temporal lobe surgery, extratemporal lobe surgery, disconnection surgeries, hemispherectomy techniques, and so forth. For example, all major hemispherectomy and hemispherotomy techniques are covered in a separate section that includes separate chapters for each surgical approach. These chapters were written by the most prominent experts in these techniques, and extensive details with a large number of illustrations and high-quality photos were used to describe the procedures. The book also, for the first time, uniquely integrates the pediatric neurosurgery and epilepsy surgery perspectives in a text dedicated to pediatric epilepsy surgery.

This book was conceived by two pediatric neurosurgeons who were privileged to be trained in pediatric neurosurgery from one of the pioneers of this field: Fred Epstein. They also share another common interest: the surgical management of children with epilepsy. One of us had an opportunity to have extensive exposure to epilepsy surgery and fellowship training under G. Rees Cosgrove at Massachusetts General Hospital and Youssef Comair at the Cleveland Clinic. The other of us took over a well-known pediatric epilepsy surgery program during the early stage of his pediatric epilepsy surgery career. This background gave us a unique opportunity to develop a subspecialty interest and to embrace both fields with equal enthusiasm. It is our sincere hope that this book will fulfill our goal to integrate both aspects of pediatric epilepsy surgery and to give some additional insights to the reader managing this complex and challenging patient group.

Acknowledgments

I would like to thank a number of people who played a significant role in shaping my professional career. I wish to express my sincere gratitude to Aykut Erbengi, Tuncalp Ozgen, and all other members of the Department of Neurosurgery at Hacettepe University Hospital where I learned the nuts and bolts of neurosurgery many years ago and first developed my subspecialty interest in pediatric neurosurgery. I would like to thank Rees G. Cosgrove and Andrew Cole at Massachusetts General Hospital for introducing me to the field of epilepsy surgery. I am grateful to Youssef Comair for his exceptional mentoring and friendship during my fellowship training in epilepsy surgery at Cleveland Clinic. I am, of course, deeply indebted to the late Fred Epstein for his guidance and support during my training in a wonderful environment that he and Rick Abbott created at the Department of Pediatric Neurosurgery at the Institute for Neurology and Neurosurgery at Beth Israel Medical Center in New York. I would also like to thank my colleagues in the Departments of Neurosurgery and Pediatrics at the University of Massachusetts Medical Center. Finally, I would be remiss if I did not give credit to Arda Çataltepe for helping and motivating me with great enthusiasm during the preparation of this book.

Oğuz Çataltepe

We would like to express our sincere gratitude to our team at Thieme Medical Publishers, New York, especially to Kay Conerly, Lauren Henry, and Chad Hollingsworth for their help and patience during the preparation and publication of this book.

We also would like to express our gratitude to all our contributors that we feel very fortunate to have worked with on this project. This book would not be possible without their expertise and their lifelong dedication to treating children with epilepsy.

Oğuz Çataltepe and George I. Jallo

Contributors

Seema Adhami, MD, MRCP
Assistant Professor
Pediatrics
Division of Neurology
University of Massachusetts Medical School
University of Massachusetts Memorial Children's
    Medical Center
Worcester, Massachusetts

Tomoyuki Akiyama, MD, PhD
Clinical Fellow
Department of Pediatrics
University of Toronto
Division of Neurology
The Hospital for Sick Children
Toronto, Canada

Erich G. Anderer, MD
Chief Resident
Department of Neurosurgery
New York University School of Medicine
New York University Langone Medical Center
New York, New York

K. Srinivasa Babu, PhD
Senior Scientist
Neurophysiology Unit
Department of Neurological Sciences
Christian Medical College
Vellore, Tamilnadu, India

Torsten Baldeweg, MD
Reader
Developmental Cognitive Neuroscience Unit
University College London Institute of Child Health
London, United Kingdom

Fabrice Bartolomei, MD, PhD
Clinical Neurophysiology Service
Timone Hospital
Marseille, France

Canan Aykut Bingöl, MD
Professor
Department of Neurosurgery
Yeditepe University Hospital
İstanbul, Turkey

Jeffrey P. Blount, MD
Associate Professor
Pediatric Neurosurgeon
Division of Neurosurgery
The University of Alabama at Birmingham
Birmingham, Alabama

Robert J. Bollo, MD
Chief Resident
Department of Neurosurgery
New York University School of Medicine
New York University Langone Medical Center
New York, New York

Katrina M. Boyer, PhD
Assistant in Neurology and Instructor
Harvard Medical School
Division of Neurology
Children's Hospital Boston
Boston, Massachusetts

Oğuz Çataltepe, MD
Associate Professor
Departments of Surgery and Pediatrics
University of Massachusetts Medical School
Chief
Pediatric Neurosurgery
Co-Director
Epilepsy Surgery
Division of Neurosurgery
UMass Memorial Medical Center
Worcester, Massachusetts

Mackenzie C. Cervenka, MD
Epilepsy and Clinical Neurophysiology Fellow
Department of Neurosurgery
Division of Neurology
The Johns Hopkins Hospital
Baltimore, Maryland

Derrick Chan, BMBS, BMedSci, MRCPCH
Adjunct Assistant Professor
Department of Pediatric Medicine
Duke-NUS Graduate Medical School Singapore
Division of Medicine
KK Women's and Children's Hospital
Singapore, Singapore

Kai-Ping Chang, MD
Division of Pediatric Neurosurgery and Pediatric Epilepsy
National Yang-Ming University
Pediatric Epilepsy Surgery Group
Neurological Institute
Taipei Veterans General Hospital
Taipei, Taiwan

Patrick Chauvel, MD
Stereotactic and Functional Neurosurgery Department
Timone Hospital
Marseille, France

Harry T. Chugani, MD
Professor
Department of Pediatrics and Department of Neurology
Wayne State University, School of Medicine
Chief
Division of Pediatric Neurology
Children's Hospital of Michigan
Detroit, Michigan

G. Rees Cosgrove, MD
Professor
Department of Neurosurgery
Tufts University School of Medicine
Lahey Clinic Medical Center
Burlington, Massachusetts

Roy Thomas Daniel, MBBS, MCh
Professor of Neurosurgery
Neurosurgery Service
University Hospital Center Vaudois
Lausanne, Switzerland

Concezio Di Rocco, MD
Professor and Chairman
Pediatric Neurosurgery
Department of Neurosciences
Institute of Neurosurgery
Catholic University School of Medicine
Pediatric Neurosurgery
University Polyclinic Agostino Gemelli
Rome, Italy

Yaman Eksioglu, MD, PhD
Clinical Assistant and Educational Instructor in Neurology
Department of Neurophysiology
Children's Hospital Boston
Boston, Massachusetts

Irene Elliott, RN, MHSC, NP
Lecturer
Faculty of Nursing
University of Toronto
Division of Neurology
The Hospital for Sick Children
Toronto, Canada

Kostas N. Fountas, MD, PhD
Assistant Professor
Neurosurgery
University Hospital of Larisa
University of Thessaly School of Medicine
Larisa, Greece

James Frazier, MD
Resident
Department of Neurosurgery
The Johns Hopkins Hospital
Baltimore, Maryland

Alexandra J. Golby, MD
Assistant Professor
Radiology
Harvard Medical School
Associate Surgeon
Department of Neurosurgery
Brigham and Women's Hospital
Boston, Massachusetts

Ronald T. Grondin, MD
Department of Neurosurgery
Children's Surgical Associates
Columbus, Ohio

Michael M. Haglund, MD, PhD
Professor
Department of Surgery
Division of Neurosurgery
Duke University Medical Center
Durham, North Carolina

Lorie D. Hamiwka, MD, FRCPC
Pediatric Neurologist and Epileptologist
Division of Child Neurology
Nationwide Children's Hospital
Pediatric Academic Association
Columbus, Ohio

Chellamani Harini, MD, MRCP
Assistant Professor of Clinical Neurosciences
Brown University School of Medicine
Hasbro Children's Hospital
Providence, Rhode Island

Adam L. Hartman, MD
Assistant Professor
Department of Neurology
The Johns Hopkins University
The Johns Hopkins Hospital
The John M. Freeman Pediatric Epilepsy Center
Baltimore, Maryland

Daryl W. Hochman, PhD
Assistant Professor
Departments of Surgery, Pharmacology, and Cancer Biology
Duke University Medical Center
Durham, North Carolina

Rebecca Jacob, MD
Department of Anesthesia
Christian Medical College
Vellore, Tamil Nadu, India

George I. Jallo, MD
Associate Professor
Departments of Neurosurgery, Pediatrics, and Oncology
Director
Neurosurgery Residency Program
The Johns Hopkins University
Clinical Director
Pediatric Neurosurgery
The Johns Hopkins Hospital
Baltimore, Maryland

Prasanna Jayakar, MBBS, MD, PhD
Chairman of the Brain Institute
Director of the Neuroscience Center
Miami Children's Hospital
Miami, Florida

Pongkiat Kankirawatana, MD
Associate Professor
Department of Pediatrics
Division of Neurology
The University of Alabama at Birmingham
Birmingham, Alabama

Ahmet Hilmi Kaya, MD
Department of Neurosurgery and Department of Neurology
Yeditepe University School of Medicine
İstanbul, Turkey

John R. W. Kestle MD
Professor
Department of Neurosurgery
University of Utah School of Medicine
Chief
Division of Pediatric Neurosurgery
University of Utah Medical Center
Primary Children's Medical Center
Salt Lake City, Utah

Hyunmi Kim, MD, PhD
Assistant Professor
Department of Pediatrics
Division Neurology
The University of Alabama at Birmingham
Birmingham, Alabama

Eric H. Kossoff, MD
Assistant Professor
Department of Neurology
The Johns Hopkins University
The Johns Hopkins Hospital
Baltimore, Maryland

Ajay Kumar, MD, PhD, DNB
Assistant Professor
Department of Pediatrics and Neurology
Wayne State University School of Medicine
Children's Hospital of Michigan
Detroit Medical Center
Detroit, Michigan

Shang-Yeong Kwan, MD
Department of Neurology
National Yang-Ming University
Pediatric Epilepsy Surgery Group
Neurological Institute
Taipei Veterans General Hospital
Taipei, Taiwan

Suncica Lah, PhD
Senior Lecturer
School of Psychology
The University of Sydney
Sydney, Australia

Sandi Lam, MD
Resident
Department of Neurosurgery
David Geffen School of Medicine
University of California–Los Angeles
Los Angeles, California

Gregory P. Lee, PhD
Professor
Department of Neurology
Medical College of Georgia
Children's Medical Center
Augusta, Georgia

Marc Lévêque, MD
Stereotactic and Functional Neurosurgery Service
Timone Hospital
Marseilles, France

Frédérique Liégeois, PhD
Lecturer
Developmental Cognitive Neuroscience Unit
University College London Institute of Child Health
London, United Kingdom

David D. Limbrick Jr., MD, PhD
Assistant Professor
Departments of Neurological Surgery and Pediatrics
St. Louis Children's Hospital
Washington University School of Medicine–St. Louis
St. Louis, Missouri

Tobias Loddenkemper, MD
Assistant Professor of Neurology
Harvard Medical School
Assistant in Neurology
Department of Neurology
Children's Hospital Boston
Boston, Massachusetts

David W. Loring, PhD
Professor
Department of Neurology
Emory University School of Medicine
Atlanta, Georgia

Joseph R. Madsen, MD
Associate Professor
Department of Neurosurgery
Children's Hospital Boston
Boston, Massachusetts

Luca Massimi, MD
Assistant Professor and Pediatric Neurosurgeon
Pediatric Neurology Department
Catholic University School of Medicine
Rome, Italy

Gary W. Mathern, MD
Professor
Department of Neurosurgery
The Brain Research Institute
The Mental Retardation Research Center
David Geffen School of Medicine
Reed Neurological Research Center
University of California–Los Angeles
Los Angeles, California

Michael L. McManus, MD, MPH
Associate Professor
Department of Anesthesia
Harvard Medical School
Division of Critical Care
Children's Hospital Boston
Boston, Massachusetts

Christoph M. Michel, PhD
Associate Professor
Clinical Neuroscience
Head
Functional Brain Mapping Laboratory
Director
EEG-Core of the Lemanic Biomedical Imaging Center
Neurology Clinics
University Hospital of Geneva
Department of Fundamental Neurosciences
University Medical School
University of Geneva
Geneva, Switzerland

Ian Miller, MD
Director
Neuroinformatics
Department of Neurology
Miami Children's Hospital Brain Institute
Miami, Florida

John M. K. Mislow, MD, PhD†
Department of Neurosurgery
Harvard Medical School
Brigham and Women's Hospital
Boston, Massachusetts

Ahsan N. V. Moosa, MD
Fellow
Pediatric Epilepsy
Department of Neurology
Epilepsy Center
Cleveland Clinic
Cleveland, Ohio

Ayako Ochi, MD, PhD
Assistant Professor
Department of Pediatrics
University of Toronto
Department of Neurology
The Hospital for Sick Children
Toronto, Canada

Jeffrey G. Ojemann, MD
Professor
Department of Neurological Surgery
University of Washington School of Medicine
Seattle Children's Hospital
Seattle, Washington

Hiroshi Otsubo, MD
Associate Professor
Department of Pediatrics
University of Toronto
Department of Neurology
The Hospital for Sick Children
Toronto, Canada

Julie Pilitsis, MD, PhD
Assistant Professor
Department of Surgery
University of Massachusetts Medical School
Division of Neurosurgery
University of Massachusetts Medical Center
Worcester, Massachusetts

Charles Raybaud, MD
Professor
Department of Medical Imaging
University of Toronto
Division of Neuroradiology
The Hospital for Sick Children
Toronto, Canada

Jean Regis, MD
Stereotactic and Functional Neurosurgery Service
Timone Hospital
Marseille, France

James J. Riviello Jr., MD
Professor of Pediatrics
Department of Pediatrics
Baylor College of Medicine
Chief
Division of Neurophysiology
Texas Children's Hospital
Houston, Texas

Curtis J. Rozzelle, MD
Assistant Professor
Department on Surgery
The University of Alabama at Birmingham
Division of Neurosurgery
Children's Hospital of Alabama
Birmingham, Alabama

James T. Rutka MD, PhD, FRCSC, FACS, FAAP
Professor
Department of Neurosurgery
University of Toronto
Division of Neurosurgery
The Hospital for Sick Children
Toronto, Canada

†deceased

Didier Scavarda, MD
Pediatric Neurosurgery
Timone Hospital
Marseille, France

Johannes Schramm, MD
Professor
Department of Neurosurgery
Bonn University Medical Center
University of Bonn
Bonn, Germany

Margitta Seeck, MD
Department of Neurology
University Hospital of Geneva
Geneva, Switzerland

Hiroyuki Shimizu
Department of Neurosurgery
Tokyo Metropolitan Neurological Hospital
Tokyo, Japan

Mary Lou Smith, PhD, CPsych
Professor and Chair
Department of Psychology
University of Toronto Mississauga
Mississauga, Canada
Department of Psychology
The Hospital for Sick Children
Toronto, Canada

Matthew D. Smyth, MD, FACS, FAAP
Associate Professor
Department of Neurosurgery
Washington University School of Medicine
St. Louis Children's Hospital
St. Louis, Missouri

O. Carter Snead III, MD
Professor
Departments of Medicine, Paediatrics, and Pharmacolgy
University of Toronto
Division Head
Department of Neurology
The Hospital for Sick Children
Toronto, Canada

Sulpicio G. Soriano, MD
Associate Professor
Department of Anaesthesia
Harvard Medical School
Senior Associate in Anesthesiology
Children's Hospital Boston
Boston, Massachusetts

Zulma Tovar-Spinoza, MD
Assistant Professor
Division of Neurosurgery
State University of New York
Upstate Medical University
Syracuse, New York

Uğur Türe, MD
Professor and Chairman
Department of Neurosurgery
Yeditepe University Hospital
Istanbul, Turkey

Ingrid Tuxhorn, MD
Professor of Medicine
Epilepsy Center
Lerner College of Medicine
Case Western Reserve University
Center for Pediatric Epilepsy
Cleveland Clinic
Cleveland, Ohio

Jean-Guy Villemure
Chief
Department of Neurosurgery
University of Montreal
Montreal, Canada

John Weaver, MD
Associate Professor
Division of Neurosurgery
University of Massachusetts Medical School
University of Massachusetts Memorial Medical Center
Worcester, Massachusetts

Howard L. Weiner, MD, FACS, FAAP
Professor
Department of Neurosurgery and Pediatrics
Division of Pediatric Neurosurgery
New York University Medical School
New York University Langone Medical Center
New York, New York

Nicholas M. Wetjen, MD
Assistant Professor
Departments of Neurosurgery and Pediatrics
Mayo Clinic College of Medicine
Pediatric Neurosurgery
Saint Mary's Hospital
Rochester Methodist Hospital
Rochester, Minnesota

Elysa Widjaja, MD, FRCR
Assistant Professor
Department of Medical Imaging
University of Toronto
The Hospital for Sick Children
Toronto, Canada

Tai-Tong Wong
Professor
Department of Medicine
National Yang-Ming University
Chief
Pediatric Neurosurgery
Pediatric Epilepsy Surgery Group
Neurological Institute
Taipei Veterans General Hospital
Taipei, Taiwan

Elaine Wyllie, MD
Director
Center for Pediatric Neurology
Cleveland Clinic
Cleveland, Ohio

1 Pediatric Epilepsy Surgery: Introduction

Oğuz Çataltepe and George I. Jallo

An estimated 10.5 million children worldwide have epilepsy. The annual incidence is reported to be 61 to 124 per 100,000 children in developing countries and 41 to 50 per 100,000 children in developed countries.[1] Epilepsy, especially pediatric epilepsy, not only causes seizures but also is frequently associated with other disabilities. Almost half of all children with epilepsy have high rates of co-morbid learning disabilities, mental retardation, developmental delay, psychiatric and behavioral difficulties, and psychosocial problems. Therefore, preventing cognitive and developmental stagnation or decline in children with epilepsy is as important as achieving seizure freedom and constitutes one of the main challenges in the management of these patients. However, despite major advances and improvements in diagnostic techniques and medical management options in pediatric epilepsy, approximately 20% of children with this disease continue to suffer from medically intractable epilepsy. Surgical management is often the single remaining treatment option for some of these children, not only to control seizures but also to prevent and improve the co-morbid conditions mentioned previously.[2–7]

It is a well-known fact that the comprehensive care of children with epilepsy is challenging. Specialized knowledge of and expertise in the medical and surgical management of such patients are required. Thus, a well-coordinated, collaborative relationship between medical and surgical teams in a multidisciplinary environment is critical for successfully managing pediatric epilepsy patients. Today, many pediatric epilepsy centers are designed and organized with this collaboration in mind, although it was not the case for many years.

■ Historical Evolution of Pediatric Epilepsy Surgery

Although surgical intervention in epilepsy patients has a relatively long history, many decades elapsed before epilepsy surgery became an established and accepted treatment option for adult epilepsy patients. Pediatric epilepsy surgery has followed an even more hesitant course. For years it was performed in only a handful of centers, remaining an option of last resort in the management of children with epilepsy.

Even children with intractable epilepsy were rarely referred to specialized epilepsy surgery centers. The outcomes data derived from an early pediatric epilepsy surgery series were also discouraging.

The historical reluctance to perform pediatric epilepsy surgery stemmed from several legitimate concerns at the time, such as the unavailability of epilepsy surgery centers in many locations, poor results, and a general lack of knowledge or misinformation about pediatric epilepsy surgery. Limited data regarding the long-term effects of epilepsy surgery on children as well as epidemiologic data showing that many childhood seizures were benign and had favorable outcomes also contributed to this reluctance to perform pediatric epilepsy surgery.[8]

As a result, it took almost two decades after publication of the results of initial surgical series with pediatric epilepsy patients to see any increase in the number of centers offering surgery as a management option for children with epilepsy.[9–12] As interest in pediatric epilepsy and its surgical management gradually increased, many pediatric neurology programs established separate pediatric epilepsy sections. Gradually, pediatric neurosurgeons, along with epilepsy surgeons, started to operate on increasing numbers of pediatric epilepsy patients. Although the initial surgical series included mostly older children, the patient age gradually decreased to the point that reports of infantile epilepsy surgical cases started appearing in medical journals.[5–7,13,14] As a result, there has been a gradual, then an exponential, increase over the past 10 years in the number of centers providing surgical management as an option for pediatric epilepsy patients.

The accumulated data and reported results from the most recent surgical series are encouraging. It is now clear that surgical intervention in children with intractable epilepsy dramatically improves outcomes, providing not only seizure reduction and freedom but also resulting in improved behavior, quality of life, language, and cognitive function.[15] Thus, in a relatively short period of time, pediatric epilepsy surgery procedures have been transformed from rarely performed interventions into an established management option for children with intractable epilepsy. These developments have led many children's hospitals to establish pediatric epilepsy surgery programs. As a result, pediatric epilepsy surgery has become a very active subspecialty interest for many pediatric neurosurgeons in these programs.

■ Epilepsy Surgery in Children as a Special Expertise

Initially, the main principles behind the surgical management of epilepsy patients, starting with the preoperative assessment and extending to the actual surgical procedures, were primarily developed for adult epilepsy patients. These principles were later extrapolated and applied to pediatric epilepsy patients.[16] However, because pediatric epilepsy patients are significantly different from their adult counterparts, pediatric epilepsy surgery should not be viewed simply as an extension of adult epilepsy surgery.

Although there are many common features in the surgical management of pediatric and adult epilepsy patients, there are also many differences. Understanding these differences is of critical importance in patient management.[4,17] For example, pediatric epilepsy patients have very diverse epileptic disorders that exhibit different electrophysiological characteristics and clinical semiology from adult epileptic disorders. In addition, pediatric epilepsy patients may have developmental and psychosocial problems that must be taken into account when considering surgery. Therefore, using appropriate pediatric neurosurgery techniques and having expertise in the surgical management of children, especially infants, are as important as having expertise in epilepsy surgery.

Among pediatric epilepsy patients, infants and young children constitute an extremely challenging subset. Awareness of age-related characteristics as well as of the special paradigms and issues related to treating this patient group is an important prerequisite for ensuring good surgical outcomes. For example, the surgical management of medically intractable seizures in children is characterized by several uniquely challenging problems and requires a special approach to presurgical assessment, surgical indications, and surgical strategy. In addition, there is significant controversy regarding issues such as patient selection criteria, presurgical assessment methods, appropriate surgical indications, and the timing of surgery, as well as the appropriate surgical techniques to be used for children of different ages.

To meet these challenges, the Subcommission for Pediatric Epilepsy Surgery was formed by the International League Against Epilepsy (ILAE) in 1998 to formulate appropriate standards for epilepsy surgery in childhood. In 2003, the subcommission organized a meeting to address the following questions[4]:

1. Are the unique characteristics of children with epilepsy and their syndromes sufficiently different to justify dedicated pediatric epilepsy centers?

2. Is adequate information available to propose guidelines regarding patient selection and surgical treatment for pediatric epilepsy surgery patients?

At the end of the meeting, the subcommission agreed that the "neurobiological aspects of epilepsy are unique to children, especially the young, and as such require specific pediatric epilepsy expertise. Collectively these features justify the unique approach necessary for dedicated pediatric epilepsy surgery centers."[4]

■ Characteristics and Special Considerations of Pediatric Epilepsy Surgery

Although many aspects of epilepsy and its surgical management in children are similar to those in adults, there are significant differences and challenges unique to children, especially infants and young children. These differences become critical during many stages of the surgical management of pediatric epilepsy, starting from the preoperative assessment and extending to the surgical intervention itself. We will briefly review these areas to provide a general perspective on the subject.

Preoperative Assessment

Pediatric Epilepsy Syndromes

The causes of epileptic seizures amenable to surgery are much more common and diverse in children[1,3]: perinatal injuries; infantile spasms; hemispheric syndromes, such as Rasmussen encephalitis; and neurocutaneous disorders, such as Sturge-Weber syndrome. Some causes are seen exclusively in children and rarely or never occur in adults. Each of these disorders has its own unique diagnostic and surgical challenges as an epilepsy syndrome.

The neuropathological substrate of epilepsy and its observed frequency in children are also significantly different from those in adults. Although cortical malformations are the most common neuropathological substrate in children (23–78%), they are much less common in adults. Although mesial temporal sclerosis (MTS) in children is seen much less frequently (17–38%) than in adults, dual pathologies associated with MTS occur much more frequently in children.[1,3,4,7]

The clinical and electrophysiological spectrum and presentation of intractable, localization-related epilepsy are often heterogeneous and wide ranging in childhood. In childhood, intractable seizures can be quite atypical and poorly defined compared with the relatively well-defined clinical and electrophysiological characteristics of epilepsy syndromes in adults. Unilateral localized or hemispheric etiologies in children may present with generalized seizures and electroencephalography (EEG) patterns, progressive neurological disorders, and bilateral congenital brain syndromes.[4,17]

Some of the pediatric epilepsy syndromes seen in infants and young children are much more than seizure disorders and can be catastrophic because of the associated cognitive and developmental delay or regression. These cases are problematic, and their management requires a great deal of expertise. The seizures in these patients are also frequently extratemporal and cover large cortical areas, including the eloquent cortex. Invasive monitoring, cortical mapping, and stimulation studies may be needed more frequently in these children than in adults.

Age of Patient

Although the age of the patient is almost never a significant topic in the treatment of adult epilepsy, it dominates the entire approach to treatment in many areas of pediatric epilepsy surgery, including preoperative assessment and testing, surgical indications, the timing of surgery, surgical approaches, and outcome measures. Rapid brain maturation during early infancy and childhood is responsible for a complex evolution of clinical seizure semiology and EEG and neuroimaging findings.[4,17] This complexity makes the assessment of the clinical, electrophysiological, and imaging findings very challenging.

The naturally lower level of cognitive maturation and language development in children can be an obstacle or a limiting factor for some preoperative tests, such as the intracarotid amobarbital procedure (Wada test) or functional magnetic resonance imaging (fMRI). Also, the harmful and sometimes catastrophic effects of seizures on the developing brain in young children are a major concern, and early surgical intervention may be considered in some infants to prevent these seizures. However, some surgical techniques, such as cortical stimulation and mapping under local anesthesia and depth electrode placement, may not be feasible in young children.

Medical Intractability of Epilepsy

The criteria used to define medical intractability in children are significantly different from those used in adults. Earlier identification of medical intractability in pediatric epilepsy patients, as opposed to adult epilepsy patients, is feasible in many cases because certain pediatric epilepsy syndromes or seizure etiologies imply intractability by their very nature. These children do not need long trial periods with every major antiepileptic drug (AED). The developing brain is also much more vulnerable to the adverse effects of AEDs, making the risk–benefit assessment for long-term trials of AEDs more critical in children than in adults. Conversely, epilepsy in childhood is often not a fixed condition, and although it may evolve toward intractability in some cases, it may remit or stop spontaneously in others. Therefore, decisions regard-

ing medical intractability can be made easily and quickly in some well-defined pediatric epilepsy syndromes. However, in some cases, great caution must be exercised before deciding whether a patient is indeed a surgical candidate.

Electrophysiological Characteristics of Epilepsy

Electrophysiological evaluation of cortical activity in infants and young children is extremely difficult because of poorly defined "normal" and "abnormal" EEG patterns of the immature brain, the absence of well-defined epileptiform discharges, rapidly spreading ictal activity, and the great variability of electrophysiological seizure patterns. These characteristics make the localizing value of EEG findings for children very controversial as opposed to those for adults. As a result, defining the epileptogenic zone in the immature brain is a daunting task in many cases, one that needs to be handled with a great deal of expertise.

Surgical Indications
Harmful Effect of Seizures on the Developing Brain

The cumulative harmful effect of frequent seizures on the developing brain can be catastrophic. In addition to frequent clinical seizures, continuous postictal state and frequent interictal epileptiform discharges may cause an irritable, dysfunctional cortex and, possibly, secondary epileptogenesis. Consequently, intractable seizures and their deleterious effect on the developing brain may result in mental retardation, debilitating behavioral problems, aggression, attention deficit disorder, and hyperactivity. Although spontaneous remission of the seizures is possible, the risk of permanent neurologic, psychosocial, and cognitive impairment from their recurrence and from the adverse effects of AEDs is significant during this crucial period of brain development. Therefore, pediatric epilepsy teams must not only consider seizures when making decisions regarding epilepsy surgery but also consider the potentially harmful effects of seizures on the developing brain.

Functional Plasticity of the Developing Brain

There is a significant amount of accumulated data regarding the functional plasticity of the young brain gleaned from experimental animal studies as well as from observation of human patients after surgical resection or cerebral insults at a young age.[8] These data show that young children have a much greater potential for recovery after a cerebral injury, including surgery, and a significant capacity for reorganization of neurological function.[15] These phenomena are especially evident in the often speedy recovery of speech-related functions in young children and constitute a remarkable asset of early childhood. The functional plasticity of the young brain also makes children more vulnerable to the deleterious effects of repeating seizures, which can result in deviant or delayed development and trigger permanent changes in developing neural circuitry. It is of utmost importance that the pediatric epilepsy surgery team members fully appreciate the functional plasticity and potential of the young brain and take these characteristics into consideration when making presurgical assessments and surgical decisions.[4]

Psychosocial Factors

The psychosocial effects of seizures are much more detrimental in young children than in adults. Although this theory has yet to be proven, successful seizure control may facilitate cognitive development and may help reduce the behavioral or psychological burden of epilepsy on the child and family.[4] Therefore, the importance of early reduction of the burden of chronic epilepsy, its psychosocial benefit, and its positive effect on the quality of life in children and their families cannot be overemphasized.

Timing of Surgery

The timing of surgery is another unique aspect of pediatric epilepsy. As discussed earlier, the cumulative harmful effects of epilepsy on early brain development are a major concern in the treatment of pediatric epilepsy patients. Although consensus is still lacking, there are strong arguments in the literature supporting emerging clinical data indicating the benefits of early surgical intervention in catastrophic epilepsy.

Because many types of pediatric epilepsy syndromes are inherently medically refractory, there is no need to "prove" medical intractability before embarking on a surgical course of action. The harmful effects of prolonged seizures and the toxic effects of AEDs on synaptogenesis, brain development, and cognitive and psychosocial development bolster the argument for early surgery in pediatric epilepsy patients. Even if seizures are successfully controlled with medical treatment, frequent interictal discharges can still cause permanent changes in synaptogenesis and cytoarchitecture in immature brains and may even create a secondary epileptogenic focus.

The potential for significant recovery is highest during the period of high synaptic and dendritic density (ages 3–7 years), when the plasticity of the brain peaks.[13] Surgery performed within this time frame may help hasten recovery, and anticipated postoperative impairments may be milder. In well-selected patients, early surgical intervention may prevent the negative cognitive, psychosocial, and developmental effects of seizures. Accumulating data show the positive effect of epilepsy surgery on clinical outcome; not only is seizure control enhanced, but so are the behavioral, cognitive, and developmental domains of life.[2,4] Thus, early surgi-

cal intervention helps children to develop without further psychosocial harm and, in many cases, to maximize their developmental potential.

Nevertheless, there are significant concerns regarding early surgical intervention in pediatric epilepsy patients. The possibility of spontaneous remission is one of the main arguments against early surgical intervention because many childhood seizure disorders spontaneously remit in adulthood. Other concerns militating against early surgical intervention include the possibility of eventually achieving seizure control with AEDs, as well as the morbidity and mortality risks associated with surgical intervention in infants and young children.

Goals of Surgery

The goals of epilepsy surgery in children are somewhat different from those for adults. In addition to controlling seizures, the goals of pediatric epilepsy surgery are to prevent the possible harmful consequences of uncontrolled seizures; to prevent continued interictal activity resulting in permanent cognitive, behavioral, and psychosocial problems; to prevent secondary epileptogenesis; and to avoid the adverse effects of AEDs. However, despite the general acceptance of and expectations regarding the benefits of seizure control on the cognitive, behavioral, and psychological development of the child, it is important to keep in mind that definitive data on this matter are still pending. Therefore, the primary goal of pediatric epilepsy surgery remains limited to the attainment of seizure freedom until further data are gathered to support the beneficial effects of surgery on the other domains of a child's life.[4]

Surgical Procedures

The type and frequency of commonly performed surgical procedures used with pediatric epilepsy patients are different from those used with adults. Some surgical procedures, such as hemispheric or multilobar resections, disconnections, or multistage resections, are performed much more commonly in pediatric epilepsy patients than in adults. Hemispheric syndromes and related procedures are frequently performed in young children, even in infants, but are very rarely performed in adults. Hemispherectomy and its variations in some large pediatric epilepsy surgery centers compose up to 30% of epilepsy surgery procedures. These are challenging and complex procedures that require considerable expertise. Hemispheric and multilobar surgical interventions in infants have a higher risk of perioperative complications than any other epilepsy surgery procedure. **Table 1.1** presents data on the frequency of pediatric epilepsy surgery procedures performed in three large centers.[2]

Multistage resective procedures performed in pediatric patients with tuberosclerosis are also almost uniquely a pe-

Table 1.1 Frequency of Pediatric Epilepsy Surgery Procedures

	Cleveland Clinic[7]	University of California, Los Angeles[19]	GOSH[2]
Number of pediatric epilepsy surgery patients, n	136	198	199
Temporal procedures, %	53%	28%	44%
Extratemporal procedures, %	35%	23%	25%
Hemispherectomy procedures, %	12%	42%	32%
Other procedures, %	N/A	7%	13%

Abbreviation: Great Ormond Street Hospital, GOSH; not applicable, N/A.
Source: Cross JH. Epilepsy surgery in childhood. Epilepsia 2002; 43(suppl 3):65–70; Wyllie E, Comair YG, Kotagal P, Bulacio J, Bingaman W, Ruggieri P. Seizure outcome after epilepsy surgery in children and adolescents. Ann Neurol 1998;44(5):740–748; Mathern GW, Giza CC, Yudovin S, et al. Postoperative seizure control and antiepileptic drug use in pediatric epilepsy surgery patients: the UCLA experience 1986–1997. Epilepsia 1999;40(2):1740–1749.

diatric epilepsy surgery procedure. Tuberosclerosis has its own diagnostic challenges from the standpoint of epilepsy surgery, and multistage procedures play a significant role in the treatment of this disease complex. Another condition seen in children, Sturge-Weber syndrome, has its unique aspects as well, with affected patients requiring urgent attention in pediatric epilepsy surgery centers because of the syndrome's potentially deleterious effects, such as developmental delays and progressive hemiparesis. Rasmussen syndrome and Landau-Kleffner syndrome also appear mainly in childhood, and their management requires considerable medical and surgical experience and expertise.[4,17,18]

■ Present Status and Future Considerations

Many advances in structural and functional neuroimaging, EEG/video monitoring technology, perioperative care, and surgical technology have occurred within the last two decades, revolutionizing the practice of pediatric epilepsy surgery. The number of pediatric epilepsy surgery centers and young epilepsy patients undergoing surgery has increased exponentially. The age distribution of these patients has drastically changed and now includes infants. Also, the availability of outcomes data for pediatric epilepsy surgery patients has significantly increased, as has the use of sophisticated neurophysiological data acquisition techniques. As a result, criteria for surgical candidacy are better defined than ever

before. Previously unimaginable improvements in preoperative planning technology, such as image fusion techniques, and in the modern neurosurgical armamentarium, such as the development of neuronavigators and intraoperative MRIs, have enabled neurosurgeons to perform more precise interventions in epilepsy patients than in the past. Advances in the neurosurgical techniques used in epilepsy cases and in the surgical skill and experience of epilepsy surgeons using these techniques have resulted in increasingly sophisticated surgical procedures. In addition, remarkable improvements in pediatric neuroanesthesiology and pediatric intensive care have had a huge impact on surgical outcomes in pediatric epilepsy patients. Refined pre- and postoperative neuropsychological assessment techniques and improved data accumulation methods have provided valuable insights into the effect of current surgical interventions on the various life domains of the pediatric epilepsy patient.

These developments have opened a unique window of opportunity for pediatric epilepsy surgery. The number of pediatric epilepsy surgery centers and children undergoing epilepsy surgery has increased dramatically over the past 10 years. The involvement of pediatric neurosurgeons in pediatric epilepsy cases has also become more common, similar to the trend seen in pediatric neurology in the previous decade. As a result, pediatric epilepsy surgery has become an established, safe, and efficacious treatment modality in carefully selected children.

However, pediatric epilepsy surgery still faces many hurdles, such as the lack of consensus for identification and selection criteria for surgical candidates as well as the lack of guidelines for determining the proper timing for the surgery. Although surgical techniques have been refined and are safer than ever, many new and potentially beneficial areas in pediatric epilepsy surgery remain open to exploration and development, including new neuromodulation procedures, such as deep brain stimulation and the application of radiosurgery in children. Data on these new procedures and similar treatment modalities are very limited or are yet to be gathered. Also, many surgery-related topics have been extensively discussed for adult epilepsy patients but not for pediatric epilepsy patients, such as the application and benefits of selective amygdalohippocampectomy in children and its long-term results compared with the application and benefits of anteromesial temporal lobectomy.

■ Conclusion

Although pediatric epilepsy surgery is a well-established management option in the treatment of this highly vulnerable patient population, the accumulated data are still far from satisfactory in terms of providing well-defined guidelines and parameters. Because children, especially young children and infants, are still developing, epilepsy in this population is not a fixed but an evolving and complex process. Therefore, the selection and referral of young patients for epilepsy surgery constitute a delicate endeavor—one that needs to be handled with great care and expertise. It is necessary to maintain an exquisite balance between avoiding unnecessary surgery and inadvertently causing a patient to experience psychosocial deterioration or the adverse effects from AEDs because of unrealistic expectations of a spontaneous remission. This is the unique challenge that the pediatric epilepsy surgery community now faces and must overcome.

References

1. Guerrini R. Epilepsy in children. Lancet 2006;367(9509):499–524
2. Cross JH. Epilepsy surgery in childhood. Epilepsia 2002;43(suppl 3):65–70
3. Spencer S, Huh L. Outcomes of epilepsy surgery in adults and children. Lancet Neurol 2008;7(6):525–537
4. Cross JH, Jayakar P, Nordli D, et al. International League Against Epilepsy, Subcommission for Paediatric Epilepsy Surgery; Commissions of Neurosurgery and Paediatrics. Proposed criteria for referral and evaluation of children for epilepsy surgery: recommendations of the Subcommission for Paediatric Epilepsy Surgery. Epilepsia 2006;47:952–959
5. Wyllie E. Catastrophic epilepsy in infants and children: identification of surgical candidates. Epileptic Disord 1999;1(4):261–264
6. Duchowny M. Epilepsy surgery in children. Curr Opin Neurol 1995;8(2):112–116
7. Wyllie E, Comair YG, Kotagal P, Bulacio J, Bingaman W, Ruggieri P. Seizure outcome after epilepsy surgery in children and adolescents. Ann Neurol 1998;44(5):740–748
8. Stafstrom CE, Lynch M, Sutula TP. Consequences of epilepsy in the developing brain: implications for surgical management. Semin Pediatr Neurol 2000;7(3):147–157
9. Falconer MA. Place of surgery for temporal lobe epilepsy during childhood. BMJ 1972;2(5814):631–635
10. Goldring S. A method for surgical management of focal epilepsy, especially as it relates to children. J Neurosurg 1978;49(3):344–356
11. Green JR, Pootrakul A. Surgical aspects of the treatment of epilepsy during childhood and adolescence. Ariz Med 1982;39(1):35–38
12. Rasmussen T. Surgical aspects. In: Lee RG, ed. Topics in Child Neurology. New York, NY: Spectrum Publications; 1977:143–157
13. Adelson PD. Temporal lobectomy in children with intractable seizures. Pediatr Neurosurg 2001;34(5):268–277
14. Duchowny M, Levin B, Jayakar P, et al. Temporal lobectomy in early childhood. Epilepsia 1992;33(2):298–303
15. Depositario-Cabacar DT, Riviello JJ, Takeoka M. Present status of surgical intervention for children with intractable seizures. Curr Neurol Neurosci Rep 2008;8(2):123–129
16. Obeid M, Wyllie E, Rahi AC, Mikati MA. Approach to pediatric epilepsy surgery: state of the art. Part I: general principles and presurgical workup. Eur J Paediatr Neurol 2009;13:102–114
17. Shewmon DA, Shields WD, Chugani HT, Peacock WJ. Contrasts between pediatric and adult epilepsy surgery: rationale and strategy for focal resection. J Epilepsy 1990;3(suppl):141–155
18. Saneto RP, Wyllie E. Surgically treatable epilepsy syndromes in infancy and childhood. In: Miller JW, Silbergeld DL, eds. Epilepsy Surgery. New York, NY: Taylor and Francis; 2006:121–141
19. Mathern GW, Giza CC, Yudovin S, et al. Postoperative seizure control and antiepileptic drug use in pediatric epilepsy surgery patients: the UCLA experience 1986–1997. Epilepsia 1999;40(2):1740–1749

2 Intractable Epilepsy in Children and Selection of Surgical Candidates

Yaman Eksioglu and James J. Riviello Jr.

Surgery for childhood epilepsy is now considered an established treatment for medically refractory seizures.[1–3] Various surgical procedures are available, the choice depending on the etiology, the location of the epileptic focus, and the function of the cortex in which the focus is located. It is of the utmost importance to consider both the control of seizures and the quality of life after epilepsy surgery. If the epileptic focus is located in a cortical area subserving a critical neurological function (typically language, motor, primary sensory, or memory, referred to as eloquent cortex), and resection sacrifices this function, the result would cause an unacceptable compromise in quality of life despite seizure freedom. The best outcome, complete seizure freedom without a deficit, is possible when a single epileptic focus exists in noneloquent cortex that can undergo complete resection. The identification of the epileptic focus and function of its underlying cortex require data from multiple modalities: clinical, neurophysiological, and neuroanatomical (**Table 2.1**).

The Commission on Neurosurgery of the International League Against Epilepsy (ILAE) developed recommended standards for epilepsy surgery.[4] The ILAE also established a Pediatric Epilepsy Surgery Subcommission, which has produced criteria for the referral and evaluation of children for epilepsy surgery[5] and completed an international survey on the practice of pediatric epilepsy surgery (The 2004 ILAE International Survey: 543 children younger than 18 years of age from 20 centers).[6] A retrospective outcome study is in progress, and a prospective study is planned. This chapter reviews the multimodal data used in the selection process of surgical candidates. Subsequent chapters will discuss each technique in detail.

■ Process of Evaluation for Selection of Surgical Candidates

The selection of surgical candidates starts with an exact description of the clinical manifestations of the seizure, called seizure semiology. This is then followed by a general physical and neurological examination, basic and computerized neurophysiological testing (electroencephalography [EEG] and magnetoencephalography [MEG]), structural (magnetic resonance imaging [MRI]) and functional neuroimaging (single photon emission computed tomography [SPECT] and positron emission tomography [PET] scans), and a neuropsychological examination. The results are analyzed to determine if there is evidence of focal, multifocal, or diffuse dysfunction. Further invasive monitoring may be needed, depending on the specifics of each case. The intracarotid amobarbital procedure (Wada test), or invasive EEG monitoring, may be needed to identify the exact location of seizure onset and to map cortical function. However, noninvasive mapping may now be accomplished with functional MRI (fMRI), EEG-guided fMRI,

Table 2.1 Modalities to Identify the Epileptic Focus

Clinical	
Semiology	
Physical and neurological examination	
Neurophysiological	
EEG (interictal)	
EEG (ictal)	
MEG	
Source analysis	
Neuroimaging	CT scan
Structural	MRI (structural)
MRI: DTI	
MRI: DWI	
MRS	
Functional	
fMRI	
SPECT (interictal/ictal)	
PET (interictal)	
Additional invasive tests	
Intracarotid amobarbital procedure (Wada test)	
Invasive monitoring: ECoG Cortical stimulation	
Evoked potentials: somatosensory	
Visual-evoked potentials	

Abbreviations: electroencephalogram; EEG; magnetoencephalography, MEG; computed tomography, CT; magnetic resonance imaging, MRI; diffusion tensor imaging, DTI; diffusion weighted imaging, DWI; magnetic resonance spectroscopy, MRS; functional magnetic resonance imaging, fMRI; single photon emission computed tomography, SPECT; positron emission tomography, PET; electrocorticography, ECoG.

Table 2.2   Cortical Zones

Epileptogenic zone	Cortical area indispensable for clinical seizure generation May include portions or all of the following
Functional deficit zone	Cortical region abnormal in the interictal period Defined by neurological examination, neuropsychological examination, EEG, and functional neuroimaging
Irritative zone	Generates interictal spikes and sharp waves
Symptomatogenic zone	Cortical area that produces the ictal symptoms when activated Primary or secondarily activated from propagation of an epileptic discharge
Ictal (seizure) onset zone	Area from which the seizure is actually generated Silent, if originates from a silent cortical area (noneloquent cortex)
Epileptogenic lesion	Neuroradiological lesion causing epilepsy. Important in the presurgical evaluation, but not all lesions are necessarily the lesion causing the refractory seizures
Eloquent cortex	Cortex related to a given function For epilepsy surgery, typically refers to primary motor, primary sensory, language, or memory functions. The term *silent cortex* is a misnomer; it really means that its function is not known because the correct paradigm has not been tested.

Abbreviations: electroencephalogram, EEG.

and MEG. The seizure focus itself can consist of several cortical zones, with each modality examining a different cortical zone (**Table 2.2**).[2,3,7,8]

Possible surgical procedures include multifocal cortical resection, hemispherectomy, corpus callosotomy, and multiple subpial transection (MST). These procedures are considered with either multifocal or generalized seizures. Multilobar resection or hemispherectomy are considered when the epileptogenic zone is primarily multifocal but unilateral, corpus callosotomy is done for either a bilateral or generalized seizure onset, and MST is considered when the epileptic focus is within eloquent cortex. Neurostimulation techniques, such as vagus nerve stimulation (VNS), can be performed for patients not considered ideal candidates for a focal resection: patients with multifocal seizures, or patients with the epileptic focus within eloquent cortex, for example, or when the patient or family are not interested in resective surgery.

The selection of the appropriate treatment is determined by the presurgical evaluation. This is divided into three phases: the noninvasive presurgical evaluation is phase 1,

invasive monitoring is phase 2, and the surgical resection is phase 3. All three phases may not be needed in every patient. There are three major aims:

1. To lateralize and localize the epileptic focus
2. To determine the function of the presumed epileptic focus (brain mapping)
3. To determine which surgical procedure has the greatest chance of controlling seizures without causing a neurological deficit

■ Presurgical Clinical Evaluation

This process begins with an initial outpatient evaluation.[9] Several questions are addressed before any invasive procedure:

1. Does the child truly have epilepsy?
2. What is its etiology?
3. Is epilepsy surgery warranted for the given seizure type or epilepsy syndrome?
4. Is the epilepsy truly refractory, or are other therapies indicated before any consideration of surgery?
5. What is the possibility of remission?
6. Are the child and family prepared for surgery, including the psychological aspects of the invasive monitoring, the resection, or even its failure? (**Table 2.3**)

We find it best to review this in an outpatient visit before the admission so that the family knows what to expect and we know how to best tailor the phase 1 evaluation to the child's individual needs and expectations.

Table 2.3   Questions for the Presurgical Evaluation

Does the child truly have epilepsy?	Have pseudoseizures, vasovagal events, periodic movement disorders, and hyperekplexia been ruled out?
Is surgery warranted for the case?	Is there a metabolic or degenerative condition or benign rolandic epilepsy?
What is the underlying etiology?	Lesional, nonlesional, channelopathies, metabolic, degenerative, tumor, infection, etc.
Is epilepsy truly refractory?	Have appropriate AEDs been used to their therapeutic maximum levels?
Is remission still a possibility?	Have all nonsurgical avenues been exhausted?
How prepared are the child and family for surgery?	(Have they been counseled on the possible side effects or psychological aspects)

Abbreviations: antiepileptic drug, AED.

The epileptologist must first determine whether the initial diagnosis of epilepsy was correct. Many nonepileptic paroxysmal events are easily mistaken for epilepsy, treated with antiepileptic drugs, and ultimately referred for a presurgical evaluation. In a study of 223 children referred to a tertiary epilepsy center, 87 (39%) did not have epilepsy.[10] We have seen children referred for refractory epilepsy with other diagnoses, especially pseudoseizures, vasovagal events, periodic movement disorders, and hyperekplexia. Capturing the habitual seizure on long-term EEG monitoring excludes these conditions. Appropriate AED treatment for the seizure type or epilepsy syndrome is needed before considering surgery. If an underlying metabolic or degenerative condition is responsible for the seizures, respective surgery may not be appropriate.

Epilepsy syndromes are divided into benign or malignant. This distinction refers to the ultimate course of the actual seizures in addition to the developmental outcome. The term *catastrophic epilepsy* applies to early onset epilepsy

Table 2.4 Definition Intractable Epilepsy

Subcommission ILAE[5]	Failure of either 2 or 3 appropriate AEDs, disabling seizure side effects, or disabling AED side effects
Connecticut[12]	Failure of more than 2 appropriate first-line AEDs, with an average of more than 1 seizure per month over 18 months and not seizure free for more than 3 consecutive months in this time interval
Halifax/ Canada[13]	Two or more seizures in each 2-month period during the last year of follow-up, despite treatment with at least 3 AEDs as monotherapy or polytherapy
Holland[14]	Failure to achieve more than 3 months seizure freedom and an epileptiform EEG at 6 months after diagnosis
Philadelphia[15]	Persistence of any seizures between 18 and 24 months after onset epilepsy and despite at least 2 maximally tolerated AEDs

Abbreviations: antiepileptic drug, AED; ILAE, International League Against Epilepsy; electroencephalogram, EEG.
Source: Cross JH, Jayakar P, Nordli D, et al., International League Against Epilepsy, Subcommission for Paediatric Epilepsy Surgery; Commissions of Neurosurgery and Paediatrics. Proposed criteria for referral and evaluation of children for epilepsy surgery: recommendations of the Subcommission for Pediatric Epilepsy Surgery. Epilepsia 2006;47(6):952–959; Berg AT, Vickrey BG, Testa FM, et al. How long does it take for epilepsy to become intractable? A prospective investigation. Ann Neurol 2006;60(1):73–79; Camfield PR, Camfield CS. Antiepileptic drug therapy: when is epilepsy truly intractable? Epilepsia 1996;37(suppl 1):S60–S65; Dlugos DJ, Sammel MD, Strom BL, Farrar JT. Response to first drug trial predicts outcome in childhood temporal lobe epilepsy. Neurology 2001;57(12):2259–2264; Arts WFM, Geerts AT, Brouwer OF, Boudewyn Peters AC, Stroink H, van Donselaar CA. The early prognosis of epilepsy in childhood: the prediction of a poor outcome. The Dutch study of epilepsy in childhood. Epilepsia 1999;40(6):726–734

Table 2.5 Potential Epileptogenic Lesions

Developmental lesions
Cortical dysplasia
Hamartoma
Heterotopia
Tumors
Low-grade glioma
Ganglioglioma
DNET
Vascular lesions
AVM
Cavernous malformations
Injury-related lesions
Gliosis (CVA, trauma)
Infectious lesions
Granuloma
Parasitic cyst

Abbreviations: DNET, dysembryoplastic neuroepithelial tumor; AVM, arteriovenous malformation; CVA, cerebrovascular accident.

syndromes in which the outcome is poor unless seizures can be controlled, commonly occurring when a structural lesion causes refractory epilepsy.[11] Alternatively, children with benign syndromes, such as rolandic epilepsy, may have seizures that, although difficult to control, will ultimately remit.

The Subcommission for Pediatric Epilepsy Surgery defined refractory epilepsy as the failure of two or three appropriate AEDs, disabling side effects of seizures, or disabling side effects of medications. However, the definition of refractory epilepsy varies (**Table 2.4**),[12–15] and children considered intractable may later achieve seizure control. In a prospective, community-based study of 613 children with epilepsy, 13% of those considered refractory ultimately became seizure free and early remission periods preceded intractability in two thirds, with catastrophic epilepsy as a risk factor.[12] Other factors contributing to refractory epilepsy include cryptogenic or symptomatic generalized epilepsy, high initial seizure frequency, early onset epilepsy, and focal EEG slowing.[16]

The subcommission listed other indications for referral to a center specialized in surgical epilepsy: seizures unable to be classified as a clearly defined electroclinical syndrome, stereotyped or lateralized seizures, other evidence of focality, or a potentially resectable epileptogenic lesion evident on MRI study (**Table 2.5**). Specific disorders considered for surgical epilepsy syndromes are cortical dysplasia, tuberous sclerosis complex, polymicrogyria, hypothalamic hamartoma, hemispheric syndromes, Sturge-Weber syndrome, Rasmussen syndrome, Landau-Kleffner syndrome, and certain lesions (tumors, infarctions).

■ Presurgical Evaluation Techniques and Modalities

The presurgical evaluation varies among centers. The subcommission recommended minimal requirements: neurophysiological studies (interictal EEG with sleep recording and ictal video-EEG), neuroimaging (MRI with specified epilepsy protocol), an age-specific neuropsychological assessment, and invasive monitoring to localize the epileptogenic region or map cortical function.[5] Some centers routinely perform functional neuroimaging in all surgical candidates. The 2004 ILAE International Survey on the practice of pediatric epilepsy surgery identified 543 children younger than 18 years of age from 20 centers. The survey showed that more studies were routinely done in the United States and Western Europe than other parts of the world. All 20 centers surveyed used scalp EEG, video EEG, and MRI; 17 (85%) used PET scan; 16 (80%) used ictal SPECT; 14 (70%) used fMRI for language lateralization; 7 (35%) used MEG; and 10 (50%) used the Wada test. Fourteen centers used both ictal SPECT and PET, three centers used all tests but only one center used only EEG and MRI.[5]

Testing and Studies

Each modality identifies areas of cortical dysfunction, and some map eloquent cortex. In the ideal epilepsy surgery patient, one localized cortical area contains the epileptic focus and has no eloquent cortex. In this ideal situation, the data are all congruent to the same cortical area, and no mapping modality demonstrates that the focus is within eloquent cortex. Congruent data imply neurological dysfunction in only one area, which predicts a better chance for seizure control. Alternatively, noncongruent data suggest multiple dysfunctional areas, possibly with multifocal seizure onset, which implies a lower chance of achieving complete seizure control.[17,18]

Seizure Semiology and Neurological Examination

The ILAE classifies seizures as focal or generalized, which refers to the seizure onset, but this dichotomy alone does not lateralize or localize the epileptogenic zone. A semiology classification system was devised to better aid this process.[19] The neurological examination along seizure semiology (**Table 2.6**) helps to lateralize and localize the functional deficit zone, with the ultimate purpose of answering the question, where is the lesion?

Neurophysiology

Spikes and sharp waves on the interictal EEG identify the irritative zone, and focal slowing on EEG identifies the functional deficit zone. The ictal EEG has been considered the sine qua non for localizing the ictal onset region. Pitfalls in this lateralization and localization process are covered in Chapter 4. MEG is analogous to EEG, because it is a neurophysiological tool that identifies the magnetic fields generated by electrical activity. The MEG dipoles can be superimposed onto MRI, which is useful for localization.

Structural Neuroimaging

The ILAE has recommendations for structural and functional neuroimaging in epilepsy patients[20,21]: the presurgical evaluation[21] and functional neuroimaging.[22] A structural lesion is considered one of the best indicators of the epileptogenic zone because specific lesions have a high association with epilepsy. However, a structural lesion may not always contain the focus, or dual pathology may be present. MRI is now the procedure of choice for imaging the patient with refractory epilepsy, although computed tomography (CT) scan shows calcified lesions better than MRI (tuberous sclerosis, cysticercosis). MRI is especially useful for identifying focal cortical dysplasia, hippocampal sclerosis, and dysembryoplastic neuroepithelial tumors,[5] which may not be visualized at all on CT scan.

Certain MRI sequences and the slice orientation and thickness are better for identifying specific epileptogenic lesions. Epileptogenic tumors are seen best on T1-weighted and T2-weighted images and the fluid attenuation inversion recovery (FLAIR) sequence; mesial temporal sclerosis is seen best with thin coronal cuts, using T2-weighted and FLAIR sequences; a cortical dysplasia may be best seen with T2-weighted FLAIR sequences, especially visualizing blurring of the gray–white junctions. Gradient-echo sequences best visualize a cavernous angioma, and tumors may be seen after administration of contrast material. A phased array surface coil study performed at 3 Tesla (3T PA MRI) is preferable, because of its ability to detect and define lesions better than the 1.5 Tesla MRI.[23]

Functional Neuroimaging

Functional neuroimaging refers to studies using either metabolic or blood flow measurements to identify dysfunctional cortex, with the data presented in an anatomical view. Functional imaging is especially helpful when MRI is negative (nonlesional). These include SPECT, both ictal and interictal, PET scan, which is usually interictal, fMRI, and MRI/PET. Localization based on functional imaging presumes that abnormal cortical areas generating seizures have abnormal perfusion or metabolism and they may also identify the functional deficit zone. The epileptogenic zone and the functional deficit zone may not always be located in the same area. fMRI and MEG may also identify eloquent cortex. Each modality has advantages and disadvantages, with none being the single best modality for localizing the epileptic focus or functional cortex.[24]

Magnetic resonance spectroscopy (MRS) is a noninvasive measurement of chemical substances, especially N–acetyl-

Table 2.6   Semiology by Lobe

Temporal	Frontal	Parietal	Occipital
Hippocampus/Amygdala: Rising epigastric sensation; nausea; fear, panic; autonomic symptoms; experiential symptoms, such as déjà vu	*Lateral Frontal*: Contralateral tonic head and eye deviation; speech arrest	Positive or negative sensory phenomenon, pain, numbness, electric feeling; spreading paresthesias (Jacksonian March); desire to move, feeling of moving or loss of awareness of a body part; palinopsia	Simple or complex visual phenomenon; sparks, flashes, phosphenes; scotoma, hemianopia, amaurosis; perceptual illusions, sensation oscillation; clonic or tonic contraversion of head and eyes; palpebral jerks, forced eyelid closure
Posterior Lateral Temporal: Auditory hallucinations or illusions; vertigo, visual misperceptions; language disturbance	*Cingulate Gyrus*: Absence seizures, with CPS and complex motor gestures, GTC seizures; autonomic signs; mood changes		
	Frontopolar: Drop attacks, tonic seizures, aversive seizures (head and eyes); secondarily GTC seizures; forced ideation		
	Orbitofrontal: CPS with motor automatisms, olfactory hallucinations and illusions, autonomic signs		
	Opercular: Simple partial seizures with clonic facial movements; mastication, salivation, swallowing; speech arrest, fear, epigastric aura, gustatory hallucinations, autonomic signs		
	Motor (central lobe): Simple partial seizures with clonic movements; epilepsia partialis continua		

Abbreviations: complex partial seizures, CPS; generalized tonic clonic, GTC.

aspartate (NAA), choline, creatine, and lactic acid, which may be abnormal within the epileptogenic zone. Diffusion tensor imaging (DTI), measuring the diffusion of water molecules, identifies white matter tracts, which is helpful in surgical planning and diffusion-weighted imaging (DWI) may identify the epileptogenic zone, if performed rapidly after a seizure. EEG-guided fMRI identifies cortical areas activated by epileptiform activity, although in clinical practice, obtaining an ictal study is difficult for most seizure types, except absence epilepsy, because of artifact.

Neuropsychological Evaluation

The neuropsychological examination may identify functional deficit zones, telling "where is the lesion" and if there is focal and multifocal dysfunction. As with other modalities, the epileptic focus may be located in this dysfunctional cortex. There are also specific neuropsychological profiles for the various focal epilepsies: frontal, temporal, parietal or occipital.[25,26] The neuropsychological evaluation also identifies the individual intellectual strengths and weaknesses so that an educational plan can be developed to optimize education and help compensate for deficits, and may predict the risk of postoperative deficits, which is especially important in determining the risk–benefit ratio for the surgery.

Neuropsychological testing done during the Wada test helps to determine cerebral dominance for language, memory, and visuospatial functions. Language or verbal memory deficits suggest dominant hemisphere dysfunction, visuospatial memory deficits suggest nondominant temporal dysfunction, and deficits in both suggest bitemporal disease. The Wada is done by a team from neurology, neuropsychology, and neurophysiology. It may be difficult to perform a successful Wada test when the child has a low IQ, is younger than 10 years, or has seizures arising from the dominant hemisphere.[27]

Epilepsy causes many stresses on the child and family. These are especially magnified when epilepsy is refractory and may be further exacerbated by presurgical evaluation and possibility of surgery. If invasive monitoring is needed, the child must be cooperative enough so that safety is not compromised, and providing for safe invasive monitoring may require psychiatric or psychological intervention. We also use the neuropsychological evaluation to detect potential psychological and psychiatric problems and decide whether therapy is needed beforehand.

■ Epilepsy Surgery Conference and Invasive Monitoring

The phase 1 results are presented at the epilepsy surgery conference, usually attended by the epileptologists, epilepsy surgeons, neuropsychologists, neuroradiologists, electroneurodiagnostic technologists, and epilepsy and neurology trainees. It is best to obtain consensus regarding the appropriate surgical procedure. If the data are congruent showing a single epileptic focus located in noneloquent cortex adjacent to a structural lesion, then no further functional imaging or invasive monitoring may be needed, and the patient may proceed to surgery. One study reviewing a "streamlined evaluation" suggested that ictal EEG or ictal SPECT are not needed if MRI shows an epileptogenic lesion,[28] although this is currently not the practice.

If the focus is not clearly identified or could be within eloquent cortex, then fMRI or MEG can be done, with these results then presented. If seizure onset or eloquent cortex is not clearly localized, invasive monitoring may be needed. Usual indications for invasive EEG monitoring include the following:

1. localizing a focal seizure onset with normal or nonlocalizing imaging,
2. defining seizure onset around a potential epileptogenic lesion,
3. gathering noncongruent, noninvasive data,

4. assessing multiple lesions or multifocal interictal epileptiform activity, and
5. identifying eloquent cortex.[29]

■ Surgical Treatment and Outcome

The 2004 ILAE International Survey identified 543 children younger than 18 years of age from 20 centers.[6] Resections were done in 440 children; these were lobar or focal resections in 261 children (48%); hemispherectomy was done in 86 (15.8%); multilobar resections were done in 70 (12.9%); and VNS was placed in 86 (15.8%). Of the lobar/focal resections, a temporal lobe resection was done in 126 (23.2%), a frontal lobe resection was done in 95 (17.5%), a parietal lobe resection was done in 15 (2.8%), a lobe resection was done in 9 (1.7%), and hypothalamic lobe resection was done in 15 (2.8%).

In an outcome study of 75 children from Miami Children's Hospital, a good outcome was achieved in 92% of patients when there was complete resection of the epileptogenic lesion, if present, and the electrographically abnormal region (prominent interictal and ictal abnormalities on intracranial EEG), compared with only 50% with an incomplete resection.[30] Even in nonlesional refractory focal epilepsy, a good outcome can be achieved after complete resection of the epileptogenic zone using a multimodality approach.[31] The ILAE outcome study is in progress.

■ Postsurgical Follow-Up

The postsurgical follow-up period, with routine visits, should last at least 5 years. Visits should assess seizure outcome using a recognized scale, AED use, quality of life, and the neuropsychological status.[22] A postoperative MRI should be performed a minimum of 3 months after surgery, especially when there is surgical failure or complications.[21] To consider tapering of AEDs, we typically see the children back at 1 month, 6 months, 12 months, and 2 years, using a modified Engel Scale; perform a complete neuropsychological examination at 1 year; and depending on case specifics, consider an EEG at 6 months.[32]

References

1. Depositario-Cabacar DT, Riviello JJ, Takeoka M. Present status of surgical intervention for children with intractable seizures. Curr Neurol Neurosci Rep 2008;8(2):123–129
2. Obeid M, Wyllie E, Rahi AC, Mikati MA. Approach to pediatric epilepsy surgery: state of the art. Part I: general principles and presurgical workup. Eur J Paediatr Neurol 2009;13(2):102–114

3. Obeid M, Wyllie E, Rahi AC, Mikati MA. Approach to pediatric epilepsy surgery: state of the art. Part II: approach to specific epilepsy syndromes and etiologies. Eur J Paediatr Neurol 2009;13(2):115–127
4. Binnie CD, Polkey CE; International League Against Epilepsy. Commission on Neurosurgery of the International League Against

Epilepsy (ILAE) 1993–1997: recommended standards. Epilepsia 2000;41(10):1346–1349

5. Cross JH, Jayakar P, Nordli D, et al., International League Against Epilepsy, Subcommission for Paediatric Epilepsy Surgery; Commissions of Neurosurgery and Paediatrics. Proposed criteria for referral and evaluation of children for epilepsy surgery: recommendations of the Subcommission for Pediatric Epilepsy Surgery. Epilepsia 2006;47(6):952–959

6. Harvey AS, Cross JH, Shinnar S, Mathern BW; ILAE Pediatric Epilepsy Surgery Survey Taskforce. Defining the spectrum of international practice in pediatric epilepsy surgery patients. Epilepsia 2008;49(1):146–155

7. Rosenow F, Lüders H. Presurgical evaluation of epilepsy. Brain 2001;124(pt 9):1683–1700

8. Sarco DP, Burke JF, Madsen JR. Electroencephalography in epilepsy surgery planning. Childs Nerv Syst 2006;22(8):760–765

9. Riviello JJ, Helmers SH, Mikati M, Holmes GL. The preoperative evaluation of the child with epilepsy. Neurosurg Clin N Am 1995;6:431–442

10. Uldall P, Alving J, Hansen LK, Kibaek M, Buchholt J. The misdiagnosis of epilepsy in children admitted to a tertiary epilepsy centre with paroxysmal events. Arch Dis Child 2006;91(3):219–221

11. Mikati MA, Andermann F, Comair YG, et al. Indications and timing of surgery of catastrophic epilepsy. In: Luders HO, Comair YG, eds. Epilepsy Surgery. 2nd ed. Philadelphia, Pa.: Lippincott Williams and Wilkins: 2001;1035–1038

12. Berg AT, Vickrey BG, Testa FM, et al. How long does it take for epilepsy to become intractable? A prospective investigation. Ann Neurol 2006;60(1):73–79

13. Camfield PR, Camfield CS. Antiepileptic drug therapy: when is epilepsy truly intractable? Epilepsia 1996;37(suppl 1):S60–S65

14. Dlugos DJ, Sammel MD, Strom BL, Farrar JT. Response to first drug trial predicts outcome in childhood temporal lobe epilepsy. Neurology 2001;57(12):2259–2264

15. Arts WFM, Geerts AT, Brouwer OF, Boudewyn Peters AC, Stroink H, van Donselaar CA. The early prognosis of epilepsy in childhood: the prediction of a poor outcome. The Dutch study of epilepsy in childhood. Epilepsia 1999;40(6):726–734

16. Ko TS, Holmes GL. EEG and clinical predictors of medically intractable childhood epilepsy. Clin Neurophysiol 1999;110(7):1245–1251

17. Labiner DM, Weinand ME, Brainerd CJ, Ahern GL, Herring AM, Melgar MA. Prognostic value of concordant seizure focus localizing data in the selection of temporal lobectomy candidates. Neurol Res 2002;24(8):747–755

18. Kurian M, Spinelli L, Delavelle J, et al. Multimodality imaging for focus localization in pediatric pharmacoresistant epilepsy. Epileptic Disord 2007;9(1):20–31

19. Lüders H, Acharya J, Baumgartner C, et al. Semiological seizure classification. Epilepsia 1998;39(9):1006–1013

20. Commission on Neuroimaging of the International League Against Epilepsy. Recommendations for neuroimaging of patients with epilepsy. Epilepsia 1997;38(11):1255–1256

21. Commission on Neuroimaging of the International League Against Epilepsy. Guidelines for neuroimaging evaluation of patients with uncontrolled epilepsy considered for surgery. Epilepsia 1998;39(12):1375–1376

22. Neuroimaging Subcommission of the International League Against Epilepsy. Commission on Diagnostic Strategies: recommendations for functional neuroimaging of persons with epilepsy. Epilepsia 2000;41(10):1350–1356

23. Knake S, Triantafyllou C, Wald LL, et al. 3T phased array MRI improves the presurgical evaluation in focal epilepsies: a prospective study. Neurology 2005;65(7):1026–1031

24. So EL. Role of neuroimaging in the management of seizure disorders. Mayo Clin Proc 2002;77(11):1251–1264

25. Lassonde M, Sauerwein HC, Jambaqué I, Smith ML, Helmstaedter C. Neuropsychology of childhood epilepsy: pre- and postsurgical assessment. Epileptic Disord 2000;2(1):3–13

26. Helmstaedter C. Neuropsychological aspects of epilepsy surgery. Epilepsy Behav 2004;5(suppl 1):S45–S55

27. Hamer HM, Wyllie E, Stanford L, Mascha E, Kotagal P, Wolgamuth B. Risk factors for unsuccessful testing during the intracarotid amobarbital procedure in preadolescent children. Epilepsia 2000;41(5):554–563

28. Patil SG, Cross JH, Kling Chong W, et al. Is streamlined evaluation of children for epilepsy surgery possible? Epilepsia 2008;49(8):1340–1347

29. Duchowny M. Surgical Evaluation. In: Pellock JM, Bourgeois BFD, Dodson WE, Nordli DR Jr., Sankar R. Demos, eds. Pediatric Epilepsy: Diagnosis and Therapy. 3rd ed. New York, NY:2008;771–784

30. Paolicchi JM, Jayakar P, Dean P, et al. Predictors of outcome in pediatric epilepsy surgery. Neurology 2000;54(3):642–647

31. Jayakar P, Dunoyer C, Dean P, et al. Epilepsy surgery in patients with normal or nonfocal MRI scans: integrative strategies offer long-term seizure relief. Epilepsia 2008;49(5):758–764

32. Lachhwani DK, Loddenkemper T, Holland KD, et al. Discontinuation of medications after successful epilepsy surgery in children. Pediatr Neurol 2008;38(5):340–344

3 Epilepsy Surgery for Congenital or Early Lesions

Ahsan N. V. Moosa, Tobias Loddenkemper, and Elaine Wyllie

Identification of candidates for epilepsy surgery was originally derived from experience in adult and adolescent patients, often with epileptogenic lesions acquired later in life.[1,2] In this patient population, the hallmark features predicting postoperative seizure freedom included focal lesion seen on neuroimaging, together with congruent focal features on ictal and interictal electroencephalography (EEG).[3] As magnetic resonance imaging (MRI) became more sensitive for identification of more subtle lesions such as malformations of cortical development[4,5] and as epilepsy surgery came into the mainstream as a treatment modality for infants and children,[6-10] certain challenges to this selection paradigm emerged. In the 1990s, with successful surgical treatment of group of children with infantile spasms caused by focal cortical dysplasia, it became accepted that in very young surgical candidates, the seizure semiology and the EEG may lack the focal features characteristic of epileptogenic lesions acquired later in life.[11] Thus, these early lesions pose unique challenges in selection of surgical candidates.

Issues related to selection of pediatric epilepsy surgical candidates are discussed in several chapters throughout the book. In this chapter, we will address the special challenges presented by early epileptogenic lesions in older children and adolescents, as well as infants, and issues related to timing of surgery in pediatric patients.

■ Types of Congenital or Early Acquired Lesions Causing Epilepsy

From the standpoint of surgical planning, congenital or early acquired lesions may be categorized into two broad groups: hemispheric lesions and focal or multifocal lesions.[12] The former group requires hemispherectomy, and the later group needs lobar or multilobar resection. In addition, localization of the epileptogenic zone, distribution of eloquent areas, age, and plasticity potential need to be considered in the equation.

Hemispheric Lesions

Epileptogenic lesions affecting the whole or most of a hemisphere are more common in pediatric than adult epilepsy surgery candidates. Malformations of cortical development (MCD), Sturge-Weber syndrome, encephalomalacia caused by a variety of insults, and Rasmussen's encephalitis constitute the four major groups. These groups are typically associated with hemiparesis, with or without hemianopsia.

Malformations of Cortical Development

MCDs can affect the whole or most of a hemisphere, referred to here as hemispheric malformations.[13] The prototype of hemispheric MCD is hemimegalencephaly. Hemimegalencephaly may occur as an isolated abnormality or with neurocutaneous syndromes such as epidermal nevus syndrome,[14] Hypomelanosis of Ito,[15] Klippel-Trénauney–Weber syndrome,[16] Proteus syndrome,[17] neurofibromatosis type 1,[18] and tuberous sclerosis.[19] Precise diagnosis is important in such cases to address other systemic problems in these syndromes. In some cases, megalencephaly may not affect the whole hemisphere and may be confined to posterior or anterior regions of affected hemisphere. Some authors refer to these cases as hemi-hemimegalencephaly.[20] Some of the hemispheric MCDs may have associated atrophy and are distinct from megalencephalic malformations.[21] Other less common malformations in surgical series include schizencephaly and polymicrogyria.[21,22] Subtle abnormalities may be present on the contralateral side.[13] Gross bilateral malformations, such as lissencephaly and subcortical band heterotopia, are excluded from this group because they are usually not amenable to epilepsy surgery currently.

Sturge-Weber Syndrome

Sturge-Weber syndrome was one of the first disorders to undergo surgery in an early series of hemispherectomy in infants.[23] This syndrome can be easily recognized by the clinical triad of facial nevus flammeus; contralateral hemiparesis; and visual field defect; along characteristic neuroradiological abnormalities including leptomeningeal and intraparenchymal angiomatosis typically in the posterior quadrant, choroid plexus hypertrophy, gyriform calcification, and progressive regional or hemispheric cerebral atrophy.[24,25]

Encephalomalacia

Extensive cystic encephalomalacia or gliosis affecting most of the hemisphere form an important group in recent pediatric surgical series.[26-28] Encephalomalacia acquired early in life is most often caused by pre- or perinatal cerebral artery infarction, intraventricular hemorrhage, or hypoxia-ischemia. Trauma and infection are important etiologies in the postnatal period, infancy, and early childhood.

Rasmussen's Syndrome

Rasmussen's syndrome is a progressive disorder characterized by severe unilateral focal epilepsy, often with epilepsia partialis continua, and progressive neurological deficits including hemiparesis, cognitive decline, and (if the dominant hemisphere is involved) aphasia.[29-31] MRI in early stages is often normal. Few patients show transiently focal cortical swelling at the onset of disease. As disease advances, progressive hemispheric atrophy, most prominent in insular and peri-insular regions with increased cortical and subcortical signal on T2 and fluid attenuation inversion recovery (FLAIR) sequences, appear.[30,32] Involvement of ipsilateral caudate head and putamen is common.[33] Rarely both hemispheres may be affected.[34]

Neoplasms

Rarely, tumors may involve a large part of one hemisphere, but surgery in this situation may not be for the sole purpose of seizure control. Gliomatosis cerebri may be misdiagnosed as hemimegalencephaly, especially when it occurs in very young children with refractory epilepsy.[35]

Focal Lesions

The single major group of early focal epileptogenic lesions requiring epilepsy surgery is focal cortical dysplasia.[7,36] Other focal malformations would include heterotopia, polymicrogyria, schizencephaly, and hypothalamic hamartomas.[37] Dysembryoplastic neuroepithelial tumors and the multifocal cortical tubers of tuberous sclerosis also fall in the spectrum of dysplasias on the border zone of neoplasms.[37] Other early tumors include ganglioglioma, gangliocytoma, and pleomorphic xanthoastrocytoma.[7,38] Focal areas of gliosis caused by remote vascular insult, trauma, and infection constitute the rest of early focal lesions.[9,39]

Mesial temporal sclerosis (MTS) is an uncommon lesion in early life,[9] although cases in patients as young as 4 months have been described.[40] In pediatric epilepsy, surgery candidates, MTS is more likely to exist as dual pathology with ipsilateral anterior temporal cortical dysplasia.[9,38,41]

Nonlesional MRI

Despite advances in structural neuroimaging, a significant number of patients with drug-resistant focal epilepsy do not have an identifiable structural lesion on MRI. Successful surgical excision has been performed in some of these apparently nonlesional patients on the basis of convergence of clinical and electrophysiological data[7] or supported by functional imaging studies such as positron emission tomography or ictal single photon emission computed tomography.[11] Histopathology revealed evidence of cortical dysplasia, neuronal heterotopia, and focal gliosis as the substrates of epilepsy in majority of MRI-negative lesions.[7,42]

■ Impact of Early Lesions

Early Lesions: Role of Adaptive Plasticity

Unlike in adults, plasticity of the young brain serves as a cushion against new postoperative neurological deficits after resection of eloquent regions, including language, motor, and primary visual cortex areas.[43-45] *Plasticity*, in simple terms, refers to the recruitment of neurons to perform an eloquent function that is otherwise not destined to. Such gain of function through plasticity is referred to as adaptive plasticity.[44] The classic example is transfer of language functions to the right hemisphere with early left hemispheric injuries.[43,46-50] Dominant handedness can also transfer effectively with early injuries. Handedness is determined by the presence of praxis center in the inferior parietal lobule rather than language areas.[51] However language and praxis centers often exist in the same hemisphere, and, hence, handedness is a surrogate marker for language dominance.[51,52] Motor, sensory, and visual functions have limited plasticity, and the contribution of neuronal plasticity to recovery is limited. Plasticity of cognitive functions is difficult to evaluate separately but likely to be significantly more than sensorimotor functions.

Plasticity and the resultant transfer of functions are best studied in the language domain. The anatomical location of Broca's area and Wernicke's area are fairly consistent in the majority of normal subjects. Epileptogenic lesions in and around these locations displace the language functions to adjacent areas or in extreme instances to the homologous area in opposite hemisphere.[49,50,53] Three major factors influence the transfer of the language functions: age at insult and the size and the nature of the lesion. Younger age at insult, large lesions, and destructive lesions are more likely to shift the language areas. Of these, the most important factor is age at insult; 6 years is generally the cut-off for effective language transfer to occur.[50] However, these early lesions may not manifest with epilepsy until later, technically beyond the period of effective plasticity. In these instances, the age at the time of brain injury is more important than the age at onset of epilepsy or age at surgery. Hence these plasticity rules may apply even in adults, provided the lesion is acquired within the period of plasticity window, typically before 6 years of age. Even though effective transfer of functions occurs when the brain injury occurs early in life, some degree of plasticity may be possible in late childhood and even in adults.[47,54,55] Large hemispheric lesions, as in perinatal stroke or hemimegalencephaly, shift language areas to the opposite hemisphere.[49,50] On the contrary, smaller lesions such as tumors tend to displace language areas to adjacent areas in the same hemisphere.[53] This information is critical when operating such lesions, because peritumoral bed may have language function.

Transferred language function is never as good as naturally acquired language, and several studies suggest that the left hemisphere is phylogenetically superior in language acquisition in most patients.[43,56] This applies more so to expressive compared with receptive language functions. Wada testing is difficult to perform in children with neurocognitive deficits but has been reported to be of help in selected cases in the past.[57] Functional MRI and child-specific language testing paradigms may soon replace Wada testing for language lateralization.[58,59]

Early Lesions: EEG Manifestations

Interactions between an early epileptogenic brain lesion and normal developmental processes may result in EEG patterns that are different from, and more diffuse than, those seen in patients with lesions acquired after brain maturity. This was first recognized in young children who presented with the generalized pattern of hypsarrhythmia and infantile spasms and had seizure-free outcome after resection of a congenital or early acquired focal or hemispheric brain lesion.[11,42] Subsequently, successful epilepsy surgery was also reported for older children and adolescents with early brain lesions and other generalized EEG patterns, including the generalized pattern of slow spike-wave complexes traditionally associated with Lennox-Gastaut syndrome **(Fig. 3.1)** or the contralesional patterns (maximum epileptiform abnormalities over the hemisphere contralateral to the lesion) seen in the setting of extensive unilateral encephalomalacia **(Fig. 3.2)**.[26,60]

Neither West syndrome with hypsarrhythmia nor Lennox-Gastaut syndrome with generalized slow spike wave complexes were recognized as surgically amenable initially.[61,62] These syndromes are not etiology specific and can occur in response to a wide variety of cerebral insults. The occurrence of identifiable focal and multifocal lesions in these disorders prompted several centers to attempt lesionectomies in these patients who otherwise had multidrug-resistant epilepsy with very high seizure burden with very few options left.[8,11,26,60,63–65] Successful surgery in these patients has widened the spectrum of epilepsy phenotypes amenable to surgery.

The key factor for manifestation of the generalized patterns in these surgical candidates appeared to be the age at the time of lesion occurrence (78% pre- or perinatal; 90% within the first 2 years of life in one series)[26] rather than the age at evaluation for epilepsy surgery (0.2 to 24 years, median 8 years). This phenomenon of "generalized patterns in focal lesions" follows the rules similar to the adaptive plasticity rules in language transfer described earlier. When we assess an individual for left hemispherectomy at any age, the important factor deciding the side of language dominance is age at lesion occurrence, not age at presurgical evaluation.[50] Generalized EEG patterns seen in focal lesions appear to follow the same rules.[26]

Although not all children or adolescents with early lesions will present with generalized or contralesional epileptiform discharges, it is important to be aware of the phenomenon so that carefully selected children with focal or unilateral epileptogenic lesions are not excluded from surgical consideration. In one series,[26] seizure-free outcome did not differ between children and adolescents with early brain lesions who had generalized EEG abnormalities (72% of patients were seizure free at last follow-up) compared with children with ipsilesional epileptiform discharges. The contralesional EEG abnormalities (24% of patients) appeared to represent an altered expression of diffuse EEG pattern, decreased on the ipsilesional side affected by large destructive lesion. Such false localizing and lateralizing EEG abnormalities are not limited to large destructive hemispheric lesions. Even in typical focal epileptic syndromes, such as temporal lobe epilepsy caused by neoplasms in childhood, may express multiregional and contralesional EEG abnormalities that disappeared after successful removal of the focal epileptogenic lesions.[66,67] Most of the patients in the latter series had early onset brain lesions.

The mechanisms underlying the generalized epileptiform abnormalities in focal cerebral lesions are unknown. Some practitioners view this as a form of maladaptive plasticity of immature brain.[44,60] The lesions in the environment of immature or maturing neural network of the young brain alter the neural circuits, leading to spontaneous hypersynchrony, resulting in generalized features.[68] Some authors suggested involvement of the thalamocortical networks.[69] Generalized epileptiform abnormalities have been described with hypothalamic hamartomas, as well.[65] In a study on the evolution of epilepsy in hypothalamic hamartomas in children, gelastic seizures were noted in infancy, followed by generalized tonic seizures at approximately 6 years of age. Early EEGs were normal but later became progressively abnormal with the emergence of generalized epileptiform abnormalities. Intraoperative EEG showed persistence of generalized interictal spike-wave, even after removal of hamartoma; however, these discharges resolved in postoperative studies. This observation suggests that the generalized epileptiform discharges may be a result of secondary epileptogenesis similar

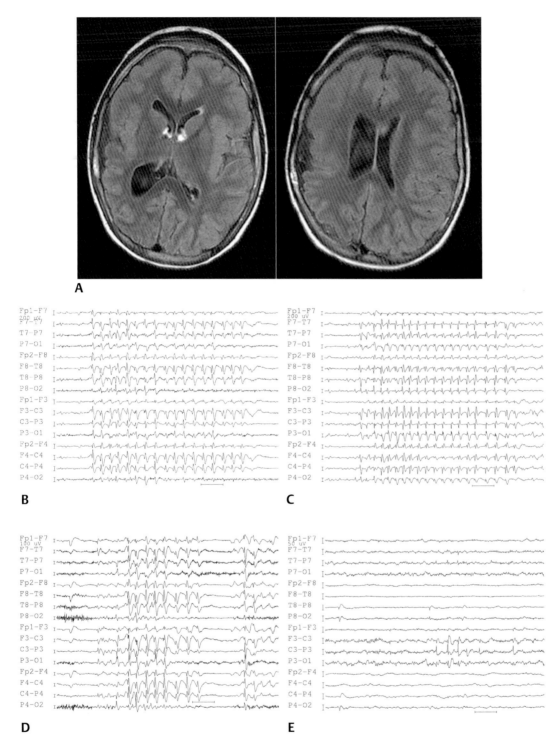

Fig. 3.1 **(A)** Axial magnetic resonance images demonstrate right hemispheric malformation of cortical development in an 8-year-old girl with left hemiparesis, mental impairment, and refractory epilepsy since 18 months of age. Seizures included daily multiple drop attacks and episodes of slumping over with unresponsiveness and head bobbing for 10 to 30 seconds, 50 to 100 times per day. **(B)** Interictal electroencephalogram (EEG) shows generalized slow-spike-wave complexes (SSWC). **(C)** Ictal EEG illustrates generalized SSWC during an episode of slumping over with unresponsiveness and head nodding. **(D)** Most of the bursts of SSWC were bilaterally synchronous at on-

set, but a few had an initial maximum or lead-in from the left (shown here) or right side. **(E)** Postoperative EEG, 6 months after right functional hemispherectomy showing expected diminished background and sharp waves on the right and persistent focal sharp waves on the left side. Follow-up EEG at 1, 2, and 3 years after surgery showed no contralateral interictal epileptiform discharges. (Reprinted with permission from: Wyllie E, Lachhwani DK, Gupta A, et al. Successful surgery for epilepsy due to early brain lesions despite generalized EEG findings. Neurology 2007;69(4):389–397. ©2007 Lippincott Williams & Wilkins.)

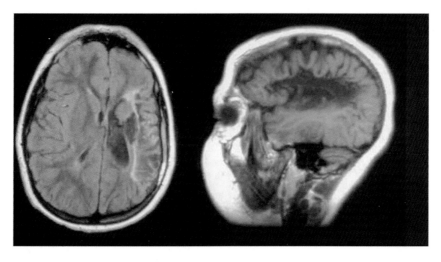

A

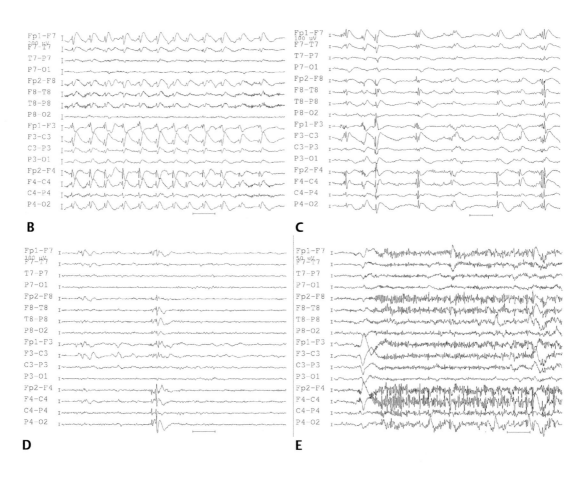

B

C

D

E

Fig. 3.2 (A) Axial and sagittal magnetic resonance images show cystic encephalomalacia caused by perinatal left middle cerebral artery infarction in a 12-year-old boy with severe right hemiparesis, mental impairment, and refractory epilepsy since 9 years of age. He had daily tonic seizures. **(B)** Interictal awake electroencephalogram (EEG) reveals a run of generalized slow-spike-wave complexes. **(C)** Interictal EEG during sleep shows generalized polyspike-and-wave complexes, sometimes maximum on the right (shown here) or left side. **(D)** Interictal EEG demonstrates a spike maximum on the right, and continuous slowing in the left frontal region. **(E)** Ictal EEG shows initial movement artifact followed by generalized polyspikes, maximum in the right frontal region. An identical pattern was seen in all 11 recorded seizures. (Reprinted with permission from: Wyllie E, Lachhwani DK, Gupta A, et al. Successful surgery for epilepsy because of early brain lesions despite generalized EEG findings. Neurology 2007;69(4):389–397. ©2007 Lippincott Williams & Wilkins.)

to the kindling phenomenon seen in animals.[70] These discharges may ultimately resolve if the kindling primary focus is removed before the secondary epileptogenic areas become completely independent.

Timing of Surgery

Intractable epilepsy within the first 2 years of life is a significant risk factor for mental handicap, especially if seizures occur daily.[71] Also, repeated episodes of prolonged status epilepticus produce more global damage. Mechanisms of brain injury may vary with etiology. For instance, in Sturge-Weber syndrome, progressive neurological deficits occur because of two processes: hypoxemia caused by thrombosis and venous stasis, which affects the ipsilesional hemisphere, and recurrent seizures that may affect the contralesional hemisphere.[72,73] Early successful surgery may prevent damage to contralesional side.

Epilepsy surgery within the period of effective neuronal plasticity window provides the best opportunity to maximize developmental potential and minimize postoperative deficit. As noted earlier, surgery involving the dominant hemisphere is less likely to result in major language deficits if performed before 6 years of age,[50] even if the eloquent areas have resided in the surgical bed. According to one study, developmental quotient may improve for children operated on in infancy.[74] In another study,[75] cognitive function improved in preschool children after epilepsy surgery, with improved catch-up development in children rendered seizure free. Shorter duration of epilepsy was significantly associated with postoperative improvement in developmental quotient.[75] Improvement in developmental outcome in these children may be caused by multiple factors including seizure control, resolution of epileptic encephalopathy, and reduction of toxic antiepileptic drugs.

As a guiding principle, the ideal age for epilepsy surgery may be the earliest age at which the usual selection criteria for surgery are met.[6,12] These criteria are built on three critical questions: Is surgery warranted? Will it work? Is it safe? If the answer is yes to all these questions, then surgery should be performed at the earliest opportunity. For catastrophic epilepsy, surgery within the first year of life may be indicated, although this entails special risks and may be most safely performed at specialized pediatric centers.

■ Selection of Surgical Candidates

In the child or adolescent with a congenital or early acquired lesion, the evaluation and decision for epilepsy surgery is no longer based on traditional unilateral or focal findings on EEG and seizure semiology. Instead it is based on the comprehensive picture of a child with severe epilepsy, a potentially epileptogenic unilateral lesion seen on MRI, and

focal or generalized EEG and seizure types. Surgical decision making is fairly straightforward in patients with focal lesions with concordant localizing seizures and EEG abnormalities, but it is more challenging when EEG is generalized. Focal clinical features during seizures are helpful when they suggest seizure onset on the side of the lesion, but these may or may not be present, even in children with subsequent seizure-free postoperative outcome.[26,60] Hemiparesis may also be helpful to surgical planning, as long as it is concordant with the side of proposed surgery.

Surgical decision making is challenging when the seizures and EEG are generalized. In the early series of generalized epilepsy phenotypes undergoing surgery, co-existing dominant focal features on EEG and semiology were taken as primary factors for determining epilepsy surgical candidacy.[8,11,63,76] However, recent experience has shown that surgery can be successful in children and adolescents with generalized EEG patterns and an early unilateral brain lesion.[26,60] The role of invasive monitoring is limited in this group and was not used to clarify the extent of the epileptogenic zone in any patients in these series,[26,60] who were seizure free after surgery. Just as hypsarrhythmia is an accepted diffuse manifestation of an early epileptogenic lesion in infants, slow-spike-wave complexes and other forms of generalized discharges may be the manifestation of such lesions later in childhood.

In children and adolescents with extensive encephalomalacia caused by an early destructive brain injury, the ipsilesional hemisphere may not express normal or abnormal EEG activity (**Fig. 3.2**). In these cases, ictal and interictal epileptiform discharges may be maximum over the contralesional hemisphere, possibly reflected by a generalized discharge that is reduced on the ipsilesional side.[26] In every case, key features for consideration of surgery include the nature, timing, and extent of the unilateral brain lesion, together with the severity and catastrophic impact of the epilepsy.[26,60] Performing preoperative video-EEG evaluation in this group of patients remains important for the following reasons:

1. To identify focal EEG features or lateralizing signs during clinical seizures that would help to build a case for surgery in complicated cases;
2. To clarify that all of the reported clinical events are in fact seizures and not nonepileptic events; and
3. To expand our understanding of such cases and their postsurgical evolution.

EEG plays an important role in children with multifocal lesions, as in tuberous sclerosis. Careful identification of the epileptogenic zone can lead to seizure freedom in some of these patients.[77,78] EEG abnormalities concordant with an isolated or the largest tuber predict good outcome. Some centers perform serial invasive monitoring in a multistaged approach to identify multiple possible epileptogenic lesions in tuberous sclerosis.[79,80] In this approach, a second surgery would include removal of the epileptogenic lesion confirmed by initial invasive monitoring and would include placing of additional electrodes for further monitoring to map additional epileptogenic zones, if any.

■ Types of Surgeries for Early Lesions

Resective epilepsy surgery for early lesions falls under three broad categories: hemispheric surgery, lesionectomy or lobar resection, and multilobar resection.[7,8,21,26] Decision making regarding the type of surgery is a multidisciplinary approach, involving pediatric epileptologists, neurosurgeons, neuropsychologists, neuroradiologists, social workers, and bioethicists. Hemispherectomies and multilobar resections are common surgeries performed in children and adolescents with early lesions,[6-9,21,26] but in some cases, lesionectomy or more limited lobar resection may be appropriate.[81,82] The decision is based on a comprehensive assessment of all lines of evidence including seizure semiology, EEG, MRI, neurological examination, and other features. Utility of intraoperative electrocorticography is unclear.

Infants and young children pose unique risks for major surgeries, such as hemispherectomy, and an experienced pediatric epilepsy surgery team is crucial for better outcome. Callosotomy, multiple subpial transaction, and vagal nerve stimulation are mostly palliative. Readers are referred to the dedicated chapters on surgeries elsewhere in this book for further details on these surgical procedures.

■ Outcome

The pediatric epilepsy population is heterogeneous, and many factors have to be taken into account before meaningful interpretation of outcome data. Outcome should emphasize not only seizure outcome but also developmental and cognitive outcome and quality of life for patients and caregivers.[83] Risks of epilepsy surgery should be weighed against the benefits of surgery and against the risk of continued uncontrolled seizures.[83,84]

Despite age-related differences in etiology, pediatric surgical results for lobar resection are comparable to adults.[85,86] Seizure outcome after resection of cortical dysplasias in children and adolescents is not significantly different from adults.[9] Surgery in infancy can yield similar results in terms of seizure outcome.[7,8,21,42] In a series of 33 patients who had undergone hemispherectomy, seizure freedom was highest in those with acquired pathology such as cystic encephalomalacia (82%), followed by those with progressive pathology such as Rasmussen encephalitis and Sturge-Weber syndrome (50%) and those with MCD (31%).[22] Similar outcome has been reported by other centers.[21,87] Although it appears counterintuitive, lesions requiring the most extensive surgery (e.g., hemispheric infarction or posterior quadrant malformations) may, in fact, be associated with a relatively better chance for seizure-free outcome than smaller lesions near eloquent cortex (e.g., frontocentral malformations associated with little or no hemiparesis). In these patients, the limitations on extent of surgery may reduce the ability to completely remove the epileptogenic zone.

Many studies have examine predictors of seizure-free outcome. In one series,[39] complete resection of the epileptogenic lesion and the electrographically abnormal region was the major determinant of good outcome. The site of resection, lesional status, and pathological diagnosis were not significant predictors of outcome.[39] Intelligence quotient alone is not a predictor of outcome, and patients with low intelligence should not be denied surgery if other presurgical data point to a resectable focus.[88] Presence of generalized EEG abnormalities does not portend to poor outcome in carefully selected patients with early unilateral brain lesions.[26,60]

Successful epilepsy surgery has been shown to improve quality of life in children with intractable seizures.[89,90] Improvement in cognition and other developmental aspects after epilepsy surgery is unclear.[91] In one series, temporal lobe resections have been shown to have a negative effect on verbal memory skills in high-functioning children.[92] However, compared with adults, greater functional recovery has been noted with both left and right temporal surgical resections in pediatric surgical candidates.[45] Cognitive improvement can be tremendous in individual cases after successful epilepsy surgery.[11] In one series, a larger increase in developmental quotient was noted after surgery in children operated at younger age and those with epileptic spasms.[74]

■ Conclusion

Drug-resistant epilepsy in children is often secondary to congenital or early acquired brain lesions that occur during the phase of rapid brain growth and development. These early lesions in the environment of an immature nervous system have special implications for the clinical and electrophysiological phenotype of epilepsy, with generalized or contralesional EEG discharges in some patients. Early surgery may be warranted in selected children with severe epilepsy to reduce the seizure and medication burden and capitalize on the period of plasticity to maximize developmental potential.

References

1. Engel J Jr. Update on surgical treatment of the epilepsies. Summary of the second international palm desert conference on the surgical treatment of the epilepsies (1992). Neurology 1993;43(8):1612–1617
2. Engel J Jr. Surgery for seizures. N Engl J Med 1996;334(10):647–652
3. Berg AT, Walczak T, Hirsch LJ, Spencer SS. Multivariable prediction of seizure outcome one year after resective epilepsy surgery: development of a model with independent validation. Epilepsy Res 1998;29(3):185–194
4. Kuzniecky R, Berkovic S, Andermann F, Melanson D, Olivier A, Robitaille Y. Focal cortical myoclonus and rolandic cortical dysplasia: clarification by magnetic resonance imaging. Ann Neurol 1988;23(4):317–325
5. Sperling MR, Wilson G, Engel J Jr, Babb TL, Phelps M, Bradley W. Magnetic resonance imaging in intractable partial epilepsy: correlative studies. Ann Neurol 1986;20(1):57–62
6. Wyllie E. Catastrophic epilepsy in infants and children: identification of surgical candidates. Epileptic Disord 1999;1(4):261–264
7. Duchowny M, Jayakar P, Resnick T, et al. Epilepsy surgery in the first three years of life. Epilepsia 1998;39(7):737–743
8. Wyllie E, Comair YG, Kotagal P, Raja S, Ruggieri P. Epilepsy surgery in infants. Epilepsia 1996;37(7):625–637
9. Wyllie E, Comair YG, Kotagal P, Bulacio J, Bingaman W, Ruggieri P. Seizure outcome after epilepsy surgery in children and adolescents. Ann Neurol 1998;44(5):740–748
10. Centeno RS, Yacubian EM, Sakamoto AC, Ferraz AF, Junior HC, Cavalheiro S. Pre-surgical evaluation and surgical treatment in children with extratemporal epilepsy. Childs Nerv Syst 2006;22(8):945–959
11. Chugani HT, Shields WD, Shewmon DA, Olson DM, Phelps ME, Peacock WJ. Infantile spasms: I. PET identifies focal cortical dysgenesis in cryptogenic cases for surgical treatment. Ann Neurol 1990;27(4):406–413
12. Engel J Jr, Cascino GD, Shields WD. Surgically remediable syndromes. In: Engel J Jr, Pedley TA, eds. Epilepsy: A Comprehensive Textbook. Vol II. Philadelphia: Lippincott-Raven Publishers;1997:1687–1696
13. Gupta A, Carreño M, Wyllie E, Bingaman WE. Hemispheric malformations of cortical development. Neurology 2004; 62(6, suppl 3)S20–S26
14. Pavone L, Curatolo P, Rizzo R, et al. Epidermal nevus syndrome: a neurologic variant with hemimegalencephaly, gyral malformation, mental retardation, seizures, and facial hemihypertrophy. Neurology 1991;41(2(pt 1)):266–271
15. Tagawa T, Futagi Y, Arai H, Mushiake S, Nakayama M. Hypomelanosis of Ito associated with hemimegalencephaly: a clinicopathological study. Pediatr Neurol 1997;17(2):180–184
16. Cristaldi A, Vigevano F, Antoniazzi G, et al. Hemimegalencephaly, hemihypertrophy and vascular lesions. Eur J Pediatr 1995;154(2):134–137
17. Griffiths PD, Welch RJ, Gardner-Medwin D, Gholkar A, McAllister V. The radiological features of hemimegalencephaly including three cases associated with proteus syndrome. Neuropediatrics 1994;25(3):140–144
18. Cusmai R, Curatolo P, Mangano S, Cheminal R, Echenne B. Hemimegalencephaly and neurofibromatosis. Neuropediatrics 1990;21(4):179–182
19. Maloof J, Sledz K, Hogg JF, Bodensteiner JB, Schwartz T, Schochet SS. Unilateral megalencephaly and tuberous sclerosis: related disorders? J Child Neurol 1994;9(4):443–446
20. D'Agostino MD, Bastos A, Piras C, et al. Posterior quadrantic dysplasia or hemi-hemimegalencephaly: a characteristic brain malformation. Neurology 2004;62(12):2214–2220
21. González-Martínez JA, Gupta A, Kotagal P, et al. Hemispherectomy for catastrophic epilepsy in infants. Epilepsia 2005;46(9):1518–1525
22. Devlin AM, Cross JH, Harkness W, et al. Clinical outcomes of hemispherectomy for epilepsy in childhood and adolescence. Brain 2003;126(pt 3):556–566
23. Hoffman HJ, Hendrick EB, Dennis M, Armstrong D. Hemispherectomy for Sturge-Weber syndrome. Childs Brain 1979;5(3):233–248
24. Krings T, Geibprasert S, Luo CB, Bhattacharya JJ, Alvarez H, Lasjaunias P. Segmental neurovascular syndromes in children. Neuroimaging Clin N Am 2007;17(2):245–258
25. Bourgeois M, Crimmins DW, de Oliveira RS, et al. Surgical treatment of epilepsy in Sturge-Weber syndrome in children. J Neurosurg 2007;106(1, suppl)20–28
26. Wyllie E, Lachhwani DK, Gupta A, et al. Successful surgery for epilepsy due to early brain lesions despite generalized EEG findings. Neurology 2007;69(4):389–397
27. Guzzetta F, Battaglia D, Di Rocco C, Caldarelli M. Symptomatic epilepsy in children with poroencephalic cysts secondary to perinatal middle cerebral artery occlusion. Childs Nerv Syst 2006;22(8):922–930
28. Carreño M, Kotagal P, Perez Jiménez A, Mesa T, Bingaman W, Wyllie E. Intractable epilepsy in vascular congenital hemiparesis: clinical features and surgical options. Neurology 2002;59(1):129–131
29. Dubeau F. Rasmussen's encephalitis (chronic focal encephalitis). In: Wyllie E, Gupta A, Lacchwani DK, eds. The Treatment of Epilepsy. 4th ed. Philadelphia: Lippincott Williams & Wilkins;2006:441–454
30. Bien CG, Granata T, Antozzi C, et al. Pathogenesis, diagnosis and treatment of Rasmussen encephalitis: a European consensus statement. Brain 2005;128(pt 3):454–471
31. Hart Y. Rasmussen's encephalitis. Epileptic Disord 2004;6(3):133–144
32. Vining EP, Freeman JM, Brandt J, Carson BS, Uematsu S. Progressive unilateral encephalopathy of childhood (Rasmussen's syndrome): a reappraisal. Epilepsia 1993;34(4):639–650
33. Rajesh B, Kesavadas C, Ashalatha R, Thomas B. Putaminal involvement in Rasmussen encephalitis. Pediatr Radiol 2006;36(8):816–822
34. Tobias SM, Robitaille Y, Hickey WF, Rhodes CH, Nordgren R, Andermann F. Bilateral Rasmussen encephalitis: postmortem documentation in a five-year-old. Epilepsia 2003;44(1):127–130
35. Maton B, Resnick T, Jayakar P, Morrison G, Duchowny M. Epilepsy surgery in children with gliomatosis cerebri. Epilepsia 2007;48(8):1485–1490
36. Sisodiya SM. Surgery for malformations of cortical development causing epilepsy. Brain 2000;123(pt 6):1075–1091
37. Raymond AA, Fish DR, Sisodiya SM, Alsanjari N, Stevens JM, Shorvon SD. Abnormalities of gyration, heterotopias, tuberous sclerosis,

focal cortical dysplasia, microdysgenesis, dysembryoplastic neuroepithelial tumour and dysgenesis of the archicortex in epilepsy. Clinical, EEG and neuroimaging features in 100 adult patients. Brain 1995;118(pt 3):629–660

38. Maton B, Jayakar P, Resnick T, Morrison G, Ragheb J, Duchowny M. Surgery for medically intractable temporal lobe epilepsy during early life. Epilepsia 2008;49(1):80–87

39. Paolicchi JM, Jayakar P, Dean P, et al. Predictors of outcome in pediatric epilepsy surgery. Neurology 2000;54(3):642–647

40. DeLong GR, Heinz ER. The clinical syndrome of early-life bilateral hippocampal sclerosis. Ann Neurol 1997;42(1):11–17

41. Mohamed A, Wyllie E, Ruggieri P, et al. Temporal lobe epilepsy due to hippocampal sclerosis in pediatric candidates for epilepsy surgery. Neurology 2001;56(12):1643–1649

42. Chugani HT, Shewmon DA, Shields WD, et al. Surgery for intractable infantile spasms: neuroimaging perspectives. Epilepsia 1993; 34(4):764–771

43. Helmstaedter C, Kurthen M, Linke DB, Elger CE. Right hemisphere restitution of language and memory functions in right hemisphere language-dominant patients with left temporal lobe epilepsy. Brain 1994;117(pt 4):729–737

44. Johnston MV. Clinical disorders of brain plasticity. Brain Dev 2004;26(2):73–80

45. Gleissner U, Sassen R, Schramm J, Elger CE, Helmstaedter C. Greater functional recovery after temporal lobe epilepsy surgery in children. Brain 2005;128(pt 12):2822–2829

46. Helmstaedter C, Kurthen M, Linke DB, Elger CE. Patterns of language dominance in focal left and right hemisphere epilepsies: relation to MRI findings, EEG, sex, and age at onset of epilepsy. Brain Cogn 1997;33(2):135–150

47. Loddenkemper T, Wyllie E, Lardizabal D, Stanford LD, Bingaman W. Late language transfer in patients with Rasmussen encephalitis. Epilepsia 2003;44(6):870–871

48. Liégeois F, Connelly A, Cross JH, et al. Language reorganization in children with early-onset lesions of the left hemisphere: an fMRI study. Brain 2004;127(pt 6):1229–1236

49. Rausch R, Walsh GO. Right-hemisphere language dominance in right-handed epileptic patients. Arch Neurol 1984;41(10):1077–1080

50. Rasmussen T, Milner B. The role of early left-brain injury in determining lateralization of cerebral speech functions. Ann N Y Acad Sci 1977;299:355–369

51. Meador KJ, Loring DW, Lee K, et al. Cerebral lateralization: relationship of language and ideomotor praxis. Neurology 1999;53(9):2028–2031

52. Papagno C, Della Sala S, Basso A. Ideomotor apraxia without aphasia and aphasia without apraxia: the anatomical support for a double dissociation. J Neurol Neurosurg Psychiatry 1993;56(3):286–289

53. DeVos KJ, Wyllie E, Geckler C, Kotagal P, Comair Y. Language dominance in patients with early childhood tumors near left hemisphere language areas. Neurology 1995;45(2):349–356

54. Hertz-Pannier L, Chiron C, Jambaqué I, et al. Late plasticity for language in a child's non-dominant hemisphere: a pre- and post-surgery fMRI study. Brain 2002;125(pt 2):361–372

55. Boatman D, Freeman J, Vining E, et al. Language recovery after left hemispherectomy in children with late-onset seizures. Ann Neurol 1999;46(4):579–586

56. de Bode S, Curtiss S. Language after hemispherectomy. Brain Cogn 2000;43(1-3):135–138

57. Jansen FE, Jennekens-Schinkel A, Van Huffelen AC, et al. Diagnostic significance of Wada procedure in very young children and children with developmental delay. Eur J Paediatr Neurol 2002;6(6):315–320

58. Gaillard WD, Balsamo LM, Ibrahim Z, Sachs BC, Xu B. fMRI identifies regional specialization of neural networks for reading in young children. Neurology 2003;60(1):94–100

59. Gaillard WD, Berl MM, Moore EN, et al. Atypical language in lesional and nonlesional complex partial epilepsy. Neurology 2007;69(18):1761–1771

60. Gupta A, Chirla A, Wyllie E, Lachhwani DK, Kotagal P, Bingaman WE. Pediatric epilepsy surgery in focal lesions and generalized electroencephalogram abnormalities. Pediatr Neurol 2007;37(1):8–15

61. Nolte R, Christen HJ, Doerrer J. Preliminary report of a multi-center study on the West syndrome. Brain Dev 1988;10(4):236–242

62. Dulac O, N'Guyen T. The Lennox-Gastaut syndrome. Epilepsia 1993;34(suppl 7):S7–S17

63. Kramer U, Sue WC, Mikati MA. Focal features in West syndrome indicating candidacy for surgery. Pediatr Neurol 1997;16(3):213–217

64. Wyllie E, Comair Y, Ruggieri P, Raja S, Prayson R. Epilepsy surgery in the setting of periventricular leukomalacia and focal cortical dysplasia. Neurology 1996;46(3):839–841

65. Freeman JL, Harvey AS, Rosenfeld JV, Wrennall JA, Bailey CA, Berkovic SF. Generalized epilepsy in hypothalamic hamartoma: evolution and postoperative resolution. Neurology 2003;60(5):762–767

66. Blume WT, Girvin JP, Kaufmann JC. Childhood brain tumors presenting as chronic uncontrolled focal seizure disorders. Ann Neurol 1982;12(6):538–541

67. Wyllie E, Chee M, Granström ML, et al. Temporal lobe epilepsy in early childhood. Epilepsia 1993;34(5):859–868

68. Sutula TP. Mechanisms of epilepsy progression: current theories and perspectives from neuroplasticity in adulthood and development. Epilepsy Res 2004;60(2-3):161–171

69. Van Hirtum-Das M, Licht EA, Koh S, Wu JY, Shields WD, Sankar R. Children with ESES: variability in the syndrome. Epilepsy Res 2006;70(suppl 1):S248–S258

70. Bertram E. The relevance of kindling for human epilepsy. Epilepsia 2007;48(suppl 2):65–74

71. Vasconcellos E, Wyllie E, Sullivan S, et al. Mental retardation in pediatric candidates for epilepsy surgery: the role of early seizure onset. Epilepsia 2001;42(2):268–274

72. Jansen FE, van der Worp HB, van Huffelen A, van Nieuwenhuizen O. Sturge-Weber syndrome and paroxysmal hemiparesis: epilepsy or ischaemia? Dev Med Child Neurol 2004;46(11):783–786

73. Comi AM. Pathophysiology of Sturge-Weber syndrome. J Child Neurol 2003;18(8):509–516

74. Loddenkemper T, Holland KD, Stanford LD, Kotagal P, Bingaman W, Wyllie E. Developmental outcome after epilepsy surgery in infancy. Pediatrics 2007;119(5):930–935

75. Freitag H, Tuxhorn I. Cognitive function in preschool children after epilepsy surgery: rationale for early intervention. Epilepsia 2005;46(4):561–567

76. Asano E, Chugani DC, Juhász C, Muzik O, Chugani HT. Surgical treatment of West syndrome. Brain Dev 2001;23(7):668–676

77. Lachhwani DK, Pestana E, Gupta A, Kotagal P, Bingaman W, Wyllie E. Identification of candidates for epilepsy surgery in patients with tuberous sclerosis. Neurology 2005;64(9):1651–1654

78. Jansen FE, van Huffelen AC, Algra A, van Nieuwenhuizen O. Epilepsy surgery in tuberous sclerosis: a systematic review. Epilepsia 2007;48(8):1477–1484
79. Romanelli P, Najjar S, Weiner HL, Devinsky O. Epilepsy surgery in tuberous sclerosis: multistage procedures with bilateral or multilobar foci. J Child Neurol 2002;17(9):689–692
80. Weiner HL, Carlson C, Ridgway EB, et al. Epilepsy surgery in young children with tuberous sclerosis: results of a novel approach. Pediatrics 2006;117(5):1494–1502
81. Çataltepe O, Turanli G, Yalnizoglu D, Topçu M, Akalan N. Surgical management of temporal lobe tumor-related epilepsy in children. J Neurosurg 2005; 102(3, suppl):280–287
82. Minkin K, Klein O, Mancini J, Lena G. Surgical strategies and seizure control in pediatric patients with dysembryoplastic neuroepithelial tumors: a single-institution experience. J Neurosurg Pediatr 2008;1(3):206–210
83. Gilliam F, Wyllie E, Kashden J, et al. Epilepsy surgery outcome: comprehensive assessment in children. Neurology 1997;48(5):1368–1374
84. Donner EJ, Smith CR, Snead OC III. Sudden unexplained death in children with epilepsy. Neurology 2001;57(3):430–434
85. Mizrahi EM, Kellaway P, Grossman RG, et al. Anterior temporal lobectomy and medically refractory temporal lobe epilepsy of childhood. Epilepsia 1990;31(3):302–312
86. Adler J, Erba G, Winston KR, Welch K, Lombroso CT. Results of surgery for extratemporal partial epilepsy that began in childhood. Arch Neurol 1991;48(2):133–140
87. Basheer SN, Connolly MB, Lautzenhiser A, Sherman EM, Hendson G, Steinbok P. Hemispheric surgery in children with refractory epilepsy: seizure outcome, complications, and adaptive function. Epilepsia 2007;48(1):133–140
88. Gleissner U, Clusmann H, Sassen R, Elger CE, Helmstaedter C. Postsurgical outcome in pediatric patients with epilepsy: a comparison of patients with intellectual disabilities, subaverage intelligence, and average-range intelligence. Epilepsia 2006;47(2):406–414
89. Sabaz M, Lawson JA, Cairns DR, et al. The impact of epilepsy surgery on quality of life in children. Neurology 2006;66(4):557–561
90. van Empelen R, Jennekens-Schinkel A, van Rijen PC, Helders PJ, van Nieuwenhuizen O. Health-related quality of life and self-perceived competence of children assessed before and up to two years after epilepsy surgery. Epilepsia 2005;46(2):258–271
91. Lah S. Neuropsychological outcome following focal cortical removal for intractable epilepsy in children. Epilepsy Behav 2004;5(6):804–817
92. Szabó CA, Wyllie E, Stanford LD, et al. Neuropsychological effect of temporal lobe resection in preadolescent children with epilepsy. Epilepsia 1998;39(8):814–819

I Preoperative Assessment

A. Electrophysiological Assessment

   4. EEG and Noninvasive Electrophysiological Monitoring

   5. Invasive Electrophysiological Monitoring

   6. Extra-operative and Intra-operative Electrical Stimulation

   7. Magnetoencephalography

B. Neuroimaging

   8. Structural Brain Imaging in Epilepsy

   9. Functional MRI in Pediatric Epilepsy Surgery

  10. Application of PET and SPECT in Pediatric Epilepsy Surgery

  11. Coregistration and Newer Imaging Techniques

C. Neuropsychological Cognitive Assessment

  12. Wada Testing in Pediatric Epilepsy

  13. Preoperative Neuropsychological Assessment

4 EEG and Noninvasive Electrophysiological Monitoring

Yaman Eksioglu and James J. Riviello Jr.

The goal of epilepsy surgery is to locate and resect the epileptic focus without losing any cortical function. The purpose of the presurgical evaluation is to lateralize and localize this focus using a combination of data: the semiology of the clinical seizure, neuroimaging, and electroencephalography (EEG). Initial EEG recording is noninvasive, with scalp surface recording, and presurgical data determine whether further invasive monitoring with intracranial recording electrodes is needed. This chapter reviews the interictal and ictal EEG data used to identify the epileptic focus and discusses pitfalls in lateralization and localization with seizure semiology and noninvasive EEG.

Seizures are classified by their initial site of cortical origin—focal or generalized[1]—determined by the seizure semiology and surface, noninvasive EEG. The seizure has several phases: the onset, or aura, that begins the ictal phase; the continuation of the ictal phase during which the discharge may spread, activating additional neurons; and the postictal phase. A focal seizure without altered awareness is called a simple partial seizure; one with altered awareness is called a complex partial seizure (CPS).

Interictal data are important, but the gold standard is to capture the habitual seizure during time-locked video-EEG monitoring and to analyze its clinical sequence along with the electrographic manifestations. This requires prolonged EEG recordings, referred to as long-term monitoring. The spatial and temporal relationships of the clinical manifestations (semiology) to the electrographic seizure are important, because the electrographic seizure may begin in one area but spread to another before any clinical manifestations are noted. The term *inverse* solution applies to using the seizure semiology and ictal surface EEG data to predict the cortical location of the epileptic focus.[2]

The concept of an *epileptogenic zone* is a practical method used to identify the epileptic focus. Data from the various modalities reviewed in Chapter 2 are used to identify its constituents. An in-depth discussion of the epileptogenic zone and its constituents can be found in several articles, especially the article by Rosenow and Lüders.[3–6]

The epileptogenic zone is the theoretical cortical area indispensable to generating a clinical seizure, and its complete removal is needed to control seizures.[7] It consists of the following constituent zones:

- The *irritative zone* is the cortical area generating epileptiform activity, defined by interictal spikes and sharp waves. This irritative zone is usually larger than the actual epileptogenic zone and can be thought of as all areas in which the epileptic focus may potentially be located. Interictal spikes may spread more in children.
- The *symptomatogenic zone* is the cortical area producing the actual ictal symptoms, when activated. It may be the origin of the epileptic discharge or may be secondarily activated by the propagation of a discharge from the ictal onset zone (seizure onset zone).
- The *ictal onset zone* is the area in which the seizure is actually generated, and if the ictal onset zone is located in a silent cortical area (noneloquent cortex), there are no associated clinical manifestations.
- The *epileptogenic lesion* is the neuroradiological lesion that causes epilepsy. Therefore, neuroimaging, usually magnetic resonance imaging (MRI), is an important modality, but not all MRI lesions seen are necessarily in the cortical area from which seizures originate.
- The *functional deficit zone* is the cortical region abnormal in the interictal period. This zone may be either focal or diffuse and is defined by several modalities: the neurological examination, the neuropsychological examination, and the EEG or functional neuroimaging [typically a single photon emission computed tomography or positron emission tomography (PET) scan]. The EEG shows slowing in the functional deficit zone but not epileptiform activity. A functional deficit zone may not be present in every patient. This zone may be focal or generalized, if there is diffuse dysfunction.
- *Eloquent cortex* refers to cortex in which a defined clinical function is located. For the purposes of epilepsy surgery, eloquent cortex refers to primary motor, primary sensory, language, or memory functions. It is sometimes referred to as the silent cortex. However, the term *silent cortex* is a misnomer because every cortical area has some function, but it may not be possible to specifically identify its function.

Seizure semiology (see **Table 2.6** on page 11) and the ictal surface EEG are important in localizing the epileptic focus, and combining these modalities improves lateralization.[8] Using these data to infer the cortical location of the epileptic focus is referred to as the *inverse problem*. The symptomatogenic zone is identified by the clinical manifestations, whereas the ictal onset zone is identified by the electrographic discharge. The exact temporal relationship between the clinical onset and the electrographic seizure must be determined. This is done by close inspection of the videotape of the recorded seizure, noting the time of the clinical onset as "Time 0" and then relating the electrographic seizure onset to this Time 0. The ictal onset and symptomatogenic zones are certainly interrelated. Ideally, these would be located in the same or contiguous cortical areas, and a focal resection removes both. But the ictal onset may occur in an area of silent cortex, causing no symptoms until it propagates and activates the symptomatogenic zone.

■ EEG Interpretation

EEG records the electrical activity generated by cortical neurons, consisting of the summation of excitatory and inhibitory postsynaptic potentials, which spread to the scalp surface where the recording electrode is placed. All structures between the generator and the electrode attenuate these signals, especially the skull, which is a high-frequency filter. Surface EEG electrodes are placed in a standard array, a montage, as designated by the American Clinical Neurophysiologic Society. A standard 10/20 International Distribution is used for diagnostic EEG, with electrode positions related to the underlying brain.[9] When localizing for epilepsy surgery, additional scalp electrodes may be required, using a 10/10,[10] or even a 10/5 array,[11] which vary by how closely spaced the scalp electrodes are (**Fig. 4.1**). Closely spaced electrodes are more precise when localizing for epilepsy surgery.[12] High-density EEG recording may better localize an epileptic focus.

Both interictal and ictal EEG are analyzed, starting with the interictal EEG background: continuity, symmetry, and the individual components in the waking and sleep states (**Fig. 4.2**). Subtle background asymmetries may be important for lateralization and localization, especially without an epileptogenic lesion (**Table 4.1**). Slow wave activity, one component of the functional deficit zone, and epileptiform activity (spikes and sharp waves), which defines the irritative zone, are identified and locations noted.

Analyzing the habitual seizures is important to determine that they are originating from one location or, in some cases, to exclude nonepileptic seizures. Even if a lesion is present, ictal recordings confirm that the seizures arise from the lesion or are not multifocal. We prefer to capture at least three habitual seizures. In a study of ictal 259 EEGs in 183 children, the seizure type was confirmed in 101 seizures, ictal EEG aided in the classification in 101 seizures, errors in classification were corrected in 37 seizures (detected 11 nonepileptic seizures), and previously undetected seizures were found in 20 seizures. Eleven children had no interictal spikes.[13] Ictal onset patterns include discharges with rhythmic frequencies (α, θ, δ), paroxysmal fast activity, suppression of activity (electrodecremental response), repetitive epileptiform activity, arrhythmic activity, or may stay obscured. The initial ictal rhythm is more predictive of the seizure origin.[7]

Anterior temporal spikes (F7/F8) are the most commonly encountered epileptiform feature in temporal lobe epilepsy (TLE). Focal sharp waves; spike and wave discharges; and slowing (especially polymorphic δ activity) or independent

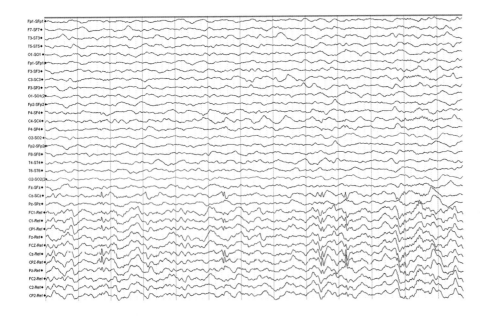

Fig. 4.1 Modified 10/10 montage. 10/10 montage demonstrating lateralization of the Cz spike to the left centroparietal–parietal midline region.

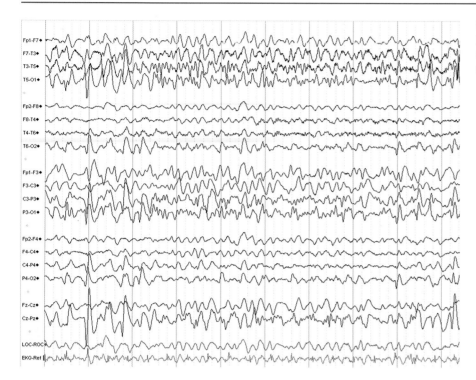

Fig. 4.2 EEG background asymmetry. Marked background asymmetry in child with left hemimegalencephaly with a more normal right hemisphere.

dent, synchronous, or time-locked (a time lag) bitemporal discharges may be seen. Synchronous bitemporal spikes indicate a generating source propagating to the two temporal lobes, whereas time-locked bitemporal discharges indicate transcallosal propagation. Generalized discharges may occur.[14] Frequent interictal discharges were present in symptomatic TLE patients and in mesial temporal sclerosis cases but in only one third of these cases they were strictly temporal.[15] In the Miami series, unilateral temporal discharges occurred in 22 EEGs (36%), unilateral multilobar or poorly localized abnormalities occurred in 23 patients EEGs, bilateral abnormalities occurred in 12 patients EEGs, and no abnormal-

ity occurred in 3 patients EEGs.[16] Spikes in the waking state or during active sleep provide the best localizing data, and sleep typically activates anterior temporal lobe discharges.[17]

For TLE, Ebersole and Pacia defined three seizure types: regular 5- to 9-Hz rhythm, irregular 2- to 5-Hz rhythm, and no distinct ictal discharge. Type 1 seizures likely originate in hippocampus. Type 2 seizures likely have a neocortical origin.[18] In children, two types of ictal discharges were seen: a rhythmic δ-θ pattern progressively increasing in amplitude, followed by a rhythmic monomorphic θ and initial temporal flattening (an electrodecrement) with a progressive appearance of fast activity, frequently spreading to surrounding areas, and finally postictal slowing with a temporal predominance[15] (**Fig. 4.3**).

The largest series after a temporal lobectomy is from Toronto, with 126 children.[19] The interictal EEG showed lateralization in only 68/126 (54%); 26 children had ipsilateral diffuse epileptiform discharges, 7 children had bitemporal discharges, 8 children had generalized activity, and 17 children had a normal interictal EEG. Ictal EEG showed ipsilateral localization in 72 children, and 3 children had a generalized pattern. Nineteen children had either no seizures or had a normal EEG. In the Miami series, a unilateral and well-localized ictal onset was seen in 33 children (54%); a lateralized but poorly localized or multilobular discharge occurred in 23 children; and an independent or a synchronous, bilateral onset was seen in 3 children.[16]

In frontal lobe epilepsy (FLE), the frontal lobe is a large area with much of its cortex inaccessible to scalp electrodes:

Table 4.1 Analysis of Interictal EEG Background

Overall background	Symmetric or asymmetric
Posterior dominant rhythm	Reactive or nonreactive
	Symmetric or asymmetric
	Slowing or speeding up
Central rhythm	Can be normally asymmetric
Sleep spindles	Symmetric or asymmetric (voltage)
	Synchronous versus asynchronous (timing)
Slowing	Focal or generalized
Epileptiform features	Spikes, sharp waves

Abbreviation: electroencephalography, EEG.

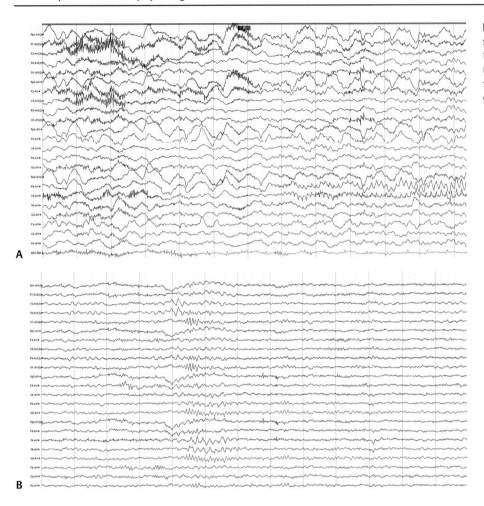

Fig. 4.3 (A) Temporal lobe seizure. Onset electrographic seizure from right temporal lobe with right mesial temporal sclerosis on MRI. **(B)** Temporal lobe seizure. Interictal slowing in same region (T4 and T6 electrodes).

mesial, inferior, and orbitofrontal regions. Seizures originating from the dorsolateral convexity demonstrated interictal activity, whereas seizures originating from the mesial frontal region either had no interictal or multifocal activity.[20] A younger age is also associated with discordant discharges.[21] Discharges from the mesial areas may be detected in the vertex electrodes: Fz, Cz, and Pz electrodes. In a series from Alberta, the interictal EEG was normal in 18 of 21 children.[22] Ictal recordings showed a frontal onset in 9 children and a bifrontal onset in 13 children. Generalized discharges may predict surgical failure.[23] The absence of interictal spikes with documented seizures suggests extratemporal epilepsy.[24]

In FLE, three patterns were reported by Battaglia et al: high-amplitude sharp transients followed by low-voltage fast activity, rhythmic fast activity/decremental activity followed by slow waves with admixed spikes, and repetitive localized θ activity with spike waves[25] (**Fig. 4.4**).

In a study of supplementary sensory–motor seizures in children, the interictal EEG was normal in 49%, and generalized slowing or background disorganization was the only finding in 19%.[26] Interictal EEG abnormalities included mid-

line spikes; both negative and positive sharp waves; and slowing that could spread unilaterally or bilaterally to the frontal, temporal, or parietal areas—all more frequent in sleep. The actual ictal EEG findings may be subtle: an abrupt attenuation of background activity (electrodecrement) accompanied by diffuse β activity followed by semirhythmic θ or δ activity in the frontal or frontocentral regions or by generalized rhythmic slowing, maximal in the midline. These may be misdiagnosed as pseudoseizures.[27]

Most of the pediatric focal resections done in the posterior cortex are on patients with a documented lesion. The surface EEG localizes poorly to the parietal lobe; only 10% of parietal lobe seizures have localized EEG changes.[28] The interictal EEG may be normal; show focal slowing; or have unilateral or bilateral parietal spikes, central spikes, or temporal synchronous or independent discharges, with a more posterior spreading, bifrontal, or even widespread discharges.[29] In a large series of all ages in both children and adults from Montreal, only 9 of 66 patients (14%) had interictal parietal spikes, and ictal discharges were predominantly lateralized, but a localized parietal onset occurred in only four.[30] The

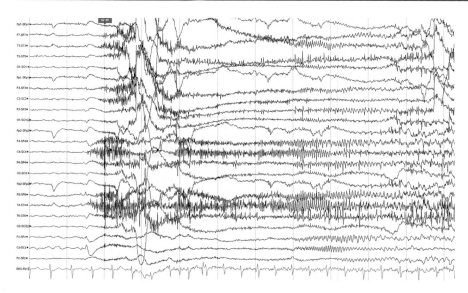

Fig. 4.4 Frontal lobe seizure. Right frontal lobe seizure with electrodecremental response followed by repetitive fast spikes from the right frontal region. Note the Cz sharp wave at onset, followed by muscle artifact, the electrodecremental response, and then the spikes. Frontal seizures typically have much movement artifact.

ictal EEG may show diffuse suppression at onset, followed by sharp waves over the parietal areas, or these may spread to other areas, especially the frontal and mesial frontal regions.[29] In a series of children from Alberta with posterior resections, nine children had parietal lobe surgery and all has lesions except for one.[31] Only two had epileptiform activity limited to the parietal lobe, one had frontal activity, five had ipsilateral diffuse activity, and one had slowing.

The surface EEG may also be misleading in occipital epilepsy, showing posterior temporal activity or bilateral, independent, or synchronous occipital spikes or sharp waves, with a lower amplitude on the contralateral side; diffuse posterior spikes or sharp waves; or involvement of the bilateral frontal, posterior temporal, or parietal regions.[29] Surface EEG may show regionalized patterns over the ipsilateral occipital lobe in 50%, with less than 20% showing focal ictal patterns.[28] Results vary; one study showed that the most active interictal area correctly identified the epileptic focus in 15 of 19 patients[32]; another study revealed that only 18% of patients had spikes limited to the occipital areas, with posterior temporo-occipital spikes seen in 46%.[33] The number was similar for ictal data (80%). There were six occipital patients in the Alberta series; one each had epileptiform activity localized to the occipital area or to the parietooccipital region, three had hemispheric activity, and one had generalized slowing.[31]

Computerized techniques for dipole mapping (source analysis) are now available and are used to identify the epileptic focus. These can be done on both ictal and interictal data.[34,35]

■ Pitfalls of Localization

Seizure semiology is critical for localization, but practitioners must be cautious regarding semiology, especially for extratemporal seizures. A given aura may originate from various cortical areas or represent a propagated discharge. In FLE, signs may localize to the frontal lobe but not to the specific areas within the frontal lobe.[36] We studied the clinical manifestations of frontal and temporal seizures, with only leg movements and hand posturing occurring specifically in frontal seizures whereas oral automatisms occurred only in TLE.[37] Ideally, if there are multiple seizure types, each should be captured and analyzed, especially with a possible multifocal onset, such as with a cortical dysplasia. Bilateral seizures generally preclude a focal cortical resection if occurring equally from both hemispheres, although we have very rarely made an exception, depending on specific case circumstances. We would consider a focal resection if the majority are from one side.

Very few cortical spikes have a surface correlate.[38] Discharges from the cortical generators, after-discharges, have very small amplitudes usually not detected on surface EEG, build up, and then spread to reach the scalp electrodes, which detect the area to which the discharge spreads. Even when the surface electrode shows well-defined spikes or sharp waves, these represent a more regionalized rather than localized phenomenon. It has been estimated that the activation of 6 cm^2 of cortex is required to generate a surface potential.[39] Data from simultaneous surface and invasive recordings show that a much larger cortical area is needed. For temporal lobe seizures, if less than 6 cm^2 was activated on the cortical surface, no recognizable scalp potentials were seen. If 6 to 10 cm^2 were activated, scalp recorded interictal spikes were seen only rarely. Greater than 10 cm^2 activation commonly resulted in recognizable scalp potentials, but prominent scalp spikes were seen only with activation of greater than 30 cm^2 of cortical surface.[38]

The aura (initial seizure onset, which should best localize the ictal onset zone, symptomatogenic zone) may not be detected by EEG. In a study of simultaneous surface and subdural EEG recordings of simple partial seizures (auras), only 6 of 55 auras were recorded on surface EEG.[40] FLE has also been misdiagnosed as pseudoseizures, because the ictal onset may be deep, or the surface EEG is obscured by movement artifact. Patients may also not remember an aura because of retrograde amnesia, or younger children may not be able to report an aura.

Invasive recordings demonstrate high-frequency oscillations (HFO) in the γ band during ictal activity.[41] HFOs are attenuated by the skull (fast frequency filter) and are not detected by surface recordings. In the diffuse electrodecremental ictal pattern EEG, seven patients who had subdural recordings showed high-frequency frontal lobe discharges at the time of the electrodecremental pattern.[42] In epileptic spasms, HFOs have been detected when the surface EEG shows high-amplitude slow waves or electrodecrements.[43]

Even a defined MRI lesion may not always correlate exactly with the interictal or ictal EEG, or the specific lesion may not be the cause of the epilepsy. For tumor-related TLE, in 29 children, interictal epileptiform activity was seen in only 63%; lateralized epileptiform activity was seen in 70% but localized in only 55%; and ictal EEG showed lateralization in 80% but localized in only 40%.[44] Early brain lesions may cause generalized EEG abnormalities. In a study from the Cleveland Clinic, 50 children with focal lesions had refractory epilepsy with either generalized or contralateral epileptiform features; after surgery, 72% were seizure free and 16% had marked improvement with only brief seizures.[45] Focal lesions can cause the generalized pattern of electrical status epilepticus of sleep.[46] They may also cause hypsarrhythmia infantile spasms, and PET scan may demonstrate a possible focus.[47]

In lesions with encephalomalacia and marked cortical atrophy, especially porencephaly, the electrographic seizure may be seen in the contralateral hemisphere: it begins on the side ipsilateral to the lesion but propagates to the contralateral side. The ipsilateral cortical volume may not be enough to generate ictal scalp findings.[48,49] We have seen this in other disorders where a hemisphere is badly damaged, such as Sturge-Weber syndrome. This has also been reported with marked hippocampal sclerosis, with propagation to the contralateral side.[50]

In epilepsy, *dual pathology* refers to the presence of different pathological abnormalities, which may be unrelated or, more likely, the propagation of discharges from the initial epileptogenic lesion. This can result in secondary injury, typically in the hippocampus that later would cause development of hippocampal sclerosis. This has been seen with temporal lobe developmental lesions and congenital abnormalities.[51,52] Even with a demonstrated focal cortical dysplasia generating seizures, there may be microdysgenesis in other areas not visualized by MRI, which could cause postoperative seizures.

If there has been previous surgery, such as prior resection with recurrent seizures, or a skull defect (breach rhythm), there may be distortion of epileptiform activity because of the skull defect, fluid-filled cavities, or distorted postoperative anatomy with adhesions.[53] Magnetoencephalography (MEG) signals are not distorted by these factors.

References

1. Commission on Classification and Terminology of the International League Against Epilepsy. Proposal for revised classification of epilepsies and epileptic syndromes. Epilepsia 1989;30(4):389–399

2. Grech R, Cassar T, Muscat J, et al. Review on solving the inverse problem in EEG source analysis. J Neuroeng Rehabil 2008;5:25–58

3. Rosenow F, Lüders H. Presurgical evaluation of epilepsy. Brain 2001;124(pt 9):1683–1700

4. Sarco DP, Burke JF, Madsen JR. Electroencephalography in epilepsy surgery planning. Childs Nerv Syst 2006;22(8):760–765

5. Obeid M, Wyllie E, Rahi AC, Mikati MA. Approach to pediatric epilepsy surgery. State of the art, Part I: general principles and presurgical workup. Eur J Paediatr Neurol 2009;13(2):102–114

6. Obeid M, Wyllie E, Rahi AC, Mikati MA. Approach to pediatric epilepsy surgery. state of the art, Part II: approach to specific epilepsy syndromes and etiologies. Eur J Paediatr Neurol 2009;13(2):115–127

7. Foldvary N, Klem G, Hammel J, Bingaman W, Najm I, Lüders H. The localizing value of ictal EEG in focal epilepsy. Neurology 2001;57(11):2022–2028

8. Serles W, Caramanos Z, Lindinger G, Pataraia E, Baumgartner C. Combining ictal surface-electroencephalography and seizure semiology improves patient lateralization in temporal lobe epilepsy. Epilepsia 2000;41(12):1567–1573

9. Blume WT, Buza RC, Okazaki H. Anatomic correlates of the ten-twenty electrode placement system in infants. Electroencephalogr Clin Neurophysiol 1974;36(3):303–307

10. Chatrian GE, Lettich E, Nelson PL. Ten percent electrode system for topographic studies of spontaneous and evoked EEG activity. Am J EEG Technol 1985;25:83–92

11. Oostenveld R, Praamstra P. The five percent electrode system for high-resolution EEG and ERP measurements. Clin Neurophysiol 2001;112(4):713–719

12. Morris HH III, Lüders H, Lesser RP, Dinner DS, Klem GH. The value of closely spaced scalp electrodes in the localization of epileptiform foci: a study of 26 patients with complex partial seizures. Electroencephalogr Clin Neurophysiol 1986;63(2):107–111

13. Yoshinaga H, Hattori J, Ohta H, et al. Utility of the scalp-recorded ictal EEG in childhood epilepsy. Epilepsia 2001;42(6):772–777

14. Holmes GL. Temporal lobe epilepsy in childhood. In: Tuxhorn I, Holthausen H, Boenigk H, eds. Paediatric Epilepsy Syndromes and Their Surgical Treatment. London: John Libbey; 1997;251–260

15. Fontana E, Negrini F, Francione S, et al. Temporal lobe epilepsy in children: electroclinical study of 77 cases. Epilepsia 2006;47(suppl 5):26–30

16. Duchowny M, Harvey AS, Jayakar P, et al. The preoperative evaluation of paediatric temporal lobe epilepsy. In: Tuxhorn I, Holthausen

H, Boenigk H, eds. Paediatric Epilepsy Syndromes and Their Surgical Treatment. London: John Libbey; 1997;261–273

17. Malow BA, Selwa LM, Ross D, Aldrich MS. Lateralizing value of interictal spikes on overnight sleep-EEG studies in temporal lobe epilepsy. Epilepsia 1999;40(11):1587–1592

18. Ebersole JS, Pacia SV. Localization of temporal lobe foci by ictal EEG patterns. Epilepsia 1996;37(4):386–399

19. Benifla M, Otsubo H, Ochi A, et al. Temporal lobe surgery for intractable epilepsy in children: an analysis of outcomes in 126 children. Neurosurgery 2006;59(6):1203–1213, discussion 1213–1214

20. Bautista RE, Spencer DD, Spencer SS. EEG findings in frontal lobe epilepsies. Neurology 1998;50(6):1765–1771

21. Vadlamudi L, So EL, Worrell GA, et al. Factors underlying scalp-EEG interictal epileptiform discharges in intractable frontal lobe epilepsy. Epileptic Disord 2004;6(2):89–95

22. Sinclair DB, Wheatley M, Snyder T. Frontal lobe epilepsy in childhood. Pediatr Neurol 2004;30(3):169–176

23. Janszky J, Jokeit H, Schulz R, Hoppe M, Ebner A. EEG predicts surgical outcome in lesional frontal lobe epilepsy. Neurology 2000;54(7):1470–1476

24. Stüve O, Dodrill CB, Holmes MD, Miller JW. The absence of interictal spikes with documented seizures suggests extratemporal epilepsy. Epilepsia 2001;42(6):778–781

25. Battaglia D, Lettori D, Contaldo I, et al. Seizure semiology of lesional frontal lobe epilepsies in children. Neuropediatrics 2007;38(6):287–291

26. Connolly MB, Langill L, Wong PK, Farrell K. Seizures involving the supplementary sensorimotor area in children: a video-EEG analysis. Epilepsia 1995;36(10):1025–1032

27. Kanner AM, Morris HH, Lüders H, et al. Supplementary motor seizures mimicking pseudoseizures: some clinical differences. Neurology 1990;40(9):1404–1407

28. Risinger MW. Noninvasive ictal electroencephalography in humans. In: Luders HO, Noachtar S, eds. Epileptic Seizures: Pathophysiology and Clinical Semiology. New York, NY: Churchill Livingstone; 2000;32–48

29. Sveinbjornsdottir S, Duncan JS. Parietal and occipital lobe epilepsy: a review. Epilepsia 1993;34(3):493–521

30. Salanova V, Andermann F, Rasmussen T, Olivier A, Quesney LF. Parietal lobe epilepsy. Clinical manifestations and outcome in 82 patients treated surgically between 1929 and 1988. Brain 1995;118(pt 3):607–627

31. Sinclair DB, Wheatley M, Snyder T, Gross D, Ahmed N. Posterior resection for childhood epilepsy. Pediatr Neurol 2005;32(4):257–263

32. Blume WT, Whiting SE, Girvin JP. Epilepsy surgery in the posterior cortex. Ann Neurol 1991;29(6):638–645

33. Salanova V, Andermann F, Olivier A, Rasmussen T, Quesney LF. Occipital lobe epilepsy: electroclinical manifestations, electrocorticography, cortical stimulation and outcome in 42 patients treated between 1930 and 1991. Surgery of occipital lobe epilepsy. Brain 1992;115(pt 6):1655–1680

34. Michel CM, Murray MM, Lantz G, Gonzalez S, Spinelli L, Grave de Peralta R. EEG source imaging. Clin Neurophysiol 2004;115(10):2195–2222

35. Sperli F, Spinelli L, Seeck M, Kurian M, Michel CM, Lantz G. EEG source imaging in pediatric epilepsy surgery: a new perspective in presurgical workup. Epilepsia 2006;47(6):981–990

36. Jobst BC, Siegel AM, Thadani VM, Roberts DW, Rhodes HC, Williamson PD. Intractable seizures of frontal lobe origin: clinical characteristics, localizing signs, and results of surgery. Epilepsia 2000;41(9):1139–1152

37. Kramer U, Riviello JJ Jr, Carmant L, Black PM, Madsen J, Holmes GL. Clinical characteristics of complex partial seizures: a temporal versus a frontal lobe onset. Seizure 1997;6(1):57–61

38. Tao JX, Ray A, Hawes-Ebersole S, Ebersole JS. Intracranial EEG substrates of scalp EEG interictal spikes. Epilepsia 2005;46(5):669–676

39. Cooper R, Winter AL, Crow HJ, Walter WG. Comparison of subcortical, cortical, and scalp activity using chronically indwelling electrodes in man. Electroencephalogr Clin Neurophysiol 1965;18:217–228

40. Devinsky O, Sato S, Kufta CV, et al. Electroencephalographic studies of simple partial seizures with subdural electrode recordings. Neurology 1989;39(4):527–533

41. Jirsch JD, Urrestarazu E, LeVan P, Olivier A, Dubeau F, Gotman J. High-frequency oscillations during human focal seizures. Brain 2006;129(pt 6):1593–1608

42. Arroyo S, Lesser RP, Fisher RS, et al. Clinical and electroencephalographic evidence for sites of origin of seizures with diffuse electrodecremental pattern. Epilepsia 1994;35(5):974–987

43. Ramachandrannair R, Ochi A, Imai K, et al. Epileptic spasms in older pediatric patients: MEG and ictal high-frequency oscillations suggest focal-onset seizures in a subset of epileptic spasms. Epilepsy Res 2008;78(2-3):216–224

44. Çataltepe O, Turanli G, Yalnizoglu D, Topçu M, Akalan N. Surgical management of temporal lobe tumor-related epilepsy in children. J Neurosurg 2005;102(3, suppl):280–287

45. Wyllie E, Lachhwani DK, Gupta A, et al. Successful surgery for epilepsy because of early brain lesions despite generalized EEG findings. Neurology 2007;69(4):389–397

46. Loddenkemper T, Cosmo G, Kotagal P, et al. Epilepsy surgery in children with electrical status epilepticus in sleep. Neurosurgery 2009;64(2):328–337, discussion 337

47. Chugani HT, Shields WD, Shewmon DA, Olson DM, Phelps ME, Peacock WJ. Infantile spasms: I. PET identifies focal cortical dysgenesis in cryptogenic cases for surgical treatment. Ann Neurol 1990;27(4):406–413

48. Sammaritano M, de Lotbinière A, Andermann F, Olivier A, Gloor P, Quesney LF. False lateralization by surface EEG of seizure onset in patients with temporal lobe epilepsy and gross focal cerebral lesions. Ann Neurol 1987;21(4):361–369

49. Chang V, Edwards J, Sagher O. False lateralization of electrographic onset in the setting of cerebral atrophy. J Clin Neurophysiol 2007;24(6):438–443

50. Mintzer S, Cendes F, Soss J, et al. Unilateral hippocampal sclerosis with contralateral temporal scalp ictal onset. Epilepsia 2004;45(7):792–802

51. Ho SS, Kuzniecky RI, Gilliam F, Faught E, Morawetz R. Temporal lobe developmental malformations and epilepsy: dual pathology and bilateral hippocampal abnormalities. Neurology 1998;50(3):748–754

52. Lawn N, Londono A, Sawrie S, et al. Occipitoparietal epilepsy, hippocampal atrophy, and congenital developmental abnormalities. Epilepsia 2000;41(12):1546–1553

53. Mohamed IS, Otsubo H, Ochi A, et al. Utility of magnetoencephalography in the evaluation of recurrent seizures after epilepsy surgery. Epilepsia 2007;48(11):2150–2159

5 Invasive Electrophysiological Monitoring

Prasanna Jayakar and Ian Miller

The primary goal of the presurgical evaluation for intractable epilepsy is to accurately define the epileptogenic region (ER). The ER is mainly conceptual and, in practical terms, translates to the minimum amount of tissue that must be resected to ameliorate all seizures. This critical mass of tissue is viewed as a function of the region of seizure onset, seizure propagation patterns, the areas that could become epileptogenic later, and the underlying structural lesion and functional abnormality. As in adults, surgical strategies in childhood are guided by diverse pieces of information obtained from clinical semiology, imaging, and neurophysiological data; the task, however, is more daunting given the greater heterogeneity of etiopathological substrates and maturational factors that significantly influence the clinical presentation and investigative findings.[1]

The role of invasive electroencephalography (EEG) monitoring (IEM) in the evaluation of childhood epilepsy has evolved. With advances in magnetic resonance imaging (MRI), single photon emission computed tomography (SPECT) and positron emission tomography (PET) imaging, presurgical evaluation in many children can be adequately performed through noninvasive means. In the International League Against Epilepsy (ILAE) study of 543 children, the 20 participating centers worldwide reported using IEM in just more than 25% of their surgeries.[2] The increasing use of magnetoencephalography, or three-dimensional EEG dipole source localization algorithms, and the advent of functional MRI to define critical cortex may further diminish the need for IEM. This trend will likely be offset as pediatric centers gain more experience in identifying subtle focal abnormalities using noninvasive tools and aggressively pursue surgical candidacy in increasingly complex cases. This chapter critically examines the continuing role of IEM in presurgical evaluation.

■ Pragmatic Considerations

IEM is inherently costly, risky, and not devoid of limitations. It is therefore prudent to first consider some practical issues as they relate to a given patient. IEM is preferably undertaken only if prior noninvasive evaluation provides sufficient information as to the side or approximate location of the ER; it should not be used as an "exploratory procedure." Also, it is prudent to ask the question if a more precise definition of ER using IEM will alter the ultimate surgical strategy and outcome. For example, IEM may be of little use if the noninvasive studies support widespread epileptogenic dysfunction that cannot all be resected and the goals of surgery are mainly palliative or when a "standard" temporal or precoronal frontal lobectomy is contemplated in a child with all noninvasive data indicating an ER contained within the planned resection. Similarly, when the intraoperative electrocorticography (ECoG) reveals almost continuous focal seizure discharges, the additional yield, if any, from IEM rarely justifies a two-stage procedure.

Because of limitations of sampling and interpretation, IEM does not always ensure a clear focality and precise demarcation of the ER. Although its yield cannot be predicted with certainty, our experience suggests that children who are neurodevelopmentally intact, who reveal a restricted focus with an otherwise normal scalp EEG, or who have relatively localized imaging findings that can be specifically targeted by electrodes are likely to accrue the greatest benefit. By contrast, IEM is unlikely to document discrete seizure onsets when patients with normal imaging studies present with spasms or diffuse patterns on the scalp EEG or in patients with multiple subcortical nodular heterotopias, large infiltrative lesions, or extensive multilobar cortical dysplasia.

Lastly, the use of IEM for defining critical cortex to "fine tune" the resection must be justified by the potential limitations of intraoperative functional mapping. Language mapping can rarely be performed intraoperatively in children. Somatosensory responses to median nerve stimulation help to define the central sulcus, but the estimate of sensory and motor regions may be inaccurate. The motor cortex can be crudely mapped by direct electrical stimulation, but general anesthesia often suppresses the ability to elicit consistent responses especially in the young child.

■ Indications

Although many centers offer IEM, there is no standard presurgical protocol, and its use is guided primarily by the availability of other noninvasive tools and the referral pattern at each center. At our center, all children undergo video EEG and MRI scanning; those revealing certain subtypes of MRI lesions with convergent video-EEG data require no further testing. In others, functional imaging (SPECT and or PET) scans, three-dimensional spike source localization, and functional MRI for language and motor regions are obtained. The data are reviewed at a multidisciplinary case conference where the surgical strategy is defined. Guided by the pragmatic considerations discussed previously, IEM is generally recommended for the following indications: inconclusive preoperative data (e.g., normal or nonspecific computed tomography [CT]/MRI scans, structural lesions), divergent preoperative data, or encroachment on eloquent cortex.

Inconclusive Preoperative Data: Each Test Has Limitations

Normal or Nonspecific CT/MRI Scans

Despite advances in MRI imaging, many children with localization-related intractable epilepsy have normal scans; approximately one in every four children in the ILAE series did not show a definite lesion on MRI.[2] IEM continues to play a significant role in this patient subgroup, especially when functional imaging data are inconclusive; removal of the entire region of significant abnormalities identified on IEM is generally required to achieve seizure freedom.[3] In our recent series,[4] 80 of the 102 patients underwent a two-stage evaluation, the rest could be adequately localized based on scalp EEG, functional imaging, and ECoG.

Structural Lesion

In general, a discrete structural abnormality on CT/MRI scans is regarded as a very reliable marker of the ER and biases the presurgical evaluation against IEM. However, there are many documented failures after lesionectomy in children,[5,6] partly because lesional epilepsy does not represent a homogeneous substrate. Whereas developmental tumors, hippocampal sclerosis, low-flow vascular lesions, or Sturge-Weber syndrome can often be successfully treated after noninvasive evaluation alone, children with ill-defined cortical dysplasia or multiple lesions such as tuberous sclerosis often reveal complex and rapid seizure propagation that make interpretation of the scalp EEG and functional imaging data difficult. IEM often helps clarify ambiguities of seizure origin and propagation, thus facilitating surgery in these difficult cases.[6-8] In some cases albeit rare, when the MRI shows widespread lesions but other noninvasive data suggest that seizures arise from only a restricted region, IEM may allow successful focal resections averting a hemispherectomy in a functional child.[9]

Divergent Preoperative Data

The criteria of what exactly constitutes divergence are variably defined by different centers; we regard divergence when the clinical semiology, EEG, and functional/structural imaging data implicate separate regions. In this scenario, IEM serves as the last resort to help define the ER and may permit successful focal resection. Since the divergence may arise from complex and rapid interaction between noncontiguous cortical sites, all suspected sites must be adequately sampled. When divergence occurs in the context of large or deep-seated lesions, a combination of subdural and strategically placed depth electrodes is recommended.

Encroachment on Eloquent Cortex

In our series of discrete perirolandic foci, aggressive resections tailored to the ER and eloquent motor cortex led to seizure freedom in more than half the cases, even in the absence of a structural lesion.[10] In some cases, a calculated decision to remove part of the motor cortex revealing face or proximal limb function enhances the chances of success without incurring risks of significant clinical deficits. Likewise, in patients with occipital foci who have intact visual fields, accurate demarcation of the ER over the occipital convexity or base may allow a restricted corticectomy preserving most of the calcarine cortex and visual pathways, making IEM a worthwhile endeavor.[11]

The issues surrounding the need to identify and preserve language cortex are more complex. Because language cortex is plastic under age 5 years, many centers opt for more aggressive large resections in the hope of forcing language transfer. Our presurgical evaluation strategy is driven by the intent to preserve predestined language sites unless they are involved at ictal onset. As illustrated in **Fig. 5.1**, we have used IEM to map and tailor resections, even in the very young, with the hope of maximizing language outcomes in those who are rendered seizure free.

■ Technical Aspects

Spatial Coverage

In general, an attempt must be made to place enough electrodes so that the site of seizure origin and the ER boundaries predicted on the basis of noninvasive testing are adequately sampled, and the drop-off of the epileptogenic field can be demonstrated. This task is not always easy because the range from which each electrode records is small[12] and the number of electrodes that can be placed in children, especially younger ones, are limited. When the ER is expected to encroach on critical cortex, additional coverage must be provided to perform functional mapping. Bilateral

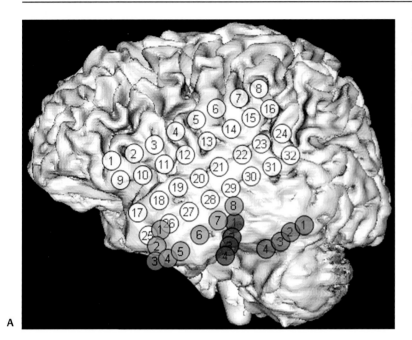

Fig. 5.1 Diagram of subdural electrodes **(A)** over the left temporal region in a 4-year-old patient with cortical dysplasia. Subdural electroencephalography recording **(B)**, showing ictal onset at contacts 3 and 4 of the anterior temporal polar strip, with early involvement of the superior temporal convexity (contacts 19–20), which were subsequently shown to be critical language areas on functional mapping. Invasive monitoring helped tailor the resection.

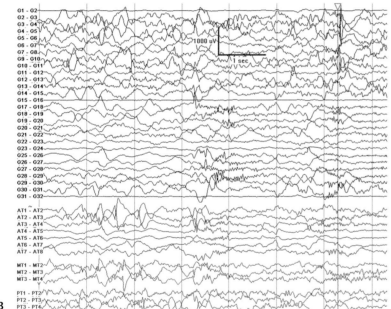

placements, commonly performed in adults, are rarely required in children.

Type of Electrodes

Foramen ovale electrodes used in adults have limited application in childhood where pure mesolimbic epilepsy is uncommon. Invasive electrodes are usually made of platinum and are configured for subdural or depth placement. Subdural electrodes spaced 5 to 10 mm apart and configured as strips (4 to 8 contacts) or grids (20 to 64 contacts) are most suited to cover large areas of the neocortical convexity and basal and interhemispheric surfaces.[13,14] They also provide the means to accurately map critical regions. Depth electrodes are designed to penetrate the brain tissue and are necessary to document seizure origin from the hippocampus or other deep-seated sites such as a lesion within a sulcus. Four to 12 contacts are arranged linearly 5 to 10 mm apart. Others may have up to 18 contacts 1.5 mm apart for closer sampling. Subdural and depth electrodes may be used in conjunction to provide comprehensive coverage of both the cortical surface and deep locations.

against the feasibility and safety of extending the resection beyond the seizure onset zone.

Interictal spikes and sharp waves, the patterns most representative of the irritative zone, show considerable variation in morphology, frequency, and distribution, and may persist after resection without adversely affecting outcome.[12,18–20] They are thus generally considered more significant if they are consistently unifocal or appear in rhythmic runs. Quantitative assessment of spike parameters, such as average frequency or amplitude, may help interpretation.[27] In some children, the discharges may be almost continuous and appear in burst or repetitive recruiting and derecruiting rhythms akin to electrographic seizures. Such patterns are regarded as a hallmark of cortical dysplasia,[7] but in our experience may be seen in other pathological substrates as well.[28]

Other patterns signifying potential epileptogenicity, albeit infrequent, may also be used in planning the extent of resection. These include focal intermittent bursts of fast activity initially described on the scalp EEG[29] and intraictal secondarily activated foci where, during the course of a seizure, a well-localized, independent ictal sequence develops at propagated sites and outlasts the primary seizure sequence.[30] In our series, three quarters of secondarily activated foci were documented as being capable of generating independent seizures.

The role of responses to electrical or pharmacologic provocation is not well studied in children. In our experience with electrical stimulation, the localization value is higher when the early manifestations of provoked seizures are similar to the patient's habitual auras; late manifestations generally tend to be less reliable. We also do not find after-discharge thresholds to be useful in defining the ER.

Functional Deficit Zone

Burst suppression activity and focal attenuation of fast activity in the background are not conventionally regarded to be epileptiform, but they closely correlate with other markers of the ER. Both patterns remain consistent over time; the focality of the β attenuation can be accentuated by administering drugs that activate fast frequencies. Polymorphic slowing, by contrast, generally shows considerable temporal variability reflecting nonspecific reactions to anesthesia or electrode implantation and may not be very useful. Postictal background abnormalities, which are shown to be reliable on the scalp EEG, have not been analyzed on invasive studies. Similarly, the role of absent or diminished evoked responses is not established.

■ Conclusion

The role of invasive monitoring in the presurgical evaluation of children continues to evolve as our experience with multimodal noninvasive techniques increases. Although a greater proportion of children now benefit from a one-stage resection, intracranial recording clearly serves as the definitive tool to accomplish outcomes successfully after resective surgery in specific subgroups and the more difficult cases.

References

1. Cross JH, Jayakar P, Nordli D, et al., International League Against Epilepsy, Subcommission for Paediatric Epilepsy Surgery; Commissions of Neurosurgery and Paediatrics. Proposed criteria for referral and evaluation of children for epilepsy surgery: recommendations of the Subcommission for Pediatric Epilepsy Surgery. Epilepsia 2006;47(6):952–959

2. Harvey AS, Cross JH, Shinnar S, Mathern BW; ILAE Pediatric Epilepsy Surgery Survey Taskforce. Defining the spectrum of international practice in pediatric epilepsy surgery patients. Epilepsia 2008;49(1):146–155

3. Jayakar P, Duchowny MS. Invasive EEG recording and functional mapping in children. In: Tuxhorn I, Holthausen H, Boenik HE, eds. Pediatric Epilepsy Syndromes and Their Surgical Treatment. London: John Libbey & Co.; 1997:547–556

4. Jayakar P, Dunoyer C, Dean P, et al. Epilepsy surgery in patients with normal or nonfocal MRI scans: integrative strategies offer long-term seizure relief. Epilepsia 2008;49(5):758–764

5. Palmini A, Andermann F, Olivier A, et al. Focal neuronal migration disorders and intractable partial epilepsy: a study of 30 patients. Ann Neurol 1991;30(6):741–749

6. Holthausen H, Teixeira VA, Tuxhorn I, et al. Epilepsy surgery in children and adolescents with focal cortical dysplasia. In: Tuxhorn

I, Holthausen H, Boenik HE, eds. Pediatric Epilepsy Syndromes and Their Surgical Treatment. London: John Libbey & Co.; 1997:199–215

7. Palmini A, Gambardella A, Andermann F, et al. Intrinsic epileptogenicity of human dysplastic cortex as suggested by corticography and surgical results. Ann Neurol 1995;37(4):476–487

8. Jayakar P. Invasive EEG monitoring in children: when, where, and what? J Clin Neurophysiol 1999;16(5):408–418

9. Duchowny MS, Jayakar P, Resnick TJ, et al. Epilepsy surgery in the first three years of life. Epilepsia 1998;39(7):737–743

10. Udani V, Jayakar P, Resnick T, Duchowny M, Alvarez LA. Excisional surgery for perirolandic epilepsy in children. Proceedings of American Epilepsy Society December 7–10, 1997. Epilepsia 1997;38(suppl 8):74

11. Kuzniecky R, Gilliam F, Morawetz R, Faught E, Palmer C, Black L. Occipital lobe developmental malformations and epilepsy: clinical spectrum, treatment, and outcome. Epilepsia 1997;38(2):175–181

12. Gloor P. Contributions of electroencephalography and electrocorticography to the neurosurgical treatment of the epilepsies. In: Purpura DP, Penry JK, Walter RD, eds. Neurosurgical Management of the Epilepsies. Advances in Neurology. Vol 8. New York, NY: Raven Press; 1975:59–105

13. Wyllie E, Lüders H, Morris HH III, et al. Subdural electrodes in the evaluation for epilepsy surgery in children and adults. Neuropediatrics 1988;19(2):80–86

14. Nespeca M, Wyllie E, Luders H, et al. EEG Recording and functional localization studies with subdural electrodes in infants and young children. J Epilepsy 1990;3:107–124

15. Burneo JG, Steven DA, McLachlan RS, Parrent AG. Morbidity associated with the use of intracranial electrodes for epilepsy surgery. Can J Neurol Sci 2006;33(2):223–227

16. Johnston JM Jr, Mangano FT, Ojemann JG, Park TS, Trevathan E, Smyth MD. Complications of invasive subdural electrode monitoring at St. Louis Children's Hospital, 1994-2005. J Neurosurg 2006; 105(5, suppl)343–347

17. Musleh W, Yassari R, Hecox K, Kohrman M, Chico M, Frim D. Low incidence of subdural grid-related complications in prolonged pediatric EEG monitoring. Pediatr Neurosurg 2006;42(5):284–287

18. Lieb JP, Joseph JP, Engel J Jr, Walker J, Crandall PH. Sleep state and seizure foci related to depth spike activity in patients with temporal lobe epilepsy. Electroencephalogr Clin Neurophysiol 1980;49(5-6): 538–557

19. Luders H, Lesser RP, Dinner DS. Commentary: chronic intracranial recording and stimulation with subdural electrodes. In: Engel J Jr, ed. Surgical Treatment of the Epilepsies. New York, NY: Raven Press; 1987:297–321

20. Ajmone-Marsan C. Chronic intracranial recording and electrocorticography. In: Daly DD, Pedley TA, eds. Current Practice of Clinical Electroencephalography. New York, NY: Raven Press; 1990:535–560

21. Jayakar P, Duchowny M, Resnick TJ, Alvarez LA. Localization of seizure foci: pitfalls and caveats. J Clin Neurophysiol 1991;8: 414–431

22. Jayakar P, Duchowny MS, Resnick TJ. Subdural monitoring in the evaluation of children for epilepsy surgery. J Child Neurol 1994;9(suppl 2):61–66

23. Ikeda A, Terada K, Mikuni N, et al. Subdural recording of ictal DC shifts in neocortical seizures in humans. Epilepsia 1996;37(7):662–674

24. Schiller Y, Cascino GD, Busacker NE, Sharbrough FW. Characterization and comparison of local onset and remote propagated electrographic seizures recorded with intracranial electrodes. Epilepsia 1998;39(4):380–388

25. Fisher RS, Webber WR, Lesser RP, Arroyo S, Uematsu S. High-frequency EEG activity at the start of seizures. J Clin Neurophysiol 1992;9(3):441–448

26. Whiting SE, Jayakar P, Resnick T, et al. The utility of subdural EEG patterns to define the epileptogenic zone in children with cortical dysplasia. American Epilepsy Society proceedings. Epilepsia 1998;39(suppl 6):65

27. Asano E, Muzik O, Shah A, et al. Quantitative interictal subdural EEG analyses in children with neocortical epilepsy. Epilepsia 2003;44(3):425–434

28. Turkdogan D, Duchowny M, Resnick T, Jayakar P. Subdural EEG patterns in children with taylor-type cortical dysplasia: comparison with nondysplastic lesions. J Clin Neurophysiol 2005;22(1): 37–42

29. Altman KD, Shewmon A. Local paroxysmal fast activity: significance interictally and in infantile spasms. American Epilepsy Society proceedings. Epilepsia 1990;31(5):623

30. Jayakar P, Duchowny M, Alvarez L, Resnick T. Intraictal activation in the neocortex: a marker of the epileptogenic region. Epilepsia 1994b;35(3):489–494

availability of other noninvasive tools and the referral pattern at each center. At our center, all children undergo video EEG and MRI scanning; those revealing certain subtypes of MRI lesions with convergent video-EEG data require no further testing. In others, functional imaging (SPECT and or PET) scans, three-dimensional spike source localization, and functional MRI for language and motor regions are obtained. The data are reviewed at a multidisciplinary case conference where the surgical strategy is defined. Guided by the pragmatic considerations discussed previously, IEM is generally recommended for the following indications: inconclusive preoperative data (e.g., normal or nonspecific computed tomography [CT]/MRI scans, structural lesions), divergent preoperative data, or encroachment on eloquent cortex.

Inconclusive Preoperative Data: Each Test Has Limitations

Normal or Nonspecific CT/MRI Scans

Despite advances in MRI imaging, many children with localization-related intractable epilepsy have normal scans; approximately one in every four children in the ILAE series did not show a definite lesion on MRI.[2] IEM continues to play a significant role in this patient subgroup, especially when functional imaging data are inconclusive; removal of the entire region of significant abnormalities identified on IEM is generally required to achieve seizure freedom.[3] In our recent series,[4] 80 of the 102 patients underwent a two-stage evaluation, the rest could be adequately localized based on scalp EEG, functional imaging, and ECoG.

Structural Lesion

In general, a discrete structural abnormality on CT/MRI scans is regarded as a very reliable marker of the ER and biases the presurgical evaluation against IEM. However, there are many documented failures after lesionectomy in children,[5,6] partly because lesional epilepsy does not represent a homogeneous substrate. Whereas developmental tumors, hippocampal sclerosis, low-flow vascular lesions, or Sturge-Weber syndrome can often be successfully treated after noninvasive evaluation alone, children with ill-defined cortical dysplasia or multiple lesions such as tuberous sclerosis often reveal complex and rapid seizure propagation that make interpretation of the scalp EEG and functional imaging data difficult. IEM often helps clarify ambiguities of seizure origin and propagation, thus facilitating surgery in these difficult cases.[6-8] In some cases albeit rare, when the MRI shows widespread lesions but other noninvasive data suggest that seizures arise from only a restricted region, IEM may allow successful focal resections averting a hemispherectomy in a functional child.[9]

Divergent Preoperative Data

The criteria of what exactly constitutes divergence are variably defined by different centers; we regard divergence when the clinical semiology, EEG, and functional/structural imaging data implicate separate regions. In this scenario, IEM serves as the last resort to help define the ER and may permit successful focal resection. Since the divergence may arise from complex and rapid interaction between noncontiguous cortical sites, all suspected sites must be adequately sampled. When divergence occurs in the context of large or deep-seated lesions, a combination of subdural and strategically placed depth electrodes is recommended.

Encroachment on Eloquent Cortex

In our series of discrete perirolandic foci, aggressive resections tailored to the ER and eloquent motor cortex led to seizure freedom in more than half the cases, even in the absence of a structural lesion.[10] In some cases, a calculated decision to remove part of the motor cortex revealing face or proximal limb function enhances the chances of success without incurring risks of significant clinical deficits. Likewise, in patients with occipital foci who have intact visual fields, accurate demarcation of the ER over the occipital convexity or base may allow a restricted corticectomy preserving most of the calcarine cortex and visual pathways, making IEM a worthwhile endeavor.[11]

The issues surrounding the need to identify and preserve language cortex are more complex. Because language cortex is plastic under age 5 years, many centers opt for more aggressive large resections in the hope of forcing language transfer. Our presurgical evaluation strategy is driven by the intent to preserve predestined language sites unless they are involved at ictal onset. As illustrated in **Fig. 5.1**, we have used IEM to map and tailor resections, even in the very young, with the hope of maximizing language outcomes in those who are rendered seizure free.

■ Technical Aspects

Spatial Coverage

In general, an attempt must be made to place enough electrodes so that the site of seizure origin and the ER boundaries predicted on the basis of noninvasive testing are adequately sampled, and the drop-off of the epileptogenic field can be demonstrated. This task is not always easy because the range from which each electrode records is small[12] and the number of electrodes that can be placed in children, especially younger ones, are limited. When the ER is expected to encroach on critical cortex, additional coverage must be provided to perform functional mapping. Bilateral

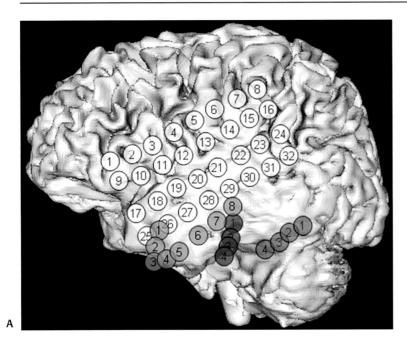

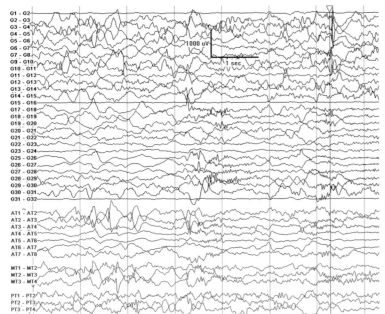

Fig. 5.1 Diagram of subdural electrodes **(A)** over the left temporal region in a 4-year-old patient with cortical dysplasia. Subdural electroencephalography recording **(B)**, showing ictal onset at contacts 3 and 4 of the anterior temporal polar strip, with early involvement of the superior temporal convexity (contacts 19–20), which were subsequently shown to be critical language areas on functional mapping. Invasive monitoring helped tailor the resection.

placements, commonly performed in adults, are rarely required in children.

Type of Electrodes

Foramen ovale electrodes used in adults have limited application in childhood where pure mesolimbic epilepsy is uncommon. Invasive electrodes are usually made of platinum and are configured for subdural or depth placement. Subdural electrodes spaced 5 to 10 mm apart and configured as strips (4 to 8 contacts) or grids (20 to 64 contacts) are most suited to cover large areas of the neocortical convexity and basal and interhemispheric surfaces.[13,14] They also provide the means to accurately map critical regions. Depth electrodes are designed to penetrate the brain tissue and are necessary to document seizure origin from the hippocampus or other deep-seated sites such as a lesion within a sulcus. Four to 12 contacts are arranged linearly 5 to 10 mm apart. Others may have up to 18 contacts 1.5 mm apart for closer sampling. Subdural and depth electrodes may be used in conjunction to provide comprehensive coverage of both the cortical surface and deep locations.

Surgical Insertion

Subdural electrodes are implanted under direct observation after craniotomy, although strips may be placed via burr holes (see Chapter 15). Depth electrodes are inserted under stereotactic MRI- or CT-guided techniques that allow accurate placement at target sites, including symmetric bilateral positioning in homotopic areas of interest; the strategy for depth placement differs somewhat in North America from that used in some European centers. Implantation may be guided by a stereotactic frame; frameless stereotactic methods are preferred in the younger child where the calvarium is thin. The exact location of the electrodes can be defined extraoperatively on MRI or high-resolution CT scans coregistered to the MR.

◼ Risks

Dedicated nursing and social intervention facilitates the perioperative care in children undergoing IEM. Prophylactic steroids help minimize the risk of reaction to the implant. Implantation is generally well tolerated, but complications, including wound infection, cerebrospinal fluid leak, intracranial bleeding, or symptomatic pneumocephalus, have all been reported.[15-17] Depth placements may lead to intracerebral microhemorrhage; subdural electrodes may cause local inflammatory reactions. Risks tend to be higher in children who are reoperated[17]; permanent neurological deficit or death associated with IEM is very rare.

◼ Recording

Current digital systems have high sampling rate capability, at 500 to 1000 Hz, allowing detection of fast frequencies that may provide useful additional information. Seizure capture may be augmented by withdrawal of antiepileptic medications; albeit rare, due consideration should be given to the chances of activating atypical seizures. Spontaneous seizures are usually captured over 4 to 10 days; longer periods of up to 1 month may occasionally be required. Generally, 3 to 10 seizures are considered adequate, although multiple factors may influence the confidence of the reader, including stereotypy of onset and evolution, and their convergence with other data. Once the capture of spontaneous seizures is deemed complete, we reinstate full medication before attempting functional mapping via electrical cortical stimulation.

◼ Interpretation

The ambiguities and complexity of intracranial EEG interpretation are well recognized,[8,12,18-22] and guidelines for its use in defining the ER are often based on empirical criteria.

Ictal Onset Zone

Defining the region of seizure onset accurately is the strongest justification for IEM, especially in children with multifocal MRI and interictal EEG abnormalities. As illustrated in **Fig. 5.2**, periodic discharges were seen independently over several regions, but ictal onset consistently occurred from a single focus. The onset zone may be regarded as the region showing the initial transformation from the interictal state—the collective area revealing a group of patterns commonly observed during the initial phase of the seizure including bursts of focal fast activity—the "beta buzz," spike/polyspikes or runs of spikes, or electrodecrement.[8,23,24] Rhythmic slow $\alpha/\theta/\delta$ range frequencies occurring discretely as the first change are considered significant but may not be included in the ictal onset zone if they are observed after onset, even when they achieve high amplitude. Very high frequencies[25] or slow direct current (DC) shifts have also been observed but may be missed with conventional filter settings.

The duration after onset in which these patterns appear is variable from patient to patient and at times even in the same subject; not all patterns are necessarily seen in every seizure. Objective definition of the onset zone can thus be challenging, especially in patients with rapid propagation in which the duration after onset that is considered significant remains arbitrary. In general, the longer the discharge remains discrete after onset, the greater the likelihood of a successful outcome will be.[23] In our experience, more than half the children with discrete ictal onset on invasive studies were rendered seizure free as opposed to fewer than 10% when the onset was diffuse.[26]

In some cases, presumably because seizures arise from lesional or severely damaged cortex, the ictal onset region does not generate a typical robust ictal sequence but merely acts as a "trigger" activating remote healthier areas.[8] The ictal trigger may be characterized by only a subtle transformation from the ongoing interictal state, such as alteration of the frequency, morphology, and distribution of interictal spikes; alteration of the frequency or content of an interictal burst suppression; or merely a further attenuation of the background. The transform may be appreciated only after the same change is consistently observed at ictal onset in several seizures. From a practical standpoint, failure to recognize the subtle transform as the true "onset zone" focuses attention on the subsequent robust buildup over remote regions, thus predisposing to false localization or apparent nonconvergence of data.

Irritative Zone

To maximize the chances of seizure freedom, the surgical resection generally also includes cortical regions, revealing "significant" potential epileptogenicity; one weighs the potential risk of seizures attributed to the observed pattern(s)

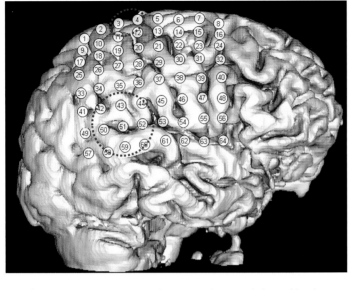

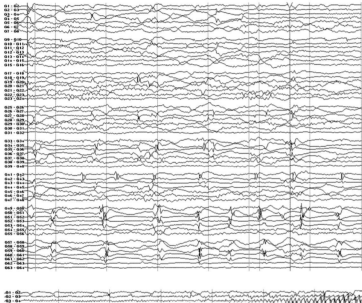

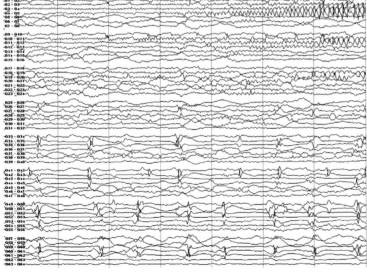

Fig. 5.2 Diagram of subdural electrodes **(A)** in a child with multifocal magnetic resonance imaging abnormalities. The subdural interictal recording **(B)** revealed independent areas of semiperiodic epileptiform discharges. The discharges over the superior part of the grid (electrodes 3 and 4) shows gradual attenuation—a subtle ictal transformation that 10 seconds later **(C)** builds up into a robust seizure discharge. This area corresponded to primary motor cortex on functional mapping. The periodic discharges over inferior region (around electrode 51) remain virtually unchanged during the seizure. The accurate identification of the ictal onset helped make the critical decision to resect the primary motor area.

6 Extra-operative and Intra-operative Electrical Stimulation

Ingrid Tuxhorn

The surgical resection of epileptic tissue is an established treatment for patients with intractable focal epilepsy and has become an important field in epilepsy and neurosurgery.[1] Pediatric epilepsy surgery is no longer a treatment of last resort.[1] There is growing evidence from expert centers that children with surgically remediable focal epilepsy syndromes should be referred and selected early for presurgical evaluation and subsequent operation to optimize seizure control and long-term psychosocial outcome.[2]

Unique pediatric aspects necessitate a specific pediatric approach for referral, diagnosis, and management, which has been outlined in the recent recommendations of the International League Against Epilepsy (ILAE) subcommission on pediatric epilepsy surgery.[3] Similarly the pediatric presurgical evaluation requires specific pediatric epilepsy expertise of experienced and knowledgeable pediatric epilepsy centers.[4] An accurate description of the phenomenology of epileptic seizures, classification of seizure types, the specific epilepsy syndromes, an etiologic diagnosis, and an optional assessment of impairments and co morbidities along the lines of the ILAE classification guidelines will be the basis of early referral and optimized management of infants and children for surgical evaluation and treatment.[5]

■ Pediatric Aspects of the Presurgical Evaluation

The presurgical evaluation should be considered as a multimodal diagnostic approach, with the goal of localizing the epileptogenic zone, defining the epileptogenic substrate, and delineating neighboring functional cortex to reduce risk for neurological deficits with surgical removal.[6] Outcome studies suggest that the cortical regions that underlie epileptogenicity must be excised entirely because residual epileptogenic tissue increases the risk for persisting postoperative seizures.[7] Compared with adults, medically resistant partial epilepsies in children are more heterogeneous in terms of anatomical localization, types and extent of pathologies, and electroclinical functional characteristics. The epileptogenic lesions may be discrete structural changes that are very amenable to surgical removal or extensive and widespread macroscopic or low-grade microscopic developmental or ac-

quired lesions.[4] The adult temporal lobe epilepsy syndrome is a well-defined, electroclinical syndrome caused by hippocampal sclerosis as its dominant etiopathological finding.[8] By contrast, seizures of temporal lobe origin in childhood are a particular diagnostic challenge because they typically involve the neocortical regions and may extend beyond the margins of the temporal lobe rather than being confined to the mesial temporolimbic structures.[9]

In addition, the seizure semiology is highly age dependent with prominent motor features (tonic, myoclonic, spasms) that are more typical of extratemporal onset and not suggestive of temporal limbic localization.[10]

Invasive electroencephalography (EEG) and functional mapping may be indicated to properly tailor a cortical resective procedure after the ictal onset zone and eloquent cortex have been clearly localized with these procedures.[11] The high incidence of extratemporal neocortical epilepsy in pediatric patients makes this an important consideration.[4]

The anatomical landmarks of cortical areas subserving important functions, such as sensation, movement, language, and vision, have been well delineated. However, there is sufficient interindividual variation that may be accentuated with associated developmental or acquired pathological conditions through a process of intrahemispheric or interhemispheric reorganization. Thus careful and individualized presurgical investigation with functional cortical mapping is essential for each patient on a case-by-case basis.

■ A Historic Note

After extensive studies in animals, cortical stimulation in humans was performed by Victor Horsely in London, Fedor Krause in Berlin, Harvey Cushing in Boston, and Ottfried Foerster in Breslau.

In the 1950s, the first pediatric patient was probably evaluated with cortical stimulation by Penfield and Jasper in Montreal. This 4 year old had tuberous sclerosis and epilepsy arising from the central region.[12] Penfield and Jasper performed intraoperative electrocorticography (ECoG) and found a well-localized spike focus in the right central region. With cortical stimulation, they reproduced the left clonic seizures of the patient before resecting that area. They also reported a 16-year-old girl who had active spontaneous spikes over the first temporal gyrus and midtemporal region and reproduced her habitual aura of fear by stimulating the anterior insula close to the junction with the uncus.[12,13] The appearance of "dreamy states" on stimulation of the uncus and other clues from animal studies and ECoG led Penfield and Jasper to believe that the mesial and inferior parts of the temporal lobe were the origin of many epileptic attacks. Resection of these regions subsequently improved the outcome significantly.

The pioneering work of Penfield and Jasper led to the mapping of the anterior and posterior language areas and visual and cortical areas and further refined the cortical map of sensory and motor representation.[12–14] Subsequently, many studies have described the utility of cortical stimulation either used extraoperatively or intraoperatively in adults and children to delineate cortical functional areas in relation to areas of epileptogenesis before surgical removal.[14]

◼ Goals of Stimulation in Presurgical Evaluation

Extraoperative stimulation is achieved with direct electrical stimulation of the cerebral cortex via subdural or depth electrodes.[11,15–17] This technique has been in use for more than 40 years, and two effects commonly observed have been described in the extensive literature. Cortical stimulation may activate cerebral function producing positive phenomena such as tonic or clonic movements, and special sensations, or cortical stimulation may inhibit function producing negative phenomena such as speech arrest or arrest of motor function. However, in the pediatric population, mapping of cortical function with direct stimulation may be less reliable because of limited patient cooperation and the absence of or inconsistent cortical responses of the immature cortex at lower stimulation thresholds compared with adults.[11,18,19]

Once interictal discharges and sufficient seizures have been recorded from intracranial electrodes, cortical stimulation is performed in a systematic fashion, usually over several days, depending on the number of electrodes, the area that needs to be mapped, and the patient's degree of cooperation. Because there is a potential to induce seizures, ECoG monitoring is essential to detect after-discharges that may herald increased epileptogenicity under the stimulated cortex. To reduce the risk of stimulation-induced seizures, anticonvulsants that may have been reduced or stopped to activate seizures for video-EEG recording and analysis should be restarted before initiating the cortical stimulation studies. In addition, temporary benzodiazepine coverage during the procedure may be useful.

◼ Physiology of Cortical Stimulation

The neurophysiological effects of extracellular neuronal stimulation has been studied extensively and was reviewed by Ranck in 1975.[20] The voltage distribution in neural tissue after electrical stimulation depends on the current density (which is a function of stimulus frequency and wave forms) applied, as well as the stimulation-induced membrane polarization. The electrical field within brain tissue produced by stimulation of a subdural electrode has a complex three-dimensional shape, and underlying neural processes may be subject to depolarizing or hyperpolarizing events from the stimulation, which may depend on stimulation parameters, the cellular geometry of cortical pyramidal neurons, and the position of the neuron in relation to the stimulating electrode.[16,21]

The effect of the applied stimulus on local neuronal cells near the stimulating electrode may be considered to result in a direct effect of the applied electrical field on the local cell or the indirect stimulation induced transsynaptic excitation and inhibition, which results from activation of a large number of axon terminals leading to increased synaptic activity on the dendritic tree of the local cells. Depending on the types and numbers of synaptic receptors activated, the transsynaptic activity induced by electrical stimulation may be excitatory, inhibitory, or a blend of both.

Generally, with appropriate stimulus conditions, the maximal current density is achieved beneath the stimulated electrodes so that the stimulus-related responses usually represent cortical function in the crown of the gyrus, whereas the banks of the sulcus are not investigated with this method. Potentially, there may be distant current spread to produce positive responses from remote areas.

Cortical excitability in children is known to be different from adults, and electrical stimulation at maximal stimulus intensity, as will be discussed later, may not elicit a positive response after stimulating functional cortex. This may result in yielding a false-negative response and the risk of removing potentially functional cortex.[11,18,19]

◼ Safety Issues and Complications in Pediatric Patients

The use of subdural or depth electrodes is an invasive procedure that may be complicated by infection, hemorrhage, edema, mass effect, or infarction. The probability of complications associated with intracranial electrodes has been reported by various centers at 2 to 4%. Patients who have undergone prior high-dose brain irradiation may be at particular risk for developing reactive cerebral edema necessitating emergent removal of subdural electrodes. This has only been reported in adult patients.[22] In the pediatric age group, the complication rate of subdural electrode implantation is also reportedly low and comparable to the adult experience.[11]

The energy applied to the surface of the brain via electrical stimulation per se may add an additional risk to damaging the cortex surface. Microscopic studies, however, have not shown gross structural damage, but mild inflammatory responses have been demonstrated in the pathology of the resected tissue.[23,24]

The use of magnetic resonance imaging (MRI) compatible platinum electrodes over stainless steel electrodes allows for coregistration imaging of the electrodes with MRI.[25] There is, however, no reported safety data on higher field strength MRI and subdural electrode (SDE) compatibility, and practitioners need to proceed with caution at this age. There is no evidence that cortical stimulation produces kindling because the after-discharge thresholds do not progressively decrease with repeated stimulation over a cortical region, although the thresholds may be variable with repeated stimulation.

■ General Principles and Techniques

The standard stimulation paradigm for extracortical cortical stimulation via subdural grid electrodes uses biphasic rectangular pulses delivered at a rate of 50/s in trains lasting 3 to 5 seconds.[11,17,18] The pulse duration is held constant at 0.3 milliseconds, whereas the stimulus intensity is increased in a stepwise fashion to a maximum of 15 mA or to a stimulus intensity that elicits a clinical response or after-discharge less than the maximal threshold of 15 mA.

The following stimulation parameters are used routinely in adult patients at the Cleveland Clinic Epilepsy Center: A stimulus is applied for a duration of 2 to 5 seconds to an active electrode with a frequency of 50 Hz as a biphasic square wave, a constant current of 300 microseconds duration with incremental steps of 1 to 2 mA over a range of 1 to 15 mA.[16] As the stimulus intensity is gradually increased to 15 mA, either positive responses are elicited or after-discharges occur. Positive motor responses are elicited at the primary and supplementary motor area; sensory responses are elicited at the primary and secondary sensory area; negative motor responses are elicited at the primary and secondary supplementary negative motor areas; and language dysfunction is elicited over Broca's, Wernicke's, and the left basal temporal language area.[15,17,26–28] Special symptoms resulting from cortical stimulation of the dominant parietal cortex may include agraphia, acalculia, finger agnosia, and left–right confusion seen in Gerstmann syndrome.[29] A variety of auras have been reproduced by cortical stimulation.[30]

A distant reference electrode over a noneloquent region of the cortex serves as a nonactive current sink. The active electrode is switched systematically from electrode to electrode across the entire grid allowing the function of the cortical area underlying each electrode to be investigated.[16]

There is a paucity of studies and reports about stimulation parameters in the pediatric population. However, conventional stimulation paradigms based on fixed pulse duration as described previously for adults rarely elicit responses in infants and young children.[11,18,19] Various pediatric centers have developed and published stimulation paradigms that rely on increments in both stimulus intensity and pulse duration. These will be discussed in more detail.

Once eloquent cortex has been identified, a resection map based on the interictal and ictal epileptiform activity, which together define the epileptogenic zone and the geography of the surrounding eloquent cortex, is designed to allow maximal resection of the epileptic and associated lesional cortex with sparing of surrounding eloquent regions.

In general, resection of primary eloquent cortex, which includes the primary motor, sensory, language, visual, and memory areas, results in neurological deficits. However, some secondary or accessory eloquent regions may be resected without significant permanent neurological deficits. These include the basal temporal language area, negative and second sensorimotor areas, and even the primary motor face area, which is bilaterally innervated.

■ Cortical Stimulation, Brain Maturation, and Special Considerations in Children

Stimulation results in the pediatric age group are highly subject to ontogenetic and maturational features. When performing cortical stimulation in children, the language and motor tasks and paradigms need to be adapted to the patient's age and neurodevelopmental status to include considerations of the individual child's ability to cooperate and performance limitations caused by attention and comprehension. This may be more time-consuming, and several sessions may be needed to obtain workable stimulation results.[11,19]

An efficient and safe paradigm for eliciting responses from immature cortex based on physiological principles of stimulation and neural maturation has been elegantly studied and described by Jayakar et al.[9,18] The response characteristics of neural tissue in relation to stimulus parameters is best described by a strength–duration (SD) curve plotting the current intensity needed to produce a response as a function of pulse duration. The minimum intensity required to elicit a response at a very long pulse duration is termed the *rheobase*, and the pulse duration required to elicit a response using stimuli at twice the intensity of the rheobase is defined as the *chronaxie*. The chronaxie represents the safest point on the SD curve for eliciting a response and is significantly affected by myelination being considerably longer in unmyelinated fibers. The SD curve thus shifts to the left as axons myelinate and the chronaxie shortens. By increasing the stimulus intensity and the pulse width from the usual 0.3 milliseconds used in adults to 1 millisecond, the longer chronaxies in children can be more effectively stimulated, and positive responses or after-discharges can be elicited.[9,18] A graphic computation of the energies delivered at all values of current intensity between 1 and 15 mA and pulse duration between 0.3 and 1.0 milliseconds has been published, and the points on the graph corresponding to progressively higher levels of energy sequentially traced.[18] A stimulation paradigm following this tracing would have the least energy increment at each step but would be extremely cumbersome for routine clinical use. The authors therefore selected three sequences of alternating increase and decrease of intensity and pulse duration that approximates the outline of the tracing. This dual-increment paradigm starts with an intensity of 1 mA and pulse duration of 0.3 milliseconds, and with each subsequent trial, the intensity and pulse duration are adjusted by 1 to 2 mA or 0.1 to 0.2 milliseconds, respectively, until clinical responses or after-discharges are obtained. In three patients aged 1,3 and 4.5 years, positive cortical responses were elicited using the dual-increment paradigm after the standard fixed pulse duration paradigm failed to elicit clinical responses or after-discharges. Thus the technique of dual-increment stimulation rather than the standard fixed-duration paradigm should be used in young children to accurately define critical cortex in the immature brain, facilitating safe excision of adjacent epileptic tissue.

There are few studies defining detailed data of sensorimotor functional maps of the developing brain in children.[11,18,31] This is partly because of the higher medical risks associated with implantation of SDE, difficulties with patient cooperation, and increased necessity for anesthesia. However, there is good evidence that the stimulation threshold to activate normal and functionally abnormal cortex is higher in infants and young children.

Clinical motor responses are frequently obtained at or above the after-discharge threshold so that the stimulation paradigm may need to "override" the after-discharge to obtain eloquent responses. Other authors have reported that they were able to elicit responses in young patients younger than 5 years of age by increasing the stimulus duration after failing to obtain any responses at the maximal fixed duration stimulation.[32]

Motor responses with tongue movement are difficult to achieve in children younger than the age of 2, and the motor responses from the lower face tend to be bilateral rather than contra- and unilateral when the lower rolandic cortex is electrically activated.[19]

Individual finger movements are usually first noted after the age of 3 years, and clonic movements appear subsequent to tonic movements in response to electrical stimulation of the central cortical hand area. This reflects maturational processes involving motor neuronal pathways in the cortical areas 4 and 6. Besides the effect of maturation on corti-

cal stimulation results, there is ample evidence for atypical functional networks in children and adults with developmental and early lesions. This will be discussed later.

■ The Effect of Pathology on Cortical Stimulation Mapping

Specific pathologies may alter cortical stimulation thresholds, resulting in a reduction of eloquent responses and false-negative results that may put the patient at risk for deficits from surgical removal of potentially eloquent cortex. Several studies report the effect of lesions on cortical stimulation results in the pediatric population.

Tumors

Intraoperative electrical stimulation was recently reported in 17 children with tumors of the central region in close relation to the motor pathways.[33] Using 0.5-millisecond pulse width, 5-second stimulus duration, and 50-Hz frequency, these authors successfully identified motor eloquent cortex in 15 patients and in all patients younger than 5 years of age with current densities between 8.5 to 12.5 mA.

These authors found intraoperative stimulation effective in mapping eloquent cortex in all patients with pre-existing motor deficits, even in patients 5 years of age and younger. However, they reported failure to evoke motor responses in two cases of retro-rolandic, low-grade tumors. Anatomical

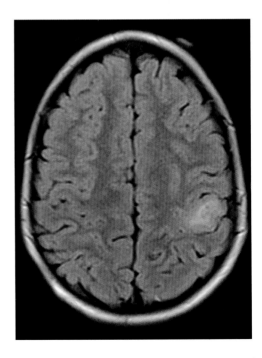

Fig. 6.1 This axial flair magnetic resonance image shows focal cortical dysplasia involving the left central rolandic region.

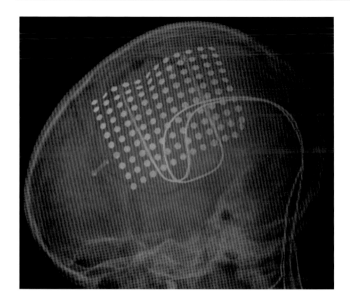

Fig. 6.2 Skull radiograph demonstrating placement of a lateral 8-cm × 8-cm subdural grid.

displacement of normally organized cortex, reorganized functional connectivity, and altered threshold responses caused by the developmental tumor lesions need to be considered when interpreting these stimulation results.

In an earlier study, intraoperative brain-mapping techniques were found to be reliable, effective, and safe in children with brain tumors.[34] Sensorimotor pathways could be reliably localized with intraoperative methods by these authors in their pediatric population with brain tumors.

Language mapping results showed variability and some anatomical unpredictability in peritumoral cortex, aiding with the operative resection of the tumors adjacent to eloquent brain regions.[34]

Brain Malformations

Newer studies with somatosensory evoked potentials and electrical stimulation of the sensorimotor cortex in pediatric patients with malformations of cortical development suggest that the overlapping of sensory and motor functions across the central sulcus is more complex and extensive.[35] This abnormal somatotopic organization in patients with cortical dysplasia supports the concept of abnormal, widespread cerebral organization in the dysgenetic cortex. This may be secondary to mechanisms leading to compensatory reorganization involving as-yet unknown processes underlying brain plasticity.[35] This type of somatotopic reorganization is demonstrated in the case seen in **Figs. 6.1, 6.2, 6.3,** and **6.4**.

A recent case report of an adolescent female further supports the notion of plastic reorganization in the proximity of these lesions.[36] The reported patient had intractable focal epilepsy caused by a mild type 1 cortical dysplasia involving eloquent hand motor cortex defined by extra- and intraoperative stimulation. The lesion was resected, followed by complete paresis, which recovered substantially after several months, leaving the patient seizure free with minimal hand weakness.

Eight pediatric and adult patients with frontal lobe cortical dysplasia involving eloquent cortex were operated on

LESION

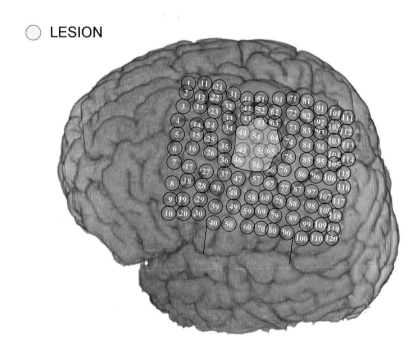

Fig. 6.3 A three-dimensional magnetic resonance imaging reconstruction of the brain with coregistration of the SDE grids demonstrates coverage of the lesion and identifies the overlying electrodes.

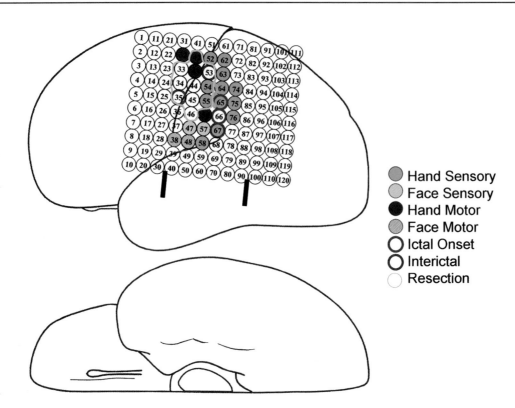

Fig. 6.4 This schematized map shows the perilesional epileptogenic zone that was defined by recording interictal and ictal discharges. ECS clearly demonstrates an abnormal somatopic homunculus with displacement in the motor hand area and redundancy of the sensory cortex of the upper extremity. A lesion-centered resection with close margins to eloquent cortex was performed with good results.

after extraoperative stimulation for medically intractable epilepsy.[37] Functional regions (language and motor) and epileptogenic areas were assessed by extraoperative electrical cortical mapping and ECOG recording and found to co-localize with epileptogenic regions and balloon cell negative dysplastic regions without fluid attenuated inversion recovery signal abnormalities on MRI.

In a further study, right-sided language localization was demonstrated with extraoperative subdural stimulation in four of six patients with known bilateral language representation.[38] The etiologies included nondominant, right-sided dysplasias, tumors, and nonlesional MRIs. The language maps were located in the analogous and classic frontal and temporal language regions of the dominant hemisphere. One patient had a silent language map in this report, and another patient had a wide distribution of single language error sites over the right temporal lobe.[38] (**Figs. 6.1, 6.2, 6.3,** and **6.4).**

Acquired Pathology

Cortical functional reorganization has also been reported in an 18-year-old patient with chronic epilepsy caused by an acquired perirolandic lesion (cavernous hemiangioma) who demonstrated expansion and redundancy of the perilesional hand and finger sensorimotor regions.[39] It has been suggested that ongoing epileptiform activity may suppress

normal cortical function overlying a lesion, whereas neighboring regions may take over function from a case studied by serial cortical stimulation mapping.[40]

■ Electrical Stimulation with Depth Electrodes in Children

Stereotactically placed intracerebral electrodes are used to define a stable, unique epileptogenic zone by several centers in France and Italy. After recording of spontaneous seizures, all patients undergo intracerebral electrical stimulation, with the goal of better defining the epileptogenic zone and providing functional mapping of eloquent brain areas.[41,42] Stimulations are usually applied between contiguous contacts of electrodes at low frequency (1 Hz, single stimulus duration 2–3 millisecond, current intensity 0.4–3 mA) or high frequency (50Hz, single stimulus duration 1 millisecond, current intensity 1–3 mA) depending on the presumed excitability of a given structure and on the type of clinical signs that are to be elicited. High-frequency stimulation is preferred as reported by these authors to assess the organization of the epileptogenic network by inducing the patient's electroclinical seizure and analyzing different ictal phenomena to gain anatomical functional correlates. Intracerebral electrical stimulation has been used to map cortical eloquent areas as well as subcortical critical bundles such as descending fibers of the corticospinal tracts. The French school has reported on the utility of mapping the somatosensory, motor, visual, and language areas in children and has found it extremely valuable in cases of cortical dysplasia involving the central region where the normal anatomy of the gyri is disrupted and the pathology may be embedded within eloquent cortex and bundles. The authors report that the information provided by intracranial functional mapping strongly contributes to the absence of postoperative motor and linguistic deficits in their series of children undergoing resections after SEEG evaluation. There are no comparative studies looking at the sensitivity and specificity of electrocortical stimulation (ECS) with SDE and stereoelectroencephalography (SEEG).

■ ECS-Induced Responses

Several robust responses have been described that define eloquent cortex with ECS. To infer that eloquent cortex has been defined, the stimulation needs to result in a reproducibly demonstrable change in neurological function that may either be a positive or negative phenomenon. Although the positive phenomena are easily observable or can be reported by older pediatric patients, the negative phenomena may go unnoticed and need to be specifically tested for, which may not be possible in the younger patient.

Primary Motor Area

A primary motor area that has been termed *area 4* according to the Brodmann's cytoarchitectural map encompasses the anterior bank of the precentral sulcus; a second premotor area, termed *area 6* encompasses the more anterior precentral gyrus and posterior portion of the superior frontal gyrus. The work of Penfield and colleagues has expanded our understanding of the somatotopic map of the body as depicted by Penfield's figurine homunculus.[12,13] The larger extension of motor responses to areas as much as 4 cm anterior and 2 cm posterior to the central sulcus and not limited to the precentral gyrus led to the appreciation of a more extensive motor representation in the central region. In addition, it has become clear that the cytoarchitectural areas 4 and 6 cannot be delineated with ECS. Stimulation parameters, including frequency, duration, and intensity, may affect the type of motor response elicited that usually first involves clonic movements of distal muscle groups.

Maximizing the resections without incurring motor deficits in lesional and nonlesional frontal lobe epilepsy that encroach on or distort the precentral area may be best achieved using detailed motor mapping. Localized reorganization of function may modify the traditional humuncular represen-

tation and put patients at increased risk for postoperative deficits on the one hand or, on the other hand, dislocation of function may allow safe and more generous resective procedures, as described in detail elsewhere in this chapter and illustrated in **Figs. 6.1–6.4**.

Supplementary Sensorimotor Area (SSMA)

Animal studies performed more than a century ago demonstrated that motor responses could be elicited by stimulation of the mesial aspect of the superior frontal gyrus just anterior to the primary motor leg area. Once implantable subdural grid electrodes and depth electrodes were developed, systematic studies of this interhemispheric mesial cortical region became possible in the 20th century.[43,44]

This region has been named the supplementary sensorimotor area (SSMA) because both sensory and motor functions are represented. The motor pattern of responses is quite distinctive from that elicited by stimulating the primary motor area. The SSMA type motor responses are characterized by predominantly tonic responses of proximal muscle groups (which are frequently bilateral), asymmetric movements of the lower and upper extremities, and head and eye deviations and vocalizations. A somatotopic organization has also been defined that is anterior-posterior in orientation with the head and eye region lying anterior and the leg region posterior. Although resection of the SSMA is generally safe, temporary contralateral weakness, difficulty in the initiation of movements, and mutism with intact comprehension has been reported. In addition, the proximity of the caudal end of the SSMA to motor and sensory control of the leg need to be appreciated.

Resection of eloquent cortex in this region therefore needs a careful risk–benefit analysis and informed consent standards involving ethics experts.

Sensory Areas

Stimulation studies have defined three distinct areas from which somatosensory sensation can be elicited: the primary sensory cortex (SI) in the postcentral gyrus, the secondary somatosensory cortex (S2) in the frontal and parietal operculum, and the supplementary sensorimotor cortical area in the mesial surface of the frontal and parietal cortex (S3).[12,13] Each region has a unique somatotopic organization—SI, located in the postcentral parietal region and consisting of Brodmann areas 3a, 3b, 2, and 1 has a clear somatotopy mirroring that of the motor strip. S2 is located on the superior bank of the sylvian fissure in proximity to the planum infraparietal of the frontal operculum and sensory responses to stimulation characteristically are somatotopically "discontiguous"—affecting the opposite whole body but also the ipsilateral side, especially simultaneous upper and lower limb involvement.[27] The S3 responses are frequently admixed with tonic motor features and may localize to the body bilaterally, ipsilaterally, and contralaterally to the brain side that is stimulated. The semiology of somatosensory auras may also give a good indication of which sensory area is the symptomatogenic zone.[45] Resections in the S1 region will lead to permanent changes in contralateral sensory perception with deficits affecting primarily position sense and fine touch, but vibration and pain sensation are not affected by S1 resections.

Language Mapping

Lesional studies in patients first defined the anterior (Broca) and posterior (Wernicke) language areas in the left inferior frontal lobe and first temporal convolution respectively. These areas were first mapped intraoperatively by Penfield and Roberts who induced speech arrest, alexia, agraphia, anomia, paraphasia, and occasional positive grunting noises with electrical interference.[12,13,46] A superior language area was also defined by them lying anterior to the rolandic motor foot area in the mesial frontal lobe.[46] A third speech area has been defined in the basal temporal region of the dominant temporal lobe.[47]

Reading aloud is a reliable screening task for mapping language area, and arrest of speech is the typical feature to look for. Importantly, negative or positive motor responses and diminished responsiveness as a cause of speech arrest need to be ruled out by checking tongue movements. If slowing of speech occurs, additional testing, including naming of objects, auditory word repetition, reading comprehension, and spontaneous speech, may be warranted. This will require good cooperation and an adequate developmental level in children to obtain reliable results. ECS usually produces interruption of verbal fluency at Broca's area and evokes comprehension deficits when stimulating Wernicke's area, but there may be a significant overlap of symptoms.

A robust negative motor response is seen when performing ECS in the inferior frontal gyrus just anterior to the primary facial motor representation, and this has been termed the *primary negative motor area*.[12,13,48] Further studies have shown a more extensive distribution of negative motor areas of the upper extremities, extending over the lateral premotor cortex. Selective removal of the primary negative motor area is possible without producing persisting speech and language deficits.

■ Studying More Specific Brain Anatomy with Stimulation

Angular Gyrus (AG)

The feasibility of intraoperative stimulation of the angular gyrus (AG) was recently studied and reported in five adult patients with circumscribed lesions (all had primary or metastatic tumors) in this region.[49] Based on human and animal studies, it is known that the AG is a higher-order supraregional center that is integrated in a neuronal network mediating movement with complex projections to the pulvinar of the thalamus and ipsi- and contralateral cortical association areas in the prefrontal, temporal, and occipital lobes. Damage to the dominant AG may result in agraphia and alexia. A previous article reported a functional Gerstmann syndrome during electrical stimulation of the dominant perisylvian cortex.[29]

In this newer study,[49] bipolar and monopolar cortical stimulation techniques were applied to the AG cortex and compound muscle action potentials (CMAPs) were recorded in the contralateral arm. The study shows that selective electrical stimulation of the AG elicits a motor response in the contralateral upper extremity. The data reported show that the technique is feasible in the intraoperative setting and that the AG cortex plays a role in bimanual motor function, which deserves further study with this technique. This technique may be of value in studying patients with Landau-Kleffner syndrome undergoing surgical epilepsy treatment.

Interhemispheric Connections of Motor Areas

Functional connectivity of the brain via various white matter tracts, which consist of the commissural fibers to the contralateral cortex, projection fibers to subcortical nuclei, and arcuate fibers to the ipsilateral cortical structures, have been studied in vitro and recently in vivo with newer MRI, especially with diffusion tensor imaging techniques as well as transcranial magnetic stimulation. In addition, newer neurophysiological techniques have been developed for the in vivo evaluation of neural fibers and their projections. A recent study to clarify interhemispheric connections of motor cortex (MC) investigated corticocortical evoked potentials in vivo using subdural grid stimulation in patients undergoing presurgical evaluation for epilepsy treatment by delivering a bipolar pulsed stimulus to two electrodes overlying one MC and recording the evoked potential (EP) contralaterally from the averaged ECoG.[50] Contralateral evoked responses with stimulation of the MC only (no responses were elicited form other stimulation sites) were recorded with interhemispheric latencies ranging from approximately 9 to 24 milliseconds for the initial positive peak and 25 to 39 milliseconds for the second negative peak. These results were felt to suggest that bilateral motor coordination is at least partially controlled at the level of the MC. In pediatric cases, this technique may shed light on the neural mechanism of associated and mirror movements seen in children with epilepsy.

Stimulation-Induced Alien Limb Phenomenon

Alien limb phenomenon was reported in a 14-year-old patient who had parietal lobe epilepsy caused by a malformation of cortical development in the left rolandic cortex.[51] Stimulation of the central cortex in proximity to the frontal operculum induced involuntary grabbing right hand movements accompanied by the perception of alienness—reported as if the arm belonged to someone else. The authors speculate that stimulation may have induced a functional disconnection or inhibition of primary sensory areas and activation of motor areas of the hand resulting in involuntary movements that were experienced as alien.

Insular Cortex

The insular cortex is not easily accessible for ECS because it is covered by the frontal, temporal, and parietal opercular cortex. Recent studies with intracerebral depth electrodes implanted transopercularly into the insular cortex have yielded more consistent responses compared with previous studies and include somatosensory responses, including painful sensations of the contralateral face, neck, hand, and upper limb (posterior insula); viscero sensitive responses (anterior insula) of the abdomen and thorax typically seen as the initial symptom in mesial temporal lobe epilepsy and a sense of pharyngeal constriction; and less frequently, simple acoustic hallucinations, experiential phenomena, olfactory, gustatory, or vegetative responses have been evoked.[52]

Laughter

Nonictal laughter has been elicited by stimulation of the mesial frontal cortex. The laughter has been reported to be involuntary and not associated with mirth or emotion. Similarly, stimulation of the cingulate cortex, orbitofrontal cortex, and mesial, basal temporal structures has been reported to produce nonepileptic laughter.[53]

Visual Cortex

ECS of Brodmann's areas 17 (primary visual cortex; also defined as the striate cortex with the lines of Gennari), 18, and 19 (visual association cortical areas) may produce either well-defined visual symptoms correlating well with epileptic visual auras, simple visual hallucinations, or visual illusions localized in the upper or lower (delineated by the calcarine fissure) contralateral quadrant.[54] Most patients with occipital lobe epilepsy will have a visual field deficit but resection of occipital cortex in the face of normal visual fields will result in a new deficit that is usually well compensated in the pediatric age group.

Auditory Cortex

The primary auditory cortex, Brodmann's area 41, is located in the posterior medial aspect of the gyrus of Heschl, whereas secondary auditory areas have been demonstrated in contiguous areas extending into the planum temporal and superior temporal sulcus (areas 42, 52, and 22). Because the stimulation response is subjective, patient cooperation is essential. Elementary crude auditory sensations, hallucinations, and illusions have been described. Unilateral lesions in this region do not appear to lead to auditory deficits.

Negative Functional Effects

Several negative responses that are stable and reproducible have been reported over the language areas (anterior, posterior, and basal temporal), primary and secondary negative motor areas, and other negative responses with stimulation of heteromodal associating cortex (supramarginal gyrus area 40, area 7, area 39), producing deficits of higher cortical functions, including a combination of deficits including alexia, anomia, apraxia, and Gerstmann syndrome).[28,29]

■ Electrical Cortical Stimulation and Other Noninvasive Functional Mapping Techniques

In the last two decades, the Wada test, neuropsychological evaluation, and 2–deoxy–2 [^{18}F] fluoro–D–glucose (FDG) PET, which allows determination of preoperative language lateralization and assessment of memory adequacy, have been supplemented with additional noninvasive mapping methods that offer a high spatial and temporal accuracy to localize sensory, motor, and language function.

Recent noninvasive techniques such as functional MRI (fMRI) and magnetoencephalography (MEG) can aid in mapping cortical function as an adjunctive method when planning invasive mapping with chronically implanted subdural electrodes. There is relatively good correlation between intraoperative ECoG and MEG, although direct measures of differences are influenced by the MEG source mapping of sulcal generators versus gyral surface maps with intracranial electrodes. The temporal course of neuronal language processing can be imaged noninvasively with millisecond resolution using MEG; however, at this stage, there is a paucity of pediatric data.[55]

Numerous studies document that fMRI is a reliable technique for lateralizing hemispheric language dominance. A recent study compared the results of fMRI language mapping with intraoperative ECS in patients with temporal lobe epilepsy. The sensitivity was 100%, and there was a high spatial accuracy with fMRI, indicating that areas not activated could be safely resected. The authors emphasize that a combination of three language tasks including verb generation, picture naming, and sentence processing was needed to ensure the high sensitivity as no single task was sufficient for this purpose. However the specificity of fMRI was low, and only 51% of fMRI activations were confirmed on ECS.[56] Motor cortex localization with fMRI is generally highly concordant with intraoperative electrocortical stimulation mapping.[57]

Several additional electrophysiological techniques besides high frequency ECS, which we described in detail previously, have been studied to map motor subareas.[58] These include slow cortical potentials termed *Bereitschaftspotential* that arise from the motor cortices and occur –1.5 seconds before the onset of self-paced voluntary movements and are recorded with a long time constant amplifier. The Bereitschaftspotential reflect excitatory postsynaptic potentials in the superficial layer of the motor cortex, occurring in the apical dendrites of the pyramidal neurons. This technique may differentiate the M1, SSMA, and aid in the functional mapping of nonprimary and association cortices. No correlative studies exist with noninvasive techniques, and there is, to date, unfortunately no body of pediatric data.

Noninvasive techniques for mapping brain function as described previously may obviate the need for invasive mapping in some cases of well-defined, single epileptogenic lesions and assist in the decision making to pursue invasive studies and potential surgery in complex cases of malformations in or near eloquent cortex.

■ Intraoperative Cortical Stimulation

Intraoperative mapping of cortical function by electrical stimulation has been used extensively in neurosurgery since it was first introduced in 1874 by Bartholow. Subsequently, Sir Victor Horsely and in 1909 Harvey Cushing used this technique to define the sensorimotor cortex surrounding a tumor.

Ideally, the patient should be awake and responsive but comfortable to perform intraoperative mapping of language cortex, which is technically challenging in pediatric patients. Anesthesia techniques are therefore of prime importance to optimize the success of intraoperative stimulation—premedication with barbiturates, benzodiazepines, and antihistamines should be avoided if ECoG is planned because these agents significantly affect the EEG and may affect the seizure threshold.

During the procedure, short-acting anesthetics such as propofol in combination with fentanyl are preferred because they permit rapid induction for the craniotomy procedure but an alert patient for subsequent functional mapping. Local analgesia with lidocaine may be used as a local field block

for the scalp incision and dural incisions. The stimulation is performed with a hand-held stimulator using either uni- or bipolar stimuli with parameters quite similar to those used with chronic extraoperative stimulation.[59] Closely spaced 5-mm and individualized stimulation points can be selected on the cortex and then tagged to generate a stimulation map and verify the reproducibility of the responses by repeating the stimulation procedure.[12–14] The ECoG will detect afterdischarges (ADs) or seizures and permit stimulation within appropriate safety limits. The application of intraoperative monitoring is quite limited in the pediatric age group because of issues of feasibility in the awake craniotomy setting and, more importantly, the specific challenges relating to higher stimulation thresholds of the immature cortex.[59] However, the value of intraoperative ECOG in children with intractable neocortical epilepsy has been recently studied and reported.[60]

■ Conclusion

Cortical stimulation is a well-established method for defining cortical functional areas subserving language and sensorimotor function in children. In children, specific features need to be considered when performing stimulation and in the interpretation of the functional maps obtained:

1. There is a higher cortical threshold, which is age dependent and reduces inversely to age. Practically, this means that higher current densities (milliamperes) are needed to elicit responses. In addition, there is a greater variability of the stimulation threshold. Stimulation currents, therefore, need to be maximal at each site and after-discharges may have to be "overridden" to obtain this. The dual-stimulation paradigm varying the stimulus duration and intensity is valuable in defining critical cortex in young children.
2. Certain pathologies may further raise the stimulation threshold of tumors so that it may be difficult to obtain evoked motor responses. After lesion removal, it has been noted that the stimulation threshold may be lowered.
3. Pathology underlying the epileptic zone as an anatomical substrate is frequently developmental and may result in altered functional plasticity. This may lead to intra- and interhemispheric reorganization with atypical regions of functional mapping (e.g., bilateral language, displaced or extended functional regions).
4. Because the immature cerebral cortex is relatively refractory to cortical stimulation with standard adult parameters, widened pulse widths (0.14–200 milliseconds), higher frequency ranges (20–50 Hz), increased current densities (0.5–20 mA), and wider train duration ranges (3–25 seconds) need to be used.

5. The invasive nature of stimulating the cortex directly should be balanced against the accuracy of mapping obtained in each patient as noninvasive imaging may be preferable in some cases. However, it still is the gold standard method for mapping eloquent cortex in proximity to the epileptogenic zone that needs to be resected to treat refractory focal epilepsy.

6. Intraoperative stimulation has limited application in the pediatric age group because of technical and feasibility issues relating to the awake craniotomy setting.

Acknowledgments I thank Tim O'Connor, head EEG technologist, for his assistance with the case illustrations.

References

1. National Institutes of Health Consensus Conference. Surgery for epilepsy. JAMA 1990;264(6):729–733

2. Aicardi J. Pediatric epilepsy surgery: how the view has changed. In: Tuxhorn I, Holthausen H, Boenigk H, eds. Pediatric Epilepsy Syndromes and Their Surgical Treatment. London: John Libby; 1997:3–7

3. Cross JH, Jayakar P, Nordli D, et al., International League against Epilepsy, Subcommission for Paediatric Epilepsy Surgery; Commissions of Neurosurgery and Paediatrics. Proposed criteria for referral and evaluation of children for epilepsy surgery: recommendations of the Subcommission for Pediatric Epilepsy Surgery. Epilepsia 2006;47(6):952–959

4. Cross JH. Epilepsy surgery in childhood. Epilepsia 2002;43(suppl 3):65–70

5. Tuxhorn I, Kotagal P. Classification. Semin Neurol 2008;28(3):277–288

6. Lueders H. Textbook of Epilepsy Surgery. London: Informa, Ltd.; 2008

7. Engel J, Van Ness PC, Rasmussen TB, Ojeman LM. Outcome with respect to epileptic seizures. In: Engel J, ed. Surgical Treatment of the Epilepsies, 2nd ed. New York: Raven Press; 2003:609–621

8. Babb TL, Brown WJ. Pathological findings in epilepsy. In: Epel J Jr, ed. Surgical Treatment of Epilepsies. Raven Press: New York; 1987: 511–540

9. Jayakar P, Duchowny M, Resnick TJ. Subdural monitoring in the evaluation of children for epilepsy surgery. J Child Neurol 1994;9(suppl 2):61–66

10. Fogarasi A, Tuxhorn I, Janszky J, et al. Age-dependent seizure semiology in temporal lobe epilepsy. Epilepsia 2007;48(9):1697–1702

11. Wyllie E, Lüders H, Morris HH III, et al. Subdural electrodes in the evaluation for epilepsy surgery in children and adults. Neuropediatrics 1988;19(2):80–86

12. Penfield W, Jasper H. Epilepsy and the Functional Anatomy of the Human Brain. Boston, Mass: Little Brown; 1954

13. Penfield W, Rasmussen T. The Cerebral Cortex of Man. A Clinical Study of Localization of Function. New York, NY: Macmillian;1957

14. Gallentine WB, Mikati MA. Intraoperative electrocorticography and cortical stimulation in children. J Clin Neurophysiol 2009;26(2): 95–108

15. Luders H. Symptomatic Areas and Electrical Cortical Stimulation. New York, NY: Churchill Livingstone; 2000

16. Nair DR, Burgess R, McIntyre CC, Lüders H. Chronic subdural electrodes in the management of epilepsy. Clin Neurophysiol 2008;119(1):11–28

17. Lesser RP, Lüders H, Klem G, et al. Extraoperative cortical functional localization in patients with epilepsy. J Clin Neurophysiol 1987;4(1):27–53

18. Jayakar P, Alvarez LA, Duchowny MS, Resnick TJ. A safe and effective paradigm to functionally map the cortex in childhood. J Clin Neurophysiol 1992;9(2):288–293

19. Lachhwani D, Dinner D. Cortical Stimulation in the Definition of Eloquent Areas. Amsterdam, The Netherlands: Elsevier; 2004

20. Ranck JB Jr. Which elements are excited in electrical stimulation of mammalian central nervous system: a review. Brain Res 1975;98(3):417–440

21. Manola L, Roelofsen BH, Holsheimer J, Marani E, Geelen J. Modelling motor cortex stimulation for chronic pain control: electrical potential field, activating functions and responses of simple nerve fibre models. Med Biol Eng Comput 2005;43(3):335–343

22. Jobst BC, Williamson PD, Coughlin CT, Thadani VM, Roberts DW. An unusual complication of intracranial electrodes. Epilepsia 2000;41(7):898–902

23. Gordon B, Lesser RP, Rance NE, et al. Parameters for direct cortical electrical stimulation in the human: histopathologic confirmation. Electroencephalogr Clin Neurophysiol 1990;75(5):371–377

24. Wyler AR, Walker G, Somes G. The morbidity of long-term seizure monitoring using subdural strip electrodes. J Neurosurg 1991;74(5):734–737

25. Hamer HM, Morris HH, Mascha EJ, et al. Complications of invasive video-EEG monitoring with subdural grid electrodes. Neurology 2002;58(1):97–103

26. Lüders H, Lesser RP, Hahn J, et al. Basal temporal language area demonstrated by electrical stimulation. Neurology 1986;36(4):505–510

27. Lüders H, Lesser RP, Dinner DS, Hahn JF, Salanga V, Morris HH. The second sensory area in humans: evoked potential and electrical stimulation studies. Ann Neurol 1985;17(2):177–184

28. Lüders HO, Dinner DS, Morris HH, Wyllie E, Comair YG. Cortical electrical stimulation in humans. The negative motor areas. Adv Neurol 1995;67:115–129

29. Morris HH, Lüders H, Lesser RP, Dinner DS, Hahn J. Transient neuropsychological abnormalities (including Gerstmann's syndrome) during cortical stimulation. Neurology 1984;34(7):877–883

30. Schulz R, Lüders HO, Tuxhorn I, et al. Localization of epileptic auras induced on stimulation by subdural electrodes. Epilepsia 1997;38(12):1321–1329

31. Chitoku S, Otsubo H, Harada Y, et al. Extraoperative cortical stimulation of motor function in children. Pediatr Neurol 2001;24(5):344–350

32. Schuele S, McIntyre C, Lueders H. General principles of cortical mapping by electrical stimulation. In: Luders H, ed. Textbook of Epilepsy Surgery. London: Informa Ltd. 2008; 963–977

33. Signorelli F, Guyotat J, Mottolese C, Schneider F, D'Acunzi G, Isnard J. Intraoperative electrical stimulation mapping as an aid for surgery of intracranial lesions involving motor areas in children. Childs Nerv Syst 2004;20(6):420–426

34. Berger MS, Kincaid J, Ojemann GA, Lettich E. Brain mapping techniques to maximize resection, safety, and seizure control in children with brain tumors. Neurosurgery 1989;25(5):786–792

35. Akai T, Otsubo H, Pang EW, et al. Complex central cortex in pediatric patients with malformations of cortical development. J Child Neurol 2002;17(5):347–352

36. Chamoun RB, Mikati MA, Comair YG. Functional recovery following resection of an epileptogenic focus in the motor hand area. Epilepsy Behav 2007;11(3):384–388

37. Marusic P, Najm IM, Ying Z, et al. Focal cortical dysplasias in eloquent cortex: functional characteristics and correlation with MRI and histopathologic changes. Epilepsia 2002;43(1):27–32

38. Jabbour RA, Hempel A, Gates JR, Zhang W, Risse GL. Right hemisphere language mapping in patients with bilateral language. Epilepsy Behav 2005;6(4):587–592

39. Kirsch HE, Sepkuty JP, Crone NE. Multimodal functional mapping of sensorimotor cortex before resection of an epileptogenic perirolandic lesion. Epilepsy Behav 2004;5(3):407–410

40. Lado FA, Legatt AD, LaSala PA, Shinnar S. Alteration of the cortical motor map in a patient with intractable focal seizures. J Neurol Neurosurg Psychiatry 2002;72(6):812–815

41. Cossu M, Cardinale F, Colombo N, et al. Stereoelectroencephalography in the presurgical evaluation of children with drug-resistant focal epilepsy. J Neurosurg 2005; 103(4, suppl)333–343

42. Cossu M, Cardinale F, Castana L, Nobili L, Sartori I, Lo Russo G. Stereo-EEG in children. Childs Nerv Syst 2006;22(8):766–778

43. Lim SH, Dinner DS, Pillay PK, et al. Functional anatomy of the human supplementary sensorimotor area: results of extraoperative electrical stimulation. Electroencephalogr Clin Neurophysiol 1994;91(3):179–193

44. Fried I, Katz A, McCarthy G, et al. Functional organization of human supplementary motor cortex studied by electrical stimulation. J Neurosci 1991;11(11):3656–3666

45. Tuxhorn IE. Somatosensory auras in focal epilepsy: a clinical, video EEG and MRI study. Seizure 2005;14(4):262–268

46. Penfield W, Roberts L. Speech and Brain Mechanisms. Princeton, NJ: Princeton Press; 1959

47. Lüders H, Lesser RP, Hahn J, et al. Basal temporal language area demonstrated by electrical stimulation. Neurology 1986;36(4): 505–510

48. Lüders HO, Lesser RP, Dinner DS, et al. A negative motor response elicited by electrical stimulation of the human frontal cortex. Adv Neurol 1992;57:149–157

49. Kombos T, Picht T, Suess O. Electrical excitability of the angular gyrus. J Clin Neurophysiol 2008;25(6):340–345

50. Terada K, Usui N, Umeoka S, et al. Interhemispheric connection of motor areas in humans. J Clin Neurophysiol 2008;25(6):351–356

51. Boesebeck F, Ebner A. Paroxysmal alien limb phenomena because of epileptic seizures and electrical cortical stimulation. Neurology 2004;63(9):1725–1727

52. Isnard J, Mauguière F. The insula in partial epilepsy[in French]. Rev Neurol (Paris) 2005;161(1):17–26

53. Hoppe M. Cortical mapping by electrical stimulation: other eloquent areas. In: Luders H, ed. Textbook of Epilepsy Surgery. London: Informa Ltd.; 2008

54. Murphey DK, Maunsell JH, Beauchamp MS, Yoshor D. Perceiving electrical stimulation of identified human visual areas. Proc Natl Acad Sci U S A 2009;106(13):5389–5393

55. Roberts TP, Zusman E, McDermott M, Barbaro N, Rowley HA. Correlation of functional magnetic source imaging with intraoperative cortical stimulation in neurosurgical patients. J Image Guid Surg 1995;1(6):339–347

56. Rutten GJ, Ramsey NF, van Rijen PC, Noordmans HJ, van Veelen CW. Development of a functional magnetic resonance imaging protocol for intraoperative localization of critical temporoparietal language areas. Ann Neurol 2002;51(3):350–360

57. Chapman PH, Buchbinder BR, Cosgrove GR, Jiang HJ. Functional magnetic resonance imaging for cortical mapping in pediatric neurosurgery. Pediatr Neurosurg 1995;23(3):122–126

58. Ikeda A, Miyamoto S, Shibasaki H. Cortical motor mapping in epilepsy patients: information from subdural electrodes in presurgical evaluation. Epilepsia 2002;43(suppl 9):56–60

59. Çataltepe O, Comair Y. Intrasurgical cortical stimulation. In: Luders H and Noachtar S, eds. Epileptic Seizures: Pathophysiology and Clinical Semiology. New York, NY: Churchill Livingstone; 2000:172–176

60. Asano E, Benedek K, Shah A, et al. Is intraoperative electrocorticography reliable in children with intractable neocortical epilepsy? Epilepsia 2004;45(9):1091–1099

7 Magnetoencephalography

Hiroshi Otsubo, Ayako Ochi, and O. Carter Snead III

Localization-related epilepsy refractory to antiepileptic drugs in children is more often associated with an extratemporal epileptogenic focus than that seen in adults. Thus invasive intracranial electroencephalography (EEG) with extraoperative subdural electrode recordings to localize the epileptogenic zone is often needed in children. These neocortical epileptic zones frequently are adjacent to eloquent cortex, and the surgical treatment requires accurate delineation of both epileptogenic and functional zones. Magnetoencephalography (MEG) has been reported to be a valuable noninvasive technique that can be used to localize both epileptogenic and eloquent cortices in children with medically refractory localization-related epilepsy undergoing evaluation for surgical treatment of their seizure disorder.[1-6] This chapter reviews the current clinical applications of MEG for pediatric epilepsy surgery.

■ Basic Principles of Magnetoencephalography and Magnetic Source Imaging

MEG is a technique for measuring the magnetic fields associated with the intracellular current flows within neurons. Source localization of epileptic spikes and evoked responses as determined by MEG are co-registered with magnetic resonance imaging (MRI) as magnetic source imaging (MSI). MEG is based on the physical phenomenon that electrical currents generate accompanying magnetic fields. The orientation of the magnetic field relative to the electrical current is described as Orsted's "right-hand rule," which states that when the thumb of the right hand is pointed in the direction of the electrical current, the surrounding magnetic flux is aligned in the direction of the other four right fingers. MEG uses highly sensitive biomagnetometers to detect extracranial magnetic fields produced by intracellular neuronal currents. On the basis of the right-hand rule, MEG is primarily sensitive to signals arising from regions in which the apical dendrites are tangentially oriented to the skull and scalp surface.

The source localization has to solve the inverse problem that calculates the three-dimensional intracranial location, orientation, and strength of the neuronal sources backward from a measured extracranial magnetic field pattern. The accuracy of a solution of the inverse problem depends on numerous factors, including the forward problem. The forward problem uses an iterative algorithm to determine the location, orientation, and strength of the equivalent current dipole that best account for the measured magnetic field pattern. The accuracy of the forward problem is critically determined by the shape and conductivity of the volume conductor of head model. MEG forward solution is more robust than that of EEG because of homogeneous conductivity in a magnetic field. Therefore, the localization of both MEG spike sources (MEGSS) and evoked responses on MSI is quite reliable for presurgical evaluation in pediatric localization-related epilepsy.[2] In short, MEG is an extremely valuable and reliable technique with which to localize the source of interictal epileptiform discharges.[7]

■ MEG Spike Sources

The Hospital for Sick Children in Toronto, Canada, has pioneered the use of MEG for clinical application in pediatric epilepsy. From August 2000 to December 2007, MEG was studied in more than 600 patients with localization-related epilepsy as part of a presurgical protocol that also includes careful definition of seizure semiology based on clinical features and prolonged scalp video-EEG (VEEG), MRI, and neuropsychological testing.[2] More than 200 of these children have undergone epilepsy surgery procedures based on the concordance of these data.

We have defined the distribution of MEGSS by number and density.[6] An MEG spike cluster is six or more spike sources with 1 cm or less between adjacent sources. A MEG spike scatters is fewer than six spike sources regardless of the distance between sources or spike sources with more than 1 cm between sources regardless of the number of sources in a group. The zone of clustered MEGSS correlates with the ictal onset zone and the prominent interictal zone as determined by extraoperative intracranial VEEG as recorded from subdural electrodes. MEG spike scatters alone should be examined by intracranial VEEG, because an epileptic zone may exist within the scatter distribution of MEGSS. We have shown the complete resection of MEG clusters to be correlated with postsurgical seizure freedom. For presurgical evaluation, concordant lateralization of the EEG spike sources on scalp VEEG and the clustered MEGSS indicate the primary epileptogenic hemisphere.[8] Discordant lateralization of EEG spike sources and MEGSS indicate an undetermined epileptogenic hemisphere and contraindicate surgery without further testing.[8]

Lesional Epilepsy

Surgical treatment of seizure disorders secondary to a lesion requires that the lesion be removed and epileptogenic tissue removed or disconnected. MSI provided accurate data on the spatial relations of lesion, epileptogenic zone, and functional cortex in children with lesional extratemporal epilepsy.[4] MEG delineates asymmetric epileptogenicity surrounding lesions and eloquent cortex. When the focal seizures are secondary to a neoplasm, complete tumor resection with resection of MEGSS marginal to the tumor is associated with favorable outcomes despite residual postexcisional electrocorticography (ECoG) spikes and extramarginal MEGSS. When the focal seizures are secondary to dysplastic brain, the cortical dysplasia as characterized by clusters of MEGSS within and extend-ing from MRI lesion should be removed completely, including both the anatomical lesion and MEGSS, to achieve seizure freedom.[9,10]

MEG has proven useful in identifying which children with tuberous sclerosis complex (TSC) may be candidates for epilepsy surgery (**Fig. 7.1**). Wu et al[11] studied six children with focal seizures secondary to TSC. In these six TSC patients with focal seizures secondary to bilateral multilobar cortical tubers, ictal VEEG predicted the region of resection with 56% sensitivity, 80% specificity, and 77% accuracy. Interictal MEG, however, fared better, with 100% sensitivity, 94% specificity, and 95% accuracy. In TSC, MEGSS tend to localize around visible tubers. MEG enabled precise localization of the epileptic foci and provided crucial information of surgical treatment in children with localization related epilepsy secondary to TSC.[12-14]

Extratemporal Lobe Epilepsy

In infants and young children, the occipital lobe frequently generates focal onset seizures and even infantile spasms.[15] In addition, more occipital spikes migrate anteriorly than

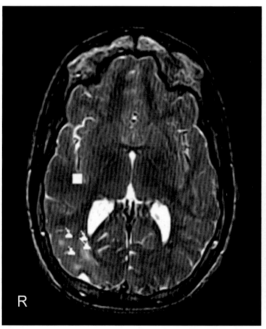
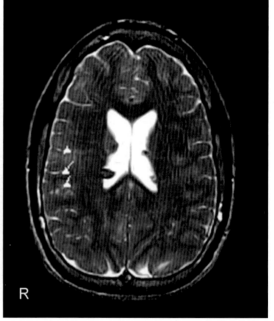

Fig. 7.1 Magnetoencephalography (MEG) in the presurgical evaluation of a child with tuberous sclerosis. Axial T2 magnetic resonance imaging (MRI) shows multiple cortical tubers, MEG spike sources (MEGSS), and auditory evoked field. This 17-year-old, right-handed boy presents intractable epilepsy secondary to tuberous sclerosis complex. His seizures consist of gagging followed by clonic movements of face and left upper extremity. MEG shows a total of 70 MEGSS consisting of two clusters over the right hemisphere. **(A)** Axial T2 MRI shows 4 of 46 clustered MEGSS over the right temporooccipital region around the occipital cortical tuber. (Closed triangles represent the location of the MEGSS and tails indicate the orientation of the MEGSS). A closed square represents auditory evoked field. **(B)** Axial T2 MRI shows 3 of 24 clustered MEGSS in the right inferior frontal to the superior rolandic region, superior and posterior to the frontal cortical tuber. The patient underwent intracranial video-electroencephalography monitoring using 103 subdural grid and depth electrodes. Cortical resection was performed over the right occipitotemporal region and inferior frontal region, which correlated to the two MEGSS clusters. He has been seizure free for 9 months with medications.

frontal spikes migrate posteriorly in children.[16] Therefore, in younger patients with extratemporal localization-related epilepsy, multiple clustered MEGSS are often seen in temporal/parietal/occipital lobes, whereas in older patients, single clusters are observed frequently with an ictal onset zone in the frontal lobe.[17] These data suggest that posteriorly dominant epilepsy can extend anteriorly to expand the epileptic network through anatomical and functional connections in developing brains, whereas frontal lobe epilepsy less frequently migrates to other lobes. Therefore, multiple clustered MEGSS associated with the posterior epileptic network may require extensive resection, especially in young children. Conversely, the single cluster that correlates with a discrete anterior epileptic region in relatively old patients may predict a successful focal resection.

The diagnosis of frontal lobe epilepsy may be compounded by poor electroclinical localization on scalp EEG, caused by deep, distributed, or rapidly propagating epileptiform activities over the bilateral hemispheres. The yield of MEGSS in terms of localization of the epileptogenic zone in frontal lobe epilepsy is superior to that of EEG because of high resolution of spatial and temporal data with the former[18] (**Fig. 7.2**). When interictal epileptiform discharges on scalp EEGs show a diffuse hemispheric distribution, or bilateral synchronous spike-waves, analysis of MEGSS at the earliest time point or

dynamic statistical parametric maps can lateralize and localize the epileptogenic zone.[19,20]

In age-related epilepsy, benign rolandic epilepsy (BRE) and Landau-Kleffner syndrome (LKS) are forms of childhood epilepsy that share particular characteristics and can be controlled with medication. Both BRE and LKS have identical orientation of MEGSS directing vertical to the rolandic[21] and sylvian.[22] However, a subgroup of patients who manifest some of the characteristic of both BRE and LKS, but who do not fulfill all criteria for these epilepsy syndromes have been designated atypical BRE and LKS variant. We have introduced the term *malignant rolandic-sylvian epilepsy* to describe this subgroup, which is characterized by fronto-centro-temporal spikes on EEG, absence of lesions on MRI, MEGSS with random orientations around rolandic and sylvian fissures, intractable sensorimotor partial seizures that progress to secondary generalization, and neurocognitive problems.[3]

■ Temporal Lobe Epilepsy

Temporal lobectomy in children for temporal lobe epilepsy has a seizure-free outcome similar to that reported in adults.[23] Unlike extratemporal localization-related epilepsy, MEGSS in temporal lobe epilepsy do not represent the exact

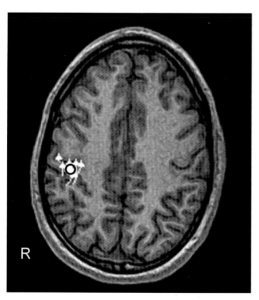

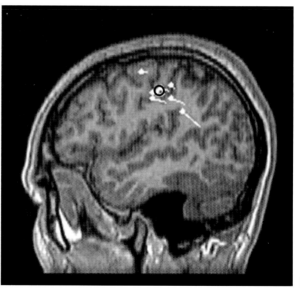

Fig. 7.2 Magnetoencephalography (MEG) in presurgical evaluation of a child with extratemporal, localization-related epilepsy. T1 magnetic resonance imaging (MRI) shows MEG spike sources (MEGSS) and somatosensory-evoked field. This 17-year-old right-handed boy presents with sensory aura with or without secondarily generalized tonic clonic seizures. MRI showed small nonspecific high fluid attenuation inversion recovery signal seen in the right perirolandic region. **(A)** Axial T1 MRI shows 6 of clustered 75 MEGSS over the postcentral gyrus. (Closed triangles represent the location of MEGSS and tails indicate the orientation of the MEGSS). Open black circle represents somatosensory evoked field by left median nerve stimulation. **(B)** Sagittal T1 MRI shows seven MEGSS around the central sulcus with predominant postcentral gyrus spreading to supramarginal gyrus. The open black circle represents somatosensory-evoked field. The patient underwent intracranial video-electroencephalography monitoring using 120 subdural electrodes over the right frontoparietal region. Corticectomy of right postcentral gyrus, including clustered MEGSS, was performed. The pathology was reported to be cortical dysplasia type IIB. He has been seizure free for 5 months with medications.

location of the source of interictal epileptiform discharges.[7] There are five reasons for the failure of MEG in this regard:

1. Mesial-temporal areas are farther from MEG sensors.[24] Because magnetic fields attenuate in square proportion to the distance from the source,[25] there are less prominent MEG spikes with mesial-temporal discharges.
2. The cylindrical architecture of hippocampal neurons cancels the generated excitatory postsynaptic potentials (closed circuit), in contrast to the linear and laminar architecture of neocortical neurons (open circuit).[24]
3. Insufficient coverage of the subtemporal magnetic fields by a whole-head MEG sensor array increases errors for dipole estimation.
4. The propagation of epileptiform discharges to surrounding temporal structures through the limbic network is not suitable for application of single dipole analysis.[26]
5. Magnetic fields from lateral and superior temporal cortices overwhelm those from mesial temporal structures.

MEG is more valuable in those cases where the temporal lobe is part of a wider circuitry in localization-related epilepsy. For example, in a child with intractable epilepsy secondary to a temporo-parieto-occipital porencephalic cyst after encephalitis, vertically oriented MEGSS were obtained without superior lateral temporal cortices. The absence of superolateral temporal cortices, prominent temporal EEG spikes, less prominent MEG spikes, and mesiobasal synthetic aperture magnetometry spikes using spatial filtering method all indicated that the vertically oriented MEGSS were projected directly from the mesiobasal temporal region.[27]

In another example, a 9-year-old boy with benign epileptiform discharges in the rolandic region, co-existing with intractable mesial temporal lobe epilepsy secondary to hippocampal sclerosis on MRI, though scalp VEEG showed left temporal rhythmic sharp waves after the clinical onset of epigastric aura, followed by staring.[28] MEG identified rolandic MEGSS, which were prominent on scalp EEG as well. MEG was unable to localize the epileptogenic sources in the temporal lobe because higher amplitude signals of rolandic spikes masked lower amplitude spikes from mesial temporal network in this case. The benign form of rolandic MEGSS in which orientation of dipoles are identical and vertical to central sulcus similar to those of BRE are often seen in children as an age-related phenomenon and occasionally seen in adults with temporal lobe epilepsy.

■ Nonlesional Epilepsy

Nonlesional epilepsy represents a challenge for epilepsy surgical evaluation in children. In a cohort of 75 children younger than 12 years who underwent resective surgery for intractable epilepsy at a pediatric epilepsy center, 35 had no identifiable focal lesion on MRI.[29] In addition, some researchers have shown that MRI does not aid in the presurgical evaluation in nearly 29% of patients in whom it is normal or shows nonspecific findings.[30] The outcome after epilepsy surgery in patients with normal brain MRI depends on the case selection criteria and expertise of the epilepsy center. Surgery for intractable epilepsy in children with normal MRI findings but clustered MEGSS provided good postsurgical outcomes in the majority.[31] Restricted ictal onset zone predicted postoperative seizure freedom. Seizure freedom was most likely to occur when there was concordance between EEG and MEG localization and least likely to occur when these results were divergent. Postoperative seizure freedom was less likely to occur in children with bilateral MEG clusters or only scatters, multiple seizure types, and incomplete resection of the proposed epileptogenic zone.

■ Recurrent or Residual Seizures after Surgery

The success rate of surgery in extratemporal epilepsies, which are particularly common in children, continues to be disappointing, with a 27 to 46% seizure-free rate in long-term follow-up.[32] Standard MRI techniques used postoperatively in patients after epilepsy surgery may miss the extent of the residual lesion. Similarly, postoperative ictal scalp EEG findings are misleading because of skull defects, dural scarring, cerebrospinal fluid-filled intracranial cavities, and alterations or distortions of brain structures from a previous surgery. In patients who have a second epilepsy surgery after the initial one failed to control seizures, the interpretation of invasive EEG as recorded from subdural electrodes becomes complicated by differences in amplitude between normal and gliotic cortical surfaces at the site of previous surgery.

Specific MEGSS patterns delineated the epileptogenic zone in 17 children with recurrent seizures after previous epilepsy surgery.[33] The clustered MEGSS occurred at the margins of previous resections within two contiguous gyri in 10 patients (group A), extended spatially from a margin by 3 cm or less in 3 patients (group B), and were remote from the resection margin by more than 3 cm in 6 patients (group C). Two patients had concomitant group A and C clusters. Eleven of 13 children who underwent repeat surgeries that included resection of the area of clustered MEGSS obtained favorable surgical outcomes. MEG is particularly advantageous in those children in whom a second epilepsy surgery is being contemplated, because in children who have had previous surgery, MEG signals are far less distorted by postoperative skull defects, subdural scarring, arachnoid adhesions, and shifting of the normal brain into resection cavities than the scalp EEG. Thus, MEG can identify the recurrent epileptogenic zone for the subgroup of patients with late recurrent seizures after epilepsy surgery.

■ Functional Mapping

A successful outcome from epilepsy surgery is generally defined as a seizure-free state with no imposition of neurological deficit.[34] To achieve these twin goals, two criteria must be fulfilled. First, precise localization of the epileptogenic zone in the brain is necessary. Second, one must determine the anatomical localization of eloquent cortex that subserves sensory, motor, language, and memory function. Therefore, the neurosurgeon requires the precise anatomical correlation between the epileptogenic zone and eloquent cortex before surgery. Noninvasive MEG studies are now used routinely in some centers to localize eloquent cortex in patients undergoing epilepsy surgery.

The somatosensory evoked magnetic field (SEF) for median nerve stimulation is now widely accepted as the most reliable method for identifying the primary somatosensory cortex and localization of the central sulcus.[35] Because the N20m component of SEF reflects the direct neuronal activity of primary sensory cortex, the SEF is generated from the posterior bank of the central sulcus.

Pihko et al[36] successfully measured the SEF in normal newborns during their frequent postprandial sleep. However, sleep recordings are less feasible in older infants because of their shortened sleep cycles. Therefore total intravenous anesthesia using propofol has been applied for MEG and MRI studies in uncooperative children.[37] We analyzed 26 infants younger than 4 years under total intravenous anesthesia using propofol and showed that SEFs can still be detected and reliably observed under these conditions.[38] MEG source localization of evoked fields can address whether functional reorganization of primary sensory modalities exists in malformations of cortical development.[39]

MEG can also identify motor cortex. Movement-related cerebral magnetic fields following voluntary finger movement have demonstrated a unique area of motor control in children.[40]

The auditory evoked magnetic field is used to identify the primary auditory cortex. The prominent components of N100m around 100 milliseconds after contralateral audio stimulation represent the auditory evoked magnetic field in the Heschl gyrus in the planum temporale.[41,42] Similarly, the visual evoked magnetic field is used to localize the primary visual cortex. P100m at around 100 milliseconds after visual stimulation produces visual evoked magnetic fields in the mesial occipital region.[43]

MEG has been reported to be useful in the lateralization and localization of language in seizure patients.[44–46] During MEG recordings, patients engaged in a word recognition task have been shown to activate language areas. Excellent agreement has been reported between MEG data and those obtained from Wada testing.[47] In addition, there is good correlation between MEG and intraoperative direct cortical mapping in terms of localization of receptive language areas.[48]

■ Conclusion

MEG provides excellent spatiotemporal resolution for localizing sources of intracranial epileptic discharges and functional representation on MRI. MEG study is a noninvasive assessment for selecting candidates with intractable epilepsy for resective surgery because they identify localization-related epilepsy and localize the cluster of epileptogenic spike sources. The cluster of MEGSSs indicate the epileptogenic zone preoperatively for maximum removal with lesion, if lesional-epilepsy, to improve seizure control. The increased clinical application of MEG can reduce the use of invasive subdural and depth electrode recordings for a subset of patients with intractable localization-related epilepsy, especially for the patients with recurrent seizures after epilepsey surgeries fail.

References

1. Wheless JW, Willmore LJ, Breier JI, et al. A comparison of magnetoencephalography, MRI, and V-EEG in patients evaluated for epilepsy surgery. Epilepsia 1999;40(7):931–941
2. Minassian BA, Otsubo H, Weiss S, Elliott I, Rutka JT, Snead OC III. Magnetoencephalographic localization in pediatric epilepsy surgery: comparison with invasive intracranial electroencephalography. Ann Neurol 1999;46(4):627–633
3. Otsubo H, Chitoku S, Ochi A, et al. Malignant rolandic-sylvian epilepsy in children: diagnosis, treatment, and outcomes. Neurology 2001;57(4):590–596
4. Otsubo H, Ochi A, Elliott I, et al. MEG predicts epileptic zone in lesional extrahippocampal epilepsy: 12 pediatric surgery cases. Epilepsia 2001;42(12):1523–1530
5. Pataraia E, Simos PG, Castillo EM, et al. Does magnetoencephalography add to scalp video-EEG as a diagnostic tool in epilepsy surgery? Neurology 2004;62(6):943–948

6. Iida K, Otsubo H, Matsumoto Y, et al. Characterizing magnetic spike sources by using magnetoencephalography-guided neuronavigation in epilepsy surgery in pediatric patients. J Neurosurg 2005; 102(2, suppl)187–196
7. Ebersole JS. Defining epileptogenic foci: past, present, future. J Clin Neurophysiol 1997;14(6):470–483
8. Ochi A, Otsubo H, Iida K, et al. Identifying the primary epileptogenic hemisphere from electroencephalographic (EEG) and magnetoencephalographic dipole lateralizations in children with intractable epilepsy. J Child Neurol 2005;20(11):885–892
9. Bast T, Oezkan O, Rona S, et al. EEG and MEG source analysis of single and averaged interictal spikes reveals intrinsic epileptogenicity in focal cortical dysplasia. Epilepsia 2004;45(6):621–631
10. Otsubo H, Iida K, Oishi M, et al. Neurophysiologic findings of neuronal migration disorders: intrinsic epileptogenicity of focal cortical dysplasia on electroencephalography, electrocorticography,

and magnetoencephalography. J Child Neurol 2005;20(4):357–363

11. Wu JY, Sutherling WW, Koh S, et al. Magnetic source imaging localizes epileptogenic zone in children with tuberous sclerosis complex. Neurology 2006;66(8):1270–1272

12. Iida K, Otsubo H, Mohamed IS, et al. Characterizing magnetoencephalographic spike sources in children with tuberous sclerosis complex. Epilepsia 2005;46(9):1510–1517

13. Xiao Z, Xiang J, Holowka S, et al. Volumetric localization of epileptic activities in tuberous sclerosis using synthetic aperture magnetometry. Pediatr Radiol 2006;36(1):16–21

14. Kamimura T, Tohyama J, Oishi M, et al. Magnetoencephalography in patients with tuberous sclerosis and localization-related epilepsy. Epilepsia 2006;47(6):991–997

15. Koo B, Hwang P. Localization of focal cortical lesions influences age of onset of infantile spasms. Epilepsia 1996;37(11):1068–1071

16. Oguni H, Hayashi K, Osawa M. Migration of epileptic foci in children. Adv Neurol 1999;81:131–143

17. Oishi M, Kameyama S, Masuda H, et al. Single and multiple clusters of magnetoencephalographic dipoles in neocortical epilepsy: significance in characterizing the epileptogenic zone. Epilepsia 2006;47(2):355–364

18. Ossenblok P, de Munck JC, Colon A, Drolsbach W, Boon P. Magnetoencephalography is more successful for screening and localizing frontal lobe epilepsy than electroencephalography. Epilepsia 2007;48(11):2139–2149

19. Hara K, Lin FH, Camposano S, et al. Magnetoencephalographic mapping of interictal spike propagation: a technical and clinical report. AJNR Am J Neuroradiol 2007;28(8):1486–1488

20. Shiraishi H, Ahlfors SP, Stufflebeam SM, et al. Application of magnetoencephalography in epilepsy patients with widespread spike or slow-wave activity. Epilepsia 2005;46(8):1264–1272

21. Ishitobi M, Nakasato N, Yamamoto K, Iinuma K. Opercular to interhemispheric source distribution of benign rolandic spikes of childhood. Neuroimage 2005;25(2):417–423

22. Sobel DF, Aung M, Otsubo H, Smith MC. Magnetoencephalography in children with Landau-Kleffner syndrome and acquired epileptic aphasia. AJNR Am J Neuroradiol 2000;21(2):301–307

23. Benifla M, Otsubo H, Ochi A, et al. Temporal lobe surgery for intractable epilepsy in children: an analysis of outcomes in 126 children. Neurosurgery 2006;59(6):1203–1213, discussion 1213–1214

24. Mikuni N, Nagamine T, Ikeda A, et al. Simultaneous recording of epileptiform discharges by MEG and subdural electrodes in temporal lobe epilepsy. Neuroimage 1997;5(4 pt 1):298–306

25. Sato S, Balish M, Muratore R. Principles of magnetoencephalography. J Clin Neurophysiol 1991;8(2):144–156

26. Alarcon G, Guy CN, Binnie CD, Walker SR, Elwes RD, Polkey CE. Intracerebral propagation of interictal activity in partial epilepsy: implications for source localisation. J Neurol Neurosurg Psychiatry 1994;57(4):435–449

27. Imai K, Otsubo H, Sell E, et al. MEG source estimation from mesiobasal temporal areas in a child with a porencephalic cyst. Acta Neurol Scand 2007;116(4):263–267

28. RamachandranNair R, Ochi A, Benifla M, Rutka JT, Snead OC III, Otsubo H. Benign epileptiform discharges in Rolandic region with mesial temporal lobe epilepsy: MEG, scalp and intracranial EEG features. Acta Neurol Scand 2007;116(1):59–64

29. Paolicchi JM, Jayakar P, Dean P, et al. Predictors of outcome in pediatric epilepsy surgery. Neurology 2000;54(3):642–647

30. Semah F, Picot MC, Adam C, et al. Is the underlying cause of epilepsy a major prognostic factor for recurrence? Neurology 1998;51(5):1256–1262

31. RamachandranNair R, Otsubo H, Shroff MM, et al. MEG predicts outcome following surgery for intractable epilepsy in children with normal or nonfocal MRI findings. Epilepsia 2007;48(1):149–157

32. Téllez-Zenteno JF, Dhar R, Wiebe S. Long-term seizure outcomes following epilepsy surgery: a systematic review and meta-analysis. Brain 2005;128(Pt 5):1188–1198

33. Mohamed IS, Otsubo H, Ochi A, et al. Utility of magnetoencephalography in the evaluation of recurrent seizures after epilepsy surgery. Epilepsia 2007;48(11):2150–2159

34. Snead OC III. Surgical treatment of medically refractory epilepsy in childhood. Brain Dev 2001;23(4):199–207

35. Kawamura T, Nakasato N, Seki K, et al. Neuromagnetic evidence of pre- and post-central cortical sources of somatosensory evoked responses. Electroencephalogr Clin Neurophysiol 1996;100(1):44–50

36. Pihko E, Lauronen L, Wikström H, et al. Somatosensory evoked potentials and magnetic fields elicited by tactile stimulation of the hand during active and quiet sleep in newborns. Clin Neurophysiol 2004;115(2):448–455

37. Sharma R, Pang EW, Mohamed I, et al. Magnetoencephalography in children: routine clinical protocol for intractable epilepsy at the Hospital for Sick Children. In: Cheyne D, Ross B, Stroink G, Weinberg H, eds. New Frontiers in Biomagnetism. International Congress Series 2007;1300. Amsterdam, The Netherlands: Elsevier; 2007:685–688

38. Bercovici E, Pang EW, Sharma R, et al. Somatosensory-evoked fields on magnetoencephalography for epilepsy infants younger than 4 years with total intravenous anesthesia. Clin Neurophysiol 2008;119(6):1328–1334

39. Burneo JG, Kuzniecky RI, Bebin M, Knowlton RC. Cortical reorganization in malformations of cortical development: a magnetoencephalographic study. Neurology 2004;63(10):1818–1824

40. Gaetz W, Cheyne D. Localization of sensorimotor cortical rhythms induced by tactile stimulation using spatially filtered MEG. Neuroimage 2006;30(3):899–908

41. Nakasato N, Kumabe T, Kanno A, Ohtomo S, Mizoi K, Yoshimoto T. Neuromagnetic evaluation of cortical auditory function in patients with temporal lobe tumors. J Neurosurg 1997;86(4):610–618

42. Pang EW, Gaetz W, Otsubo H, Chuang S, Cheyne D. Localization of auditory N1 in children using MEG: source modeling issues. Int J Psychophysiol 2003;51(1):27–35

43. Nakasato N, Yoshimoto T. Somatosensory, auditory, and visual evoked magnetic fields in patients with brain diseases. J Clin Neurophysiol 2000;17(2):201–211

44. Pataraia E, Simos PG, Castillo EM, et al. Reorganization of language-specific cortex in patients with lesions or mesial temporal epilepsy. Neurology 2004;63(10):1825–1832

45. Breier JI, Castillo EM, Simos PG, et al. Atypical language representation in patients with chronic seizure disorder and achievement deficits with magnetoencephalography. Epilepsia 2005;46(4):540–548

46. Lee D, Sawrie SM, Simos PG, Killen J, Knowlton RC. Reliability of language mapping with magnetic source imaging in epilepsy surgery candidates. Epilepsy Behav 2006;8(4):742–749

47. Papanicolaou AC, Simos PG, Castillo EM, et al. Magnetocephalography: a noninvasive alternative to the Wada procedure. J Neurosurg 2004;100(5):867–876

48. Papanicolaou AC, Simos PG, Breier JI, et al. Magnetoencephalographic mapping of the language-specific cortex. J Neurosurg 1999;90(1):85–93

8 Structural Brain Imaging in Epilepsy

Charles Raybaud and Elysa Widjaja

Epilepsy is a common problem, with a prevalence of 0.4 to 1% of the population. Epilepsies and epileptic syndromes are classified into focal and generalized epilepsies. Focal epilepsies account for 40 to 60% of all newly diagnosed cases. Up to 30% of these patients develop intractable epilepsy, despite medical therapy.[1,2] In some patients, surgical treatment may lead to cessation or significant improvement in seizure control. The role of structural imaging is to identify the pathological substrate responsible for the epilepsy and to demonstrate the relation of lesion to eloquent areas of the brain. Any epilepsy that is not a benign, idiopathic form of epilepsy requires neuroimaging, including symptomatic focal epilepsy, specific epileptic syndromes pointing to structural brain abnormalities such as Ohtahara or West syndromes, status epilepticus, the so-called catastrophic epilepsies, and progressive deterioration.

Computed tomography (CT) scan is not the first line investigation for epilepsy, but may supplement magnetic resonance imaging (MRI) in the detection of focal area of calcification, such as with tuberous sclerosis or Sturge-Weber syndrome. The main imaging modality for detecting the pathological substrate responsible for epilepsy is MRI. In children with newly diagnosed epilepsy, MRI detected an abnormality in 62/388 (16%).[3] In patients with intractable epilepsy, MRI detected an abnormality in 82 to 86% of cases.[4,5] MRI has excellent soft tissue contrast, better spatial resolution, multiplanar capability, and higher sensitivity than CT and is therefore the imaging modality of choice. With advances in techniques, previously undetectable subtle structural abnormalities can now be demonstrated by MRI. It is, however, crucial to correlate MRI-identified substrate with clinical and electrophysiological data to avoid false localization. MRI also has prognostic implications: failure to detect a lesion on MRI leads to a worse surgical outcome compared with when a lesion is identified.[6–8]

■ MRI Techniques

The sensitivity of MRI for detecting abnormalities depends on the MRI techniques used, the pathological substrate, and the experience of the interpreting physician. Visual assessment of MRIs should be done by experts in epilepsy imaging,

with knowledge of the clinical semiology and electroencephalography (EEG) findings. An optimal MRI technique for assessing the pathological substrate should include a variety of imaging sequences, including T1-weighted imaging (WI), T2WI, proton density, and fluid attenuation inversion recovery (FLAIR) sequences. These need to be acquired in at least two orthogonal planes covering the whole brain, using the minimum slice thickness. In patients with temporal lobe epilepsy, the coronal plane should be perpendicular to the long axis of the hippocampus to optimize visualization of the hippocampus and mesial temporal lobe structures. For extratemporal epilepsy, the bicommissural plane (i.e., parallel to the anterior commissure-posterior commissure plane) is the standard method used. A three-dimensional T1 volume sequence with slice thickness of 1.5 mm or less should be included because this sequence provides excellent gray/white matter contrast and can be reformatted into any orthogonal or nonorthogonal planes. The three-dimensional volume T1WI can also be subjected to additional postprocessing without the penalty of additional imaging time. Gadolinium does not improve the sensitivity of MRI in patients with epilepsy and should be used only to characterize selective intracerebral lesions, such as tumors. A systematic approach should be used to evaluate MRIs to optimize detection of subtle lesions and dual pathologies.

MRI Spectroscopy

MRI spectroscopy may be used to better characterize a lesion (mostly between tumors, or tumor vs. dysplasia according to the spectral profile), or, by showing a decreased N-acetylaspartate (NAA), to locate the epileptogenic area. However, the changes may reflect both the structural abnormalities and the metabolic alterations related to the seizures, making the interpretation of the results difficult.[9-11]

Diffusion Imaging

Diffusion imaging has shown striking abnormalities during status epilepticus, reflecting cytotoxic edema, both locally and remotely in the ipsilateral pulvinar[12,13]; ipsilateral hippocampus[13]; and contralateral cerebellum (diaschisis-like response)[12] as well as in the corpus callosum.[12] This brain response to repeated or prolonged seizures may be useful in locating a focus. In addition to conventional MRI, diffusion tensor imaging (DTI) better depicts the structure of the white matter. Although it is not currently used for diagnosis, it may help in understanding the abnormalities of white matter associated with cortical malformations.[14] It also helps in preparing the surgical approach to a lesion[15] (**Fig. 8.1B**). Perfusion imaging in the setting of epilepsy is still in an experimental stage.

Structural Image Analyses

Structural image analyses describe various computer-assisted methods devised to improve the rate of detection of subtle brain abnormalities in epilepsy. Most use segmentation methods and postprocessing algorithms aimed at quantifying the volume of various compartments of the brain (such as gray and white matter) or specific lobes or structures (such as the hippocampus) or to evaluate the thickness of the cortex or blurring of the cortical–subcortical junction. Unfortunately, these methods are not fully automated, are time-consuming, and are difficult to use in clinical practice.

Multimodal integration of the anatomical data from MRI, functional data from interictal positron emission tomography (PET) or ictal/interictal single photon emission computed tomography (SPECT), and electrophysiological data from cortical or stereo-EEG or from magnetoencephalography (MEG) may also help in identifying the epileptogenic focus with its underlying structural abnormalities.

■ Epileptogenic Substrates

Although the range of pathological substrates responsible for intractable partial epilepsy in children is similar to that of adults, malformations of cortical development (MCD) and developmental tumors are more commonly detected in surgical specimens of pediatric epilepsy patients. MCD constitute 10 to 50% of pediatric epilepsy cases being evaluated for surgery and 4 to 25% of adult cases of intractable epilepsy.[16] By contrast, hippocampal sclerosis is less common in pediatric patients compared with adults. In a series of 126 children undergoing temporal lobectomy for intractable epilepsy, the reported prevalence of hippocampal sclerosis was 13%.[6] However, in another cohort of the 109 children, a higher prevalence (45%) of hippocampal sclerosis was reported.[17] By contrast, hippocampal sclerosis is the most common epileptogenic substrate in adults with intractable epilepsy and accounts for 50 to 70% of cases.

■ Epilepsy-Associated Tumors

Epilepsy-associated developmental tumors may account for up to two thirds of the surgical pathological substrate.[6,17–19] These tumors originate in and develop from the cortex and, therefore, clinically present with seizures. They are slow-growing tumors, with well-defined margin, without associated edema or necrosis. Complete removal results in good seizure control or renders the patients seizure free. These tumors may developmentally be related to focal cortical dys-

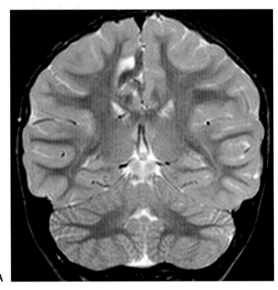
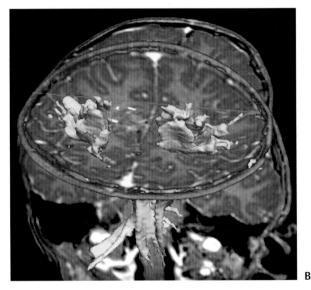

Fig. 8.1 (A) Coronal T2 image demonstrates a lesion in the right supplementary motor area, which is of low T2 signal in the cortex because of the presence of calcification and high T2 signal in the subcortical white matter from gliosis (*arrowhead*). Histology of the lesion confirms meningioangiomatosis. **(B)** Corticospinal tracts from diffusion tensor imaging overlaid onto oblique coronal and axial T1 postcontrast sequences. The lesion lies immediately anterior and medial to the right corticospinal tract.

plasia (FCD).[20] They may all derive from the same precursor cells and may have originated from the dysplastic tissue.[20,21] FCD may be present in the cortex adjacent to the developmental tumors. The epilepsy-associated tumors include ganglioglioma and its variants, dysembryoplastic neuroepithelial tumor (DNET), pleomorphic xanthoastrocytoma (PXA), and low grade astrocytoma. More glioneuronal tumors have recently been described, but they are uncommon.[22]

Gangliogliomas

Gangliogliomas are slightly more common in male patients and are 10 times more common in children than in adults.[20] They are macroscopically observed to be up to eight times larger in children than in adults.[23] They are associated with chronic epilepsy in 85% of cases, and are located mostly in the temporomesial (50%) or temporolateral (29%) location.[24] Gangliogliomas and low-grade astrocytomas were found to be the most common tumors in a temporal lobectomy series.[6] Gangliogliomas may present as a solid mass in 43%, a cyst in 5%, and a mixed lesion in 52% of patients[25] (**Fig. 8.2A,B**). They involve the cortex, usually broaden the gyri, and may cause remodeling of the adjacent bone. On CT, gangliogliomas may present as hypo- (38%), iso- (15%), hyperattenuating (15%), or mixed masses (32%). Calcification may be seen in approximately 30 to 50% of cases. On MRI, the tumor may appear hypo- or isointense to gray matter on T1WI and hyperintense on T2WI. Some may demonstrate intrinsic high T1 signal.[25] Enhancement after gadolinium administration is common in up to 60% of cases. It can be nodular, ring-like, or solid. Leptomeningeal involvement may rarely be seen.[25] Gangliogliomas histologically consist of two cellular populations: one neuronal and one glial. The neuronal component does not expand, and the glial component may evolve to become anaplastic tumor or glioblastoma multiforme in approximately 6% of cases.[25] Patients

with ganglioglioma had the best outcome compared with other types of epilepsy associated tumors (92% Engel class I and II).[6,18,24]

Gangliocytoma

Gangliocytoma is uncommon and affects older children and young adults. It involves the cortex and consists of neurons without glial tissue. It usually has solid and cystic components. On MRI, gangliocytoma demonstrates low T1 and high T2 signals and enhances on the postgadolinium scans.

Desmoplastic Infantile Ganglioglioma

Desmoplastic infantile ganglioglioma (DIG) is a rare, likely congenital tumor that develops in infants. It is usually huge and more often suprasylvian in location. The mass is partly cystic and partly solid. The solid portion incorporates the cortex and is diffusely attached to the dura; it is strongly desmoplastic, and this, together with the age of the patient, characterizes the tumor. In approximately half the cases, the infant presents with macrocephaly, neurological deficits, and seizures. The imaging features are relatively specific when observed in an infant: huge cystic and solid mass involving more often the frontal and parietal lobes, less commonly the temporal lobe, with cranial asymmetry and expansion of the vault. The solid portion, attached to the dura, is mildly hyperattenuating on CT and may be calcified.[26] The cystic portion extends into the white matter. On MRIs, the solid portion is isointense to gray matter on T1WI and hyper-, iso-, or hypointense on T2WI, usually heterogeneously. Contrast-enhancement of the solid portion is intense and extends to the dura. The wall of the cystic component does not enhance.[26] In spite of the spectacular appearance of the tumor, the prognosis is good.[25,26]

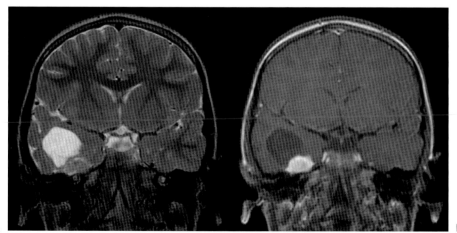

A   B

Fig. 8.2 (A) Coronal T2 and **(B)** coronal T1 postcontrast images demonstrate a cystic tumor with an enhancing eccentric nodule in the right temporal lobe. MRI appearance suggests ganglioglioma, which is confirmed on histology.

Dysembryoplastic Neuroepithelial Tumor

DNET was first described by Daumas-Duport et al in 1988.[27] It affects the temporal and frontal lobes predominantly. DNET (14%) is less common in children compared with ganglioglioma (43%).[18] The lesion may have a well-demarcated margin (50%), or the margins may be slightly blurred.[28] The tumor may cause broadening of the gyri, effacement of the sulci, and distortion of the ventricles.[28] The tumor may also result in remodeling of the overlying skull vault in 44% of cases.[29] On CT, the tumor is hypoattenuating with cystic appearance.[30] Calcification has been reported in 20 to 36% of cases.[18,29] On MRI, the tumor is of low T1/high T2 signal, often with multicystic, multinodular changes and "bubbly" appearance,[28] and it may have a thin rim of high signal on FLAIR sequence (**Fig. 8.3A**). The tumor appears wedge shaped and extends to the ventricle in 30% of cases. One third of cases show faint punctate or ring enhancement. Spontaneous hemorrhage has been reported in DNET.[31] The tumor is usually stable over the years. However, a significant increase in size has been documented in a few cases.[28,32] DNET has less favorable outcome compared with ganglioglioma, with 70% of patients with DNET having Engel class I and II surgical outcomes.[6] Long-term follow-up of DNET has reported reduced seizure-free surgical outcome,[33] which may be attributed to incomplete resection of the tumor or the presence of cortical dysplasia beyond the margins of the resected DNET.[34] The cortical dysplasia is usually not visible on MRI. The differential diagnoses of DNET include ganglioglioma, low-grade glioma, and FCD. FCD does not enhance and usually does not have mass effect. Gangliogliomas usually have more mass effect. MRI spectroscopy is reported to be normal in DNET,[35] whereas high choline and low NAA are observed in gliomas and gangliogliomas.

Another tumor has been described both as a "nonspecific DNET" and as a cortical oligodendroglioma (World Health Organization [WHO] grade II). It is an intracortical hemispheric tumor that presents with isolated epilepsy without neurological deficit or increased intracranial pressure. It has a DNET-like appearance on imaging: triangular cortical lesion with septa, low T1/high T2 signals, without surrounding edema or mass effect, and no enhancement.[36] By contrast with the deep oligodendroglioma, this peripheral epilepsy-associated tumor has a good prognosis.[36,37]

Pleomorphic Xanthoastrocytoma

PXA is a rare tumor affecting children and young adults. Like the other epilepsy-associated tumors, PXA is slow growing, located in the cortex, and highly epileptogenic. It is supratentorial in 98% of cases; mostly temporal (49%) in location; and less commonly parietal, frontal, and occipital.[38] The tumor is located in the cortex, has cystic and solid components, and may demonstrate continuity with the dura (**Fig. 8.4B**). On CT, the tumor is predominantly hypodense with mixed density nodule. On MRI, the tumor is hypo- to isointense to gray matter on T1WI and hyper- to isointense on T2WI, and the cystic portion is isointense to cerebrospinal fluid (CSF). Postgadolinium scans demonstrate enhancement of the nodular solid component as well as enhancement of the adjacent meninges (dural "tail"). The enhancing nodule often abuts the pial surface. Calcification is rare, and the tumor is well circumscribed without peritumoral edema.[25,39] Hemorrhage has been reported. It contains predominantly glial component but may also contain neuronal elements.[40,41] Like

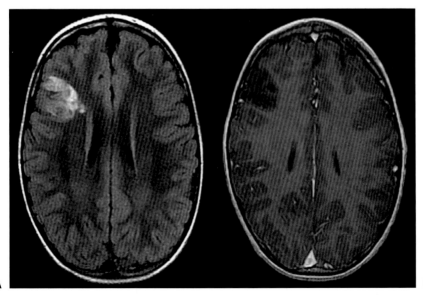

A   B

Fig. 8.3 **(A)** Axial FLAIR and **(B)** axial T1 post-contrast images demonstrate a "bubbly" appearance of a cortically based tumor in the right frontal lobe. The tumor has a wedge shape with a rim of high FLAIR signal medially and "nodular" signal intensity medial to the tumor that extends toward the margin of the ventricle. Histology of the lesion confirms dysembryoplastic neuroepithelial tumor.

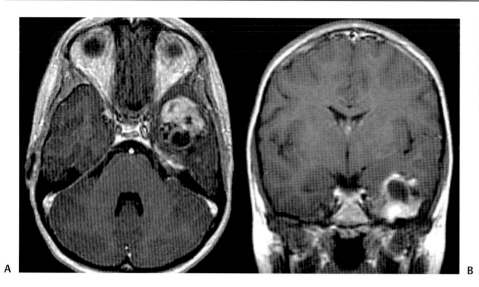

A

B

Fig. 8.4 (A) Axial and **(B)** coronal post-contrast T1 weighted images show a complex solid cystic tumor in the left temporal lobe. The tumor is cortically based with extension to the dura. Histology of the lesion shows pleomorphic xanthoastrocytoma.

DNET, PXA is also associated with cortical dysplasia.[40,42] The prognosis is generally good, but it may recur and malignant degeneration occurs in 20% of cases.[38]

Low-Grade (Fibrillary) Astrocytomas

Low-grade astrocytomas are usually ill-defined infiltrative tumor located predominantly in the frontal or temporal lobes and invading the cortex. They do not contain ganglionic cells. CT demonstrates ill-defined homogeneous hypodense or isodense mass. MRI demonstrates a homogenous mass that is hypointense on T1 and hyperintense on T2 and may expand the adjacent cortex (**Fig. 8.5B**). The tumor usu-

ally does not show enhancement. Calcification and cysts are uncommon, and hemorrhage or surrounding edema is rare. The tumor has an inherent tendency for malignant progression to anaplastic astrocytoma.

■ Malformations of Cortical Development

Of the different subtypes of malformations of cortical development, the lesions that more commonly undergo surgical management of epilepsy are FCD, hemimegalencephaly, and tuberous sclerosis.

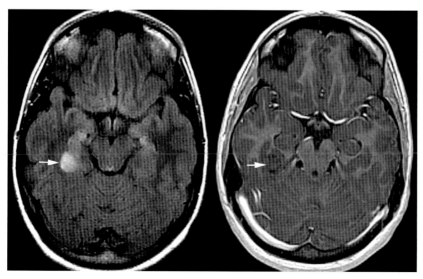

A

B

Fig. 8.5 (A) Axial FLAIR and **(B)** axial T1 postcontrast images demonstrate a well-circumscribed tumor (*arrow*) in the right parahippocampal gyrus with no evidence of contrast enhancement. Imaging appearance is in keeping with a low-grade tumor and histology of the lesion is that of a low-grade glioma.

Focal Cortical Dysplasia

FCD is intrinsically epileptogenic and is a frequent cause of epilepsy in children.[43,44] Palmini et al.[43] have shown selective occurrence of ictal or continuous epileptogenic discharges in FCD compared with other epileptic pathologies such as tumors or arteriovenous malformations. The mechanism of the epilepsy is still unclear. Several possibilities have been proposed, including abnormal firing from the dysplastic neurons rather than from the balloon cells,[45] dysfunction of synaptic circuits with abnormal synchronization of the neuronal population, and abnormal organization of the inhibitory interneurons.[46] FCD is identified in 18 to 40% of localization-related epilepsy.[47-51] There has been a suggestion that FCD has been more frequently reported in the pediatric population than in adult series[52]: 18% of FCD in surgical specimens of a series of 216 adult patients with intractable epilepsy,[49] versus 30 to 39% of FCD in pediatric patients.[47,48]

Classification and Origin of FCD

The term *FCD* was originally coined by Taylor et al[53] to describe a specific cortical abnormality found in patients who presented with refractory partial epilepsy and who were cured by excision of the affected cortical area. The dysplastic cortex was characterized by disorganized "bizarre neurons" and giant dysmorphic "balloon cells." Since then, the term FCD has been used extensively in the literature to refer to a wide range of derangements of the cortex, and various classifications have been proposed.[50,54-58]

The classification proposed by Palmini et al is based on neuropathological findings[58]:

- Mild malformations of cortical development, previously known as microdysgenesis, consist of heterotopic or excess neurons in or outside layer I.
- Type IA FCD consists of cortical dyslamination without giant or immature neurons, whereas type IB consists of cortical dyslamination with giant or immature neurons but no dysmorphic neurons.
- Type IIA FCD consists of cortical dyslamination with dysmorphic neurons but no balloon cells, whereas type IIB consists of cortical dyslamination with balloon cells.

Both type IIA and IIB FCD have been considered to represent the most severe end of the histopathological spectrum of FCD,[56,58] and type IA, type IB, and mild MCD have been considered as the milder end of the spectrum.

Other classifications have been based on the stage at which abnormal development occurred[54]: FCD with balloon cells has been classified as malformation because of abnormal neuronal proliferation or apoptosis, whereas FCD without balloon cells as well as microdysgenesis has been classified as malformation because of abnormal cortical or-

ganization (including late neuronal migration). Work by Englund et al[59] suggested that cortical dysplasia with balloon cells was the result of very early disturbance of glialneuronal differentiation and therefore supported its inclusion in malformations of cellular proliferation or apoptosis. Colombo et al[60] and Urbach et al[61] found that Taylor's FCD was more likely to demonstrate abnormal signal in the white matter that tapers from the cortex toward the ventricles (transmantle dysplasia).[62] During development, cells migrate from the germinal matrix to the cortex along radial glial fibers; abnormal cellular proliferation may in turn affect cellular migration and cortical organization and potentially be responsible for this transmantle abnormal signal. This supports the suggestion that FCD with balloon cells occurs at an earlier stage of cortical development compared with FCD without balloon cells. By contrast, Andres et al[63] found an increased number of neurons in layer I of the cortex and the white matter and abnormal morphology of neurons in Taylor's FCD. They suggested that excessive neurogenesis of late-generated neurons and possible retention of radial glial and subplate neurons may account for the development of Taylor's FCD, which would then indicate that Taylor's FCD occurs in the later stage of cortical development.[63]

Type IA and IB FCD and mild malformations of cortical development are classified as malformations because of abnormal cortical organization.[54] These lesions are thought to arise secondary to insults occurring later in the development of the cortex, during late gestation, and they may be acquired up to 2 years postnatally.[64-68] Histological findings of dysplastic neurons with giant neurons have been seen after severe perinatal injury such as ventricular hemorrhage in the premature neonate,[65] white matter hypoxic-ischemic injury in premature[66] and term neonates,[67] early perinatal closed head injury,[64] and in nonaccidental injury.[68]

Imaging Appearance of FCD

FCD more commonly involves the frontal lobe. In half of the cases, two adjacent gyri are involved; less commonly, one gyrus or the depth of a sulcus is involved.[61] Two discrete FCDs may be found in the same patient.[61,69] On MRI, the features of FCD include thick cortex, blurring of the cortical–subcortical junction, abnormal signal in the white matter, and deep sulci. The cortex may demonstrate mildly high T1/low T2 signal. Contrast enhancement is rare but has been reported in FCD.[61,70] Taylor's FCD (IIA and IIB) more commonly involves the extratemporal cortex. Taylor's FCD is more likely to demonstrate high T2/ FLAIR signal that extends to and tapers toward the ventricle[50,60,61] (**Fig. 8.6A,B**). By contrast, non-Taylor's FCD (IA and IB) is more likely to be located in the temporal lobe, to demonstrate mild increased signal and hypoplasia or atrophy of the white matter (**Fig. 8.6C,D**), and to be associated with hippocampal sclerosis.[60]

The MRI appearance of FCD may change with brain maturation. In longitudinal MRI studies in infants with FCD, the early study may be normal, but repeat imaging at a later date may demonstrate high T2 signal in the white matter, high T1 signal in the cortex, and blurring of the cortical–subcortical white matter junction.[71] A repeat study is recommended at a later stage when the MRI appears initially normal in an infant with refractory partial seizures or infantile spasm.[71] Also, in contrast to the high T2/FLAIR signal in the white matter of FCD in children, the white matter adjacent to the dysplastic cortex may demonstrate low T2/high T1 signal in neonates and infants. This is postulated to be secondary to early myelination because of repeated seizures. Experimental study in the mouse has shown that repeated neuronal electrical activity such as those occurring in seizures induces myelination.[72]

Surgical Outcome of FCD

EEG abnormalities of FCD usually exceed the limits of MRI-visible abnormality. Similarly, the extent of FCD as defined by histopathology usually exceeds that visualized on MRI. The surgical results are dependent on resecting both the MRI-visible lesion and the cortical areas of abnormal EEG activity.[73] Earlier studies on surgical outcomes of FCD have reported that only 38 to 40% of patients achieved Engel class I outcome 1 or more years after surgery.[74] Subsequent studies have shown that up to 50 to 70% seizure-free outcome may be obtained after wider surgical resection[75-78]; Otsubo et al found that of 10 patients whose preoperative imaging showed FCD and who had MEG examination, 7 experienced good seizure outcome after resection of the MRI-visible lesion and of areas with MEG spike sources.[79] This finding compares favorably with outcome of patients with hippocampal sclerosis[80] and low-grade neoplasm.[81]

There is no consensus on the surgical outcome of subtypes of FCD. Some authors have reported a better surgical outcome for Taylor's FCD, whereas others have reported mild MCD and type I FCD have better surgical outcome.[50,52,73,82-85] The better surgical outcome of mild MCD and type I FCD

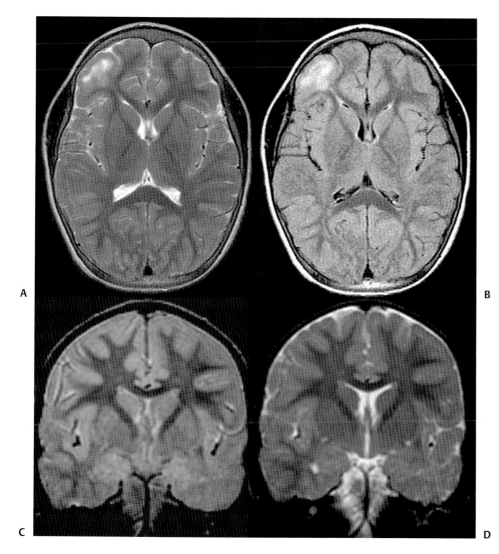

A

B

C

D

Fig. 8.6 Axial **(A)** T2 and **(B)** FLAIR images showing a lesion of high T2 and FLAIR signal involving the cortex and subcortical white matter associated with mild gyral expansion. There is tapering of the abnormal signal toward the ventricle, a feature that is very suggestive of Taylor's focal cortical dysplasia. Coronal **(C)** proton density and **(D)** T2-weighted imaging show high signal in the white matter of the left temporal lobe with blurring of the gray–white matter junction and slight reduction in the size of the left temporal lobe. The imaging findings are in keeping with focal cortical dysplasia. Histologically, there is evidence of lack of well-defined laminar cortical layering, neuronal clustering in the cortex, and heterotopic neurons in the white matter, in keeping with microdysgenesis.

could either be because of the lesser degree of histopathologic abnormalities or a preponderance of lesion location in the temporal lobe.

Hemimegalencephaly

Hemimegalencephaly (HME) may be sporadic or be associated with neurocutaneous syndromes (tuberous sclerosis, epidermal nevus syndrome, linear nevus sebaceous syndrome, hypomelanosis of Ito, Proteus syndrome, Klippel-Trénaunay syndrome, and encephalocraniocutaneous lipomatosis). The sporadic form is considered a hemispheric variant of FCD.[86] Histologically, the appearance is similar to FCD with abnormal gyration of the cortex, dyslamination, blurring of gray–white matter junction, giant neurons in both gray and white matter, and balloon cells in 50% of cases. Clinically, it may present early with intractable epilepsy; other clinical presentations include hemiparesis, hemianopia, and mental retardation. On imaging, one hemisphere is large with expanded calvarium, and this may be associated with enlarged lateral ventricle of the affected side.[87,88] The cortex is usually thick with broad gyri. The white matter usually has low T1/high T2 signal with possible cystic changes and calcification. In infants, the white matter of the affected hemisphere may show high T1/low T2 signal, suggesting early myelination,[89] possibly caused by seizure activity.[72] HME may involve the cerebellum[90] or may be limited to part of the hemisphere, usually its posterior portion.[91] With recurrent seizures or refractory status epilepticus, the enlarged hemisphere may later become atrophic.[92] Because of the intractable seizures, which are often poorly controlled by medications, and progressive deterioration, functional or anatomical hemispherectomy may be required to control the seizures.

Tuberous Sclerosis

Brain abnormalities in tuberous sclerosis (TSC) may be considered as a syndromic variant of FCD. The giant astrocytes that are present in cortical tubers correspond to the balloon cells present in Taylor's FCD. On imaging, TSC is characterized by the presence of multiple cortical/subcortical tubers distributed in both hemispheres and subependymal nodules along the margins of the ventricles. Cortical/subcortical tubers have broad gyri, thick cortex, and abnormal signal in the cortex and subcortical white matter and may occasionally demonstrate calcification. The subependymal nodules are more commonly calcified. In the region of the foramen of Monro, subependymal nodules may grow gradually to form the giant cell astrocytomas. The cerebellar cortex is often dysplastic as well. Surgery is not commonly performed in these patients because of the multiplicity of the lesions and the multiple seizure types, but it is occasionally possible if electrophysiology and imaging with PET or SPECT demonstrate a focal abnormality in keeping with an epileptogenic focus and if there is a large discrete tuber.

Other Malformations of Cortical Development

Beside FCD, malformations of cortical development (MCD) include disorders of cellular proliferation, such as microcephaly with simplified gyral pattern (for which epilepsy, when it occurs, is only part of a globally severe condition), migration disorders such as the nodular and band heterotopia, organization disorders such as the polymicrogyria, and schizencephaly.[54,93] Surgery is not commonly indicated in these conditions.

Gray Matter Heterotopia

Gray matter heterotopia are masses of apparently normal gray matter located in abnormal places. They are assumed to be disorders of migration. They are presumed to be epileptogenic because they are made of active neurons with abnormal connections between themselves as well as with the overlying cortex. This overlying cortex also is somewhat dysplastic, typically in proportion to the size of the heterotopia. On MRI, heterotopia have the same signal as the central or cortical gray matter. Depending on their location, they are designated as periventricular nodular heterotopia (PNH; isolated, multiple or diffuse; never on the basal ganglia or corpus callosum), subcortical nodular heterotopia (often huge, transcerebral), and band heterotopia; the latter correspond to the lesser end of the agyria/pachygyria spectrum. Most cases of heterotopia are not indications for epilepsy surgery.

Polymicrogyria and Schizencephaly

Both disorders are classified as disorders of late organization of the cortex[54] and may be sporadic, familial, or acquired (often associated with cytomegalovirus [CMV]). In approximately 50% of cases, the patients present with neurological deficits and epilepsy. Polymicrogyria (PMG)[93] is characterized by multiple small gyri below a continuous molecular layer. The sulcal pattern in the affected area is disorganized with aberrant sulci. The lesion is usually located around the insula, with a variable extent toward the hemispheric convexities. It may be unilateral or bilateral but usually not absolutely symmetrical. The corresponding white matter and the brainstem are atrophic. Areas of high T2 signal may be present, suggesting previous CMV infection. Typically, the abnormal cortex is still functional, and the surrounding normal-appearing cortex is often epileptogenic,[94] probably because of abnormal connectivity.[94-97] For these reasons, and because of the large extent of the lesion, PMG is a poor indication for epilepsy surgery, except for hemispherectomy. In rare cases, PMG may be focal and can be resected.

Schizencephaly is characterized by a transcerebral cleft lined with polymicrogyric cortex joining the ependyma. The cleft may be small or large, unilateral or bilateral, and not perfectly symmetrical. The septum pellucidum is absent when the cleft is frontal or central. There are reports of successful surgery of closed lip schizencephaly[98-100]; the epileptogenic cortex surrounding the cleft was described as dysplastic with giant neurons.[99] Surgical indications for schizencephaly associated epilepsy are, nevertheless, uncommon.

Hypothalamic Hamartomas

Hypothalamic hamartomas (HH) are abnormal masses of normal-appearing gray matter located in or attached to the tuber cinereum. Their clinical features are epilepsy (mostly refractory gelastic seizures in the initial stage of the disease) and central precocious puberty. The epilepsy is severe, and over time results in cognitive deterioration and behavioral problems. A morphological distinction of HH has been proposed between the intrahypothalamic hamartomas that encroach on the third ventricle and would be characterized by the early occurrence of epilepsy, and the parahypothalamic hamartomas, pedunculated or sessile but not encroaching on the third ventricle, which would be characterized by a central precocious puberty.[101] Using the displacement of the white matter bundles and the mammillary bodies, it has been suggested that epilepsy-associated HH are invariably located behind the postcommissural fornix, in front of the mammillothalamic tract, and above the mammillary bodies.[102] Epileptogenic HH therefore are intrahypothalamic masses that encroaches on the third ventricle. Their T1WI signal is mildly inferior to that of the central gray matter (74%); their T2WI signal is superior to that of central gray matter (93%), and the FLAIR signal is always high.[102] This signal might reflect some degree of gliosis related to the seizure activity,[102] and it can be used to demarcate the lesion from the surrounding hypothalamus.[102] There is no enhancement and no calcification. Cystic components may be found.[102,103] The mass usually does not increase in size over the years, but a decrease in size during the first months of life has been reported in one case.[102] Small epileptogenic lesions are typically intraventricular, whereas large lesions extend both into the ventricular lumen and the interpeduncular fossa; strictly inferior masses are rarely epileptogenic. The mass may splay the cerebral peduncles apart and displace the basilar artery. Epileptogenic HH always involve the mamillary bodies, and it involves the tuber cinereum in 90% of cases. They may involve the chiasm (22%), lamina terminalis (17%), or the pituitary stalk (20% and associated with central precocious puberty).[102] The mass may be bilateral and symmetrical (37%) or predominantly or entirely unilateral (63%); it may distort the mammillary bodies on one side (68%) or on both (19%) sides; intraventricular expansion is usual.[102] MRI spec-

troscopy shows increased myoinositol and decreased NAA compared with the thalami or the frontal lobes; this correlates with the presence of gliosis on histology.[102] In 25% of patients, other brain abnormalities are found. High signal of the anterior temporal white matter and blurring of the cortical–subcortical junction are seen in 16% of patients on the side of the hamartoma when it is lateralized or in both temporal lobes when the hamartoma is bilateral; this may relate to epilepsy-related gliosis rather than dysplasia.[102] A dysplastic appearance of the hippocampus was reported in four cases[102]. "Arachnoid" cysts have been observed in relation with HH.[102,103] These might represent predominantly cystic hamartomas. Ependymal remnants have been observed in otherwise solid HH,[101] and we have observed that closed suprasellar cysts without apparent HH are occasionally found in patients with refractory epilepsy or precocious puberty. Epilepsy-associated HH can be treated with surgical disconnection or radiosurgery.

Hippocampal Sclerosis

Although hippocampal sclerosis is the most common epileptogenic substrate seen in adult surgical epilepsy series, it is less common in children.[6] Hippocampal sclerosis is characterized by neuronal loss and gliosis in CA1, CA3, and dentate hilus.[104] On MRI, the findings include high T2/FLAIR signal and atrophy of the hippocampus[8,104] (**Fig. 8.7A,B**). Other findings include loss of internal architecture, loss of hippocampal head interdigitations,[105] atrophy of ipsilateral mamillary body and fornix,[106] dilatation of the ipsilateral temporal horn, volume loss of the temporal lobe, and atrophy of the collateral white matter between the hippocampus and collateral sulcus.[107] The sensitivity of MRI in detecting hippocampal sclerosis by qualitative assessment is on the order of 80 to 90%. Visual assessment of MRI may reliably detect hippocampal volume asymmetry of more than 20%. Lesser degrees of asymmetry require quantitative volumetric analysis.[108-110] Hippocampal volume reduction correlates with the severity of neuronal cell loss.

Rasmussen Encephalitis

Rasmussen encephalitis is a chronic, progressive encephalitis of unknown etiology that results in severe intractable epilepsy. There is a suggestion of possible autoimmune basis for the disease. An antibody that reacted to glutamate receptor subunit GluR3 produced features similar to Rasmussen's disease when injected into rabbits.[111] Pathological examinations of surgical specimens have supported evidence of immune system involvement by demonstration of complement deposition along blood vessel wall.[112] An inciting event with breakdown of the blood–brain barrier, thereby exposing the

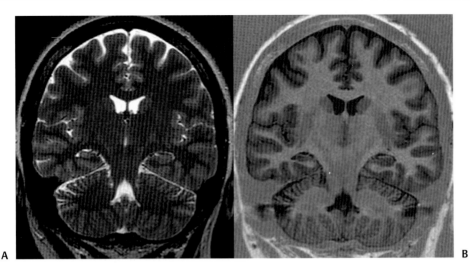

A   B

Fig. 8.7 Oblique **(A)** coronal T2 and **(B)** coronal inversion recovery sequences showing atrophy and high T2 signal in the right hippocampus, features in keeping with mesial temporal sclerosis.

brain to antigens, provides the basis for an autoimmune response and results in the clinical development of Rasmussen encephalitis.[113,114] Clinically, the seizures begin abruptly in previously normal children and include partial seizures and epilepsia partialis continua. With disease progression, the patients develop hemiparesis or hemiplegia and cognitive decline. The histological findings are those of chronic, nonspecific encephalitis with perivascular lymphocytic cuffing, gliosis, microglial nodules, and neuronal loss. At a later stage of the disease, biopsy may show nonspecific findings of atrophy and residual gliosis with minimal inflammatory cellular infiltrate, referred to as "burned out encephalitis" by Aguilar and Rasmussen.[115] Early in the course of the disease, CT and MRI may be entirely normal[116] or may show swelling of the cortex.[117] With disease progression, MRI demonstrates progressive atrophy and progressive abnormal signal in the white matter and cortex[117] (**Fig. 8.8A,B**). Serial MRI of 10 patients revealed a step-like evolution, with successive fo-

cal areas becoming involved.[118] Frontal and frontotemporal lobes involvement are common, and there may be associated ipsilateral atrophy of striate and hippocampus.[117] Proton MRI spectroscopy reveals decreased NAA concentration in patients with Rasmussen encephalitis, and this finding has been found to correlate with brain atrophy and neuronal loss.[119] Treatment options include medical treatment such as intravenous immunoglobulin, plasmapheresis, or immunosuppressant medications.[120,121]

■ Other Causes for Partial or Catastrophic Epilepsies in Children

It is generally agreed on that the intellectual and neurological development of children suffering from Sturge-Weber disease depends on the occurrence of repeated seizures. If

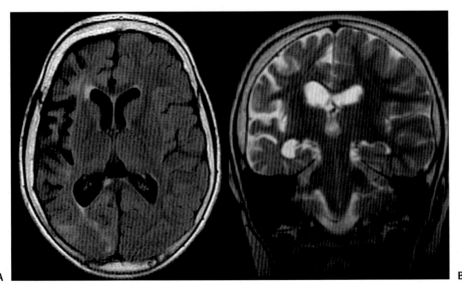

A   B

Fig. 8.8 (A) Axial FLAIR and **(B)** coronal T2 images demonstrate right hemiatrophy and abnormal signal in the subcortical and periventricular white matter in a child with intractable seizures. There is associated right hippocampal atrophy. The imaging findings are suspicious of Rasmussen encephalitis.

medical treatment fails, the intractable epilepsy may require treatment with hemispherectomy; the absence of contralateral involvement should therefore be ascertained. The characteristic brain MRI features of Stürge-Weber disease are diffuse enhancement of the surface of one hemisphere, typically over its posterior portion, reflecting the pial angioma. A contrast-enhanced FLAIR sequence better demonstrates the angioma.[122] A T1 sequence with fat saturation may show associated abnormalities of the ocular choroid and of the calvarium. Other usual findings are a large choroid plexus in the ipsilateral ventricle and prominent, developmental venous anomalies (DVA)-like transmedullary veins. Hemispheric swelling from prolonged seizure activity may be demonstrated. Acute ischemia may also occur, with focal edema and possibly bleed. In infants, the white matter may present with a low T2 signal[123] that has been tentatively explained by the venous congestion,[124] but early myelination induced by seizure activity may be an alternative explanation.[72] Calcification is unusual in infants. The angiomatous hemisphere may already show atrophy, either because of previous seizure activity or to a perfusion defect.

Arteriovenous Malformations

Arteriovenous malformations (AVMs) are usually not epileptogenic in children, except for the large AVMs. Cavernomas are often located at the cortical–subcortical junction and are often epileptogenic[125]; they may be small, and they are best depicted on T2*GE imaging, which should always be done when no other cause is found for partial seizures. The rare sporadic meningioangiomatosis is characterized by meningovascular proliferation and calcification[126,127]; the underlying brain tissue may appear dysplastic, and the affected cortex as well as the perilesional cortex may be intrinsically epileptogenic.[126] The cortex is high T1/low T2 because of the calcification; the white matter is dark on T1WI and bright on

T2/FLAIR. There may be slight meningeal enhancement. The treatment is surgical.[127]

Others

Refractory epilepsy and epileptic encephalopathies are common complications of destructive brain lesions. These may be nonspecific (atrophy) or specific (porencephalies, focal scars). They typically relate to late gestational, perinatal or early infantile events such as hemorrhages, ischemia, infection, trauma, hypoxic ischemic encephalopathy (HIE)-related ulegyria,[128] and hypoglycemia.[129] Obviously, the scar itself does not generate epilepsy, but in a developing brain, a distorted plasticity with abnormal neuronal networks may develop in the surrounding preserved cortex. There is still controversy on whether a loss of gray–white matter contrast reflects a cortical dysplasia or some gliotic changes.[130]

Finally, refractory status epilepticus also may need urgent surgical treatment. MRI may help demonstrate a structural epileptogenic lesion or, in generalized status epilepticus, demonstrate focal cortical edema, such as in the cornu ammonis, which together with the electrophysiological data, locate the epileptogenic area.[131,132]

■ Conclusion

In addition to the substrates mentioned previously, any kind of brain malformation (including Chiari II, or the classic commissural agenesis) may present with focal epilepsy. Over the last decade, thanks to better signal-to-noise ratio (high field, better coils) and sequences such as FLAIR, the efficacy of MRI in detecting and assessing the epilepsy-associated focal lesions and preparing the surgical strategy when surgery is needed has improved considerably. MRI has become the primary diagnostic tool and, in conjunction with the clinical assessment, assists in identifying the epileptogenic substrate and classifying the epilepsy syndromes in a vast majority of cases.

References

1. Arroyo S. [Evaluation of drug-resistant epilepsy]. Rev Neurol 2000;30(9):881–886
2. Kwan P, Brodie MJ. Early identification of refractory epilepsy. N Engl J Med 2000;342(5):314–319
3. Berg AT, Testa FM, Levy SR, Shinnar S. Neuroimaging in children with newly diagnosed epilepsy: a community-based study. Pediatrics 2000;106(3):527–532
4. Bronen RA, Fulbright RK, Spencer DD, et al. Refractory epilepsy: comparison of MR imaging, CT, and histopathologic findings in 117 patients. Radiology 1996;201(1):97–105
5. Scott CA, Fish DR, Smith SJ, et al. Presurgical evaluation of patients with epilepsy and normal MRI: role of scalp video-EEG telemetry. J Neurol Neurosurg Psychiatry 1999;66(1):69–71
6. Benifla M, Otsubo H, Ochi A, et al. Temporal lobe surgery for intractable epilepsy in children: an analysis of outcomes in 126 children. Neurosurgery 2006;59(6):1203–1213, discussion 1213–1214
7. Berkovic SF, McIntosh AM, Kalnins RM, et al. Preoperative MRI predicts outcome of temporal lobectomy: an actuarial analysis. Neurology 1995;45(7):1358–1363
8. Jack CR Jr, Sharbrough FW, Cascino GD, Hirschorn KA, O'Brien PC, Marsh WR. Magnetic resonance image-based hippocampal volumetry: correlation with outcome after temporal lobectomy. Ann Neurol 1992;31(2):138–146
9. Woermann FG, McLean MA, Bartlett PA, Barker GJ, Duncan JS. Quantitative short echo time proton magnetic resonance spectroscopic

imaging study of malformations of cortical development causing epilepsy. Brain 2001;124(pt 2):427–436

10. Guye M, Le Fur Y, Confort-Gouny S, et al. Metabolic and electrophysiological alterations in subtypes of temporal lobe epilepsy: a combined proton magnetic resonance spectroscopic imaging and depth electrodes study. Epilepsia 2002;43(10):1197–1209

11. Wu WC, Huang CC, Chung HW, et al. Hippocampal alterations in children with temporal lobe epilepsy with or without a history of febrile convulsions: evaluations with MR volumetry and proton MR spectroscopy. AJNR Am J Neuroradiol 2005;26(5):1270–1275

12. Wall CJ, Kendall EJ, Obenaus A. Rapid alterations in diffusion-weighted images with anatomic correlates in a rodent model of status epilepticus. AJNR Am J Neuroradiol 2000;21(10):1841–1852

13. Alsop DC, Connelly A, Duncan JS, et al. Diffusion and perfusion MRI in epilepsy. Epilepsia 2002; 43(suppl 1):69–77

14. Widjaja E, Blaser S, Miller E, et al. Evaluation of subcortical white matter and deep white matter tracts in malformations of cortical development. Epilepsia 2007;48(8):1460–1469

15. Nilsson D, Starck G, Ljungberg M, et al. Intersubject variability in the anterior extent of the optic radiation assessed by tractography. Epilepsy Res 2007;77(1):11–16

16. Raymond AA, Fish DR, Sisodiya SM, Alsanjari N, Stevens JM, Shorvon SD. Abnormalities of gyration, heterotopias, tuberous sclerosis, focal cortical dysplasia, microdysgenesis, dysembryoplastic neuroepithelial tumour and dysgenesis of the archicortex in epilepsy. Clinical, EEG and neuroimaging features in 100 adult patients. Brain 1995;118(pt 3):629–660

17. Mittal S, Montes JL, Farmer JP, et al. Long-term outcome after surgical treatment of temporal lobe epilepsy in children. J Neurosurg 2005; 103(5, suppl)401–412

18. Luyken C, Blümcke I, Fimmers R, et al. The spectrum of long-term epilepsy-associated tumors: long-term seizure and tumor outcome and neurosurgical aspects. Epilepsia 2003;44(6):822–830

19. Clusmann H, Kral T, Gleissner U, et al. Analysis of different types of resection for pediatric patients with temporal lobe epilepsy. Neurosurgery 2004;54(4):847–859, discussion 859–860

20. Blümcke I, Löbach M, Wolf HK, Wiestler OD. Evidence for developmental precursor lesions in epilepsy-associated glioneuronal tumors. Microsc Res Tech 1999;46(1):53–58

21. Pasquier B, Péoc'H M, Fabre-Bocquentin B, et al. Surgical pathology of drug-resistant partial epilepsy. A 10-year-experience with a series of 327 consecutive resections. Epileptic Disord 2002;4(2):99–119

22. Rosenblum MK. The 2007 WHO Classification of Nervous System Tumors: newly recognized members of the mixed glioneuronal group. Brain Pathol 2007;17(3):308–313

23. Provenzale JM, Ali U, Barboriak DP, Kallmes DF, Delong DM, McLendon RE. Comparison of patient age with MR imaging features of gangliogliomas. AJR Am J Roentgenol 2000;174(3):859–862

24. Luyken C, Blümcke I, Fimmers R, Urbach H, Wiestler OD, Schramm J. Supratentorial gangliogliomas: histopathologic grading and tumor recurrence in 184 patients with a median follow-up of 8 years. Cancer 2004;101(1):146–155

25. Koeller KK, Henry JM; Armed Forces Institute of Pathology. From the archives of the AFIP: superficial gliomas: radiologic-pathologic correlation. Radiographics 2001;21(6):1533–1556

26. Tamburrini G, Colosimo C Jr, Giangaspero F, Riccardi R, Di Rocco C. Desmoplastic infantile ganglioglioma. Childs Nerv Syst 2003;19(5–6):292–297

27. Daumas-Duport C, Scheithauer BW, Chodkiewicz JP, Laws ER Jr, Vedrenne C. Dysembryoplastic neuroepithelial tumor: a surgically curable tumor of young patients with intractable partial seizures. Report of thirty-nine cases. Neurosurgery 1988;23(5):545–556

28. Ostertun B, Wolf HK, Campos MG, et al. Dysembryoplastic neuroepithelial tumors: MR and CT evaluation. AJNR Am J Neuroradiol 1996;17(3):419–430

29. Stanescu Cosson R, Varlet P, Beuvon F, et al. Dysembryoplastic neuroepithelial tumors: CT, MR findings and imaging follow-up: a study of 53 cases. J Neuroradiol 2001;28(4):230–240

30. Shin JH, Lee HK, Khang SK, et al. Neuronal tumors of the central nervous system: radiologic findings and pathologic correlation. Radiographics 2002;22(5):1177–1189

31. Thom M, Gomez-Anson B, Revesz T, et al. Spontaneous intralesional haemorrhage in dysembryoplastic neuroepithelial tumours: a series of five cases. J Neurol Neurosurg Psychiatry 1999;67(1):97–101

32. Raybaud C, Shroff M, Rutka JT, Chuang SH. Imaging surgical epilepsy in children. Childs Nerv Syst 2006;22(8):786–809

33. Nolan MA, Sakuta R, Chuang N, et al. Dysembryoplastic neuroepithelial tumors in childhood: long-term outcome and prognostic features. Neurology 2004;62(12):2270–2276

34. Sakuta R, Otsubo H, Nolan MA, et al. Recurrent intractable seizures in children with cortical dysplasia adjacent to dysembryoplastic neuroepithelial tumor. J Child Neurol 2005;20(4):377–384

35. Bulakbasi N, Kocaoglu M, Ors F, Tayfun C, Uçöz T. Combination of single-voxel proton MR spectroscopy and apparent diffusion coefficient calculation in the evaluation of common brain tumors. AJNR Am J Neuroradiol 2003;24(2):225–233

36. Lena G, Mottolese C, Paz-Paredes A, et al. Pediatric supratentorial oligodendrogliomas: Marseilles and Lyons experiences [in French]. Neurochirurgie 2005;51(3–4 pt 2):400–409

37. Peters O, Gnekow AK, Rating D, Wolff JEA. Impact of location on outcome in children with low-grade oligodendroglioma. Pediatr Blood Cancer 2004;43(3):250–256

38. Giannini C, Scheithauer BW, Burger PC, et al. Pleomorphic xanthoastrocytoma: what do we really know about it? Cancer 1999;85(9):2033–2045

39. Lipper MH, Eberhard DA, Phillips CD, Vezina LG, Cail WS. Pleomorphic xanthoastrocytoma, a distinctive astroglial tumor: neuroradiologic and pathologic features. AJNR Am J Neuroradiol 1993;14(6):1397–1404

40. Im SH, Chung CK, Kim SK, Cho BK, Kim MK, Chi JG. Pleomorphic xanthoastrocytoma: a developmental glioneuronal tumor with prominent glioproliferative changes. J Neurooncol 2004;66(1–2):17–27

41. Powell SZ, Yachnis AT, Rorke LB, Rojiani AM, Eskin TA. Divergent differentiation in pleomorphic xanthoastrocytoma. Evidence for a neuronal element and possible relationship to ganglion cell tumors. Am J Surg Pathol 1996;20(1):80–85

42. Lach B, Duggal N, DaSilva VF, Benoit BG. Association of pleomorphic xanthoastrocytoma with cortical dysplasia and neuronal tumors. A report of three cases. Cancer 1996;78(12):2551–2563

43. Palmini A, Gambardella A, Andermann F, et al. Intrinsic epileptogenicity of human dysplastic cortex as suggested by corticography and surgical results. Ann Neurol 1995;37(4):476–487

44. Otsubo H, Ochi A, Elliott I, et al. MEG predicts epileptic zone in lesional extrahippocampal epilepsy: 12 pediatric surgery cases. Epilepsia 2001;42(12):1523–1530

45. Cepeda C, André VM, Vinters HV, Levine MS, Mathern GW. Are cytomegalic neurons and balloon cells generators of epileptic activity in pediatric cortical dysplasia? Epilepsia 2005;46(suppl 5):82–88

46. Guerrini R, Sicca F, Parmeggiani L. Epilepsy and malformations of the cerebral cortex. Epileptic Disord 2003;5(suppl 2):S9–S26
47. Farrell MA, DeRosa MJ, Curran JG, et al. Neuropathologic findings in cortical resections (including hemispherectomies) performed for the treatment of intractable childhood epilepsy. Acta Neuropathol 1992;83(3):246–259
48. Jay V, Becker LE, Otsubo H, Hwang PA, Hoffman HJ, Harwood-Nash D. Pathology of temporal lobectomy for refractory seizures in children. Review of 20 cases including some unique malformative lesions. J Neurosurg 1993;79(1):53–61
49. Wolf HK, Wiestler OD. Surgical pathology of chronic epileptic seizure disorders. Brain Pathol 1993;3(4):371–380
50. Kuzniecky R, Murro A, King D, et al. Magnetic resonance imaging in childhood intractable partial epilepsies: pathologic correlations. Neurology 1993;43(4):681–687
51. Tassi L, Colombo N, Garbelli R, et al. Focal cortical dysplasia: neuropathological subtypes, EEG, neuroimaging and surgical outcome. Brain 2002;125(pt 8):1719–1732
52. Keene DL, Jimenez CC, Ventureyra E. Cortical microdysplasia and surgical outcome in refractory epilepsy of childhood. Pediatr Neurosurg 1998;29(2):69–72
53. Taylor DC, Falconer MA, Bruton CJ, Corsellis JA. Focal dysplasia of the cerebral cortex in epilepsy. J Neurol Neurosurg Psychiatry 1971;34(4):369–387
54. Barkovich AJ, Kuzniecky RI, Jackson GD, Guerrini R, Dobyns WB. A developmental and genetic classification for malformations of cortical development. Neurology 2005;65(12):1873–1887
55. Kuzniecky R, Garcia JH, Faught E, Morawetz RB. Cortical dysplasia in temporal lobe epilepsy: magnetic resonance imaging correlations. Ann Neurol 1991;29(3):293–298
56. Mischel PS, Nguyen LP, Vinters HV. Cerebral cortical dysplasia associated with pediatric epilepsy. Review of neuropathologic features and proposal for a grading system. J Neuropathol Exp Neurol 1995;54(2):137–153
57. Palmini A, Lüders HO. Classification issues in malformations caused by abnormalities of cortical development. Neurosurg Clin N Am 2002;13(1):1–16, vii
58. Palmini A, Najm I, Avanzini G, et al. Terminology and classification of the cortical dysplasias. Neurology 2004; 62(6, suppl 3)S2–S8
59. Englund C, Folkerth RD, Born D, Lacy JM, Hevner RF. Aberrant neuronal-glial differentiation in Taylor-type focal cortical dysplasia (type IIA/B). Acta Neuropathol 2005;109(5):519–533
60. Colombo N, Tassi L, Galli C, et al. Focal cortical dysplasias: MR imaging, histopathologic, and clinical correlations in surgically treated patients with epilepsy. AJNR Am J Neuroradiol 2003;24(4):724–733
61. Urbach H, Scheffler B, Heinrichsmeier T, et al. Focal cortical dysplasia of Taylor's balloon cell type: a clinicopathological entity with characteristic neuroimaging and histopathological features, and favorable postsurgical outcome. Epilepsia 2002;43(1):33–40
62. Barkovich AJ, Kuzniecky RI, Bollen AW, Grant PE. Focal transmantle dysplasia: a specific malformation of cortical development. Neurology 1997;49(4):1148–1152
63. Andres M, Andre VM, Nguyen S, et al. Human cortical dysplasia and epilepsy: an ontogenetic hypothesis based on volumetric MRI and NeuN neuronal density and size measurements. Cereb Cortex 2005;15(2):194–210
64. Lombroso CT. Can early postnatal closed head injury induce cortical dysplasia. Epilepsia 2000;41(2):245–253
65. Marín-Padilla M. Developmental neuropathology and impact of perinatal brain damage. I: hemorrhagic lesions of neocortex. J Neuropathol Exp Neurol 1996;55(7):758–773
66. Marín-Padilla M. Developmental neuropathology and impact of perinatal brain damage. II: white matter lesions of the neocortex. J Neuropathol Exp Neurol 1997;56(3):219–235
67. Marín-Padilla M. Developmental neuropathology and impact of perinatal brain damage. III: gray matter lesions of the neocortex. J Neuropathol Exp Neurol 1999;58(5):407–429
68. Marín-Padilla M, Parisi JE, Armstrong DL, Sargent SK, Kaplan JA. Shaken infant syndrome: developmental neuropathology, progressive cortical dysplasia, and epilepsy. Acta Neuropathol 2002;103(4):321–332
69. Lee BC, Schmidt RE, Hatfield GA, Bourgeois B, Park TS. MRI of focal cortical dysplasia. Neuroradiology 1998;40(10):675–683
70. Bronen RA, Vives KP, Kim JH, Fulbright RK, Spencer SS, Spencer DD. Focal cortical dysplasia of Taylor, balloon cell subtype: MR differentiation from low-grade tumors. AJNR Am J Neuroradiol 1997;18(6):1141–1151
71. Yagishita A, Arai N, Maehara T, Shimizu H, Tokumaru AM, Oda M. Focal cortical dysplasia: appearance on MR images. Radiology 1997;203(2):553–559
72. Demerens C, Stankoff B, Logak M, et al. Induction of myelination in the central nervous system by electrical activity. Proc Natl Acad Sci U S A 1996;93(18):9887–9892
73. Palmini A, Gambardella A, Andermann F, et al. Operative strategies for patients with cortical dysplastic lesions and intractable epilepsy. Epilepsia 1994;35(suppl 6):S57–S71
74. Sisodiya SM. Surgery for malformations of cortical development causing epilepsy. Brain 2000;123(pt 6):1075–1091
75. Bautista JF, Foldvary-Schaefer N, Bingaman WE, Lüders HO. Focal cortical dysplasia and intractable epilepsy in adults: clinical, EEG, imaging, and surgical features. Epilepsy Res 2003;55(1–2):131–136
76. Edwards JC, Wyllie E, Ruggeri PM, et al. Seizure outcome after surgery for epilepsy due to malformation of cortical development. Neurology 2000;55(8):1110–1114
77. Hong SC, Kang KS, Seo DW, et al. Surgical treatment of intractable epilepsy accompanying cortical dysplasia. J Neurosurg 2000;93(5):766–773
78. Kral T, Clusmann H, Blümcke I, et al. Outcome of epilepsy surgery in focal cortical dysplasia. J Neurol Neurosurg Psychiatry 2003;74(2):183–188
79. Otsubo H, Iida K, Oishi M, et al. Neurophysiologic findings of neuronal migration disorders: intrinsic epileptogenicity of focal cortical dysplasia on electroencephalography, electrocorticography, and magnetoencephalography. J Child Neurol 2005;20(4):357–363
80. Sperling MR, O'Connor MJ, Saykin AJ, Plummer C. Temporal lobectomy for refractory epilepsy. JAMA 1996;276(6):470–475
81. Britton JW, Cascino GD, Sharbrough FW, Kelly PJ. Low-grade glial neoplasms and intractable partial epilepsy: efficacy of surgical treatment. Epilepsia 1994;35(6):1130–1135
82. Chassoux F, Devaux B, Landré E, et al. Stereoelectroencephalography in focal cortical dysplasia: a 3D approach to delineating the dysplastic cortex. Brain 2000;123(pt 8):1733–1751
83. Fauser S, Schulze-Bonhage A, Honegger J, et al. Focal cortical dysplasias: surgical outcome in 67 patients in relation to histological subtypes and dual pathology. Brain 2004;127(pt 11):2406–2418

84. Kloss S, Pieper T, Pannek H, Holthausen H, Tuxhorn I. Epilepsy surgery in children with focal cortical dysplasia (FCD): results of long-term seizure outcome. Neuropediatrics 2002;33(1):21–26

85. Widdess-Walsh P, Kellinghaus C, Jeha L, et al. Electro-clinical and imaging characteristics of focal cortical dysplasia: correlation with pathological subtypes. Epilepsy Res 2005;67(1-2):25–33

86. Robain O, Gelot A. Neuropathology of hemimegalencephaly. In: Guerrini R, Andermann F, Canapicchi R, Roger J, Zifkin BG, Pfanner P, eds. Dysplasias of Cerebral Cortex and Epilepsy. Philadelphia, Pa: Lippincott-Raven; 1996:89–92

87. Barkovich AJ, Chuang SH. Unilateral megalencephaly: correlation of MR imaging and pathologic characteristics. AJNR Am J Neuroradiol 1990;11(3):523–531

88. Broumandi DD, Hayward UM, Benzian JM, Gonzalez I, Nelson MD. Best cases from the AFIP: hemimegalencephaly. Radiographics 2004;24(3):843–848

89. Yagishita A, Arai N, Tamagawa K, Oda M. Hemimegalencephaly: signal changes suggesting abnormal myelination on MRI. Neuroradiology 1998;40(11):734–738

90. Di Rocco F, Novegno F, Tamburrini G, Iannelli A. Hemimegalencephaly involving the cerebellum. Pediatr Neurosurg 2001;35(5):274–276

91. D'Agostino MD, Bastos A, Piras C, et al. Posterior quadrantic dysplasia or hemi-hemimegalencephaly: a characteristic brain malformation. Neurology 2004;62(12):2214–2220

92. Wolpert SM, Cohen A, Libenson MH. Hemimegalencephaly: a longitudinal MR study. AJNR Am J Neuroradiol 1994;15(8):1479–1482

93. Barkovich AJ, Raybaud CA. Malformations of cortical development. Neuroimaging Clin N Am 2004;14(3):401–423

94. Jacobs KM, Kharazia VN, Prince DA. Mechanisms underlying epileptogenesis in cortical malformations. Epilepsy Res 1999;36(2-3):165–188

95. Giannetti S, Gaglini P, Granato A, Di Rocco C. Organization of callosal connections in rats with experimentally induced microgyria. Childs Nerv Syst 1999;15(9):444–448, discussion 449–450

96. Giannetti S, Gaglini P, Di Rocco F, Di Rocco C, Granato A. Organization of cortico-cortical associative projections in a rat model of microgyria. Neuroreport 2000;11(10):2185–2189

97. Di Rocco F, Giannetti S, Gaglini P, Di Rocco C, Granato A. Dendritic architecture of corticothalamic neurons in a rat model of microgyria. Childs Nerv Syst 2002;18(12):690–693

98. Leblanc R, Tampieri D, Robitaille Y, Feindel W, Andermann F. Surgical treatment of intractable epilepsy associated with schizencephaly. Neurosurgery 1991;29(3):421–429

99. Maehara T, Shimizu H, Nakayama H, Oda M, Arai N. Surgical treatment of epilepsy from schizencephaly with fused lips. Surg Neurol 1997;48(5):507–510

100. Cascino GD, Buchhalter JR, Sirven JI, et al. Peri-ictal SPECT and surgical treatment for intractable epilepsy related to schizencephaly. Neurology 2004;63(12):2426–2428

101. Arita K, Kurisu K, Kiura Y, Iida K, Otsubo H. Hypothalamic hamartoma. Neurol Med Chir (Tokyo) 2005;45(5):221–231

102. Freeman JL, Coleman LT, Wellard RM, et al. MR imaging and spectroscopic study of epileptogenic hypothalamic hamartomas: analysis of 72 cases. AJNR Am J Neuroradiol 2004;25(3):450–462

103. Booth TN, Timmons CT, Shapiro K, Rollins NK. Pre- and postnatal MR imaging of hypothalamic hamartomas associated with arachnoid cysts. AJNR Am J Neuroradiol 2004;25(7):1283–1285

104. Bronen RA. Epilepsy: the role of MR imaging. AJR Am J Roentgenol 1992;159(6):1165–1174

105. Oppenheim C, Dormont D, Biondi A, et al. Loss of digitations of the hippocampal head on high-resolution fast spin-echo MR: a sign of mesial temporal sclerosis. AJNR Am J Neuroradiol 1998;19(3):457–463

106. Baldwin GN, Tsuruda JS, Maravilla KR, Hamill GS, Hayes CE. The fornix in patients with seizures caused by unilateral hippocampal sclerosis: detection of unilateral volume loss on MR images. AJR Am J Roentgenol 1994;162(5):1185–1189

107. Meiners LC, Witkamp TD, de Kort GA, et al. Relevance of temporal lobe white matter changes in hippocampal sclerosis. Magnetic resonance imaging and histology. Invest Radiol 1999;34(1):38–45

108. Jack CR Jr, Sharbrough FW, Twomey CK, et al. Temporal lobe seizures: lateralization with MR volume measurements of the hippocampal formation. Radiology 1990;175(2):423–429

109. Jack CR Jr. MRI-based hippocampal volume measurements in epilepsy. Epilepsia 1994;35(suppl 6):S21–S29

110. Bronen RA, Anderson AW, Spencer DD. Quantitative MR for epilepsy: a clinical and research tool? AJNR Am J Neuroradiol 1994;15(6):1157–1160

111. Rogers SW, Andrews PI, Gahring LC, et al. Autoantibodies to glutamate receptor GluR3 in Rasmussen's encephalitis. Science 1994;265(5172):648–651

112. Whitney KD, Andrews PI, McNamara JO. Immunoglobulin G and complement immunoreactivity in the cerebral cortex of patients with Rasmussen's encephalitis. Neurology 1999;53(4):699–708

113. He XP, Patel M, Whitney KD, Janumpalli S, Tenner A, McNamara JO. Glutamate receptor GluR3 antibodies and death of cortical cells. Neuron 1998;20(1):153–163

114. McNamara JO, Whitney KD, Andrews PI, He XP, Janumpalli S, Patel MN. Evidence for glutamate receptor autoimmunity in the pathogenesis of Rasmussen encephalitis. Adv Neurol 1999;79:543–550

115. Aguilar MJ, Rasmussen T. Role of encephalitis in pathogenesis of epilepsy. Arch Neurol 1960;2:663–676

116. Geller E, Faerber EN, Legido A, et al. Rasmussen encephalitis: complementary role of multitechnique neuroimaging. AJNR Am J Neuroradiol 1998;19(3):445–449

117. Chiapparini L, Granata T, Farina L, et al. Diagnostic imaging in 13 cases of Rasmussen's encephalitis: can early MRI suggest the diagnosis? Neuroradiology 2003;45(3):171–183

118. Bien CG, Urbach H, Deckert M, et al. Diagnosis and staging of Rasmussen's encephalitis by serial MRI and histopathology. Neurology 2002;58(2):250–257

119. Matthews PM, Andermann F, Arnold DL. A proton magnetic resonance spectroscopy study of focal epilepsy in humans. Neurology 1990;40(6):985–989

120. Andrews PI, Dichter MA, Berkovic SF, Newton MR, McNamara JO. Plasmapheresis in Rasmussen's encephalitis. Neurology 1996;46(1):242–246

121. Granata T, Fusco L, Gobbi G, et al. Experience with immunomodulatory treatments in Rasmussen's encephalitis. Neurology 2003;61(12):1807–1810

122. Griffiths PD, Coley SC, Romanowski CA, Hodgson T, Wilkinson ID. Contrast-enhanced fluid-attenuated inversion recovery imaging for leptomeningeal disease in children. AJNR Am J Neuroradiol 2003;24(4):719–723

123. Jacoby CG, Yuh WT, Afifi AK, Bell WE, Schelper RL, Sato Y. Accelerated myelination in early Sturge-Weber syndrome demonstrated by MR imaging. J Comput Assist Tomogr 1987;11(2):226–231

124. Porto L, Kieslich M, Yan B, Zanella FE, Lanfermann H. Accelerated myelination associated with venous congestion. Eur Radiol 2006;16(4):922–926

125. Lee JW, Kim DS, Shim KW, et al. Management of intracranial cavernous malformation in pediatric patients. Childs Nerv Syst 2008;24(3):321–327

126. Wiebe S, Munoz DG, Smith S, Lee DH. Meningioangiomatosis. A comprehensive analysis of clinical and laboratory features. Brain 1999;122(pt 4):709–726

127. Jallo GI, Kothbauer K, Mehta V, Abbott R, Epstein F. Meningioangiomatosis without neurofibromatosis: a clinical analysis. J Neurosurg 2005; 103(4, suppl)319–324

128. Villani F, D'Incerti L, Granata T, et al. Epileptic and imaging findings in perinatal hypoxic-ischemic encephalopathy with ulegyria. Epilepsy Res 2003;55(3):235–243

129. Caraballo RH, Sakr D, Mozzi M, et al. Symptomatic occipital lobe epilepsy following neonatal hypoglycemia. Pediatr Neurol 2004;31(1):24–29

130. Mitchell LA, Harvey AS, Coleman LT, Mandelstam SA, Jackson GD. Anterior temporal changes on MR images of children with hippocampal sclerosis: an effect of seizures on the immature brain? AJNR Am J Neuroradiol 2003;24(8):1670–1677

131. Kim JA, Chung JI, Yoon PH, et al. Transient MR signal changes in patients with generalized tonicoclonic seizure or status epilepticus: periictal diffusion-weighted imaging. AJNR Am J Neuroradiol 2001;22(6):1149–1160

132. Scott RC, Gadian DG, King MD, et al. Magnetic resonance imaging findings within 5 days of status epilepticus in childhood. Brain 2002;125(pt 9):1951–1959

9 Functional MRI in Pediatric Epilepsy Surgery

Torsten Baldeweg and Frédérique Liégeois

Functional magnetic resonance imaging (fMRI) has rapidly entered the armory of imaging methods available for the management of patients with focal epilepsy who may be surgery candidates. This is particularly true for presurgical investigations of cognitive and motor functions. The factors that have contributed to its success are chiefly its noninvasiveness, reproducibility, and wide availability. fMRI can reveal clinically useful information about the functional status of cortical tissue in relation to eloquent functions and, more recently, about origin and spread of epileptic activity.

In this chapter we will outline some of the basic principles of application of fMRI for complementing the neuropsychological evaluation of children and adolescents undergoing neurosurgical treatment. We will focus on two main issues that have received most attention so far: does fMRI provide a noninvasive means to reliably estimate hemispheric dominance of language and memory functions and localization of eloquent cortex? Finally, we will briefly mention recent developments in the mapping of blood flow changes associated with epileptic activity. The use of fMRI in mapping sensorimotor cortex before surgery has been reviewed previously[1,2] and will not be covered in this chapter. Several recent reviews cover different aspects relevant to fMRI application to epilepsy surgery evaluation[3-5] and its use in pediatric populations.[1,6,7]

■ Instrumentation and Methods

Basic Principles of fMRI

fMRI is based on the dependence of T2-weighted signal on the oxygenation status of hemoglobin, and the derived signal is called blood oxygen dependent (BOLD) signal. The fMRI signal is delayed with respect to the onset of neuronal activity by approximately 6 seconds and shows a more temporally protracted time course, lasting approximately 20 seconds before returning to baseline. Neurophysiological studies in the monkey visual cortex have shown that neuronal excitation results in enhanced (positive) BOLD signal, whereas reduction in net neural excitation results in reduced (negative) BOLD signal.[8] The spatial resolution is in the order of several mm (typical voxel size: $3 \times 3 \times 3$ mm^3), and its effective resolution will depend on the spatial filtering used during signal processing.

Experimental Designs

fMRI activation is detected using one of two experimental paradigms: block designs consisting of repeated activation–baseline state cycles and event-related designs, in which discrete events are analyzed separately, allowing for control of behavioral task performance during data analysis. The later is used for studies of memory (e.g., comparing recalled versus forgotten/new items), whereas the former is commonly used with language and motor activation studies. Block designs have been used most consistently in children and adolescents, because their higher signal-to-noise ratio reduces the scanning time required to obtain robust fMRI activation.

Stimulation tasks are tailored to the cognitive domains under investigation, using visual or auditory stimulus presentation. Language tasks may include story comprehension, but the most commonly used task to assess hemispheric dominance for expressive language is silent word generation to letters (fluency) or words (verb or synonym generation). Memory tasks commonly use visually presented words, pictures, or human faces.

Response Monitoring

Earlier language fMRI studies have instructed patients to covertly generate verbal responses to avoid head movements caused by overt speech. Although this has generally worked well with most patients, it has the disadvantage of being prone to ambiguous results if activation patterns are atypical or in loss of activation in less cooperative patients. More recent studies have used experimental protocols that require patients to respond using button presses to indicate a choice between different stimulus categories or presence of certain target items.[9] An alternative, yet relatively unexplored, method uses gaps in the image acquisition to allow for overt verbal responses.[10]

Assessment of Laterality of fMRI Activation

The term *fMRI lateralization* is commonly used to refer to the hemispheric asymmetry of fMRI activation in a given region of interest and may refer to extent of activation, level of activation, or both. Some epilepsy centers successfully rely on a qualitative judgment of laterality, performed by fMRI experienced neuroradiologists,[9,11,12] whereas others use a combination of qualitative and statistical measures[13,14] as converging evidence.

■ Applications for Presurgical Evaluation

The majority of published studies have been conducted on adults, and only a small number of pediatric studies have been reported.[14-18] We therefore review here the evidence from both adult and childhood epilepsy studies combined while attempting to point out issues that may have specific significance for pediatric practice.

Preoperative Assessment of Language Lateralization

Language fMRI tasks are used in candidates for epilepsy surgery with a view to improve the prognosis for postsurgical speech and language deficits. The main questions are whether surgery is planned in the language-dominant hemisphere and whether language cortex is located near the planned resection. The increased frequency of atypical language lateralization (i.e., right-sided or bilateral) in patients with focal epilepsy or lesions of the left hemisphere has been known for more than 30 years.[19] These early studies, using the intracarotid amobarbital test (IAT, or Wada test), also suggested that mainly lesions within classic language cortex (Broca's and Wernicke's regions) are responsible for inducing a shift

of language to the right hemisphere. More recent investigations, with the benefit of modern neuroimaging, have, nevertheless, shown that a considerable proportion of patients with early acquired or developmental left-sided perisylvian lesions showed evidence of intrahemispheric reorganization of language (i.e., retain typical left-sided lateralization, see example in **Fig. 9.1A**), often near the lesion.[17,18,20] Furthermore, patients with epilepsy arising from pathology in regions remote from classic language cortex, especially in the mesial temporal cortex, often show atypical, often bilateral, language representation[17,21,22] (see example in **Fig. 9.1B**). A recent study in a large cohort of patients with a left hemisphere epileptogenic focus (including children) identified the following factors associated with atypical language lateralization[12,23]: left-handedness, onset of epilepsy before age 6, and MRI type. Regarding the latter pathology factor, it is notable that patients with stroke showed a very high rate of reorganization and that approximately 35% of patients with a normal MRI had atypical language. This finding points to the possibility that epileptic activity drives functional reorganization.[24] In summary, localization-related epilepsies are associated with widespread changes in the structural and functional organization of the brain.

Assessment of Language Lateralization: fMRI and IAT

Studies on Adults

Although the IAT remains the gold standard for determining hemispheric dominance for speech and language, many epilepsy centers now routinely use fMRI.[5,25] Comparative studies

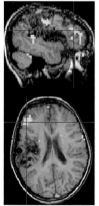
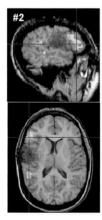
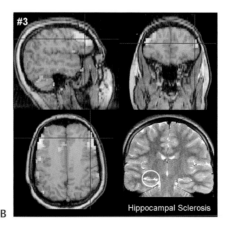
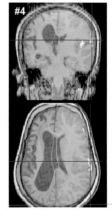
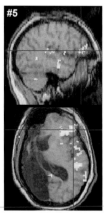

A   B   C

Fig. 9.1 Examples of functional magnetic resonance imaging (fMRI) language reorganization patterns in children with focal lesions of the left hemisphere using a silent verb generation task. **(A)** Intrahemispheric reorganization in two patients with extensive perisylvian developmental lesions (cases #1 and #2; for more details see Liégeois et al[17]). **(B)** Interhemispheric language reorganization in a child (case #3) with hippocampal sclerosis (*circled*, see also Weber et al[22]). The bilateral fMRI language representation was confirmed by intracarotid amobarbital test. **(C)** Tracking of interhemispheric language reorganization in patients with progressive neurodegenerative conditions, such as Rasmussen encephalitis, as shown in cases #4 and #5 (pre- and postoperatively, respectively; see Liégeois et al[10] for further details). Note: the crosshair indicates local maximum activation in the inferior frontal region. Left hemisphere is on the left.

using both methods[11,12,26] in adults have found agreement in approximately 80 to 90% of cases. Notwithstanding the obvious difference between an observation-based method (fMRI) and an inhibition procedure (IAT),[2] multiple other factors are likely to cause disparity,[9,11,27] including differences between fMRI and IAT tasks[12,28] and variability in the regions of interest chosen for fMRI lateralization analysis.[27,29] Finally, in contrast to the IAT, fMRI will also detect activation in regions that are not essential for the performance of a task (redundant activation). If these regions are localized in the nondominant hemisphere, this is likely to render fMRI findings more bilateral (see Woermann et al[12] for examples). No method is currently available that could distinguish essential from redundant activation foci on fMRI. The contralesional activation detected on fMRI may also indicate the potential for postsurgical reorganization of function. Indeed, two studies that have used both fMRI and IAT have found fMRI to be a better predictor of postoperative cognitive outcome. The study by Sabsevitz et al[30] in 24 patients who underwent left anterior lobe lobectomy (L-ATL) showed the fMRI lateralization index to be 100% sensitive and 73% predictive of significant visual naming decline. A recent study by Binder et al[31] corroborates this finding for verbal memory outcome after L-ATL and will be discussed in more detail later.

Although the direct comparison of fMRI with IAT was an obvious first step in validating this new method, the IAT itself is not free of potential problems,[32] such as lack of standardization and reproducibility, agitation and obtundation in some patients, potential cross-flow between the hemispheres, and many others (see Chapter 12). Indeed, there are reports of erroneous lateralization using the IAT, as evidenced by electrocortical stimulation[33] or postsurgical dysphasia[34] in which functional neuroimaging had indicated the correct lateralization. Therefore, only further postoperative outcome studies of the kind reported by Sabsevitz et al[30] and Binder et al[31] can demonstrate the true predictive value of fMRI-derived language lateralization.

In summary, a review of all available studies[35] concluded that fMRI increases importantly the probability of correctly predicting language dominance in multiple subgroups of surgery patients with and without epilepsy.

Pediatric Studies

Only a few studies have specifically investigated the role of fMRI in pediatric epilepsy surgery candidates,[14–16,18] commonly comparing fMRI with a mixture of invasive investigations (IAT, electrocortical stimulation [ECS]) or clinical observations. These studies have confirmed the feasibility and accuracy of fMRI in estimating language dominance in children, with the proviso that in some bilateral fMRI cases, only unilateral corroborating evidence was available.[14,18] A study involving a small series of children who also underwent ECS and IAT reported bilateral fMRI activation more often than suggested by IAT[36]; however, details of the procedure were not given. Longitudinal fMRI studies are particularly useful for investigating children with epilepsy caused by extensive left hemispheric injury or progressive neurodegenerative conditions, such as Rasmussen encephalitis (**Fig. 9.1C**), in revealing the gradual process of language reorganisation,[37] which can be used to optimize the timing of surgery and perhaps also for predicting the level of language proficiency after surgery.[10]

Localization of Language Cortex: fMRI and ECS

Studies on Adults

ECS is the gold standard method for mapping eloquent cortex before surgery. However, the majority of ECS sites tested intraoperatively are not associated with language-associated deficits.[38] Given also the large variability in the location of individual ECS language sites, it is, therefore, desirable to be able to selectively target critical regions preoperatively. This is particularly true when ECS is applied to children where cooperation and motivation during lengthy testing sessions can be an issue, even when performed extraoperatively. The first studies have shown some promising results,[39–41] with sensitivity of fMRI in predicting ECS language sites ranging from 80 to 100%, especially if multiple fMRI language tasks, both auditory and visual, were combined. These studies also showed that the correlation is confounded by fMRI activation in redundant (noncritical) language sites, usually leading to decreased specificity of approximately 50% for fMRI identifying positive ECS sites.

The study by Roux et al[42] showed less encouraging results (maximal sensitivity 66% for combined verb generation and naming tasks) and highlighted the challenges in combining both modalities. By necessity, different stimulations tasks are used for fMRI and ECS, often using different response modes (covert versus overt). There are inherent spatial inaccuracies in both fMRI and ECS, amounting up to approximately 1 cm each. Furthermore, the fMRI signal-to-noise ratio may not be sufficient if very short scanning sessions are used.[42] Indeed, the reports with consistent correlations[39,41] used at least three different fMRI language tasks of sufficient length to achieve good signal-to-noise ratio and convergence of activation in critical language regions. It also appears that tasks that involve sentence comprehension are better suited to activate temporoparietal language areas than those that use single-word or item processing.[40,41]

The issue of statistical threshold for the display of fMRI activation foci is particularly critical because the strength of activation may vary considerably across individuals.[13] FitzGerald et al[39] suggested using variable thresholds so the activation results in approximately 1 cm^2 or larger extent of cluster size at the cortical surface, which would be in agreement with the estimated extent of ECS language foci. By contrast, Rutten et al[41] used an operator-independent, fixed threshold—perhaps favored by a good signal-to-noise ratio in their study.

Pediatric Studies

Our own experience with extraoperative language ECS in pediatric patients is in agreement with the previously mentioned conclusions. ECS sites are commonly found in proximity to major fMRI activation foci (see example in **Fig. 9.2A**); however, in agreement with other authors, the presence of fMRI activation does not predict an ECS site with certainty. The use of a single fMRI task (auditory verb generation[14,17]), although resulting in robust and reproducible activations, is clearly insufficient to map essential ECS sites if elicited by a different task during ECS (see **Fig. 9.2B**). In addition, fMRI can indicate atypical locations of eloquent cortex, which may escape detection by ECS, especially when located deep in the vicinity of cortical sulci. This has been documented by Rutten et al[43] in a 14-year-old patient with a tumor displacing Broca's region.

In summary, although the first comparative studies were motivated by the desire to replace ECS with fMRI, currently this does not appear to be a realistic expectation. Nevertheless, the evidence accumulated so far suggests that fMRI language mapping can help in planning the extent of craniotomy, guiding the placement of subdural electrodes, and in targeting of sites for ECS.

Preoperative Assessment of Memory Lateralization

Surgical resection of the anterior temporal lobe is an established treatment for medication-resistant temporal lobe epilepsy (TLE) in both adults and children. A major clinical concern is the risk of verbal memory deficits as a consequence of ATL in the language-dominant hemisphere. Although the memory effects of ATL are well understood in adult TLE patients, few data are available for children. Individual case reports and group studies in children with mixed etiology[44] nevertheless suggest a risk for significant memory deficits in some children. Given that IAT asymmetries can predict verbal memory decline in children,[45]

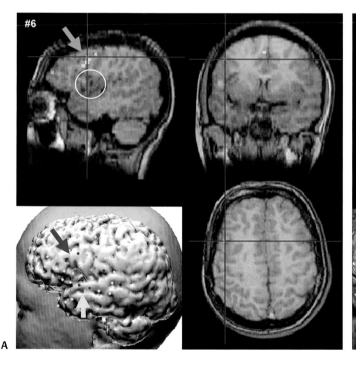
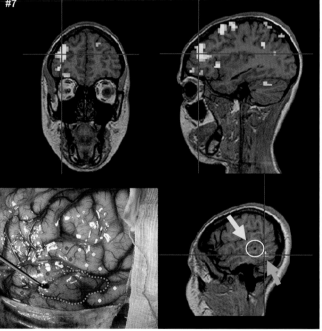

Fig. 9.2 Illustrations of possible caveats in correlating language functional magnetic resonance imaging (fMRI) and electrocortical stimulation (ECS) mapping. **(A)** Case #6: Frontal activation (*green arrow*) was displaced dorsally by focal cortical dysplasia (*circle*) within classic Broca's region and confirmed using extraoperative ECS (*red arrow and red dots* on cortical reconstruction, bottom left). A second ECS site in the anterior superior temporal gyrus (*yellow arrow*) was not visible on fMRI. **(B)** Case #7: Intraoperative mapping identified multiple ECS sites to auditory (*blue dots*) and visual (*yellow dots*) con- frontation naming in a child with a focal cortical dysplasia (circled on MRI and delineated on the photograph). fMRI failed to identify the extent of eloquent cortex (*yellow arrow*) in the posterior superior temporal (Wernicke's) region. Only a small fMRI activation focus was found posteriorly to the lesion (*green arrow*), suggesting that an additional fMRI task may have been useful. fMRI correctly identified the language dominant hemisphere in both cases. Note: the crosshair indicates the local maximum activation using silent verb generation task. Left hemisphere is on the left.

researchers hope that fMRI will one day replace this invasive procedure.

So far only a few studies have demonstrated the feasibility of conducting memory fMRI studies at group level in healthy children,[46] and there are currently no reports from clinical pediatric populations. We will therefore review fMRI studies in adult TLE that have focused on the following aspects relevant to epilepsy surgery (see review in Powell et al[47]):

Have fMRI studies:

1. demonstrated evidence for material-specific lateralization and localization of memory processes in the medial temporal lobe (MTL)?
2. revealed the impact of TLE on MTL memory organization?
3. helped to predict postsurgical memory outcome?

The material-specific lateralization of memory processes in the MTL has been shown using a variety of tasks, including incidental encoding, recognition memory, and subsequent memory tasks. Typically, verbal memory for words is associated with left MTL activation and memory for faces with right MTL; memory for visual objects results in bilateral activation.[47] There is also evidence for associated material-specific lateralization in prefrontal activation, suggesting important functional interactions with ipsilateral MTL structures. Furthermore, functional imaging studies have hinted at regional specializations within MTL with respect to different memory operations, such as encoding and retrieval, recognition, and recall.[47]

fMRI studies in adult patients have uncovered how unilateral TLE affects the organization of the MTL memory systems. Typically, patients with left-sided TLE (mostly caused by hippocampal sclerosis) show fMRI evidence for reorganization of verbal memory functions to the right MTL (focused on the hippocampus), whereas patients with right-sided TLE show greater lateralization to the left MTL.[48] Nonverbal tasks, such as mental navigation or visual scene encoding, show bilateral MTL activation in control subjects and asymmetric activation shifted contralaterally to the side of TLE seizure focus.[49-51] fMRI lateralization of memory was concordant with IAT memory scores in the majority of patients, but studies are still limited to small numbers of cases.[50,52] Furthermore, hippocampal volume loss was correlated with MTL activation in a material and side-specific way: verbal encoding-correlated activation in the left MTL with left hippocampal volume and picture encoding-correlated activation in the right MTL with right hippocampal volume.[53] It is therefore not surprising that fMRI activation within the sclerotic hippocampus correlated with memory scores: for the left side with verbal memory, and for the right side with nonverbal memory. Conversely, activation within the contralesional hippocampus was negatively correlated with memory performance, suggesting that reorganized MTL function did not positively contribute to preoperative memory function.

The critical question is whether these fMRI findings are relevant to prediction of postoperative memory changes after ATL. Indeed, correlations of preoperative memory fMRI with postoperative memory changes have been demonstrated in small groups of ATL patients. The consistent finding across these studies in exclusively adult patient groups is that the stronger the ipsilesional MTL activation is or the larger its activation asymmetry is,[48,54] the larger the postoperative memory loss will be. This is true for verbal memory change[48] as well as nonverbal memory loss.[48,51] These findings are consistent with the functional adequacy model of memory deficits following ATL in adults[55] and the fact that higher preoperative memory performance is a predictor of larger postoperative decline. Contralesional MTL fMRI activations, which can be seen as evidence for functional reorganization caused by unilateral TLE, have not been found to correlate with postoperative memory performance, at least at the short postoperative follow-up periods reported so far.

Although memory fMRI is technically challenging and the resulting activation strength within MTL regions is usually low, an alternative approach is the use of fMRI language lateralization in predicting the memory effect of ATL. Indeed, Binder and colleagues[31] reported that fMRI improved the prediction of verbal memory outcome in comparison with IAT memory lateralization in a large cohort of adult left ATL patients. This important study demonstrated how a new non-invasive imaging method should be integrated with existing clinical protocols. Future studies should establish whether memory fMRI will truly add predictive power in addition to neuropsychological evaluation, hippocampal volumetry, and language lateralization.

Given the developmental nature of many of the pathologies that give rise to TLE, we expect that reorganization of memory functions can be readily detected in children using fMRI. In the absence of evidence, one would speculate that contralesional MTL activations, unlike in adults, are more likely to predict a positive memory outcome, given the greater memory recovery after ATL in childhood.[56]

Localization of Epileptic Discharge Activity Using fMRI

Studies on Adults

Because the first description of BOLD changes during a focal seizure in a child,[57] fMRI has been increasingly used to study brain blood flow changes associated with normal and abnormal electroencephalography (EEG) activity.[58] EEG-spike associated BOLD responses have been localized in the absence of structural MRI abnormalities,[59] which has led to the expectation that EEG-fMRI may help in identifying potential surgical candidates in whom other source localization techniques have failed to localize a single focus. Only a variable proportion of adult patients show significant fMRI activation correlated with focal EEG discharges; however, a degree of topographical concordance between the two modalities is found in the majority of those cases. Recent studies have demonstrated that EEG-fMRI during ictal and interictal events in patients with malformations of cortical development can determine the involvement of the lesion in epileptogenesis and may help determine the potential surgical target.[60]

Zijlmans et al[61] evaluated EEG-fMRI in adult surgical candidates who were considered ineligible because of unclear EEG foci or multifocality. EEG-fMRI either improved source localization leading to reevaluation of surgical candidacy or corroborated the initial negative decision. The following guidelines for the application of EEG-fMRI have been proposed by those authors:

1. The best indication is for source localization in extratemporal (MRI-negative) epilepsy and when questions about the depth of the source arise.
2. In the case of presumed multifocality, EEG-fMRI will likely confirm this hypothesis, but, incidentally, it can favor one of the putative sources.
3. A priori allocation of a region of interest is crucial: topographically unrelated co-(de)activation may lack a clinical relevance.
4. EEG-fMRI can guide invasive electrode placement.

Pediatric Studies

Encouraging findings have recently been obtained in a cohort of children with pharmacoresistant focal epilepsy[62]: fMRI co-localization with EEG discharges was found in four of six children, with one confirmed by intracranial EEG. So far, patients have been preselected to have frequent interictal discharges and to be able to be scanned without sedation, and further evaluation is required to before this technique can be applied to younger patients.

■ Conclusion

fMRI examinations already play an important role within a multidisciplinary epilepsy surgery workup. In combination with comprehensive neuropsychological assessments of intellectual, language, and memory abilities; handedness; and dichotic listening performance, fMRI language lateralization findings help to estimate the risk for postoperative cognitive changes. It is also expected that in the near future, fMRI evaluations of memory functions will be possible in children, much like in adult TLE patients. Despite the existing caveats, in particular in relation to its ability in localizing eloquent cortex, it is important to stress that the fMRI methods are still undergoing rapid development. Improvements in image acquisition and stimulation paradigms as well as data analysis are likely to enhance the predictive validity of fMRI. Higher field strengths will result in better signal-to-noise ratio, thus reducing scanning time and benefiting identification of seizure foci in EEG–fMRI studies. Monitoring of task performance during scanning can reduce ambiguity of nontypical language activation patterns. Finally, statistical methods that reduce the dependence of fMRI lateralization indexes on statistical thresholds are especially welcome. Despite these existing methodological challenges, fMRI has already been proven to be an important diagnostic tool for neurosurgical practice at four key stages:

1. assessing the feasibility of surgical resection,
2. refining the extent and location of the resection in surgical candidates,
3. selecting patients for invasive functional mapping procedures, and
4. visualizing functional areas intraoperatively.[63]

In many pediatric epilepsy centers, including our own, the need for invasive IAT studies has dramatically declined since the introduction of fMRI.

References

1. Liégeois F, Cross JH, Gadian DG, Connelly A. Role of fMRI in the decision-making process: epilepsy surgery for children. J Magn Reson Imaging 2006;23(6):933–940
2. Tharin S, Golby A. Functional brain mapping and its applications to neurosurgery. Neurosurgery 2007;60(4, suppl 2)185–201, discussion 201–202
3. Detre JA. Clinical applicability of functional MRI. J Magn Reson Imaging 2006;23(6):808–815
4. Bartsch AJ, Homola G, Biller A, Solymosi L, Bendszus M. Diagnostic functional MRI: illustrated clinical applications and decision-making. J Magn Reson Imaging 2006;23(6):921–932
5. Bargalló N. Functional magnetic resonance: new applications in epilepsy. Eur J Radiol 2008;67(3):401–408
6. Sachs BC, Gaillard WD. Organization of language networks in children: functional magnetic resonance imaging studies. Curr Neurol Neurosci Rep 2003;3(2):157–162

7. O'Shaughnessy ES, Berl MM, Moore EN, Gaillard WD. Pediatric functional magnetic resonance imaging (fMRI): issues and applications. J Child Neurol 2008;23(7):791–801
8. Logothetis NK, Pauls J, Augath M, Trinath T, Oeltermann A. Neurophysiological investigation of the basis of the fMRI signal. Nature 2001;412(6843):150–157
9. Gaillard WD, Balsamo L, Xu B, et al. fMRI language task panel improves determination of language dominance. Neurology 2004; 63(8):1403–1408
10. Liégeois F, Connelly A, Baldeweg T, Vargha-Khadem F. Speaking with a single cerebral hemisphere: fMRI language organization after hemispherectomy in childhood. Brain Lang 2008;106(3):195–203
11. Benke T, Köylü B, Visani P, et al. Language lateralization in temporal lobe epilepsy: a comparison between fMRI and the Wada Test. Epilepsia 2006;47(8):1308–1319

12. Woermann FG, Jokeit H, Luerding R, et al. Language lateralization by Wada test and fMRI in 100 patients with epilepsy. Neurology 2003;61(5):699–701

13. Wilke M, Lidzba K. LI-tool: a new toolbox to assess lateralization in functional MR-data. J Neurosci Methods 2007;163(1):128–136

14. Liégeois F, Connelly A, Salmond CH, Gadian DG, Vargha-Khadem F, Baldeweg T. A direct test for lateralization of language activation using fMRI: comparison with invasive assessments in children with epilepsy. Neuroimage 2002;17(4):1861–1867

15. Hertz-Pannier L, Gaillard WD, Mott SH, et al. Noninvasive assessment of language dominance in children and adolescents with functional MRI: a preliminary study. Neurology 1997;48(4):1003–1012

16. Stapleton SR, Kiriakopoulos E, Mikulis D, et al. Combined utility of functional MRI, cortical mapping, and frameless stereotaxy in the resection of lesions in eloquent areas of brain in children. Pediatr Neurosurg 1997;26(2):68–82

17. Liégeois F, Connelly A, Cross JH, et al. Language reorganization in children with early-onset lesions of the left hemisphere: an fMRI study. Brain 2004;127(pt 6):1229–1236

18. Anderson DP, Harvey AS, Saling MM, et al. FMRI lateralization of expressive language in children with cerebral lesions. Epilepsia 2006;47(6):998–1008

19. Rasmussen T, Milner B. The role of early left-brain injury in determining lateralization of cerebral speech functions. Ann N Y Acad Sci 1977;299:355–369

20. Duchowny M, Jayakar P, Harvey AS, et al. Language cortex representation: effects of developmental versus acquired pathology. Ann Neurol 1996;40(1):31–38

21. Adcock JE, Wise RG, Oxbury JM, Oxbury SM, Matthews PM. Quantitative fMRI assessment of the differences in lateralization of language-related brain activation in patients with temporal lobe epilepsy. Neuroimage 2003;18(2):423–438

22. Weber B, Wellmer J, Reuber M, et al. Left hippocampal pathology is associated with atypical language lateralization in patients with focal epilepsy. Brain 2006;129(pt 2):346–351

23. Gaillard WD, Berl MM, Moore EN, et al. Atypical language in lesional and nonlesional complex partial epilepsy. Neurology 2007;69(18):1761–1771

24. Janszky J, Mertens M, Janszky I, Ebner A, Woermann FG. Left-sided interictal epileptic activity induces shift of language lateralization in temporal lobe epilepsy: an fMRI study. Epilepsia 2006;47(5):921–927

25. Szaflarski JP, Holland SK, Jacola LM, Lindsell C, Privitera MD, Szaflarski M. Comprehensive presurgical functional MRI language evaluation in adult patients with epilepsy. Epilepsy Behav 2008;12(1):74–83

26. Binder JR, Swanson SJ, Hammeke TA, et al. Determination of language dominance using functional MRI: a comparison with the Wada test. Neurology 1996;46(4):978–984

27. Rutten GJ, Ramsey NF, van Rijen PC, Alpherts WC, van Veelen CW. FMRI-determined language lateralization in patients with unilateral or mixed language dominance according to the Wada test. Neuroimage 2002;17(1):447–460

28. Risse GL, Gates JR, Fangman MC. A reconsideration of bilateral language representation based on the intracarotid amobarbital procedure. Brain Cogn 1997;33(1):118–132

29. Lehéricy S, Cohen L, Bazin B, et al. Functional MR evaluation of temporal and frontal language dominance compared with the Wada test. Neurology 2000;54(8):1625–1633

30. Sabsevitz DS, Swanson SJ, Hammeke TA, et al. Use of preoperative functional neuroimaging to predict language deficits from epilepsy surgery. Neurology 2003;60(11):1788–1792

31. Binder JR, Sabsevitz DS, Swanson SJ, Hammeke TA, Raghavan M, Mueller WM. Use of preoperative functional MRI to predict verbal memory decline after temporal lobe epilepsy surgery. Epilepsia 2008;49(8):1377–1394

32. Abou-Khalil B. An update on determination of language dominance in screening for epilepsy surgery: the Wada test and newer noninvasive alternatives. Epilepsia 2007;48(3):442–455

33. Kho KH, Leijten FS, Rutten GJ, Vermeulen J, Van Rijen P, Ramsey NF. Discrepant findings for Wada test and functional magnetic resonance imaging with regard to language function: use of electrocortical stimulation mapping to confirm results. Case report. J Neurosurg 2005;102(1):169–173

34. Hunter KE, Blaxton TA, Bookheimer SY, et al. (15)O water positron emission tomography in language localization: a study comparing positron emission tomography visual and computerized region of interest analysis with the Wada test. Ann Neurol 1999;45(5):662–665

35. Medina LS, Bernal B, Ruiz J. Role of functional MR in determining language dominance in epilepsy and nonepilepsy populations: a Bayesian analysis. Radiology 2007;242(1):94–100

36. Kadis DS, Iida K, Kerr EN, et al. Intrahemispheric reorganization of language in children with medically intractable epilepsy of the left hemisphere. J Int Neuropsychol Soc 2007;13(3):505–516

37. Hertz-Pannier L, Chiron C, Jambaqué I, et al. Late plasticity for language in a child's non-dominant hemisphere: a pre- and post-surgery fMRI study. Brain 2002;125(Pt 2):361–372

38. Sanai N, Mirzadeh Z, Berger MS. Functional outcome after language mapping for glioma resection. N Engl J Med 2008;358(1):18–27

39. FitzGerald DB, Cosgrove GR, Ronner S, et al. Location of language in the cortex: a comparison between functional MR imaging and electrocortical stimulation. AJNR Am J Neuroradiol 1997;18(8):1529–1539

40. Carpentier A, Pugh KR, Westerveld M, et al. Functional MRI of language processing: dependence on input modality and temporal lobe epilepsy. Epilepsia 2001;42(10):1241–1254

41. Rutten GJ, Ramsey NF, van Rijen PC, Noordmans HJ, van Veelen CW. Development of a functional magnetic resonance imaging protocol for intraoperative localization of critical temporoparietal language areas. Ann Neurol 2002;51(3):350–360

42. Roux FE, Boulanouar K, Lotterie JA, Mejdoubi M, LeSage JP, Berry I. Language functional magnetic resonance imaging in preoperative assessment of language areas: correlation with direct cortical stimulation. Neurosurgery 2003;52(6):1335–1345, discussion 1345–1347

43. Rutten GJ, van Rijen PC, van Veelen CW, Ramsey NF. Language area localization with three-dimensional functional magnetic resonance imaging matches intrasulcal electrostimulation in Broca's area. Ann Neurol 1999;46(3):405–408

44. Jambaqué I, Dellatolas G, Fohlen M, et al. Memory functions following surgery for temporal lobe epilepsy in children. Neuropsychologia 2007;45(12):2850–2862

45. Lee GP, Westerveld M, Blackburn LB, Park YD, Loring DW. Prediction of verbal memory decline after epilepsy surgery in children: effectiveness of Wada memory asymmetries. Epilepsia 2005;46(1):97–103

46. Chiu CY, Schmithorst VJ, Brown RD, Holland SK, Dunn S. Making memories: a cross-sectional investigation of episodic memory

encoding in childhood using FMRI. Dev Neuropsychol 2006;29(2):321–340

47. Powell HW, Koepp MJ, Richardson MP, Symms MR, Thompson PJ, Duncan JS. The application of functional MRI of memory in temporal lobe epilepsy: a clinical review. Epilepsia 2004;45(7):855–863

48. Powell HW, Richardson MP, Symms MR, et al. Preoperative fMRI predicts memory decline following anterior temporal lobe resection. J Neurol Neurosurg Psychiatry 2008;79(6):686–693

49. Jokeit H, Okujava M, Woermann FG. Memory fMRI lateralizes temporal lobe epilepsy. Neurology 2001;57(10):1786–1793

50. Detre JA, Maccotta L, King D, et al. Functional MRI lateralization of memory in temporal lobe epilepsy. Neurology 1998;50(4):926–932

51. Rabin ML, Narayan VM, Kimberg DY, et al. Functional MRI predicts post-surgical memory following temporal lobectomy. Brain 2004;127(pt 10):2286–2298

52. Golby AJ, Poldrack RA, Illes J, Chen D, Desmond JE, Gabrieli JD. Memory lateralization in medial temporal lobe epilepsy assessed by functional MRI. Epilepsia 2002;43(8):855–863

53. Powell HW, Richardson MP, Symms MR, et al. Reorganization of verbal and nonverbal memory in temporal lobe epilepsy due to unilateral hippocampal sclerosis. Epilepsia 2007;48(8):1512–1525

54. Frings L, Wagner K, Halsband U, Schwarzwald R, Zentner J, Schulze-Bonhage A. Lateralization of hippocampal activation differs between left and right temporal lobe epilepsy patients and correlates with postsurgical verbal learning decrement. Epilepsy Res 2008;78(2-3):161–170

55. Chelune GJ. Hippocampal adequacy versus functional reserve: predicting memory functions following temporal lobectomy. Arch Clin Neuropsychol 1995;10(5):413–432

56. Gleissner U, Sassen R, Schramm J, Elger CE, Helmstaedter C. Greater functional recovery after temporal lobe epilepsy surgery in children. Brain 2005;128(pt 12):2822–2829

57. Jackson GD, Connelly A, Cross JH, Gordon I, Gadian DG. Functional magnetic resonance imaging of focal seizures. Neurology 1994;44(5):850–856

58. Krakow K, Woermann FG, Symms MR, et al. EEG-triggered functional MRI of interictal epileptiform activity in patients with partial seizures. Brain 1999;122(pt 9):1679–1688

59. Hamandi K, Salek-Haddadi A, Fish DR, Lemieux L. EEG/functional MRI in epilepsy: The Queen Square Experience. J Clin Neurophysiol 2004;21(4):241–248

60. Tyvaert L, Hawco C, Kobayashi E, LeVan P, Dubeau F, Gotman J. Different structures involved during ictal and interictal epileptic activity in malformations of cortical development: an EEG-fMRI study. Brain 2008;131(pt 8):2042–2060

61. Zijlmans M, Huiskamp G, Hersevoort M, Seppenwoolde JH, van Huffelen AC, Leijten FS. EEG-fMRI in the preoperative work-up for epilepsy surgery. Brain 2007;130(pt 9):2343–2353

62. De Tiège X, Laufs H, Boyd SG, et al. EEG-fMRI in children with pharmacoresistant focal epilepsy. Epilepsia 2007;48(2):385–389

63. Krishnan R, Raabe A, Hattingen E, et al. Functional magnetic resonance imaging-integrated neuronavigation: correlation between lesion-to-motor cortex distance and outcome. Neurosurgery 2004;55(4):904–914, 914–915

10 Application of PET and SPECT in Pediatric Epilepsy Surgery

Ajay Kumar and Harry T. Chugani

Epilepsy is the most common neurological disorder, with a prevalence of 1 to 2% and cumulative lifetime incidence exceeding 3%. Almost 25% of epileptic patients do not respond to multiple antiepileptic treatments and will have intractable (i.e., medically refractory) seizures. These patients can be helped by surgically removing the epileptogenic region of the cerebral cortex. However, to accomplish this, the epileptogenic region has to be precisely delineated before surgery. Indeed, the most important aspect of presurgical evaluation is to identify the discrete epileptogenic region that can be resected without causing an unacceptable loss of neurological function and that will lead to complete seizure control. Functional neuroimaging, such as positron emission tomography (PET) and single photon emission computed tomography (SPECT), combined with electroencephalography (EEG), can play a very important role by providing noninvasive presurgical localization of epileptogenic foci in the patient with no brain lesion on computed tomography (CT) or magnetic resonance imaging (MRI; i.e., nonlesional cases), with multiple structural lesions of which only one or two are epileptogenic, or in cases with discordant or inconclusive EEG findings. PET and SPECT can be very useful in cases by identifying the epileptogenic regions.

■ Rationale for PET and SPECT

SPECT and PET are imaging techniques that use radioisotopes or radiolabeled molecules (the term *radiotracer* will be used for both of them) to study the perfusion or function of an organ, even at the cellular or molecular level. With both methods, a very small amount of a selected radiotracer is injected into the patient. The radiotracer is selected on the basis of desired purpose, that is, which organs and what functions the physician is interested in exploring. The gamma rays emitted by the radiotracers are detected externally with the help of suitable detectors, and an image of the spatial distribution of these radiotracers is generated. Therefore, theoretically, any organ or its function can be studied, provided appropriate radiotracers are available. The reason for applying PET and SPECT in epilepsy is based on the fact that the metabolism (particularly of glucose), receptor density and neurotransmission, and cerebral blood flow in the epileptic region (as

well as in the associated seizure propagation network) are altered and can be detected by these imaging techniques.

■ Principle and Techniques of PET and SPECT

PET

PET is an imaging technique used to noninvasively image and measure the function of various organs. In PET, positron-emitting radionuclides, such as ^{18}F, ^{11}C, ^{15}O, and ^{13}N, are used to label various natural biological substrates and drugs or pharmaceuticals. These all contain hydrogen, carbon, oxygen, or nitrogen, which can be replaced with their radioactive positron-emitting counterpart. The resulting radioactive substance, also known as a radiotracer or PET tracer, will have similar behavior and will follow the same physiological pathways by emitting paired high-energy (511 Kev) photons. These photons can be detected by external detectors, and the whole process can be traced or imaged. Any physiological or metabolic process, such as glucose metabolism, protein synthesis, enzymatic processes, or receptor–ligand interaction, can be studied using an appropriate radiotracer and various kinetic models.[1]

The most commonly used PET tracer in epilepsy is 2-deoxy-2[^{18}F]fluoro-D-glucose (FDG; half-life: 110 minutes), which measures glucose metabolism. FDG is transported in tissue and phosphorylated to FDG-6-phosphate in the same manner as glucose. However, FDG-6-phosphate is not a substrate for the next step of glycolysis. Because it cannot immediately leave the cell, phosphorylated FDG gets trapped within the cell, and its location and quantity can be measured by PET. Under steady-state conditions, FDG uptake reflects the glucose metabolic rate. In the brain, this rate is highly related to the synaptic density and functional activity of the brain tissue.

Because brain glucose metabolism undergoes age-related changes, particularly in the early childhood, practitioners should be aware of this pattern while interpreting pediatric FDG PET scans. Metabolic rates of glucose in cerebral cortex at the time of birth are usually approximately 30% less than those of adult values. They reach adult values by the second year of life, exceeding them by the third year, and reach the peak values (almost double the adult values) by 3 to 4 years of age, when a plateau is reached. This plateau persists until approximately 10 years of age, then gradually the glucose metabolic rates decline to reach adult values by the age of approximately 16 to 18 years. The glucose metabolism pattern and visual appearance on PET scans also changes with age. In the newborn, glucose metabolic activity is most prominent in primary sensory and motor cortex, thalamus, brain stem and cerebellar vermis, cingulate cortex, amygdala, and hippocampus. Between ages 2 and 4 months, glucose use increases in parietal, temporal, and primary visual cortex (medial occipital or calcarine cortex), as well as in the basal ganglia and cerebellar hemispheres. Between 6 and 8 months of age, glucose use increases in the lateral and inferior prefrontal regions, with medial and dorsal frontal cortex becoming active between 8 and 12 months of age. The adult pattern is seen by 1 year of age.[2,3]

Interictal FDG PET typically shows reduced radiotracer uptake (hypometabolism) in the epileptogenic region (**Fig. 10.1**). The hypometabolism can result from a variety of mechanisms, including neuronal loss, diaschisis, or reduction in synaptic density. It appears that cortical hypometabolism may be associated with duration, frequency, and severity of the seizures, hypometabolism is usually found in only one fourth of children with new onset epilepsy compared with 80 to 85% of adults with intractable seizures.[4] Persistent or increased seizure frequency may lead to enlargement of the hypometabolic area, whereas seizure control may be associated with decrease in the size of hypometabolic cortex or even its resolution.[5] The time interval between PET acquisition and the most recent seizure also may affect the extent and severity of the cortical abnormality, with shorter duration having a positive effect on the extent and severity of the hypometabolism.[6]

During the ictal phase, metabolism increases many fold in the epileptic region; however, because FDG PET shows cumulative FDG uptake over a period of 30 to 45 minutes, the final images can be variable and complex, depending on the exact nature of the underlying pathology, seizure duration, seizure evolution, and net summation effects of ictal, postictal, and interictal metabolism. Therefore, ictal FDG PET is not very reliable and is often difficult to interpret, and EEG monitoring should be performed during the FDG uptake period to rule out any clinical or subclinical seizure. Because ictal FDG PET is virtually not done, in all the subsequent discussion, we use the term *FDG PET* in place of interictal FDG PET.

Because FDG PET usually shows a larger area of hypometabolism extending beyond the epileptogenic region, it cannot be reliably used to precisely determine the surgical margin. However, it can be used for lateralization and general localization of the seizure focus. Further, this information can help in making an a priori hypothesis about subsequent subdural electrode placement, which may be very useful, particularly in cases of normal MRI (**Fig. 10.2A**). However, use of more specific tracers, as discussed here, can help in providing a more precise delineation of the epileptogenic tissue; this becomes particularly important in a developing pediatric brain and when the epileptic focus potentially involves eloquent brain regions (primary motor, speech, or visual areas).

Other PET tracers with the potential for detecting epileptic brain regions include ^{11}C-flumazenil (FMZ), which binds to α subunits of the $GABA_A$-benzodiazepine receptor and ^{11}C-alphamethyl-L-tryptophan (AMT), which measures tryptophan metabolism. FMZ binding or FMZ VD (volume of distribution) is high at 2 years of age and then decreases exponentially with age until adult values are reached at approximately age 20 years. The order of brain region (from highest to lowest FMZ binding) at 2 years of age is as follows: primary visual cortex, superior frontal cortex, medial temporal cortex, temporal lobe, prefrontal cortex, cerebellum, basal ganglia, and thalamus. FMZ binding in medial temporal lobe is robust enough for its good visualization (compared

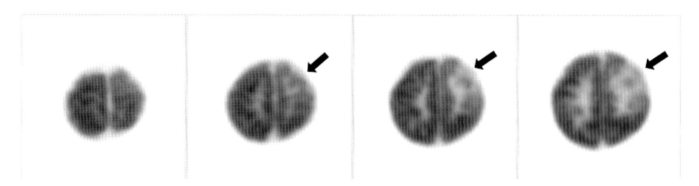

Fig. 10.1 2-deoxy-2[^{18}F]fluoro-D-glucose positron emission tomography scan showing an area of hypometabolism in the left frontal lobe (*arrows*) in an 8-year-old child with intractable seizures and normal magnetic resonance imaging. Postsurgical histopathology revealed cortical dysplasia.

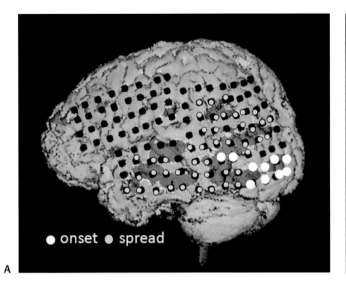

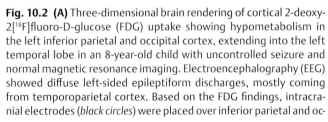

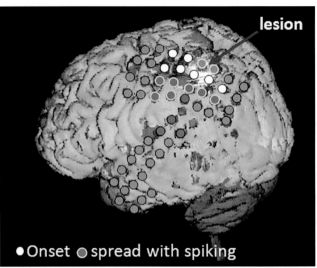

Fig. 10.2 **(A)** Three-dimensional brain rendering of cortical 2-deoxy-2[^{18}F]fluoro-D-glucose (FDG) uptake showing hypometabolism in the left inferior parietal and occipital cortex, extending into the left temporal lobe in an 8-year-old child with uncontrolled seizure and normal magnetic resonance imaging. Electroencephalography (EEG) showed diffuse left-sided epileptiform discharges, mostly coming from temporoparietal cortex. Based on the FDG findings, intracranial electrodes (*black circles*) were placed over inferior parietal and occipital cortex also, which found most of the epileptiform discharges coming from the occipital region. The rest of the hypometabolic area coincided with the electrodes showing seizure spread. **(B)** Three-dimensional brain rendering of FDG uptake, showing glucose hypometabolism extending beyond the structural lesion. Intracranial EEG monitoring revealed most of the epileptiform discharges emanating from adjacent to the lesion.

with FDG PET, in which the medial temporal region, particularly hippocampus, is often not well visualized). This is one of the main reasons for an important role of FMZ PET in epileptic patients in whom medial temporal lobe abnormalities are suspected. AMT is an analog of tryptophan, the precursor for serotonin synthesis, but, unlike tryptophan, AMT is not incorporated into protein in significant amounts. AMT is converted to α-methyl-serotonin (AM-5HT) by tryptophan hydroxylase, and it accumulates in neurons and nerve terminals along with the releasable pool of serotonin. After intravenous injection, AMT accumulates in the brain for the first 20 minutes (less than 2% of the injected dose is present in the brain at peak values), after which a plateau is reached and maintained for up to 60 minutes, with no right–left asymmetry in normal subjects.

SPECT

In SPECT, rotating γ cameras (detectors) are used to image the distribution of the injected radiotracer in the organ of interest. For this purpose, 1 to 3 detectors and only γ ray emitting radioisotopes are used. For the purpose of brain and particularly for epilepsy, SPECT is mostly used to study brain perfusion, with hexamethyl propylene amine oxime (HMPAO) and ethylene cysteine dimer (ECD) labeled with 99mTc being the most common radiotracers used for this

purpose. HMPAO readily crosses the blood–brain barrier and approximately 80% is extracted by brain during the first pass. Once inside the neurons and glial cells, HMPAO gets trapped because it is oxidized by glutathione into a nondiffusible compound. A total of 4 to 7% of the injected activity is trapped within the brain, reaching its peak in 1 to 2 minutes. ECD is another lipophilic compound that, like HMPAO, gets trapped inside neurons because of its transformation into a hydrophilic compound that cannot diffuse back. Its first pass extraction is 60 to 70%, with a maximum of 6 to 7% injected activity accumulating in the brain 1 to 2 minutes after the injection. The brain can be imaged subsequently, and the resulting image provides a snapshot of perfusion immediately after the injection. This is the basis for applying brain SPECT in epilepsy, because the ictal and interictal phases are usually associated with increased or decreased blood flow, respectively, in the epileptic foci. However, during seizure, the cerebral blood flow changes rapidly with time, depending on the seizure type and its mode of propagation. Therefore, early radiotracer injection is imperative to catch the blood flow changes in the epileptic zone, during seizure. Similarly, knowledge of the exact time of injection (because it takes approximately 20 to 30 seconds for the radiotracer to reach the brain from an arm vein) and seizure duration is very important for the correct interpretation of the SPECT images. Delayed injection of radiotracer may show a variable pattern of blood flow changes associated with seizure evolution in the epileptic zone and mode and pattern of seizure propagation, depending on the time of injection. Also, because seizure propagation is usually from the temporal to the frontal lobe or from posterior (parietooccipital lobes) to anterior cortical regions (temporal and frontal lobe),[7–10] interpretation of ictal SPECT can be very challenging if the exact timing of radiotracer injection and seizure onset is not known, unless injection is synchronized with video-EEG monitoring.

During the ictal phase, blood flow in the epileptic region can increase up to 300%, which can be seen as an area of hyperperfusion in ictal SPECT.[11] A true ictal SPECT (tracer injected immediately after the onset of the seizure and SPECT images showing perfusion at that point of time) shows an area of hyperperfusion in the epileptogenic region, surrounded by an area of hypoperfusion, which becomes more prominent at the end of the ictal phase. This surrounding area of hypoperfusion may be caused by steal syndrome (shift of blood flow to the seizure focus) or this area may function as an inhibitory zone trying to limit the seizure spread.[12] Interictal SPECT (tracer is injected when patient is not having any clinical or subclinical seizure and SPECT images show the baseline perfusion pattern) shows hypoperfusion or normal perfusion in the epileptogenic region. Even when present, hypoperfusion may be very mild and sometimes difficult to distinguish from the surrounding normal brain on visual examination. The main role of interictal SPECT currently is to assist in the evaluation of ictal SPECT, visually or quantitatively, using statistical parametric mapping (SPM) or SISCOM (subtraction ictal SPECT co-registered to MRI, i.e., the interictal SPECT images are subtracted from the ictal images and the results are displayed on co-registered MR images), by providing a baseline blood flow. Use of these registration techniques can increase the sensitivity and specificity of ictal SPECT. Studies have shown that SPM can increase the sensitivity of SPECT scan over visual analysis.[13–15] However, lack of age-matched control subjects can make its use difficult, particularly in children younger than 6 years of age.[16] SISCOM, conversely, appears to be very useful in children. The probability of localizing an ictal onset zone has been reported higher with SISCOM, compared with ictal EEG and MRI.[17,18] Use of SISCOM can help in revisiting and detecting subtle changes in MRI, which were initially reported normal.[19] Studies have shown that the area of the resected SISCOM abnormality is associated with the surgical outcome; the larger the area of resected SISCOM abnormality is, better the outcome will be.[17,20]

The major limitation of SPECT in the pediatric population is that it is difficult to acquire good interictal or ictal brain SPECT because children may have very frequent and short-lasting seizures (such as infantile spasms or myoclonic epilepsy). Another limitation is the poor spatial resolution (10–15 mm) of SPECT, compared with FDG PET (~5–6mm), which becomes even more crucial in small pediatric brains.

■ Role of PET and SPECT in Pediatric Epilepsy Surgery

The role of PET and SPECT can be summarized as follows:

1. Detection of epileptogenic cortex
2. Determination of dual pathology (i.e., medial temporal involvement)
3. Assessment for secondary epileptic focus
4. Evaluation of the functional status outside the epileptogenic zone
5. Evaluation of eloquent cortex
6. Postsurgical evaluation

Epileptogenic Region

Temporal Lobe Epilepsy

In temporal lobe epilepsy, interictal hypometabolic regions are not strictly confined to the presumed temporal epileptogenic zone or to the brain tissue showing pathological changes. They usually extend beyond temporal structures to ipsilateral parietal and frontal cortex as well as thalamus and also occasionally to the contralateral temporal lobe.[21–24] Although this may represent the epileptic network involved in seizure propagation and may be related to behavioral and neuropsychological changes seen with chronic epilepsy, these extratemporal hypometabolic regions should be further investigated. FMZ PET is highly sensitive in temporal lobe epilepsy and shows decreased FMZ binding in the sclerotic hippocampus,[22,25] and the reduction in FMZ binding is usually more than can be accounted for by the loss of hippocampal volume.[26] Contrary to FDG PET, which usually shows extratemporal hypometabolism in parietal and frontal cortex in cases of temporal lobe epilepsy (probably associated with cognitive dysfunction or reflecting diaschisis), decreased FMZ binding usually represents neuronal loss or receptor changes related to epileptogenicity and, therefore, should be more closely scrutinized.[22] The sensitivity of FMZ in detection of unilateral hippocampal sclerosis has been reported to be up to 100% with contralateral abnormalities in one third of patients.[22,25] In MRI-negative patients, FMZ PET has been found to be abnormal in up to 85% patients with temporal lobe epilepsy.[27–29] FMZ PET appears to be more sensitive than FDG PET in identifying an epileptogenic region and is associated with better surgical outcome, even when the MRI is normal. Use of SPM can further increase the accuracy of FMZ PET, with detection of subtle changes in FMZ binding, which is difficult to appreciate visually.[25,30] These SPM studies sometimes found increased FMZ binding also,[31–34] which, in some cases, indicated cortical developmental malformations.[32] Use of SPM also revealed increased FMZ binding in the normal appearing temporal lobe white matter, which was found to be microdysgenesis on histopathological examination.[35] This is an interesting finding, because these ectopic neuronal clusters may lead to epileptogenesis by providing an aberrant circuitry. Another PET tracer, AMT does not appear to be very useful in cases of medial temporal lobe epilepsy, particularly with hippocampal sclerosis.

In temporal lobe epilepsy, the pattern of perfusion on ictal SPECT depends on the origin of seizures. Although cases with medial temporal lesions usually show well-localized area of hyperperfusion involving ipsilateral medial and lateral temporal lobe, in cases of lateral temporal lesions, bilateral hyperperfusion is usually seen with higher increase in the ipsilateral side.[36,37] This can be explained on the basis of different mechanisms of seizure propagation depending on the neuronal connectivity. The timing of tracer injection is also important in the case of temporal lobe epilepsy, because ictal, postictal, and peri-ictal SPECT scans have different perfusion patterns, which also depend on the area of temporal lobe involved. In the case of medial temporal lobe epilepsy, ictal scan (tracer injection within 20 seconds of the seizure onset) typically will show hyperperfusion of the entire medial temporal lobe along with surrounding hypoperfusion of orbital cortex or the entire frontal lobe. Peri-ictal scan (slightly delayed injection, 20–60 seconds after the seizure onset) will show hyperperfusion in lateral temporal cortex, orbital cortex, basal ganglia, or in contralateral temporal lobe, probably because of rapid seizure propagation. Postictal scan (injection within 4 minutes from the end of seizure) will show persistent hyperperfusion in medial temporal lobe with hypoperfusion in lateral temporal lobe gradually extending to surrounding hyperperfused areas. The medial temporal lobe remains isoperfused for another 10 to 15 minutes and then gradually becomes hypoperfused, resembling the interictal scan.

Although an extensive experience regarding SPECT is available for adults, not much data exist for the pediatric population. Overall, interictal SPECT has very low sensitivity (less than 50%) in the detection of epileptogenic regions in pediatric temporal lobe epilepsy, with false-positive or false-negative findings in 20 to 75% cases. However, ictal SPECT can correctly localize the epileptogenic foci in 70 to 90% of cases with unilateral temporal lobe epilepsy.[38–41] As alluded to previously, various registration techniques, such as SPM or SISCOM, can further increase the sensitivity and specificity of ictal SPECT. In children, SISCOM was found to be helpful in identifying the epileptogenic region in up to 95% of cases.[19] Compared with intracranial EEG findings, ictal SPECT was found to correctly localize the seizure onset zone in 80% of children with intractable epilepsy.[42] False localization was caused by rapid seizure propagation or subclinical seizure onset. In addition, in the majority (70%) of children with favorable outcome of resective epilepsy surgery, the surgical margin coincided with the SPECT focus. Postictal SPECT is also more sensitive (70–90%) than interictal SPECT and can improve further with use of SISCOM.[18,43] SISCOM can be par-

ticularly useful in cases of dysembryoplastic neuroepithelial tumor (DNET), which is more prevalent in the pediatric population. SISCOM can demonstrate some additional dysplastic areas around the DNET, and removal of these areas is essential for better surgical outcome. The use of SISCOM can increase the focus detection rate up to 93%, compared with 74% without it.[1,19,44]

Extratemporal Lobe Epilepsy

FDG PET can play an important role in the presurgical evaluation of extratemporal lobe epilepsy in the pediatric population by providing important lateralizing and localizing information that will guide intraoperative electrode placement (**Fig. 10.2B**). Because frontal lobe epilepsy in young children is usually associated with subtle structural changes not apparent in MRI, such as cortical dysplasia or heterotopias, FDG PET is more informative in children compared with adults. Even in cases of abnormal MRI, FDG PET can sometimes be very useful. It may show hypometabolism extending beyond the lesion. These areas should be sampled with intracranial EEG during surgery, because perilesional cortex also may be epileptogenic, and lesionectomy alone may lead to surgical failure. In frontal lobe epilepsy, the sensitivity of FDG PET in localizing the epileptogenic zones is in the range of 45 to 73%.[45–49] However, using a high-resolution PET scanner, we found a sensitivity of 92% and a specificity of 62.5% of FDG PET in the detection of the epileptic foci in children with frontal lobe epilepsy.[45] In cases of occipital lobe epilepsy, a lower localization value of FDG PET has been reported.[50]

In neocortical epilepsy, FMZ PET has been reported to have 60 to 100% sensitivity compared with intracranial ictal EEG.[51–54] FMZ abnormalities usually extend beyond the lesions in an eccentric fashion. However, these extensions are usually smaller than the large perilesional hypometabolism seen with FDG PET and show good correlation with intracranial EEG.[51,55,56] In MRI-negative patients, FMZ PET is abnormal in 70% of patients with extratemporal lobe epilepsy.[28] FMZ PET appears to be more sensitive than FDG PET in identifying an epileptogenic region and complete resection of the FMZ abnormality is associated with excellent surgical outcome, even when the MRI is normal[52,57] (**Fig. 10.3**). Use of SPM can further increase the usefulness of FMZ PET in patients with neocortical epilepsy, including those with or without normal MRI.[33,58]

Another PET tracer, C-alpha-methyl trytophan (AMT), appears to have strong clinical applications in selected cases of extratemporal lobe epilepsy. We found that histologically verified (macroscopic or microscopic) cortical dysplasia is associated with a higher occurrence of increased AMT uptake compared with cases with nonspecific gliosis.[57] Also, the area of increased AMT uptake is significantly more restricted than the extent of corresponding glucose hypometabolism.

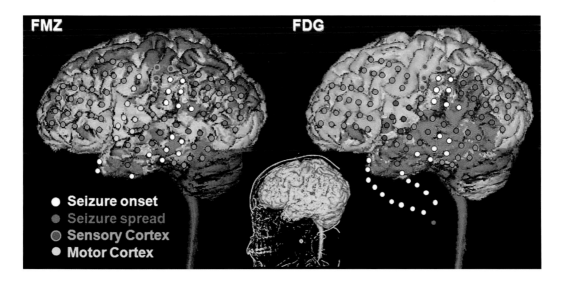

Fig. 10.3 Three-dimensional brain rendering of flumazenil (FMZ) binding (*left*) and 2-deoxy-2[¹⁸F]fluoro-D-glucose (FDG) uptake (*right*) showing much smaller area of reduced FMZ binding compared with extensive area of reduced FDG uptake in the left temporal and frontal lobe.

In some instances, AMT PET can identify the epileptogenic cortex even when FDG and FMZ PET scans are normal.

SPECT can provide a basis for the placement of intracranial electrodes in extratemporal lobe epilepsy. However, because of the very short duration of some seizures in children, it may be difficult to acquire an ictal SPECT. Postictal scans are also less helpful because, unlike temporal lobe epilepsy, seizure induced perfusion changes do not always extend into the postictal phase. Although ictal SPECT generally is not as successful in extratemporal lobe epilepsy as in temporal lobe epilepsy, nevertheless, a success rate of 70% has been reported.[59] Again, the use of SISCOM can further increase its localizing value up to 93%.[17,60]

Infantile Spasms

PET can play an important role in the evaluation of infantile spasms. For example, on PET scanning of glucose metabolism, most infants diagnosed with cryptogenic infantile spasms will have focal or multifocal cortical hypometabolism, corresponding to the areas of ictal and interictal EEG abnormalities.[61,62] In a study of 140 children with infantile spasms, we found unifocal and multifocal cortical metabolic abnormalities in 95% of children with an initial diagnosis of cryptogenic infantile spasms.[63] In cases of intractable spasms and a single focal PET abnormality, corresponding to the EEG focus, resective surgery can be planned with not only good seizure control but also complete or partial reversal of associated developmental delay. When the pattern of glucose hypometabolism is generalized and symmetric, a lesional etiology is not likely, and neurometabolic or neuro-

genetic disorders should be considered in further evaluation and management. PET findings in infants with spasms also suggest complex cortical–subcortical interactions by showing prominent glucose metabolism in lenticular nuclei and brain stem, believed to be important in the secondary generalization of focal cortical discharges resulting in spasms that account for the bilateral motor involvement and relative symmetry of the majority of spasms even in the presence of a discrete focal lesion.[64]

Tuberous Sclerosis

FDG PET shows hypometabolism in tubers, both epileptic and nonepileptic; therefore, it is not very useful as such in the evaluation of children with tuberous sclerosis. However, another PET tracer, AMT, can be used to differentiate epileptogenic from nonepileptogenic tubers in children with tuberous sclerosis, because it shows increased AMT uptake interictally in only epileptogenic tubers (**Fig. 10.4**). In epileptogenic tubers, there is increased uptake and subsequent intracellular accumulation of the AMT, because of activation of the kynurenine pathway,[65] which leads to the production of neurotoxic and convulsant metabolites, such as quinolinic acid.[66] AMT PET can identify epileptogenic tuber(s) in almost two thirds of children with tuberous sclerosis and intractable epilepsy.[65,67,68] Although the specificity of AMT PET is very high, its sensitivity is suboptimal and appears to be related to the underlying pathology as well as the method of image analysis. In patients with tuberous sclerosis and intractable epilepsy, we found that MRI-based quantitative assessment increases the sensitivity of AMT PET to 79% from

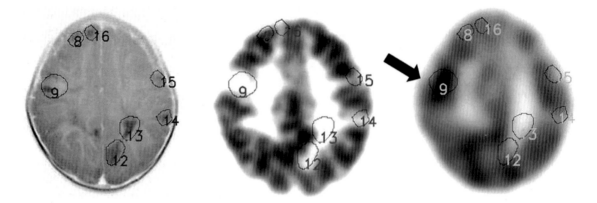

Fig. 10.4 Magnetic resonance imaging (left) showing multiple tubers in a child with tuberous sclerosis and intractable seizures with the majority of seizures coming from the right frontal lobe. Whereas 2-deoxy-2[¹⁸F]fluoro-D-glucose positron emission tomography (PET) showed glucose hypometabolism in tubers (center), α-methyl-L-tryptophan PET scan showed intense uptake in a right frontal tuber (right image), corresponding to the electroencephalography focus.

44.4% with visual assessment.[69] This apparent discrepancy is because nonepileptogenic tubers typically show decreased AMT uptake and some epileptogenic tubers showing relatively increased AMT uptake cannot be easily differentiated from adjacent normal cortex without quantitative analysis. We also found good correlation between resection of epileptogenic tubers suggested by AMT PET and seizure outcome.[70] Tubers with at least 10% increase of AMT uptake were all found to be epileptogenic. A cutoff threshold of 1.02 for AMT uptake ratio provided 83% accuracy for detecting tubers that need to be resected to achieve a seizure-free outcome.[67,70] Our own studies using FMZ PET have not found binding differences between epileptogenic and nonepileptogenic tubers (unpublished data). SPECT also may play some role in identifying epileptic tubers. One small study, in 15 children, found a good correlation between ictal SPECT and ictal scalp EEG.[71]

Lennox-Gastaut Syndrome

Children with Lennox-Gastaut syndrome (a triad of multiple seizure types including tonic seizures, developmental delay, and 1–2.5 Hz generalized "slow" spike and wave EEG pattern), may have four metabolic patterns on FDG PET scan: unilateral focal, unilateral diffuse, and bilateral diffuse hypometabolism, as well as normal patterns.[72–74] Interictal SPECT usually shows multiple areas of hypoperfusion.[75] Patients with unilateral focal and unilateral diffuse patterns may be occasionally considered for cortical resection, provided there is concordance between PET and ictal EEG findings.

Sturge-Weber Syndrome

In children with Sturge-Weber syndrome, FDG PET reveals hypometabolism ipsilateral to the facial nevus and usually identifies additional areas of abnormal cortex extending beyond the lesion visible on MRI.[76,77] However, infants may show a paradoxical pattern of increased glucose metabolism interictally in the cortex underlying the leptomeningeal angioma; as the disease progresses, the hypermetabolic area becomes hypometabolic.[76] In some patients, serial FDG PET scans show rapidly progressing and severe hypometabolism in the affected area, probably because of rapid demise of the brain tissue associated with the angioma; these patients will have improvement in seizure status and cognitive function and therefore may not require surgical intervention. Early and rapid progression in unilateral cases of Sturge-Weber leads to early and more efficient reorganization in the contralateral cortex. Conversely, persistent mild hypometabolism of the lesion may indicate ongoing functional disturbance, and these patients may show persistent seizures and developmental arrest.[78] These are the patients who require surgical intervention for seizure control and possible cognitive improvement by promoting effective reorganization in the contralateral hemisphere while brain plasticity is still at a maximum during development. In Sturge-Weber, detrimental metabolic changes occur before 3 years of age[77] coinciding with a sharp increase in developmentally regulated cerebral metabolic demand.[3] Progressive hypometabolism is associated with high seizure frequency in these children. However, metabolic abnormalities may remain limited or even partially recover later in some children with well-controlled seizures. Metabolic recovery accompanied by neurological improvement suggests a window for therapeutic intervention in children with unilateral Sturge-Weber.[77]

Perfusion SPECT shows hyperperfusion in the lesion even before seizure onset,[79] analogous to the transient hypermetabolism seen on PET.[76,77] After 1 year of age, these areas typically show hypoperfusion.[80] In a single case report on a patient with failed functional hemispherectomy, ictal SPECT showed hyperperfusion in the residual lesion with falsely lateralized EEG; further surgery resulted in seizure freedom.[81]

Rasmussen's Syndrome and Other Epilepsy of Inflammatory Origin

Neuroinflammation may be the underlying cause for intractable epilepsy in some cases, such as in Rasmussen's disease. Neuroinflammation is mediated by activated microglia, which secrete several proinflammatory molecules such as cytokines (IL-1, IL-6, TNF-α), chemokines (MIP-1α, β, MCP-1) and neurotoxins, free radicals, nitric oxide, proteinases, eicosanoids, and excitotoxins, which may play an important role in epileptogenesis. Although the exact mechanisms are unclear, it appears that the inflammatory mediators act by increasing glutamatergic neurotransmission, decreasing gamma-aminobutyric acid (GABA) mediated currents and inducing neovascularization, and damaging the blood–brain barrier. Detection of microglia is not possible with current radiological methods or biochemical techniques but requires histopathological examination of central nervous system tissues, which is quite invasive or possible only postmortem. Because activated microglia express peripheral-type benzodiazepine receptors, they can be imaged with PET using ^{11}C-PK11195, a radioligand that binds specifically to the peripheral-type benzodiazepine receptors, thus making the in vivo detection of neuroinflammation possible. PET scanning using ^{11}C-PK-11195 can help in the early diagnosis of Rasmussen's syndrome or other inflammatory conditions with intractable seizures, where CT and MRI are often normal for several months after the clinical manifestation of the disease. Localization of the most affected brain regions may also provide a guide in deciding the site of brain biopsy to avoid sampling errors and can help in the surgical removal of that region.[82]

Dual Pathology

Undiagnosed dual pathology (co-existence of neocortical lesion and hippocampal sclerosis) can be a source of surgical failure, because resection of both the cortical lesion and the affected hippocampus is necessary to optimize the surgical results. Although FDG PET can be used to evaluate for an abnormally functioning hippocampus, the higher sensitivity of FMZ PET makes it more useful in such cases, particularly when the MRI does not reveal an abnormal signal or atrophy in the hippocampus. This can be very useful because resection of both the lesions is necessary for good surgical outcome.[83]

Secondary Epileptic Foci

"Secondary" epileptic foci have been defined by Morrell[84,85] as "trans-synaptic and long-lasting alterations in nerve cell behavior characterized by paroxysmal electrographic manifestations and clinical seizures" induced by seizures from a primary epileptic focus. The secondary epileptic focus is usually located at a different site from the primary focus along the path of seizure propagation. Histopathological examination of these secondary foci usually shows gliosis.[86] FMZ PET can play a very important role in the detection of secondary epileptic foci, as shown by our experience.[51,86] It appears that complete removal of both primary and secondary foci is required to achieve the best surgical results.

■ Functional Status of the Rest of the Brain

FDG PET can be very valuable in assessing the integrity of brain regions outside of the epileptogenic zone during the surgical planning process and allows certain prognostic implications. These nonepileptogenic dysfunctional areas are often associated with specific clinical manifestations.

In children with hemimegalencephaly, FDG PET often shows additional less-pronounced abnormalities in the opposite hemisphere, which probably accounts for the suboptimal cognitive outcome even with complete seizure control after surgical removal of the profoundly abnormal hemisphere. Thus, FDG PET can be useful in such cases to assess the functional integrity of the contralateral hemisphere before hemispherectomy and help predict cognitive outcome.

Eloquent Cortex

Although ^{15}O-water PET has been used in the past to assess eloquent cortex (e.g., motor and language cortex), this type of evaluation has been, for the most part, replaced by functional MRI. The latter can be repeated and offers the advantage of no radiation exposure. As a result, PET or SPECT has a very limited role in activation studies for presurgical evaluation of epileptic patients. Epileptic subjects with implanted metallic devices, which are not MRI-compatible and who require noninvasive functional brain mapping, may be candidates for ^{15}O-water PET activation studies.

■ Postsurgical Evaluation

In surgical failures where a second surgery is being considered, very few neuroimaging options are available to pinpoint remaining epileptic tissue. Occasionally, ictal SPECT may be helpful in this regard, but, in most cases, the epileptologist is left with the scalp EEG and seizure semiology to guide placement of intracranial electrodes. In one study, SISCOM revealed a localized area of hyperperfusion in almost 80% of patients undergoing reoperation, and in 70% of cases they were concordant with EEG findings.[87] Resection of these concordant lesions led to good surgical outcome. We have found AMT PET to be particularly useful in this setting, and, unlike MRI, interictal FDG or FMZ PET, AMT PET can differentiate epileptogenic cortex from nonepileptic tissue damage caused by the initial surgery in approximately half of the cases.[88] The best results are obtained if the scan is performed between 2 months and 2 years after the first surgery. However, more work is required in this difficult group of patients undergoing reoperation.

FDG PET can be also useful in the postsurgical evaluation and monitoring of previously hypometabolic nonepileptogenic brain regions (which had no EEG correlate) in the presurgical FDG scan. Resolution of this hypometabolism, which occurs in some of these cases, will suggest the functional nature of the suppression. Conversely, persistence of a remote, but connected, region or appearance of a new area of hypometabolism (not suspected to be diaschisis) may suggest a secondary potentially epileptogenic focus.

◼ Experience with Other PET Tracers in Epilepsy

Clinical experience with opiate, histamine, N-methyl-D-aspartate (NMDA) acetylcholine, dopamine, and other neuroreceptor PET tracers is limited. They either show increased binding [^{11}C-Carfentanyl (μ-opioid receptor agonist), ^{11}C-Methylnaltrindole (δ-opioid receptor antagonist), ^{18}F-Cyclofoxy (μ,κ-opioid receptor antagonist), ^{11}C-Doxepin (H1 receptor antagonist), ^{11}C-L-Deprenyl (MAO-B inhibitor)] or decreased binding [^{11}C-Diprenorphine (μ,δ,κ-Opioid receptor antagonist), ^{11}C/^{18}F-FCWAY ($5HT_{1A}$ receptor antagonist), ^{18}F-MPPF ($5HT_{1A}$ receptor antagonist), ^{18}F-Altanserin ($5HT_{2A}$ receptor antagonist), ^{11}C-(S)-[N-methyl]-Ketamine (NMDA receptor antagonist), ^{11}C-NMBP ($_m$Ach receptor antagonist), ^{123}I-Iododexetimide ($_m$Ach receptor antagonist)]. However, because of paucity of data, their current role in presurgical evaluation is not yet established.

References

1. Carson RE. Precision and accuracy considerations of physiological quantitation in PET. J Cereb Blood Flow Metab 1991;11(2):A45–A50

2. Chugani HT, Phelps ME. Maturational changes in cerebral function in infants determined by 18FDG positron emission tomography. Science 1986;231(4740):840–843

3. Chugani HT, Phelps ME, Mazziotta JC. Positron emission tomography study of human brain functional development. Ann Neurol 1987;22(4):487–497

4. Gaillard WD, Kopylev L, Weinstein S, et al. Low incidence of abnormal (18)FDG-PET in children with new-onset partial epilepsy: a prospective study. Neurology 2002;58(5):717–722

5. Benedek K, Juhász C, Chugani DC, Muzik O, Chugani HT. Longitudinal changes in cortical glucose hypometabolism in children with intractable epilepsy. J Child Neurol 2006;21(1):26–31

6. Bouvard S, Costes N, Bonnefoi F, et al. Seizure-related short-term plasticity of benzodiazepine receptors in partial epilepsy: a [11C]flumazenil-PET study. Brain 2005;128(pt 6):1330–1343

7. Lee SK, Yun CH, Oh JB, et al. Intracranial ictal onset zone in nonlesional lateral temporal lobe epilepsy on scalp ictal EEG. Neurology 2003;61(6):757–764

8. Noachtar S, Arnold S, Yousry TA, Bartenstein P, Werhahn KJ, Tatsch K. Ictal technetium-99m ethyl cysteinate dimer single-photon emission tomographic findings and propagation of epileptic seizure activity in patients with extratemporal epilepsies. Eur J Nucl Med 1998;25(2):166–172

9. Williamson PD, Boon PA, Thadani VM, et al. Parietal lobe epilepsy: diagnostic considerations and results of surgery. Ann Neurol 1992;31(2):193–201

10. Williamson PD, Thadani VM, Darcey TM, Spencer DD, Spencer SS, Mattson RH. Occipital lobe epilepsy: clinical characteristics, seizure spread patterns, and results of surgery. Ann Neurol 1992;31(1):3–13

11. Hougaard K, Oikawa T, Sveinsdottir E, Skinoj E, Ingvar DH, Lassen NA. Regional cerebral blood flow in focal cortical epilepsy. Arch Neurol 1976;33(8):527–535

12. Prince DA, Wilder BJ. Control mechanisms in cortical epileptogenic foci. "Surround" inhibition. Arch Neurol 1967;16(2):194–202

13. Bruggemann JM, Som SS, Lawson JA, Haindl W, Cunningham AM, Bye AM. Application of statistical parametric mapping to SPET in the assessment of intractable childhood epilepsy. Eur J Nucl Med Mol Imaging 2004;31(3):369–377

14. Lee JD, Kim HJ, Lee BI, Kim OJ, Jeon TJ, Kim MJ. Evaluation of ictal brain SPET using statistical parametric mapping in temporal lobe epilepsy. Eur J Nucl Med 2000;27(11):1658–1665

15. Tae WS, Joo EY, Kim JH, et al. Cerebral perfusion changes in mesial temporal lobe epilepsy: SPM analysis of ictal and interictal SPECT. Neuroimage 2005;24(1):101–110

16. Muzik O, Chugani DC, Juhász C, Shen C, Chugani HT. Statistical parametric mapping: assessment of application in children. Neuroimage 2000;12(5):538–549

17. O'Brien TJ, So EL, Mullan BP, et al. Subtraction ictal SPECT co-registered to MRI improves clinical usefulness of SPECT in localizing the surgical seizure focus. Neurology 1998;50(2):445–454

18. O'Brien TJ, So EL, Mullan BP, et al. Subtraction SPECT co-registered to MRI improves postictal SPECT localization of seizure foci. Neurology 1999;52(1):137–146

19. Chiron C, Véra P, Kaminska A, et al. Ictal SPECT in the epileptic child. Contribution of subtraction interictal images and superposition of with MRI [in French]. Rev Neurol (Paris) 1999;155(6–7):477–481

20. O'Brien TJ, So EL, Mullan BP, et al. Subtraction peri-ictal SPECT is predictive of extratemporal epilepsy surgery outcome. Neurology 2000;55(11):1668–1677

21. Gaillard WD, Bhatia S, Bookheimer SY, Fazilat S, Sato S, Theodore WH. FDG-PET and volumetric MRI in the evaluation of patients with partial epilepsy. Neurology 1995;45(1):123–126

22. Henry TR, Frey KA, Sackellares JC, et al. In vivo cerebral metabolism and central benzodiazepine-receptor binding in temporal lobe epilepsy. Neurology 1993;43(10):1998–2006

23. Swartz BE, Halgren E, Delgado-Escueta AV, et al. Neuroimaging in patients with seizures of probable frontal lobe origin. Epilepsia 1989;30(5):547–558

24. Van Bogaert P, Massager N, Tugendhaft P, et al. Statistical parametric mapping of regional glucose metabolism in mesial temporal lobe epilepsy. Neuroimage 2000;12(2):129–138

25. Koepp MJ, Richardson MP, Brooks DJ, et al. Cerebral benzodiazepine receptors in hippocampal sclerosis. An objective in vivo analysis. Brain 1996;119(pt 5):1677–1687

26. Koepp MJ, Labbé C, Richardson MP, et al. Regional hippocampal [11C]flumazenil PET in temporal lobe epilepsy with unilateral and bilateral hippocampal sclerosis. Brain 1997;120(pt 10):1865–1876

27. Koepp MJ, Hammers A, Labbé C, Woermann FG, Brooks DJ, Duncan JS. 11C-flumazenil PET in patients with refractory temporal lobe epilepsy and normal MRI. Neurology 2000;54(2):332–339

28. Koepp MJ, Woermann FG. Imaging structure and function in refractory focal epilepsy. Lancet Neurol 2005;4(1):42–53

29. Lamusuo S, Pitkänen A, Jutila L, et al. [11 C]Flumazenil binding in the medial temporal lobe in patients with temporal lobe epilepsy: correlation with hippocampal MR volumetry, T2 relaxometry, and neuropathology. Neurology 2000;54(12):2252–2260

30. Bouilleret V, Dont S, Spelle L, Baulac M, Samson Y, Semah F. Insular cortex involvement in mesiotemporal lobe epilepsy: a positron emission tomography study. Ann Neurol 2002;51(2):202–208

31. Hammers A, Koepp MJ, Labbé C, et al. Neocortical abnormalities of [11C]-flumazenil PET in mesial temporal lobe epilepsy. Neurology 2001;56(7):897–906

32. Richardson MP, Friston KJ, Sisodiya SM, et al. Cortical grey matter and benzodiazepine receptors in malformations of cortical development. A voxel-based comparison of structural and functional imaging data. Brain 1997;120(pt 11):1961–1973

33. Richardson MP, Koepp MJ, Brooks DJ, Duncan JS. 11C-flumazenil PET in neocortical epilepsy. Neurology 1998;51(2):485–492

34. Richardson MP, Koepp MJ, Brooks DJ, Fish DR, Duncan JS. Benzodiazepine receptors in focal epilepsy with cortical dysgenesis: an 11C-flumazenil PET study. Ann Neurol 1996;40(2):188–198

35. Hammers A, Koepp MJ, Hurlemann R, et al. Abnormalities of grey and white matter [11C]flumazenil binding in temporal lobe epilepsy with normal MRI. Brain 2002;125(pt 10):2257–2271

36. Ho SS, Berkovic SF, McKay WJ, Kalnins RM, Bladin PF. Temporal lobe epilepsy subtypes: differential patterns of cerebral perfusion on ictal SPECT. Epilepsia 1996;37(8):788–795

37. Ho SS, Newton MR, McIntosh AM, et al. Perfusion patterns during temporal lobe seizures: relationship to surgical outcome. Brain 1997;120(pt 11):1921–1928

38. Benifla M, Otsubo H, Ochi A, et al. Temporal lobe surgery for intractable epilepsy in children: an analysis of outcomes in 126 children. Neurosurgery 2006;59(6):1203–1213, discussion 1213–1214

39. Harvey AS, Bowe JM, Hopkins IJ, Shield LK, Cook DJ, Berkovic SF. Ictal 99mTc-HMPAO single photon emission computed tomography in children with temporal lobe epilepsy. Epilepsia 1993;34(5):869–877

40. Lee JJ, Kang WJ, Lee DS, et al. Diagnostic performance of 18F-FDG PET and ictal 99mTc-HMPAO SPET in pediatric temporal lobe epilepsy: quantitative analysis by statistical parametric mapping, statistical probabilistic anatomical map, and subtraction ictal SPET. Seizure 2005;14(3):213–220

41. Rowe CC, Berkovic SF, Austin MC, McKay WJ, Bladin PF. Patterns of postictal cerebral blood flow in temporal lobe epilepsy: qualitative and quantitative analysis. Neurology 1991;41(7):1096–1103

42. Kaminska A, Chiron C, Ville D, et al. Ictal SPECT in children with epilepsy: comparison with intracranial EEG and relation to postsurgical outcome. Brain 2003;126(pt 1):248–260

43. Rowe CC, Berkovic SF, Austin M, McKay WJ, Bladin PF. Postictal SPET in epilepsy. Lancet 1989;1(8634):389–390

44. Valenti MP, Froelich S, Armspach JP, et al. Contribution of SISCOM imaging in the presurgical evaluation of temporal lobe epilepsy related to dysembryoplastic neuroepithelial tumors. Epilepsia 2002;43(3):270–276

45. da Silva EA, Chugani DC, Muzik O, Chugani HT. Identification of frontal lobe epileptic foci in children using positron emission tomography. Epilepsia 1997;38(11):1198–1208

46. Henry TR, Sutherling WW, Engel J Jr, et al. Interictal cerebral metabolism in partial epilepsies of neocortical origin. Epilepsy Res 1991;10(2–3):174–182

47. Kim YK, Lee DS, Lee SK, Chung CK, Chung JK, Lee MC. (18)F-FDG PET in localization of frontal lobe epilepsy: comparison of visual and SPM analysis. J Nucl Med 2002;43(9):1167–1174

48. Lee SK, Lee SY, Kim KK, Hong KS, Lee DS, Chung CK. Surgical outcome and prognostic factors of cryptogenic neocortical epilepsy. Ann Neurol 2005;58(4):525–532

49. Swartz BW, Khonsari A, Vrown C, Mandelkern M, Simpkins F, Krisdakumtorn T. Improved sensitivity of 18FDG-positron emission tomography scans in frontal and "frontal plus" epilepsy. Epilepsia 1995;36(4):388–395

50. Patil S, Biassoni L, Borgwardt L. Nuclear medicine in pediatric neurology and neurosurgery: epilepsy and brain tumors. Semin Nucl Med 2007;37(5):357–381

51. Juhász C, Chugani DC, Muzik O, et al. Electroclinical correlates of flumazenil and fluorodeoxyglucose PET abnormalities in lesional epilepsy. Neurology 2000;55(6):825–835

52. Muzik O, da Silva EA, Juhasz C, et al. Intracranial EEG versus flumazenil and glucose PET in children with extratemporal lobe epilepsy. Neurology 2000;54(1):171–179

53. Ryvlin P, Bouvard S, Le Bars D, et al. Clinical utility of flumazenil-PET versus [18F]fluorodeoxyglucose-PET and MRI in refractory partial epilepsy. A prospective study in 100 patients. Brain 1998;121(pt 11):2067–2081

54. Savic I, Thorell JO, Roland P. [11C]flumazenil positron emission tomography visualizes frontal epileptogenic regions. Epilepsia 1995;36(12):1225–1232

55. Arnold S, Berthele A, Drzezga A, et al. Reduction of benzodiazepine receptor binding is related to the seizure onset zone in extratemporal focal cortical dysplasia. Epilepsia 2000;41(7):818–824

56. Szelies B, Sobesky J, Pawlik G, et al. Impaired benzodiazepine receptor binding in peri-lesional cortex of patients with symptomatic epilepsies studied by [(11)C]-flumazenil PET. Eur J Neurol 2002;9(2):137–142

57. Juhász C, Chugani DC, Muzik O, et al. Alpha-methyl-L-tryptophan PET detects epileptogenic cortex in children with intractable epilepsy. Neurology 2003;60(6):960–968

58. Richardson MP, Hammers A, Brooks DJ, Duncan JS. Benzodiazepine-GABA(A) receptor binding is very low in dysembryoplastic neuroepithelial tumor: a PET study. Epilepsia 2001;42(10):1327–1334

59. Hwang SI, Kim JH, Park SW, et al. Comparative analysis of MR imaging, positron emission tomography, and ictal single-photon emission CT in patients with neocortical epilepsy. AJNR Am J Neuroradiol 2001;22(5):937–946

60. Véra P, Kaminska A, Cieuta C, et al. Use of subtraction ictal SPECT co-registered to MRI for optimizing the localization of seizure foci in children. J Nucl Med 1999;40(5):786–792

61. Chugani HT, Shewmon DA, Shields WD, et al. Surgery for intractable infantile spasms: neuroimaging perspectives. Epilepsia 1993;34(4):764–771

62. Chugani HT, Shields WD, Shewmon DA, Olson DM, Phelps ME, Peacock WJ. Infantile spasms: I. PET identifies focal cortical dysgenesis in cryptogenic cases for surgical treatment. Ann Neurol 1990;27(4):406–413

63. Chugani HT, Conti JR. Etiologic classification of infantile spasms in 140 cases: role of positron emission tomography. J Child Neurol 1996;11(1):44–48

64. Chugani HT, Shewmon DA, Sankar R, Chen BC, Phelps ME. Infantile spasms: II. Lenticular nuclei and brain stem activation on positron emission tomography. Ann Neurol 1992;31(2):212–219

65. Chugani DC, Muzik O, Chakraborty P, Mangner T, Chugani HT. Human brain serotonin synthesis capacity measured in vivo with alpha-[C-11]methyl-L-tryptophan. Synapse 1998;28(1):33–43

66. Stone TW. Kynurenines in the CNS: from endogenous obscurity to therapeutic importance. Prog Neurobiol 2001;64(2):185–218

67. Asano E, Chugani DC, Muzik O, et al. Multimodality imaging for improved detection of epileptogenic foci in tuberous sclerosis complex. Neurology 2000;54(10):1976–1984

68. Fedi M, Reutens DC, Andermann F, et al. alpha-[11C]-Methyl-L-tryptophan PET identifies the epileptogenic tuber and correlates with interictal spike frequency. Epilepsy Res 2003;52(3):203–213

69. Juhász C, Chugani DC, Asano E, et al. Alpha[11C]methyl-L-tryptophan positron emission tomography scanning in 176 patients with intractable epilepsy. Ann Neurol 2002;S118 (abstract)

70. Kagawa K, Chugani DC, Asano E, et al. Epilepsy surgery outcome in children with tuberous sclerosis complex evaluated with alpha-[11C]methyl-L-tryptophan positron emission tomography (PET). J Child Neurol 2005;20(5):429–438

71. Koh S, Jayakar P, Resnick T, Alvarez L, Liit RE, Duchowny M. The localizing value of ictal SPECT in children with tuberous sclerosis complex and refractory partial epilepsy. Epileptic Disord 1999;1(1):41–46

72. Chugani HT, Mazziotta JC, Engel J Jr, Phelps ME. The Lennox-Gastaut syndrome: metabolic subtypes determined by 2-deoxy-2[18F]fluoro-D-glucose positron emission tomography. Ann Neurol 1987;21(1):4–13

73. Iinuma K, Yanai K, Yanagisawa T, et al. Cerebral glucose metabolism in five patients with Lennox-Gastaut syndrome. Pediatr Neurol 1987;3(1):12–18

74. Theodore WH, Rose D, Patronas N, et al. Cerebral glucose metabolism in the Lennox-Gastaut syndrome. Ann Neurol 1987;21(1):14–21

75. Heiskala H, Launes J, Pihko H, Nikkinen P, Santavuori P. Brain perfusion SPECT in children with frequent fits. Brain Dev 1993;15(3):214–218

76. Chugani HT, Mazziotta JC, Phelps ME. Sturge-Weber syndrome: a study of cerebral glucose utilization with positron emission tomography. J Pediatr 1989;114(2):244–253

77. Juhász C, Batista CE, Chugani DC, Muzik O, Chugani HT. Evolution of cortical metabolic abnormalities and their clinical correlates in Sturge-Weber syndrome. Eur J Paediatr Neurol 2007;11(5):277–284

78. Lee JS, Asano E, Muzik O, et al. Sturge-Weber syndrome: correlation between clinical course and FDG PET findings. Neurology 2001;57(2):189–195

79. Pinton F, Chiron C, Enjolras O, Motte J, Syrota A, Dulac O. Early single photon emission computed tomography in Sturge-Weber syndrome. J Neurol Neurosurg Psychiatry 1997;63(5):616–621

80. Chiron C, Raynaud C, Tzourio N, et al. Regional cerebral blood flow by SPECT imaging in Sturge-Weber disease: an aid for diagnosis. J Neurol Neurosurg Psychiatry 1989;52(12):1402–1409

81. Bilgin O, Vollmar C, Peraud A, la Fougere C, Beleza P, Noachtar S. Ictal SPECT in Sturge-Weber syndrome. Epilepsy Res 2008;78(2–3):240–243

82. Kumar A, Chugani HT, Luat A, Asano E, Sood S. Epilepsy surgery in a case of encephalitis: use of 11C-PK11195 positron emission tomography. Pediatr Neurol 2008;38(6):439–442

83. Juhász C, Nagy F, Muzik O, Watson C, Shah J, Chugani HT. [11C]Flumazenil PET in patients with epilepsy with dual pathology. Epilepsia 1999;40(5):566–574

84. Morrell F. Secondary epileptogenesis in man. Arch Neurol 1985;42(4):318–335

85. Morrell F, deToledo-Morrell L. From mirror focus to secondary epileptogenesis in man: an historical review. Adv Neurol 1999;81:11–23

86. Juhász C, Asano E, Shah A, et al. Focal decreases of cortical GABAA receptor binding remote from the primary seizure focus: what do they indicate? Epilepsia 2009;50(2):240–250

87. Wetjen NM, Cascino GD, Fessler AJ, et al. Subtraction ictal single-photon emission computed tomography coregistered to magnetic resonance imaging in evaluating the need for repeated epilepsy surgery. J Neurosurg 2006;105(1):71–76

88. Juhász C, Chugani DC, Padhye UN, et al. Evaluation with alpha-[11C]methyl-L-tryptophan positron emission tomography for reoperation after failed epilepsy surgery. Epilepsia 2004;45(2):124–130

11 Coregistration and Newer Imaging Techniques

John M. K. Mislow and Alexandra J. Golby

In presurgical evaluation of medically intractable epilepsy, knowledge of the precise location of the seizure focus is of paramount importance. Despite advances in imaging technologies, it is difficult to evaluate data from multiple structural and functional imaging modalities in an integrated fashion. Thus, clinicians may not be able to synthesize all of the available data in the most effective fashion. As such, coregistration of multiple modalities has proven to be an invaluable tool in the armementarium of the surgical team and has led to an increase in the number of patients offered surgery for epilepsy in the United States.[1] In addition, as coregistration has improved neurosurgical efficacy, newer imaging techniques have improved presurgical lesion detection as well as demonstrating abnormalities in nonlesional epilepsy, such as hippocampal atrophy or sclerosis, cortical dysplasia, or small vascular lesions or tumors.[2]

■ Coregistration

Direct data fusion technique superimposes multiple images and presents the surgeon with a coarse approximation of the location of functional regions. This may be adequate when the surgical target is single, discrete, and in noneloquent territory. However, if the target is multifocal, indistinct, or in eloquent cortex, an understanding of the correlation between structure and function is very helpful.

Coregistration is the process of volumetrically fusing processed functional images onto a structural image by using imaging data shared by all images[3,4] and as such offers a significant advantage over direct image overlay. Image-to-image coregistration commonly relies on the identification of mutual points in both images known as tie-points. As such, software packages designed to coregister images, such as Statistical Parametric Mapping (SPM, The Mathworks, Inc. Natick, MA) FreeSurfer (A.A. Martinos Center for Biomedical Imaging, Boston, MA), 3D Slicer (Boston, MA), AFNI (Bethesda, MD), Computerized anatomical reconstruction and editing toolkit (Caret, St Louis, MS), commonly use an automated, area-based technique for identifying image tie-points. Coregistration software executes either a linear or nonlinear transformation; linear transformation is technically easier and faster than nonlinear transformation but

yields significantly lower-quality image coregistration.[5] Initially, functional data derived from positron emission tomography (PET) single photon emission computed tomography (SPECT) would be volumetrically coregistered with a standardized stereotaxic brain atlas such as that of Talairach and Tournoux,[6,7] but variations in gross morphology and microstructure of the human brain[8] make an atlas-based methodology unreliable in presurgical planning for individual patients.[9] As a result, clinical coregistration generally implies that all data involved in volumetric fusion are derived entirely from the individual patient.

One of the first efforts to address the challenge of image data fusion for surgical planning was Mountz and colleagues' description of the fusion of SPECT and computed tomography (CT) images of patients' brains as a method of providing an accurate and noninvasive method for correlating function (in the form of blood flow) and neuroanatomy.[10] The authors demonstrate lesion/pathology in clinical examples of tumor, developmental abnormality (autism), cerebrovascular disease, and, notably, in epilepsy via injection of tracer during ictal phase of seizure.[10]

The arrival of magnetic resonance imaging (MRI) heralded clinicians' ability to define neuroanatomical targets with high precision. As such, MRI replaced CT for surgical planning, and MRI–PET coregistration eclipsed PET–CT coregistration as standard of care in presurgical planning (see **Fig. 11.1**). Evidence of this evolution was borne out by Viñas and colleagues' study of MRI–PET coregistration in presurgical planning for epilepsy surgery in eloquent cortex.[11] Twelve patients underwent preoperative MRI–PET coregistration with motor, visual, and language mapping and subsequently underwent an awake craniotomy with MRI-assisted image guidance and intraoperative cortical stimulation or visual evoked potentials. The researchers found that PET was reliable in identifying most (but not all) motor, visual, and language cortex, leading to their conclusion that MRI–PET coregistration is a useful tool for identification of eloquent cortex in the setting of neurosurgical preplanning.[11] Although the authors concluded that intraoperative cortical stimulation and visual evoked potential remained the gold standard for cortical mapping,[11] further refinements of SPECT, PET, and MRI have given this type of coregistration increased precision and reliability in presurgical planning for epilepsy (see **Fig. 11.2**).[12,13]

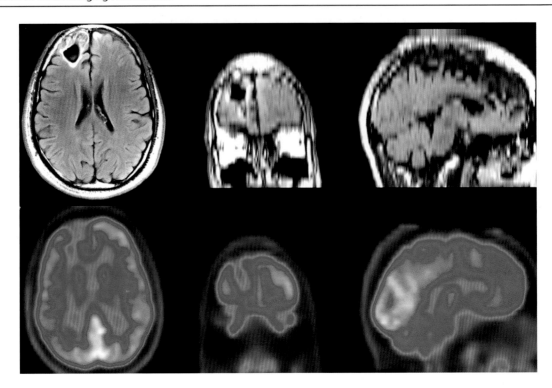

Fig. 11.1 Positron emission tomography–magnetic resonance imaging coregistration in a patient with new-onset epilepsy. The region of hypometabolism in the right frontal lobe corresponds to the site of a previously drained abscess, indicating that this is the lesion causing the patient's symptoms. *Image courtesy of Dr. Laura Horky.*

A particularly effective refinement was that of "fuzzy modeling" in which Boussion and colleagues were able to demonstrate results in accordance with the "gold standard" investigation (deep electrodes or postsurgical outcome) in 11 of 12 patients in a clinical study when fuzzy logic was applied to modeling PET and MRI coregistration.[14] With further refinements, PET–MRI coregistration has proven to be clinically valuable in patients outside the purview of medically refractory epilepsy: by differentiating actual hypoperfusion from artifactual hypoperfusion resulting from partial volume effects and also to improve the accuracy of asymmetry indexes in interictal patients, the use broadened to patients with partial epilepsy.[12] Another challenge during the infancy of coregistration was speed—significant off-line processing and manual registration work was necessary to achieve acceptably accurate coregistered PET–MRI images.[15] By combining a multiresolution approach with an automatic segmentation of input image volumes into areas of interest and background, Cízek and colleagues demonstrated that with suitable preprocessing, the time to coregister PET and MRI images with robust accuracy could be reduced by ten-fold.[16]

The next step in coregistration was the combination of MRI, CT, and PET coregistration to assist in image-guided placement of subdural electrodes and then using the information gathered by the subdural electrodes (combined with the precise location of the electrodes by CT) to aid in surgical resection of the suspected epileptogenic focus in patients undergoing image-guided surgical treatment of epilepsy.[17–20] The advent of readily available digital cameras has ushered in an even higher level of certainty in epilepsy surgery; because coregistration of digital photographs of the brain cortex with the results of three-dimensional MRI datasets is now possible,[21,22] it allows for identification of anatomical details underlying the subdural grid electrodes and enhances the intraoperative certainty and precision of the neurosurgeon. In addition, surgical navigation systems found in most modern neurosurgical operating theaters allow for coregistration of preoperative datasets to intraoperative head position of the patient.[23,24]

The clinical effectiveness of multimodal coregistration has been borne out in several studies. In 2004, Murphy and colleagues evaluated the outcomes of 22 patients selected to undergo multimodal coregistration [PET–MRI, SPECT–MRI, or fluid attenuation inversion recovery (FLAIR)–MRI] for presurgical planning because of no lesion visible on conventional MRI sequences, multiple lesions, or one very large lesion that could not be completely resected without the risk of significant postoperative morbidity.[1] Another group with lesions within eloquent cortex was included in the study and underwent further coregistration with subdural electrocorticography grids.[1,17] After an average of 27 months postsurgical follow-up, the authors found that 77% of the patients

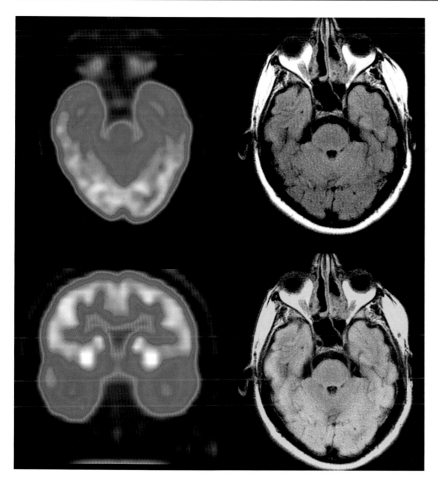

Fig. 11.2 Positron emission tomography–magnetic resonance imaging coregistration demonstrating left temporal hypometabolism, which can prove vital in lateralizing and localizing a seizure focus in nonlesional epilepsy. *Image courtesy of Dr. Laura Horky.*

had excellent outcomes for their seizures, and 86% had favorable outcomes. One patient suffered a permanent major deficit, whereas three other patients suffered permanent minor deficits. In light of the fact that all of these patients would have been poor surgical candidates without presurgical multimodal coregistration, this study provides a strong argument that this approach may allow the reevaluation of patients previously denied surgery because of the selection criteria outlined by the paper's authors.

Murphy et al's findings were confirmed in 2007 when Doelken et al studied 49 temporal lobe epilepsy (TLE) patients with coregistration of MRI, MRI spectroscopy, and SPECT and compared the imaging results with that of traditional noninvasive EEG-video monitoring and evaluated lateralization of affected hemisphere with regard to bilateral affection and postoperative outcome.[25] The authors found that EEG and MRI had a high concordance in establishing unilaterality or bilaterality for TLE and epileptogenic focus and, under the circumstances of ambiguous laterality on MRI or EEG, SPECT and MR spectroscopy, aided in identifying an epileptogenic focus, and, if so, if the lesion was unilateral or bilateral.[25] As a result, the study demonstrated that multimodal imaging for epilepsy helps in identifying bilateral involvement, which is important to identify the patients who will not benefit from epilepsy surgery.

■ Newer Imaging Technologies

Functional MRI (fMRI) has been used in surgical epilepsy patients to lateralize and localize language function[26,27] and to lateralize memory function in mesial temporal lobe (MTL) epilepsy[28] as well as for localization of sensorimotor function in extratemporal epilepsy.[24] However, using the statistical parametric mapping (SPM) or other approaches to create functional maps from the acquired images do not provide real time information to the clinician. This obstacle appears to have been overcome by Kesavadas and colleagues by using real-time fMRI instead of offline analysis; in a 10-patient study where a comparison of real-time fMRI and offline SPM processing was performed, significant concordance between the two techniques was noted, effectively demonstrating that real-time fMRI could be performed easily and effectively for pre-surgical evaluation of pediatric epilepsy.[29]

Diffusion tensor imaging (DTI) is an emerging imaging technology that offers great promise in reducing morbidity and mortality in neurosurgery, as well as increasing intraoperative precision in removal of epileptogenic targets. By evaluating the motion of water at the voxel level via quantitative measures of diffusion and fractional anisotropy, DTI can provide data on the structural integrity of brain tissue.[3,30] This radiological evaluation of the orientation of the preferential diffusion of water can create images of major white matter pathways in the brain, and as a result, can deduce the structural basis of cerebral networks.[3,30,31] (see **Fig. 11.3**). By collecting both functional and anatomical connectivity data via high-resolution neuroimaging methods such as MRI, fMRI, and DTI, the neurosurgeon may now visualize the three-dimensional structure of the patient's brain and evaluate what pathways may be disrupted or displaced by a lesion (e.g., sclerosis from TLE, tumor).[3,23,32]

Magnetoencephalography (MEG) is another emerging imaging technology in the field of epilepsy. In MEG, arrays of superconducting quantum interference devices detect magnetic fields (10^{-12} Tesla) generated by intraneuronal currents of the human brain in real time.[33] MEG offers a direct measurement neural electrical activity with high temporal resolution but relatively low spatial resolution.[33] An advantage of cogregistering MEG data over EEG data

with MRI or fMRI is absence of magnetic field distortion and attenuation by conductivities between scalp and EEG electrodes.[33] Recent clinical data from RamachandranNair and colleagues indicate that presurgical planning with MEG yielded good prediction of which patients would be appropriate surgical candidates, because postoperative seizure freedom was less likely to occur in children with bilateral MEG dipole clusters or only scattered dipoles.[34] In addition, the authors demonstrated that MEG may be accompanied by EEG data to determine which patients may or may not be good surgical candidates, because seizure freedom in the clinical study was most likely to occur when there was concordance between EEG and MEG localization and least likely to occur when these results were divergent.[34]

Lastly, intraoperative MRI within the surgical suite provides real-time acquisition of MRI scans without moving the patient, online image-guided stereotaxy without preoperative imaging, and "real-time" tracking of instruments in the operative field registered to the MRI.[35] This imaging modality helps surgeons compensate for the architectural distortion from "brain shift" after craniotomy and lesion resection, and, with newer imaging algorithms, coregistered preoperative images such as fMRI, PET, and DTI can be altered and reregistered with the new intraoperative MRI to negotiate eloquent territories.[36–38]

All these imaging modalities, in particular those that image neurological function (e.g., fMRI, MEG, DTI) have great potential for improvement in spatial and temporal resolution. As device resolution increases (e.g., 3+ Tesla for MRI, faster image acquisition for fMRI and DTI, higher spatial accuracy for MEG) the accuracy in detecting and localizing epileptogenic foci promises to greatly expand these modalities' clinical value and efficacy.

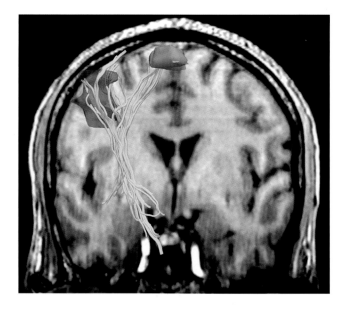

Fig. 11.3 Diffusion tensor imaging–functional magnetic resonance imaging (DTI–fMRI) coregistration. DTI illustrates the corticospinal tract and fMRI represents hand and foot movement. Coregistration of these two modalities demonstrates that it is the corticospinal tract of the hand and foot regions, illustrating that the combination of image modalities is more useful than either modality alone. *Image courtesy of Dr. Ali Radmanesh.*

■ Conclusion

Accuracy and precision remain the hallmarks of neurosurgery, and recent advances in image guidance technology represent a considerable asset to the armamentarium of tools at the disposal of the neurosurgeon. With the advent of image coregistration and introduction of newer imaging modalities, multiple images including intraoperative MRI, fMRI, CT, PET, SPECT, DTI, EEG, and MEG can all be volumetrically fused to paint an extraordinarily intricate and precise portrait of a patient's functional neuroanatomy. These accurate visual renderings contribute significantly to enable surgeons to navigate delicate neurosurgical procedures with increasing safety and efficacy. Further improvements in functional neuroimaging devices and coregistration software will continue to increase the ease and efficacy of neuronavigation in functional neurosurgery.

Acknowledgments The authors gratefully acknowledge the following grant support: NIH F32-NS061483-01A1 (John M. K. Mislow); NIH P01-CA67165, U41-RR 019703, K08 NS48063-01 (Alexandra J. Golby); and the Brain Science Foundation.

This chapter is dedicated in memory of John Mislow, MD, PhD, with great affection and admiration. His creative intellect and sparkling manner are greatly missed.

References

1. Murphy MA, O'Brien TJ, Morris K, Cook MJ. Multimodality image-guided surgery for the treatment of medically refractory epilepsy. J Neurosurg 2004;100(3):452–462

2. Brázdil M, Mikl M, Chlebus P, et al. Combining advanced neuroimaging techniques in presurgical workup of non-lesional intractable epilepsy. Epileptic Disord 2006;8(3):190–194

3. Rykhlevskaia E, Gratton G, Fabiani M. Combining structural and functional neuroimaging data for studying brain connectivity: a review. Psychophysiology 2008;45(2):173–187

4. Wells WM III, Viola P, Atsumi H, Nakajima S, Kikinis R. Multi-modal volume registration by maximization of mutual information. Med Image Anal 1996;1(1):35–51

5. Sugiura M, Kawashima R, Sadato N, et al. Anatomic validation of spatial normalization methods for PET. J Nucl Med 1999;40(2):317–322

6. Talairach J, Tournoux P. Co-planar Stereotaxic Atlas of the Human Brain: 3-Dimensional Proportional System—an Approach to Cerebral Imaging. New York, NY: Thieme Medical; 1988

7. Collins DL, Neelin P, Peters TM, Evans AC. Automatic 3D intersubject registration of MR volumetric data in standardized Talairach space. J Comput Assist Tomogr 1994;18(2):192–205

8. Fischl B, Sereno MI, Tootell RB, Dale AM. High-resolution intersubject averaging and a coordinate system for the cortical surface. Hum Brain Mapp 1999;8(4):272–284

9. Brett M, Johnsrude IS, Owen AM. The problem of functional localization in the human brain. Nat Rev Neurosci 2002;3(3):243–249

10. Mountz JM, Zhang B, Liu HG, Inampudi C. A reference method for correlation of anatomic and functional brain images: validation and clinical application. Semin Nucl Med 1994;24(4):256–271

11. Viñas FC, Zamorano L, Mueller RA, et al. [15O]-water PET and intraoperative brain mapping: a comparison in the localization of eloquent cortex. Neurol Res 1997;19(6):601–608

12. Shiga T, Morita K, Takano A, et al. Clinical advantages of interictal SPECT coregistered to magnetic resonance imaging in patients with epilepsy. Clin Nucl Med 2001;26(4):334–339

13. Shin WC, Hong SB, Tae WS, Seo DW, Kim SE. Ictal hyperperfusion of cerebellum and basal ganglia in temporal lobe epilepsy: SPECT subtraction with MRI coregistration. J Nucl Med 2001;42(6):853–858

14. Boussion N, Cinotti L, Barra V, Ryvlin P, Mauguiere F. Extraction of epileptogenic foci from PET and SPECT images by fuzzy modeling and data fusion. Neuroimage 2003;19(3):645–654

15. Pietrzyk U. Registration of MRI and PET images for clinical applications. In: Hajnal J, Hawkes D, Hill D, eds. Medical Image Registration. Boca Raton, Fla.: CRC Press; 2001:199–216

16. Cízek J, Herholz K, Vollmar S, Schrader R, Klein J, Heiss WD. Fast and robust registration of PET and MR images of human brain. Neuroimage 2004;22(1):434–442

17. Hogan RE, Lowe VJ, Bucholz RD. Triple-technique (MR imaging, single-photon emission CT, and CT) coregistration for image-guided surgical evaluation of patients with intractable epilepsy. AJNR Am J Neuroradiol 1999;20(6):1054–1058

18. Kovalev D, Spreer J, Honegger J, Zentner J, Schulze-Bonhage A, Huppertz HJ. Rapid and fully automated visualization of subdural electrodes in the presurgical evaluation of epilepsy patients. AJNR Am J Neuroradiol 2005;26(5):1078–1083

19. Ken S, Di Gennaro G, Giulietti G, et al. Quantitative evaluation for brain CT/MRI coregistration based on maximization of mutual information in patients with focal epilepsy investigated with subdural electrodes. Magn Reson Imaging 2007;25(6):883–888

20. Zhang Y, van Drongelen W, Kohrman M, He B. Three-dimensional brain current source reconstruction from intra-cranial ECoG recordings. Neuroimage 2008;42(2):683–695

21. Dalal SS, Edwards E, Kirsch HE, Barbaro NM, Knight RT, Nagarajan SS. Localization of neurosurgically implanted electrodes via photograph-MRI-radiograph coregistration. J Neurosci Methods 2008;174(1):106–115

22. Mahvash M, König R, Wellmer J, Urbach H, Meyer B, Schaller K. Coregistration of digital photography of the human cortex and cranial magnetic resonance imaging for visualization of subdural electrodes in epilepsy surgery. Neurosurgery 2007; 61(5, suppl 2)340–344, discussion 344–345

23. O'Shea JP, Whalen S, Branco DM, Petrovich NM, Knierim KE, Golby AJ. Integrated image- and function-guided surgery in eloquent cortex: a technique report. Int J Med Robot 2006;2(1):75–83

24. Tharin S, Golby A. Functional brain mapping and its applications to neurosurgery. Neurosurgery 2007; 60(4, suppl 2)185–201, discussion 201–202

25. Doelken MT, Richter G, Stefan H, et al. Multimodal coregistration in patients with temporal lobe epilepsy—results of different imaging modalities in lateralization of the affected hemisphere in MR imaging positive and negative subgroups. AJNR Am J Neuroradiol 2007;28(3):449–454

26. Gabrieli JD, Poldrack RA, Desmond JE. The role of left prefrontal cortex in language and memory. Proc Natl Acad Sci U S A 1998;95(3):906–913

27. Wagner AD, Desmond JE, Glover GH, Gabrieli JD. Prefrontal cortex and recognition memory. Functional-MRI evidence for context-dependent retrieval processes. Brain 1998;121(pt 10):1985–2002

28. Golby AJ, Poldrack RA, Illes J, Chen D, Desmond JE, Gabrieli JD. Memory lateralization in medial temporal lobe epilepsy assessed by functional MRI. Epilepsia 2002;43(8):855–863

29. Kesavadas C, Thomas B, Sujesh S, et al. Real-time functional MR imaging (fMRI) for presurgical evaluation of paediatric epilepsy. Pediatr Radiol 2007;37(10):964–974

30. Duncan JS. Imaging the brain's highways—diffusion tensor imaging in epilepsy. Epilepsy Curr 2008;8(4):85–89

31. Karis JP; Expert Panel on Neurologic Imaging. Epilepsy. AJNR Am J Neuroradiol 2008;29(6):1222–1224

32. Archip N, Clatz O, Whalen S, et al. Non-rigid alignment of pre-operative MRI, fMRI, and DT-MRI with intra-operative MRI for enhanced visualization and navigation in image-guided neurosurgery. Neuroimage 2007;35(2):609–624

33. Knowlton RC. Can magnetoencephalography aid epilepsy surgery? Epilepsy Curr 2008;8(1):1–5

34. RamachandranNair R, Otsubo H, Shroff MM, et al. MEG predicts outcome following surgery for intractable epilepsy in children with normal or nonfocal MRI findings. Epilepsia 2007;48(1):149–157

35. Moriarty TM, Kikinis R, Jolesz FA, Black PM, Alexander E III. Magnetic resonance imaging therapy. Intraoperative MR imaging. Neurosurg Clin N Am 1996;7(2):323–331

36. Nimsky C, Ganslandt O, Cerny S, Hastreiter P, Greiner G, Fahlbusch R. Quantification of, visualization of, and compensation for brain shift using intraoperative magnetic resonance imaging. Neurosurgery 2000;47(5):1070–1079, discussion 1079–1080

37. Upadhyay UM, Golby AJ. Role of pre- and intraoperative imaging and neuronavigation in neurosurgery. Expert Rev Med Devices 2008;5(1):65–73

38. Archip N, Clatz O, Whalen S, et al. Compensation of geometric distortion effects on intraoperative magnetic resonance imaging for enhanced visualization in image-guided neurosurgery. Neurosurgery 2008; 62(3, suppl 1)209–215, discussion 215–216

12 Wada Testing in Pediatric Epilepsy

David W. Loring and Gregory P. Lee

The Wada test is an essential component of the preoperative evaluation of epilepsy patients at most epilepsy surgery centers. In addition to establishing cerebral language representation preoperatively, Wada memory results may be used to establish risk for postoperative memory decline and to assist in identification of focal functional deficits associated with a unilateral seizure focus.[1-4] Although a substantial Wada clinical literature in adults exists, there have been relatively few reports describing Wada test experience in pediatric epilepsy surgery candidates.

Wada introduced his technique of intracarotid injection of amobarbital in the 1950s to establish cerebral language representation in adult patients who were undergoing evaluation for epilepsy surgery.[5] The procedure relies on a short-acting barbiturate introduced into the internal carotid artery that temporarily anesthetizes the anterior two thirds of a cerebral hemisphere during which language testing is conducted. The most common anesthetic agent is amobarbital, although other drugs are successfully used, including etomidate,[6] methohexital,[7] and propofol.[8] These newer agents have a shorter duration of action than amobarbital, and, in the case of etomidate, a constant infusion of drug is necessary to produce a sufficient length of anesthesia to permit language and memory testing.

After observing several cases of unanticipated significant decline in memory function after temporal lobectomy, a memory component was introduced as part of the Wada test to provide a reversible model of temporal lobe surgery in which the risk of developing severe anterograde amnesia could be estimated.[9] The Wada test thus creates a reversible pharmacologic lesion in which induced behavioral deficits are thought to reflect surgical risk of including these areas in a surgical resection. At most centers performing the Wada, both language and memory functions are assessed.

Language results often guide specific clinical decision making. When surgery is planned in a hemisphere dominant for language, generally more conservative surgical approaches are used, and additional measures to protect eloquent language cortex such as electrocortical stimulation mapping are performed. Although the goals of Wada memory testing vary across epilepsy centers, the test's primary purpose is to establish risk for postoperative memory decline. In addition, however, interhemispheric memory asymmetry scores may be used to help confirm seizure onset laterality in patients with less clearly established seizure onset. Patients in whom both structural and functional measures of unilateral mesial temporal lobe dysfunction are in agreement tend to have superior surgical efficacy, as well as decreased cognitive morbidity, in comparison with patients in whom there is incomplete agreement regarding lateralized impairment.

The majority of clinical experience with Wada testing has been derived from adults. However, because neurodevelopment in pediatric patients is incomplete, patterns of expected performance in adults cannot necessarily be generalized to pediatric groups, and the predictive ability of Wada testing to accurately forecast long-term cognitive outcomes may be altered by neuroplasticity and cognitive maturation.

■ Special Considerations for Pediatric Wada Testing

Testing of pediatric epilepsy patients presents unique challenges compared with adults. The Wada test is often a physically uncomfortable and emotionally frightening procedure for younger children to undergo, and they sometimes lack the appropriate maturity to participate fully in all aspects of the evaluation. Even before the potential effects of drug-induced behavioral deficits, which themselves may be frightening, the surgical aspects of catheter placement for medication delivery often exceed a child's capacity to tolerate and cooperate with the procedure. Coaching and developing behavioral intervention techniques may be useful in decreasing the anxiety associated with the procedure, but these approaches are often of limited utility, are labor and time intensive, and are less useful in younger patients or in children with decreased cognitive abilities and less insight. Pre-Wada baseline assessment is more extensive and carefully constructed in children than adults because the stimulus materials selected for use during the Wada must be tailored to the developmental and cognitive level of each child. Because of these constraints, children younger than 7 or 8 years old are generally considered unsuitable candidates for the procedure.

In youngsters who are unusually sensitive to pain or who may have difficulties cooperating for other reasons, sedation may be administered by an anesthesiologist to assist with catheter placement.[10] Propofol, for example, is sufficiently short acting that anesthesia recovery is rapid, and Wada testing can be performed within 15 to 25 minutes after propofol cessation. Thus, anxiety and discomfort associated with catheter insertion can be avoided using propofol in appropriate cases, thereby maximizing the likelihood of obtaining valid Wada behavioral results. Unfortunately, some children awaken from the anesthesia disoriented or overly emotional and require much soothing before they are capable of proceeding with Wada testing. In some cases, a parent may be an asset in helping to calm the child in the immediate post-anesthesia period. Parents may then be escorted out of the angiography suite after they have quieted their children but before amobarbital injection.

■ Wada Language Testing in Pediatrics

Because children who are evaluated for epilepsy surgery have extratemporal lobe epilepsy more often than adults, the critical information derived from Wada testing is often language laterality and representation, and Wada memory findings assume less importance. The need for valid determination of language lateralization by Wada testing is clear, if the gold standard of language localization is electrocortical stimulation mapping. Although stimulation mapping has reportedly been successfully performed in children as young as 4 years of age,[11] in addition to the greater difficulties involved in stimulation language mapping with children, language cortex is less likely to be identified with mapping in children under 10 years of age.[12] In one recent study, the presence of positive language results from stimulation language mapping was no different in children 10 years or older than it was in adults. Although these authors also described less reliable Wada language results for children younger than 10 years compared with older children, the magnitude of this difference was not as marked. Thus, Wada language testing appears more likely to succeed in identifying language representation in children than electrocortical stimulation mapping does.

Overall level of cognitive ability has been associated with the likelihood of obtaining useful Wada information in children.[13] In a small series of 22 pediatric patients (ages 5–12 years), language testing was successful in all of the children with IQs of at least 70, whereas only 57% of the children studied satisfactorily completed Wada language testing if their IQs were below 70. A similar pattern was seen with Wada memory results. Children with IQs of 70 or higher had good retention scores after injection ipsilateral to seizure onset but impaired retention after contralateral injection, whereas children with IQs of at least 70 were much less likely to show

this lateralized discrepancy. In another pediatric series, the Wada procedure successfully established hemispheric language dominance and memory representation in fewer than two thirds of 42 preadolescent candidates for epilepsy surgery.[14] Risk factors for unsuccessful testing included low Full-Scale IQ (especially < 80), young age (especially < 10 years), and left hemisphere seizure onset. The symptoms of aphasia seen in children during Wada testing also differ from those typically seen in adults, which may complicate interpretation. Many times, children simply become mute during Wada testing, and hence, there are often no positive signs of aphasia, such as paraphasic substitution errors or circumlocutions, to help confirm that language has been affected.

■ Wada Memory Testing in Pediatrics

The role of Wada memory testing has evolved since its introduction. The need to identify patients at risk for the development of a persistent frank amnesia by identifying significant contralateral mesial temporal lobe damage to the proposed temporal lobe surgery has been a significant topic in preoperative assessment of epilepsy surgery patients. Wada memory results are used to counsel patients regarding the likelihood of memory decline, which, even if not frank amnesia, is of sufficient severity to interfere with quality of life, cognitive development, and other factors that may affect school performance.[15]

Wada memory testing is intended to assess the functional integrity of the mesial temporal lobe and, to a smaller degree, the entire hemisphere being perfused with the anesthetic. This procedure differs significantly from other functional assessments in that it assesses each hemisphere in isolation, thereby helping to disentangle the effects of parallel distributed brain networks. The functional reserve capacity of the contralateral temporal lobe to sustain memory function in isolation is assessed when the hemisphere ipsilateral to a mesial temporal lobe focus is anesthetized[16] and was the original goal of Wada memory testing when the procedure was first designed to avoid postoperative global amnesia. Because there are varying degrees of residual function in the diseased temporal lobe, the potential mnemonic contributions of the mesial temporal lobe structures ipsilateral to the seizure focus also must be assessed. This evaluates the functional adequacy of the diseased temporal lobe. Functional adequacy is assessed during injection contralateral to seizure onset. The relative differences between the memory performance of each hemisphere are termed *Wada memory asymmetry* (WMA).

Although Wada memory results are not a primary measure to lateralize seizure onset, WMAs may help clinical decision making when interpreted in the context of other clinical findings. The complex process of clinical determination of seizure onset laterality often relies on the convergence of findings from multiple sources. Thus, WMAs have clinical implications that can either increase or decrease the confidence of unilateral seizure onset in cases with difficult to lateralize seizures. Patients with clinical findings that are not in complete agreement regarding seizure onset laterality or location are often thought to be less ideal candidates, with decreased likelihood of becoming seizure free and an increased risk of postoperative cognitive morbidity.

WMAs in pediatric populations correspond to seizure onset laterality both on the group level and on individual patient basis.[17] In a series of 87 children from three different institutions, Wada memory testing was able to accurately lateralize seizure onset in 69% of the sample, a rate that is somewhat lower than the rate of 70 to 88% correct classification in studies of adult surgical candidates. This slightly worse rate of seizure lateralization prediction in children is probably caused by the lower prevalence of temporal lobe seizures in the pediatric population.

Because Wada protocols are not standardized, it is sometimes difficult to estimate to what degree method variance contributes to some of the reported variability in memory outcome prediction. We have shown that factors such as stimulus type (pictures versus real objects),[18] timing of stimulus presentation,[19] mixed stimuli requiring a verbal response, and amobarbital dose[20] are related to Wada memory correlations with seizure onset laterality. The potential confound of aphasia on certain verbal memory stimuli is well recognized,[21] and generalizations of specific results to other Wada memory protocols must necessarily be made cautiously.[22]

As is the case in the adult Wada experience, a specific Wada protocol is used for assessment involves the likelihood of obtaining lateralized findings.[23] Wada memory testing involved the presentation of information to be remembered after the introduction of medication, and this material may include line drawings, pictures, real objects, words, or designs. Compared with real objects, however, mixed stimulus Wada memory testing appears less sensitive to unilateral seizures in children and adolescents. This method discrepancy is greater in children with left-sided seizure onset and is seen on both the group and individual patient level. Further, the risk of incorrect classification based on Wada memory asymmetries is greater in the mixed stimulus method compared with real object. For example, when using the mixed stimulus Wada memory testing, approximately one third of children in both the temporal and nontemporal groups had seizure onset laterality incorrectly lateralized. The mixed stimulus method also incorrectly predicted the side of seizure onset in 25% of right-hemisphere seizure patients. This finding contrasts with WMAs obtained using real objects in which 18% of children with focal seizures arising in the left hemisphere, and no (0%) child with left temporal lobe seizures had their seizure onset laterality incorrectly classified.

Several approaches have been used to validate Wada memory testing in adults. Although memory outcome might be considered the ideal variable for validation, Wada memory findings are used to establish surgical candidacy, which confounds the predicative and outcome variables. Although there are reports of successful memory outcomes after Wada memory failure,[24] there are also cases of amnesia in which Wada memory results appeared to predict that outcome.[25] In addition to memory outcome studies, there have been numerous reports suggesting a relationship between Wada memory scores and hippocampal volume or cell counts.[1,26–29] Both hippocampal volumes and WMAs are related to postoperative verbal memory decline.[1,3,4,30–33]

Prediction of postoperative memory change remains among the most important aspects of Wada memory testing. Postoperative risk, whether for cognitive change or efficacy in treating seizures, depends in part on concurrence of preoperative clinical findings. Children without WMAs or with WMAs in the direction opposite of that predicted based on clinical semiology are considered to be at higher risk of postoperative memory decline compared with children with WMAs in the predicted direction. In a retrospective review of 132 children who received resective epilepsy surgery, approximately 70% had WMAs corresponding to the side of surgery. Children without WMAs corresponding to seizure onset laterality demonstrated significant postoperative verbal memory decline, whereas children with appropriate WMAs showed significantly improved verbal memory scores after surgery. When examined on the individual patient level, 77% of children with WMAs in predicted direction showed no verbal memory decline after surgery, whereas 80% of children without correct WMAs had lower postoperative verbal memory for story recall tasks. WMAs had no value in predicting postoperative changes in visual–spatial memory.

Our series found greater sensitivity of story memory for assessing verbal decline in children, whereas in adults, the decline in verbal memory is best captured with word list tasks.[3,31] Whether these findings for story memory result from a greater number of nontemporal cases in unknown. However, because the neural and cognitive systems are in the process of development in children, the brain–memory test associations established for adults may be less applicable to children. It has been suggested that children recruit more neural tissue to perform certain linguistic tasks on functional imaging, for example, than do adults. This difference may be reflected in a different pattern of memory test failure after focal cortical resection in children.

■ Conclusion

Wada testing is a valuable tool to establish language representation and memory function in children. Although the procedure is often technically more difficult to perform in children than adults (e.g., need for anesthesia during angiography), and the results are more difficult to interpret (e.g., mutism, behavior problems, wider range of skill levels), Wada testing has clearly been validated for use in the preoperative evaluation of pediatric epilepsy surgery candidates. The likelihood of obtaining satisfactory results depends on many factors such as the maturity of the individual child. Factors that have been associated with the likelihood of obtaining valid Wada results include age (Wada testing of children younger than 10 years of age is much less likely to provide useful results) and general cognitive function (children with IQs less than 70–80 are less likely to be good candidates).

Although Wada memory testing is less likely to yield helpful lateralizing information compared with adult studies, WMAs are able to indicate which patients may be at higher risk for postoperative memory decline. Whether Wada testing provides incremental prediction of memory decline "above and beyond" other readily available clinical data (e.g., laterality of seizure focus, age at onset, mesial temporal sclerosis in magnetic resonance imaging, and preoperative neuropsychological assessment, especially memory and language test scores) has not been proven yet.

References

1. Cohen-Gadol AA, Westerveld M, Alvarez-Carilles J, Spencer DD. Intracarotid Amytal memory test and hippocampal magnetic resonance imaging volumetry: validity of the Wada test as an indicator of hippocampal integrity among candidates for epilepsy surgery. J Neurosurg 2004;101(6):926–931

2. Loring DW, Meador KJ. Wada and fMRI testing. In: Fisch B, ed. Principles and Practices of Electrophysiological and Video Monitoring in Epilepsy and Intensive *Care*. New York, NY: Demos Medical Publishing; 2008

3. Sabsevitz DS, Swanson SJ, Morris GL, Mueller WM, Seidenberg M. Memory outcome after left anterior temporal lobectomy in patients with expected and reversed Wada memory asymmetry scores. Epilepsia 2001;42(11):1408–1415

4. Stroup E, Langfitt J, Berg M, McDermott M, Pilcher W, Como P. Predicting verbal memory decline following anterior temporal lobectomy (ATL). Neurology 2003;60(8):1266–1273

5. Wada JA. Youthful season revisited. Brain Cogn 1997;33(1):7–10

6. Jones-Gotman M, Sziklas V, Djordjevic J, et al. Etomidate speech and memory test (eSAM): a new drug and improved intracarotid procedure. Neurology 2005;65(11):1723–1729

7. Buchtel HA, Passaro EA, Selwa LM, Deveikis J, Gomez-Hassan D. Sodium methohexital (brevital) as an anesthetic in the Wada test. Epilepsia 2002;43(9):1056–1061

8. Takayama M, Miyamoto S, Ikeda A, et al. Intracarotid propofol test for speech and memory dominance in man. Neurology 2004;63(3):510–515

9. Milner B, Branch C, Rasmussen T. Study of short-term memory after intracarotid injection of sodium Amytal. Trans Am Neurol Assoc 1962;87:224–226

10. Masters LT, Perrine K, Devinsky O, Nelson PK. Wada testing in pediatric patients by use of propofol anesthesia. AJNR Am J Neuroradiol 2000;21(7):1302–1305

11. Chitoku S, Otsubo H, Harada Y, et al. Extraoperative cortical stimulation of motor function in children. Pediatr Neurol 2001;24(5):344–350

12. Schevon CA, Carlson C, Zaroff CM, et al. Pediatric language mapping: sensitivity of neurostimulation and Wada testing in epilepsy surgery. Epilepsia 2007;48(3):539–545

13. Szabó CA, Wyllie E. Intracarotid amobarbital testing for language and memory dominance in children. Epilepsy Res 1993;15(3):239–246

14. Hamer HM, Wyllie E, Stanford L, Mascha E, Kotagal P, Wolgamuth B. Risk factors for unsuccessful testing during the intracarotid amobarbital procedure in preadolescent children. Epilepsia 2000;41(5):554–563

15. Loring DW, Meador KJ, Lee GP, Smith JR. Structural versus functional prediction of memory change following anterior temporal lobectomy. Epilepsy Behav 2004;5(2):264–268

16. Chelune GJ. Hippocampal adequacy versus functional reserve: predicting memory functions following temporal lobectomy. Arch Clin Neuropsychol 1995;10(5):413–432

17. Lee GP, Park YD, Hempel A, Westerveld M, Loring DW. Prediction of seizure-onset laterality by using Wada memory asymmetries in pediatric epilepsy surgery candidates. Epilepsia 2002a;43(9):1049–1055

18. Loring DW, Hermann BP, Perrine K, Plenger PM, Lee GP, Meador KJ. Effect of Wada memory stimulus type in discriminating lateralized temporal lobe impairment. Epilepsia 1997;38(2):219–224

19. Loring DW, Meador KJ, Lee GP, et al. Stimulus timing effects on Wada memory testing. Arch Neurol 1994b;51(8):806–810

20. Loring DW, Meador KJ, Lee GP. Amobarbital dose effects on Wada memory testing. J Epilepsy 1992;5:171–174

21. Kirsch HE, Walker JA, Winstanley FS, et al. Limitations of Wada memory asymmetry as a predictor of outcomes after temporal lobectomy. Neurology 2005;65(5):676–680

22. Meador KJ, Loring DW. The Wada test for language and memory lateralization. Neurology 2005;65(5):659

23. Lee GP, Park YD, Westerveld M, Hempel A, Loring DW. Effect of Wada methodology in predicting lateralized memory impairment in pediatric epilepsy surgery candidates. Epilepsy Behav 2002b;3(5):439–447

24. Loring DW, Lee GP, Meador KJ, et al. The intracarotid amobarbital procedure as a predictor of memory failure following unilateral temporal lobectomy. Neurology 1990;40(4):605–610

25. Loring DW, Hermann BP, Meador KJ, et al. Amnesia after unilateral temporal lobectomy: a case report. Epilepsia 1994a;35(4):757–763

26. Baxendale SA, Van Paesschen W, Thompson PJ, Duncan JS, Shorvon SD, Connelly A. The relation between quantitative MRI measures of hippocampal structure and the intracarotid amobarbital test. Epilepsia 1997;38(9):998–1007

27. Davies KG, Hermann BP, Foley KT. Relation between intracarotid amobarbital memory asymmetry scores and hippocampal sclerosis in patients undergoing anterior temporal lobe resections. Epilepsia 1996;37(6):522–525

28. Loring DW, Murro AM, Meador KJ, et al. Wada memory testing and hippocampal volume measurements in the evaluation for temporal lobectomy. Neurology 1993;43(9):1789–1793

29. Sass KJ, Lencz T, Westerveld M, Novelly RA, Spencer DD, Kim JH. The neural substrate of memory impairment demonstrated by the intracarotid amobarbital procedure. Arch Neurol 1991;48(1):48–52

30. Lee GP, Westerveld M, Blackburn LB, Park YD, Loring DW. Prediction of verbal memory decline after epilepsy surgery in children: effectiveness of Wada memory asymmetries. Epilepsia 2005;46(1):97–103

31. Loring DW, Meador KJ, Lee GP, et al. Wada memory asymmetries predict verbal memory decline after anterior temporal lobectomy. Neurology 1995;45(7):1329–1333

32. Perrine K, Westerveld M, Sass KJ, et al. Wada memory disparities predict seizure laterality and postoperative seizure control. Epilepsia 1995;36(9):851–856

33. Sperling MR, Saykin AJ, Glosser G, et al. Predictors of outcome after anterior temporal lobectomy: the intracarotid amobarbital test. Neurology 1994;44(12):2325–2330

13 Preoperative Neuropsychological and Cognitive Assessment

Katrina M. Boyer

Neuropsychological assessment has become standard practice in preparation for epilepsy surgery, although the reasons for such assessment have changed over time and the aims of neuropsychological evaluation of children are somewhat different from those of adults. Neuropsychological assessment provides unique information regarding the integrity of functions in specific brain regions. In the case of preoperative neuropsychological assessment of children with epilepsy, additional objectives include prediction of emotional and behavioral adjustment after surgery and the establishment of a baseline from which to evaluate postoperative outcome and target interventions as needed.

Neurocognitive functions do not operate in isolation but are interdependent and develop in the context of environmental and health-related influences. Thus, a full-profile analysis is crucial in interpretation of neuropsychological findings even when the primary functions of concern are quite specific. In children, the developmental context is a significant factor in the interpretation of neuropsychological findings because neurological development has disrupted the standard (adult data driven) rules of localization of neurocognitive function.

Neuropsychological Assessment of Children

Various approaches to pediatric neuropsychological assessment are applied to the pediatric population; some involve cognition as the core unit of analysis with developmental considerations playing a supplementary role, whereas others place greater importance on development in a broader sense, along with the environmental and contextual influences on brain–behavior relationships.[1] A developmental neuropsychological approach involves assessment of current cognitive skills and abilities within the context of environmental and developmental influences to construct a model of not only how but also why a child functions in his or her world. The latter model allows for hypotheses to be generated about future function in light of ongoing development and potential disruptions to development. This approach is particularly applicable in the assessment of children with epilepsy before surgical intervention. Understanding the developmental trajectory of a child and the various factors that serve to support as well as threaten developmental progress are necessary in predicting outcomes.

The tools of the trade for the developmental neuropsychologist include trained observation skills, developmental history gathering, psychological tests to assess cognitive abilities, and integrative analysis and interpretation of findings.

Neuropsychological assessment of the child is not merely a collection of results from various cognitive tests. Although important, quantitative test results alone are not sufficient to assess an individual child's cognitive function. Careful observation of how a child uses his or her skills to arrive at conclusions, solve problems, and provide answers is crucial for interpretation of findings. Furthermore, a child's individual skills do not operate in isolation but in a context of other neurobehavioral functions. Thus, a neuropsychological profile is carefully interpreted rather than simply providing a list of test scores.

Standardized Psychological Tests

Psychological tests to assess cognitive abilities are most often standardized, norm-referenced tools. This means that the administration directions are specific and that children should be presented materials and questions in a structured way so that responses can be compared with a sample of typically developing children in the same age range (normative reference sample). Choosing tests that are appropriate to the child's developmental level is necessary for the assessment to be valid. Current normative data are also important, as is information regarding the reliability and validity of the measure for specific purposes. Psychological tests are designed to measure specific constructs; however, it is impossible to completely isolate neurobehavioral constructs, particularly in children. As such, knowledge of the natural development of cognitive functions and well-honed observation skills are essential in interpreting psychological test scores and integrating these findings in the context of the child's social, developmental, and neurological histories.

■ Domains of Neuropsychological Assessment

Neuropsychological assessment of children can take on different forms, depending on the theoretical approach taken by the neuropsychologist and the specific goals of the evaluation. The majority of neuropsychological evaluations involve gathering information from several domains of function including general cognitive ability (a.k.a. intelligence), language, visual–perceptual, motor, sensory, memory, attention, and executive functions (*executive functions* typically include regulation of behavior as well as planning, organization, and integrative problem-solving skills) as well as assessment of emotional, social, and adaptive function.

General Cognitive Ability

The ability to reason, solve novel problems, form concepts, and demonstrate acquired knowledge are all factors related to general cognitive ability. Standardized test batteries are designed to quantify intelligence and provide structured opportunities to observe how a child thinks. Numerous test batteries are available to assess cognition in children; the choice of which test to use is not only a matter of professional preference but also is influenced by the developmental status of the child and the child's ability to respond to testing demands.

Language

Language assessment as part of a neuropsychological evaluation involves several sources of information including specific language tests, parent questionnaire data regarding communication skills, history of language development, and direct observations. Assessment of expressive and receptive language skills typically includes tests of picture naming, immediate repetition, verbal fluency, receptive vocabulary, and the ability to follow verbal directions.

Memory

Detailed memory assessment is a core feature of neuropsychological assessment. Direct assessment typically consists of both verbal and nonverbal memory measures. Furthermore, semantic verbal memory is often divided into story memory and list memory, with both immediate and delayed recall as well as delayed recognition trials. Nonverbal memory assessment often involves visual recognition, typically of faces, and constructional memory skills (recall of complex figure drawing), each with immediate and delayed recall or recognition assessment.

Visual–Spatial

Nonverbal problem-solving skills assessed as part of a neuropsychological evaluation include visual–motor integration,

constructional skills, spatial judgment, and visual perception. Spatial judgment is assessed with the patient matching lines of various orientations. Visual–motor integration assessment consists of copying geometric shapes and complex figures that integrate multiple basic geometric forms. Observation of the child's approach to constructional tasks provides information about perceptual, organization, planning, and integration functions.

Executive Functions

It is helpful to subdivide executive control skills into two subcategories known as metacognitive skills and behavioral regulation. Parental report in interview and on questionnaires designed to measure these skills are essential features of neuropsychological assessment.

Observation of the child's engagement in goal-directed behavior and online problem-solving approaches provide important information about metacognitive functions in addition to results on tests designed to measure skills such as auditory working memory, spatial planning, sequencing, and set-shifting skills.[2] Behavioral regulation includes self-monitoring of internal states and thought processes as well as outward displays of emotion, response inhibition, and physical activity level.[2]

Motor and Function

Typically, neuropsychological assessments will gather information regarding basic motor function from observations of gait, posture, and manipulation of objects, as well as from medical records. Specific tests of fine-motor speed and dexterity are used as well to make finer differentiations between the relative integrity of left and right fine-motor cortical areas.

Psychosocial Adjustment

Assessment of behavioral and emotional regulation and social adjustment are important elements of neuropsychological evaluations. Evaluation of a child's emotional and social adjustment involves interview of parents and the patient, observation, and questionnaire data gathered from parents, patients, and teachers regarding social development, peer and family relationships, emotional regulation, mood, and behavior management.

Academic Skills

Assessment of academic achievement in the context of neuropsychological evaluations will vary depending on age and the reason for referral. In all cases, the child's educational history will be an element of the information-gathering process.

Adaptive Function

Assessment of activities of daily living and adaptation to environment are routinely a part of neuropsychological assessment of children because these factors are important indicators of quality of life. Parent interview and questionnaires provide much of the data in this domain.

■ Epilepsy in Children and Its Effect on Neuropsychological Function

The developmental impact of epilepsy in childhood is highly diverse, which is not surprising given that the etiologies of pediatric epilepsy are numerous and often unknown. Moreover, the clinical presentations of patients with seizure disorders are wide ranging. As a group, children with epilepsy are vulnerable to neurodevelopmental dysfunction; however, various developmental trajectories occur in this population, and it is not possible to make broad generalizations. Specific and well-characterized epileptic syndromes are associated with relatively specific neuropsychological profiles. For example, children with Lennox-Gastaut syndrome almost invariably function within the range of moderate to severe mental retardation, whereas children with benign rolandic epilepsy most often have cognitive strengths and weaknesses that do not fall far outside normal limits for age.[3] However, most children with epilepsy do not have clearly defined syndromes such as these, and often the cause of seizures is unknown.

Significant limitations in cognitive development resulting in mental retardation occur in approximately 15 to 30% of patients with epilepsy and autism spectrum disorders occur in 20 to 30% of this population.[4] That said, the majority of children with epilepsy will have good seizure control on antiepileptic drugs and do not demonstrate substantial intellectual impairment.[5]

The specific cause of epilepsy often places the child at risk for neuropsychological dysfunction. Earlier onset of seizures has been associated with poorer cognitive outcome; however, this may be because of the likelihood of early onset epilepsy to occur when cortical malformations are present or in the setting of catastrophic epilepsy syndromes that present early in life, such as West syndrome.[5] Risk for declines in intellectual function is of concern in children with epilepsy and varies as a function of many factors, not all of which are well understood.[6] The primary risks to overall cognitive development in children with epilepsy appear to be the presence of status epilepticus, early onset of seizures in the setting of malformations of brain development, intractable seizures, and drug toxicity.[5]

Specific patterns of neuropsychological strength and weakness may be related to the neuroanatomical focality of localization-related epilepsy.

The same contributing factors that lead to cognitive limitations, such as neurodevelopment, seizure-related factors

(age of onset, syndrome, seizure severity), and medication side effects also place children at risk for academic underachievement. Specific neuropsychological impairments of skills, such as attention or memory, have substantial contributions to school performance as well. The role of psychosocial influences on academic achievement is very important to consider, including self-esteem, sense of personal effectiveness, and socioeconomic status.[5]

Children with epilepsy are three to nine times more likely to experience psychiatric disturbance than children without neurological conditions.[4] Approximately one third of pediatric epilepsy patients have affective or anxiety disorders.[7] Given the morbidity associated with depression, it is not surprising that it is a significant predictor of quality of life even when controlling for seizure frequency.[8] Risk is great for increase in mood disturbance after surgery, particularly with temporal lobe resections; however, patients with extratemporal resection and past history of mood problems are at risk of reoccurrence as well.[9]

■ Goals of Neuropsychological Assessment in Pediatric Epilepsy Surgery

The goals of preoperative neuropsychological assessment in pediatric epilepsy surgery are threefold. First, determining baseline neuropsychological function level before surgery is necessary to detect and quantify any change in function after surgery. Second, the neuropsychological evaluation provides information about localization of cognitive function. The distribution of cognitive strengths and weaknesses may correspond to functional and dysfunctional brain systems and provide clues about the location of the epileptogenic area as well as identify brain systems that are supporting well-developing cognitive function. Finally, risks to surgical intervention are highlighted; depending on the patient, these may include potential exacerbation of emotional and behavioral difficulties and risks to cognitive function should surgery proceed.

In general, if the cognitive functions assumed to be localized to the epileptogenic region are impaired in the context of an otherwise intact neuropsychological profile, and the findings are consistent with other neurodiagnostic studies, then the risks associated with resection are likely to be minimal because the region to be resected does not appear to function as intended. Alternatively, if deficits observed are associated with the region of interest within the context of a generally limited neuropsychological profile, the neuropsychological profile is thought to be nonlocalizing. In this case, risk to postsurgical function may be limited but likelihood of seizure freedom may also be reduced given the generalized nature of dysfunction. However, if no localizing deficits are found and the neuropsychological profile is largely one of competencies, the stakes are quite high because concerns about postoperative dysfunction are raised.

Special Considerations Regarding Neuropsychological Assessment of Children with Epilepsy

A desire to surgically intervene in intractable epilepsy as early in life as possible has led to increasing numbers of infants and toddlers presenting as epilepsy surgery candidates. As such, the pediatric neuropsychologist on the epilepsy surgery team must have the training and experience to evaluate the neurodevelopment of individuals from the toddler (if not infant) stage through young adulthood. Neuropsychological tools and practical approaches to assessment change with different stages of development and the knowledge base of the practitioner must be comprehensive and flexible. When working with a pediatric neurology population, many factors influencing the child's development must be considered, including timing of neurological insults and the impact on future development, behavioral and structural plasticity, and the effect of the child's social and familial context.[10] Children with intractable epilepsy may have seizures during neuropsychological assessments or may arrive for the evaluation in a postictal state; having a plan for dealing with such circumstances is necessary.

The communication or sensory functions of children with epilepsy may be compromised, and modifications to typical assessment approaches will be needed. Careful assessment planning is needed when children have communication dysfunction so that minimal demands are placed on communication function when assessing nonverbal skills. Patients with lesions along the optic radiations or in primary visual cortex may have visual field cuts necessitating presentation of information in the preserved visual field. Hemiparesis poses specific challenges because tests of constructional skills require coordinated use of both hands for optimal performance. Thus the choice of tests and normative comparison groups is crucial in the assessment of nonverbal cognition.

Neuropsychological Data for Localizing and Lateralizing the Epileptogenic Area

Long has been the tendency to extend theories of functional brain organization and neurocognitive research findings derived from adult populations to the developing brain. However, the nature and course of cognitive development has proven to be quite complex and far from understood at the present time. Plasticity of specific functions is variable so that some functions appear more likely to reorganize than others. It is likely that the timing of a neurological insult can differentially affect the development of separate cognitive functions. Moreover, reorganization of functions does not always follow predictable rules.

Language

Language lateralization and localization to the left lateral frontotemporal region in the mature brain has been well established. Although damage to cortex in and around Broca's area in the inferior frontocentral region or Wernicke's area in the superior temporal gyrus sustained in adulthood reliably result in aphasia, young children who sustain similar insults rarely demonstrate language disturbance of the same magnitude.[11] The developing brain can demonstrate remarkable plasticity to reorganize language functions if damage to the left hemisphere is sustained early in life, generally before the age of 6 years, although occasionally later reorganization can occur.[12] Such reorganization can occur within the healthy remainder of the left hemisphere or transfer of language functions to the right hemisphere is possible. Outside of near complete devastation of the left hemisphere early in life, we cannot predict whether intra- or interhemispheric transfer of functions will occur given our current state of knowledge in this area.

It has been assumed that interhemispheric transfer of function occurs when lesions are either very large or encroach on language cortex, such as Broca's and Wernicke's areas, whereas intrahemispheric reorganization occurs in the context of left hemisphere lesions more remote from primary language cortex.[11] Functional imaging research is shedding light on the normal development of language skills and neuroplasticity of these functions in the event of disruptions to typical neurodevelopment. Reorganization of language functions within the developing brain is not as predictable as once assumed as demonstrated by a recent functional magnetic resonance imaging (fMRI) study of children with developmental left hemisphere lesion and intractable epilepsy.[11]

Reorganization of language after lesions or surgery following a period of relatively normal language development has also been documented. Pre- and postsurgical fMRI of a boy with Rasmussen's syndrome document a shift from left hemisphere language lateralization at age 5½ years before significant cognitive regression to right hemisphere dominance after left hemispherotomy.[12] After surgery, this patient was densely aphasic and although he had not fully recovered language function 1 year after surgery, fMRI postoperatively documented a right-sided language network in typical primary language cortex. Other studies document recovery, at least in part, after hemispherectomy in middle and late childhood.[13,14]

Memory

Much of the adult literature on memory function, although not all, suggests that verbal memory deficits are associated with left temporal lobe epilepsy and right temporal lobe epilepsy is associated with nonverbal memory deficits.[15] The body of pediatric epilepsy literature is quite small in comparison; however, findings frequently indicate that material-specific memory is not well lateralized in childhood onset epilepsy.[16] Verbal memory has been consistently shown to be an area of limitation among children with temporal lobe epilepsy, particularly with mesial temporal lobe seizure onset, but right and left side seizure foci both have the propensity to produce verbal memory impairments. By contrast, facial recognition is more consistently lateralized to the right temporal lobe.[16] Other types of nonverbal memory are not clearly lateralizing, such as geometric figure memory or location memory.

Verbal and nonverbal memory plasticity findings give clues to the development of material specific memory. Language processing develops over the first few years of life, whereas faces are arguably the first stimuli a human infant actively processes. The brain systems involved in language processing and verbal memory can be reorganized if disrupted before development is complete and if healthy brain structures equipped to take on language functions are available. Because facial processing comes on line earlier, there is less opportunity for reorganization.[17]

Visual–Spatial

Primary visual processing takes place in the occipital lobes, whereas the parietal lobes analyze and integrate spatial information and coordinate with the frontal lobes to navigate space interact with objects. The temporal lobes are involved in recognition of known forms. These two processing pathways are commonly referred to as the "where" and "what" streams of visual processing, respectively.[18] Thus, children with parietal lobe seizure foci may demonstrate visual motor integration deficits in which they are able to copy simple and recognizable shapes, such as triangles and circles, but unable to accurately copy these same shapes when combined to form more complicated and abstract figures given the high spatial demand of the visual scene. These same children may be able to recognize common objects well, no matter how visually complex, because the parietal system demands are decreased under such circumstances. It has been commonly thought that such visual motor integration problems are associated primarily with right parietal damage, but dysfunction in either parietal lobe can produce such deficits.

Executive Functions

For the purpose of preoperative neuropsychological assessment in children, a more narrow focus on executive control skills that can be localized to the frontal lobes and, in some cases lateralized, is the goal. This goal is notoriously difficult to achieve with neuropsychological assessment; performance on tests designed to measure these skills is often not predictive of executive control impairments in daily functioning. These skills are not easy to divide conceptually, nor are they independent neuroanatomically.

Regulatory skills involve medial aspects of the prefrontal cortex and medial subcortical pathways at a basic level. Such regulatory skills include focusing and shifting attention, inhibition, emotional response modulation, and self-management of physical activity level. These skills are often impaired in children with intractable epilepsy and likely reflect a broad functional network that is easily disrupted.

Metacognitive aspects of executive control skills generally involve the lateral prefrontal cortex. Such metacognitive skills include working memory (the active manipulation of information held in immediate memory), planning, and organization. Functional imaging data of children and adults documents working memory function involving the dorsolateral prefrontal cortex, typically on the left side.[19] Spatial planning skills also involve lateral prefrontal cortices bilaterally. There is some evidence that the right prefrontal cortex is involved in generating a plan to solve spatial problems, whereas the left frontal network is involved in monitoring and carrying out the plan.[20]

Patients often present with a variable executive function profile, which is not surprising because the construct is so broad. Analysis of patterns of performance and observations of behavior may differentiate between lateral and mesial frontal system dysfunction, but neuropsychologists are not able to lateralize dysfunction based on executive function data alone.

Special Tests for Localization and Lateralization of Cognitive Function

We are far from having clear rules for the prediction of the nature of reorganization of language and memory functions in children. Functional tests are needed to identify eloquent cortex. Preoperative activation (fMRI) and deactivation (Wada and cortical mapping) studies remain essential before epilepsy surgery in frontal and temporal regions. Please refer to other chapters in this book that review functional assessment.

■ Advice to Parents and Teachers Regarding Potential Postoperative Issues

After surgery, much focus will understandably be placed on seizure outcome. Other aspects of recovery in the postoperative period also need to be a focus of attention. Neuropsychologists can help patients, parents, and teachers anticipate and minimize potential difficulties in the postoperative period. In the case of focal resections, patients often are able to walk and talk and look like they are fully recovered fairly soon after surgery and should be encouraged to return to school and other typical activities as soon as possible. However, planning for a gradual return to prior expectations is strongly advised because cognitive and physical fatigue can last many weeks and recovery of cognitive skills can be a slow and sometimes discouraging process.[2] Emotional fatigue and lability can also be expected as regulatory capacities may be strained as the child recovers from neurosurgery.

In the case of hemispherectomy or resection of eloquent cortex, depending on the child's presurgical function, more significant rehabilitation needs can be anticipated, including vision therapy to address visual filed cuts, physical and occupational therapy to address hemiparesis, and speech and language therapy to address any new challenges in communication.

The neuropsychological evaluation can be tremendously useful in educating parents, teachers, and patients themselves about their learning style, strengths, and cognitive limitations. Armed with this knowledge, caregivers can be more empathic and responsive to the child's needs.

Identification of psychological dysfunction before surgical intervention is necessary to support the child and family through the adjustments that lie ahead. Given the possibility of exacerbation of psychiatric symptoms after surgery, identification of risk before surgery and having a behavioral health treatment team in place to manage changes in presentation is very valuable. Inclusion of an experienced social worker as part of the epilepsy team can be an invaluable resource to families and patients as they prepare for and live through the epilepsy surgery process and recovery period.

■ Follow-up Assessment and Neuropsychological Outcome

Follow-up neuropsychological evaluation after surgery is needed to assess cognitive and behavioral outcomes, to identify any new problems that may be amenable to rehabilitation, and to generate more extensive recommendations to support the child's development. Initial follow-up at 6 months after operation is often appropriate because acute recovery has passed and neuropsychological function is relatively stable, yet long-term recovery is still under way and cognitive rehabilitation can potentially be effective. Long-term follow-up varies significantly and may depend on the age and needs of the patient. Please refer to the neuropsychological outcomes of pediatric epilepsy surgery chapter in this book for more information on this topic.

■ Conclusion

Although the aims of the preoperative neuropsychological evaluation are primarily to establish baseline function level, determine localization of function, and identify risks related to surgery, secondary aims include identification of academic and psychosocial needs of the patient. Along with other neurodiagnostic information, the neuropsychological profile can guide the surgical process by shedding light on the potential epileptogenic zone as well as appropriately developing cortical functions to be preserved. Establishing baseline neuropsychological function is critical for identification of cognitive or behavioral problems postoperatively that may be a target of rehabilitation. Predicting risks to cognitive function and psychosocial adjustment allows care providers to prepare for and minimize problems in the postoperative period, thus supporting the development and quality of life of the epilepsy surgery patient.

Acknowledgments   Special thanks are offered to Shannon Lundy-Krigbaum and Philip Rotella.

References

1. Bernstein JH. Developmental neuropsychological assessment. In: Yeats KO, Ris MD, Taylor HG, eds. Pediatric Neuropsychology: Research, Theory, and Practice. New York, NY: The Guilford Press; 2000;405–438
2. Bernstein JH, Prather PA, Rey-Casserly C. (1995). Neuropsychological assessment in preoperative and postoperative evaluation. In: Adelson PD, Black PM, eds. Neurosurgery Clinics of North America: Surgical Treatment of Epilepsy in Children. Philadelphia, Pa: W.B. Saunders Company, a division of Harcourt Brace & Company; 1995;443–454
3. Besag FMC. Cognitive and behavioral outcomes of epileptic syndromes. implications for education and clinical practice. Epilepsia 2006;47(2, suppl 2):119–125
4. Plioplys S, Dunn DW, Caplan R. 10-year research update review: psychiatric problems in children with epilepsy. J Am Acad Child Adolesc Psychiatry 2007;46(11):1389–1402
5. Williams J, Sharp GB. (2000). Epilepsy. In Yeats KO, Ris MD, Taylor HG, eds. Pediatric Neuropsychology: Research, Theory, and Practice. New York, NY: The Guilford Press; 2000;47–73
6. Seidenberg M, Pulsipher DT, Hermann B. Cognitive progression in epilepsy. Neuropsychol Rev 2007;17(4):445–454
7. Caplan R, Siddarth P, Gurbani S, Hanson R, Sankar R, Shields WD. Depression and anxiety disorders in pediatric epilepsy. Epilepsia 2005;46(5):720–730
8. Boylan LS, Flint LA, Labovitz DL, Jackson SC, Starner K, Devinsky O. Depression but not seizure frequency predicts quality of life in treatment-resistant epilepsy. Neurology 2004;62(2):258–261
9. Wrench J, Wilson SJ, Bladin PF. Mood disturbance before and after seizure surgery: a comparison of temporal and extratemporal resections. Epilepsia 2004;45(5):534–543
10. Lassonde M, Sauerwein HC, Jambaqué I, Smith ML, Helmstaedter C. Neuropsychology of childhood epilepsy: pre- and postsurgical assessment. Epileptic Disord 2000;2(1):3–13
11. Liégeois F, Connelly A, Cross JH, et al. Language reorganization in children with early-onset lesions of the left hemisphere: an fMRI study. Brain 2004;127(pt 6):1229–1236

12. Hertz-Pannier L, Chiron C, Jambaqué I, et al. Late plasticity for language in a child's non-dominant hemisphere: a pre- and post-surgery fMRI study. Brain 2002;125(pt 2):361–372

13. Vargha-Khadem F, Carr LJ, Isaacs E, Brett E, Adams C, Mishkin M. Onset of speech after left hemispherectomy in a nine-year-old boy. Brain 1997;120(pt 1):159–182

14. Boatman D, Freeman J, Vining E, et al. Language recovery after left hemispherectomy in children with late-onset seizures. Ann Neurol 1999;46(4):579–586

15. Bell BD, Davies KG. Anterior temporal lobectomy, hippocampal sclerosis, and memory: recent neuropsychological findings. Neuropsychol Rev 1998;8(1):25–41

16. Gonzalez LM, Anderson VA, Wood SJ, Mitchell LA, Harvey AS. The localization and lateralization of memory deficits in children with temporal lobe epilepsy. Epilepsia 2007;48(1):124–132

17. Jocic-Jakubi B, Jovic NJ. Verbal memory impairment in children with focal epilepsy. Epilepsy Behav 2006;9(3):432–439

18. Dutton GN. Cognitive vision, its disorders and differential diagnosis in adults and children: knowing where and what things are. Eye 2003;17(3):289–304

19. Dowker A. What can functional brain imaging studies tell us about typical and atypical cognitive development in children? J Physiol (Paris) 2006;99(4–6):333–341

20. Newman SD, Carpenter PA, Varma S, Just MA. Frontal and parietal participation in problem solving in the Tower of London: fMRI and computational modeling of planning and high-level perception. Neuropsychologia 2003;41(12):1668–1682

II Surgical Approaches and Techniques

14 Anesthetic Considerations and Postoperative ICU Care

Sulpicio G. Soriano and Michael L. McManus

The surgical management of intractable epilepsy has evolved owing to advances in intraoperative neuroimaging and electroencephalography (EEG). Recent advances in pediatric neurosurgery have exploited these technologies and dramatically improved the outcome in infants and children. The chapters in this section highlight the age-dependent aspects of the perioperative management of the pediatric neurosurgical patient.

■ Physiological Differences in Pediatrics

Age-dependent differences in cerebrovascular physiology have a significant impact on the perioperative management of neurosurgical patients. Cerebral blood flow (CBF) is coupled tightly to metabolic demand, and both increase proportionally immediately after birth. Wintermark and colleagues determined the effect of age on CBF.[1] Using computed tomography (CT) perfusion techniques, they reported that CBF peaked between 2 and 4 years of age and settled at 7 to 8 years of age. These changes mirror changes in neuroanatomical development. The autoregulatory range of blood pressure in a normal newborn lies between 20 and 60 mm Hg,[2] reflecting the relatively low cerebral metabolic requirements and blood pressure of the perinatal period. Although children younger than 2 years have lower baseline mean arterial pressures, they have lower autoregulatory reserve and can theoretically be at greater risk of cerebral ischemia.[3] These factors place the infant at risk for significant hemodynamic instability during neurosurgical procedures compared with adults.

■ Preoperative Evaluation and Preparation

A thorough preoperative, organ system–based evaluation of the pediatric patient is essential to minimize perioperative morbidity because infants are at higher risk for perioperative morbidity and mortality than any other age group.[4] Respiratory- and cardiac-related events account for a major-

ity of these complications and necessitate a thorough history and physical examination. First, a complete airway examination is essential, because some craniofacial anomalies may require specialized techniques to secure the airway.[5] Next, a thorough cardiovascular evaluation should be completed with an eye toward congenital heart disease that may not be apparent immediately after birth. A pediatric cardiologist should be consulted to evaluate all patients with suspected problems to identify any lesions and assess cardiac function before surgery. Optimal cardiac function is crucial intraoperatively because massive blood loss, swings in blood pressure, electrolyte shifts, and aggressive fluid administration may lead to depression of myocardial contractility and acute myocardial failure. Finally, a variety of medical conditions often accompany pediatric patients with epilepsy, and these need to be addressed when formulating the anesthetic plan.

Tuberous sclerosis (TS) is a hamartomatous disease that usually presents with cutaneous and intracranial lesions, the latter leading to medically intractable epilepsy.[6] Hamartomatous lesions frequently infiltrate and disturb the cardiac, renal, and pulmonary systems as well. Cardiac rhabdomyomas can be detected in a majority of these patients and can lead to dysrhythmias, obstruction of intracardiac blood flow, and abnormal conduction through the bundle of His. Therefore, all patients with TS should have a preoperative echocardiogram and electrocardiograph to detect any functional defects. Renal lesions often result in hypertension and azotemia, both of which may complicate the conduct of anesthesia.

Sturge-Weber syndrome, or encephalotrigeminal angiomatosis, is another of the phakomatoses and is characterized by port-wine facial stains and ipsilateral leptomeningeal angiomas. Intracranial angiomata with calcification ("railroad sign") produce cerebral atrophy, mental retardation, and seizures that are often refractory to medical management. Extracranial angiomata, including lesions involving the airway, have been reported, and congenital glaucoma is present in a third of patients. Thus, airway management, intraocular pressure, and intraoperative hemorrhage are important considerations.

Preoperative laboratory tests should be tailored to the proposed neurosurgical procedure. Hypercoagulation develops early after resection of brain tissue in pediatric neurosurgical patients, as assessed by thromboelastography.[7] Given the risk of significant blood loss associated with craniotomies, a hematocrit, prothrombin time, and partial thromboplastin time should be obtained to uncover any insidious hematological or coagulation disorders. Type- and cross-matched blood should be available before all craniotomies.

All patients presenting for epilepsy surgery have undergone drug treatment of their seizures. Each drug class has side effects that can affect the conduct of anesthesia. The traditional anticonvulsant drugs—phenobarbital, phenytoin, and carbamazepine—are potent inducers of hepatic microsomal p450 enzymes. Cerebyx (fosphenytoin) and Carbatrol (oxcarbazepine) are recent reformulations of the latter two drugs. The hepatic p450 enzymes mediate biotransformation and enhanced elimination of many drugs. Long-term administration of these specific anticonvulsant drugs results in drug resistance and increases requirements for both nondepolarizing muscle relaxants and opioids administered during general anesthesia.[8] Patients on chronic anticonvulsant drug therapy with phenobarbital, phenytoin, and carbamazepine need to be closely monitored for drug effect, and dosage should be increased accordingly. In general, the newer classes of anticonvulsant drugs do not appear to alter the metabolism of anesthetic drugs. However, other side effects have been reported with chronic administration of these new drugs. Topiramate has been shown to cause an asymptomatic anion gap metabolic acidosis because of inhibition of carbonic anhydrase.[9] This can exaggerate the metabolic acidosis that often occurs as a result of hypoperfusion because of massive blood loss. Sodium valproate is associated with platelet abnormalities and can cause bleeding disorders. Sodium valproate and felbamate can induce liver failure, and patients receiving these drugs should have the appropriate laboratory tests to determine the baseline line platelet and liver function before surgery.

The ketogenic diet is a high fat, low carbohydrate, low protein regime that promotes a chronic metabolic state of ketosis and acidosis. For reasons that remain unclear, this diet has proven to be a very useful adjunct in the treatment of many children with intractable epilepsy.[10] Although adequate calories are provided with fat, carbohydrate intake is limited to 5 to 15 g/day and hypoalbuminemia is common. Because the target metabolic state can be disrupted by administration of carbohydrate-containing intravenous (IV) solutions or by ingestion of the sweetened syrups contained in some premedications, these should be avoided by the anesthesiologist. Although both normal saline and lactated Ringer's are acceptable fluid choices, there is limited margin for additional acidosis, and the acid–base status must be monitored closely during surgery. Bicarbonate, plasma glucose, and serum ketone levels should be measured preoperatively, then sampled regularly to avoid hypoglycemia or excessive ketosis (serum or urine ketones > 160 mg/dL).

■ Anesthetic Management

Premedication

Separation from parents and perioperative anxiety play a significant role in the care of the pediatric patient and are related to the cognitive development and age of the child. Preoperative sedatives given before the induction of anesthesia can ease the transition from the preoperative holding area to the operating room.[11] Midazolam administered orally is particularly effective in relieving anxiety and producing amnesia. If an indwelling IV catheter is in place, midazolam can be slowly titrated to achieve sedation. If intraoperative electrocorticography (ECoG) is planned, the dosage of midazolam and other benzodiazepines should be reduced to minimize the depressant effects on the electroencephalogram (EEG).

Induction of Anesthesia

The patient's neurological status and co-existing medical conditions will dictate the appropriate technique and drugs for induction of anesthesia. In infants and young children, general anesthesia can be induced with inhalation of sevoflurane and nitrous oxide in oxygen. Sevoflurane has been shown to have epileptogenic potential.[12] However, the mechanism of this phenomenon is unclear. Alternatively, if the patient already has an IV catheter, anesthesia can be induced with sedative/hypnotic drugs such as thiopental (5–8 mg/kg) or propofol (3–4 mg/kg). These drugs rapidly induce unconsciousness and can blunt the hemodynamic effects of tracheal intubation. A nondepolarizing muscle relaxant is then administered after induction of general anesthesia to facilitate intubation of the trachea. Patients with nausea or gastroesophageal reflux disorder are at risk for aspiration pneumonitis and should have a rapid-sequence induction of anesthesia performed with thiopental or propofol immediately followed by a rapid-acting muscle relaxant and cricoid pressure. Rocuronium can be used when succinylcholine is contraindicated, such as for patients with spinal cord injuries or paretic extremities. In these instances, succinylcholine can result in sudden, catastrophic hyperkalemia.

Airway Management

Given the high incidence of respiratory morbidity and mortality in pediatric patients, a thorough examination of the airway and the use of appropriate equipment and techniques are mandatory. Because the trachea is relatively short, an endotracheal tube can easily migrate into a mainstem bronchus if an infant's head is flexed or turned. Therefore, great care should be devoted to assuring proper position of the endotracheal tube during tracheal intubation. Patients undergoing awake craniotomies are always at risk for airway compromise caused by sedation, seizure, or obstruction from positioning. Therefore, the patient's face should be accessible to the anesthesiologist for manipulation of the airway and ventilation of the lungs.

Positioning

Patient positioning for surgery requires careful preoperative planning to allow adequate access to the patient for both the neurosurgeon and anesthesiologist. This issue is especially important in patients undergoing awake craniotomies. In this case, the patient has to be in a comfortable position throughout the surgical procedure. A clear channel should be created in front of the patient's face to facilitate communication and facial observation during the neuropsychological assessment. If cortical stimulation or induction of the seizure is planned, the patient's limbs must be easily visualized.

Frequently, neurosurgical procedures are performed with the head slightly elevated to facilitate venous and cerebrospinal fluid (CSF) drainage from the surgical site. However, superior sagittal sinus pressures decrease with increasing head elevation, and this situation increases the likelihood of venous air embolus.[13] Extreme rotation of the head can impede venous return through the jugular veins and lead to impaired cerebral perfusion and increased intracranial pressure (ICP) and venous bleeding.

Vascular Access

Because of limited access to the patient (especially small children) during neurosurgical procedures, optimal IV access is mandatory before the start of surgery. Typically two large bore venous cannulae are sufficient for most craniotomies. Should initial attempts fail, central venous cannulation may be necessary. Use of the femoral vein avoids the risk of pneumothorax associated with subclavian catheters and does not interfere with cerebral venous return as may be the case with jugular catheters. Because significant blood loss and hemodynamic instability can occur during craniotomies, cannulation of the radial artery would provide direct blood pressure monitoring and sampling for blood gas analysis. Other useful arterial sites in infants and children include the dorsalis pedis and posterior tibial artery.

Maintenance of Anesthesia

Several classes of drugs are used to maintain general anesthesia. Potent, volatile anesthetic agents (i.e., sevoflurane, isoflurane, and desflurane) are administered by inhalation. These drugs are potent cerebrovascular dilators and cerebral metabolic depressants, which can mediate dose-dependent uncoupling of cerebral metabolic supply and demand and increase cerebral blood volume and intracranial pressure. Moreover, the use of these agents can be associated with a

significant decrease in cerebral perfusion pressure, primarily because of a dose-dependent reduction in arterial blood pressure.[14] They depress the EEG and may interfere with intraoperative ECoG. Given these issues, volatile anesthetics are rarely used as the sole anesthetic for neurosurgery.

Intravenous anesthetics are categorized as sedative/hypnotics and opioids. These drugs are also potent cerebral metabolic depressants but do not cause cerebral vasodilation. The sedative/hypnotics, propofol, midazolam, and thiopental, rapidly induce anesthesia and attenuate the EEG.[15] Opioid drugs can depress the EEG but not as severely as the sedative hypnotics. Fentanyl and other related synthetic opioids, including sufentanil, have their context-sensitive half times increase with repeated dosing or prolonged infusions and require hepatic metabolism. As a result, the narcotic effects, such as respiratory depression and sedation, of these drugs may be prolonged. Remifentanil is a unique opioid that is rapidly cleared by plasma esterases. This makes it, when administered at a rate of 0.2 to 1.0 mcg/kg/min, an ideal opioid for rapid emergence from anesthesia.[16] However, this rapid recovery is frequently accompanied by delirium and inadequate analgesia. Deep neuromuscular blockade with a nondepolarizing muscle relaxant is maintained to avoid patient movement and minimize the amount of anesthetic agents needed. Muscle relaxants should be withheld or permitted to wear off when assessment of motor function during neurosurgery is planned.

Intraoperative Fluid and Electrolyte Management

Given the unexpected nature of sudden blood loss, normovolemia should be maintained throughout the procedure. Estimation of the patient's blood volume is essential in determining the amount of allowable blood loss and when to transfuse blood. Blood volume depends on the age and size of the patient. Normal saline is commonly used as the maintenance fluid during neurosurgery, because it is mildly hyperosmolar (308 mosm/kg). However, rapid infusion of large quantities of normal saline (> 60 mL/kg) can be associated with hyperchloremic acidosis.[17] Given the relatively large blood volume of the neonate and infant, the maintenance rate of fluid administration depends on the weight of the patient. The maximum allowable blood loss should be determined in advance to determine when blood should be transfused to the patient. Initially, blood losses should be replaced with 3 mL of normal saline for 1 mL of blood loss or a colloid solution such as 5% albumin equal to the blood loss. Hematocrits of 21 to 25% should provide some impetus for blood transfusion. Massive transfusion of packed red blood cells can lead to dilutional thrombocytopenia.

Brain swelling can be initially managed by hyperventilation and elevating the head above the heart. Should these maneuvers fail, mannitol can be given at a dose of 0.25 to 1.0 g/kg intravenously. However, repeated dosing can lead to extreme hyperosmolality, renal failure, and further brain edema.[18] Furosemide is a useful adjunct to mannitol in decreasing acute cerebral edema and has been shown in vitro to prevent rebound swelling caused by mannitol.

■ Anesthetic Considerations for Specific Procedures

Vagal Nerve Stimulation

Vagal nerve stimulation is another therapeutic option for intractable seizures.[19] Placement of these devices is commonly performed under general anesthesia as same-day surgical patients. However, some groups have advocated the use of regional anesthesia in cooperative patients. Intraoperative bradycardia and transient asystole have been reported during initial stimulation and positioning of the electrodes. However, these events were short lived, and no morbidity evolved. Possible mechanisms for the bradycardia/asystole include stimulation of cervical cardiac branches of the vagus nerve either by collateral current spread or directly by inadvertent placement of the electrodes on one of these branches. Close observation of the electrocardiogram (ECG) is mandated during testing of the vagus nerve.

Anesthesia for Placement of Grids and Strips

Placement of the intracranial grids and strips carries the same operative risks noted previously. The recording derived from the cortical grids and strips is tested and requires the level of anesthesia to be decreased to minimize its depressant effects on the EEG. Because anticonvulsant drug therapy is usually removed to detect and characterize the seizure, postoperative monitoring of the patient should focus on bleeding and uncontrolled status epilepticus. The patient typically returns within 1 week for a repeat craniotomy for removal of the grids and strips and resection of the seizure focus/foci. It is important to avoid administration of nitrous oxide until the dura is opened, because intracranial air can persist up to 3 weeks after a craniotomy, and nitrous oxide in these situations can cause rapid expansion of air cavities and result in tension pneumocephalus.[20]

Resection of Seizure Focus

The depressant effects of many anesthetic agents limit the utility of intraoperative neurophysiological monitoring to be used during the surgical procedure. In general, ECoG and EEG can be used during low levels of volatile anesthetics. Cortical stimulation of the motor cortex necessitates observation of motor movement of the specific area of the homunculus. Therefore, muscle relaxation should be avoided or permitted to dissipate during the monitoring period. Because some epileptogenic foci are near cortical areas that control speech, memory, motor function, or sensory function, monitoring of patient and electrophysiological responses is frequently used to minimize iatrogenic injury to these areas.[21,22]

Awake Craniotomy

Neurological function is best assessed in an awake and cooperative patient. Positioning of the patient is critical for the success of this technique. The patient should be in a semilateral position to allow both patient comfort as well as surgical and airway access to the patient. A variety of techniques have been advocated to facilitate intraoperative assessment of motor-sensory function and speech. These range from no sedation with local anesthesia to "asleep–awake–asleep" techniques in which the general anesthesia is induced before and after functional testing.[23] Propofol does not interfere with the ECoG, when discontinued 20 minutes before monitoring in children undergoing an awake craniotomy.[24] Other drug regimens include remifentanil and dexmedetomidine.[25,26] However, it is imperative that candidates for an awake craniotomy be mature and psychologically prepared to participate in this procedure.

Corpus Callosotomy

Because intraoperative EEG is not required during corpus callosotomy, any anesthetic regiment can be used. However, the risk for uncontrolled hemorrhage and venous air embolus still exists because the surgical approach encroaches on the sagittal sinus. Lethargy and somnolence occur after complete division of the corpus callosum and place patients at risk for aspiration pneumonitis and airway obstruction during the immediate postoperative period. Therefore, the patient's trachea should be left intubated and mechanically ventilated until the patient fully regains consciousness.

Hemispherectomy

Hemispherectomies have the highest morbidity of all surgical procedures for intractable epilepsy. These procedures result in the loss of more than one blood volume and are associated with coagulopathy, hypokalemia, and hypothermia.[27] The use of central venous and pulmonary artery catheters for monitoring intravascular volume has been advocated by some groups for surgical procedures associated with large blood loss and fluid shifts. However, this practice is not universally accepted. This is primarily because of significantly higher volume of blood loss when compared with older children and those undergoing functional resections.[28] Sustained bleeding and subsequent transfusions can progress into a low cardiac output state characterized by hypotension and limited response to administration of fluid and inotropic drugs. Given the continuous blood loss, administration of tranexamic acid has been shown to significantly reduced blood loss in children undergoing cardiac and spinal surgery.[29,30] Because the prothrombotic effect of tranexamic acid is unknown, a reduced dose of 50 mg/kg load followed by an infusion of 5 mcg/kg/h may be effective. Low cardiac output states can be temporized by instituting a dopamine infusion (5–10 mcg/kg/min). If this is ineffective, an epinephrine infusion (0.05–1.0 mcg/kg/min) along with aggressive fluid resuscitation may be necessary. Given the large fluid shifts and somnolence that ensues, it may be prudent to leave a patient's trachea intubated and institute mechanical ventilation for the first postoperative day.

■ Postoperative Management

Close observation in an intensive care unit with serial neurological examinations and invasive hemodynamic monitoring is helpful for the prevention and early detection of postoperative problems. It is important to recognize that postoperative seizures can still occur in these patients and lead to significantly increased morbidity. When seizures do occur, the response must be prompt[31]: first with basic life support algorithms addressing airway, breathing, and circulation, then with administration of sufficient anticonvulsant drug to stop the seizure. A common approach involves lorazepam 0.1 mg/kg IV (repeated after 10 minutes if necessary) for immediate control, followed by fosphenytoin 20 mg/kg, phenobarbital 20 mg/kg, or levetiracetam 10 mg/kg on a regular schedule for more lasting coverage.

Postoperative nausea and vomiting can result from surgery, anesthesia, or postoperative medications. Because retching will cause sudden increases in intracranial pressure, nausea should be treated with a nonsedating antiemetic. Although the efficacy of intraoperative administration of antiemetic drugs as a prophylactic measure is controversial,[32] ondansetron (50 mcg/kg), dexamethasone (0.25 mg/kg), or metoclopramide (150 mcg/kg) can effectively treat nausea and vomiting in the postoperative period.

Fluid and electrolyte derangements are common in the postoperative neurosurgical patient. Hyponatremia can develop because of excessive free water administration (hypotonic fluids given in the setting of high antidiuretic hormone levels) or to abnormal losses of sodium (cerebral salt wasting). The syndrome of inappropriate anti-diuretic

hormone (ADH) secretion is marked by low sodium and hypervolemia, whereas cerebral salt wasting is marked by low sodium and hypovolemia. Sudden falls in serum sodium concentration can precipitate seizures that resist conventional drug therapy but respond to modest volumes of hypertonic saline (3% saline, 4 mL/kg). Hypernatremia occurs less frequently but can result from increased insensible losses (especially in infants) or the presence of diabetes insipidus. In the latter, urine volumes in excess of 4 mL/kg are usually observed, and infusion of arginine vasopressin is necessary for correction.[33]

Postoperative mechanical ventilation is uncommon but can occasionally be necessary after epilepsy surgery. Intraoperative events that most commonly necessitate postoperative tracheal intubation and mechanical ventilation include neurological dysfunction and massive blood loss followed by volume resuscitation with fluid shifts. In these patients, continuous infusions of a narcotic (fentanyl, morphine) and a benzodiazepine (midazolam) provide effective sedation. Although propofol infusion can provide reliable sedation with quick wakeups, in pediatric patients it may lead to a syndrome of metabolic acidosis and progressive multiorgan failure (the "propofol infusion syndrome").[34] When propofol must be used, it is prudent to minimize infusion rates to less than 3.0 mg/kg/h and durations to less than 12 hours. A newer agent, dexmedetomidine, offers many of the advantages of propofol as an ultra–short-acting, single-agent sedative. Unlike propofol, it does not cause apnea, so spontaneous breathing is easily maintained. Our early experience suggests that both hypotension and hypertension can be associated side effects.

The treatment of postoperative pain is a significant component of the perioperative management of the neurosurgical patient. Because most craniotomies are observed in a critical care unit, IV opioids (morphine 0.1 mg/kg IV every 2–4 hours as needed) can be carefully titrated to blunt pain but not to the point of oversedation. Patients recovering in an unmonitored setting may receive acetaminophen (10–15 mg/kg) and codeine (0.5 mg/kg) with minimal side effects.

■ Conclusion

The perioperative management of pediatric patients for epilepsy surgery should focus on the specific problems unique to the disease state, age of the child, and operative conditions. Thorough preoperative evaluation and open communication between members of the epilepsy team are important. A basic understanding of age-dependent variables and the interaction of anesthetic and surgical procedures are essential in minimizing perioperative morbidity.

References

1. Wintermark M, Lepori D, Cotting J, et al. Brain perfusion in children: evolution with age assessed by quantitative perfusion computed tomography. Pediatrics 2004;113(6):1642–1652

2. Pryds O, Edwards AD. Cerebral blood flow in the newborn infant. Arch Dis Child Fetal Neonatal Ed 1996;74(1):F63–F69

3. Vavilala MS, Lee LA, Lam AM. The lower limit of cerebral autoregulation in children during sevoflurane anesthesia. J Neurosurg Anesthesiol 2003;15(4):307–312

4. Murat I, Constant I, Maud'huy H. Perioperative anaesthetic morbidity in children: a database of 24,165 anaesthetics over a 30-month period. Paediatr Anaesth 2004;14(2):158–166

5. Nargozian CD. The difficult airway in the pediatric patient with craniofacial anomaly. Anesthesiol Clin North America 1998;16:839–852

6. Shenkman Z, Rockoff MA, Eldredge EA, Korf BR, Black PM, Soriano SG. Anaesthetic management of children with tuberous sclerosis. Paediatr Anaesth 2002;12(8):700–704

7. Goobie SM, Soriano SG, Zurakowski D, McGowan FX, Rockoff MA. Hemostatic changes in pediatric neurosurgical patients as evaluated by thrombelastograph. Anesth Analg 2001;93(4):887–892

8. Soriano SG, Martyn JA. Antiepileptic-induced resistance to neuromuscular blockers: mechanisms and clinical significance. Clin Pharmacokinet 2004;43(2):71–81

9. Groeper K, McCann ME. Topiramate and metabolic acidosis: a case series and review of the literature. Paediatr Anaesth 2005;15(2):167–170

10. Valencia I, Pfeifer H, Thiele EA. General anesthesia and the ketogenic diet: clinical experience in nine patients. Epilepsia 2002;43(5):525–529

11. McCann ME, Kain ZN. The management of preoperative anxiety in children: an update. Anesth Analg 2001;93(1):98–105

12. Constant I, Seeman R, Murat I. Sevoflurane and epileptiform EEG changes. Paediatr Anaesth 2005;15(4):266–274

13. Grady MS, Bedford RF, Park TS. Changes in superior sagittal sinus pressure in children with head elevation, jugular venous compression, and PEEP. J Neurosurg 1986;65(2):199–202

14. Sponheim S, Skraastad O, Helseth E, Due-Tønnesen B, Aamodt G, Breivik H. Effects of 0.5 and 1.0 MAC isoflurane, sevoflurane and desflurane on intracranial and cerebral perfusion pressures in children. Acta Anaesthesiol Scand 2003;47(8):932–938

15. Modica PA, Tempelhoff R, White PF. Pro- and anticonvulsant effects of anesthetics (Part I). Anesth Analg 1990;70(3):303–315

16. German JW, Aneja R, Heard C, Dias M. Continuous remifentanil for pediatric neurosurgery patients. Pediatr Neurosurg 2000;33(5):227–229

17. Scheingraber S, Rehm M, Sehmisch C, Finsterer U. Rapid saline infusion produces hyperchloremic acidosis in patients undergoing gynecologic surgery. Anesthesiology 1999;90(5):1265–1270

18. McManus ML, Soriano SG. Rebound swelling of astroglial cells exposed to hypertonic mannitol. Anesthesiology 1998;88(6):1586–1591

19. Valencia I, Holder DL, Helmers SL, Madsen JR, Riviello JJ Jr. Vagus nerve stimulation in pediatric epilepsy: a review. Pediatr Neurol 2001;25(5):368–376

20. Reasoner DK, Todd MM, Scamman FL, Warner DS. The incidence of pneumocephalus after supratentorial craniotomy. Observations on the disappearance of intracranial air. Anesthesiology 1994;80(5):1008–1012

21. Adelson PD, Black PM, Madsen JR, et al. Use of subdural grids and strip electrodes to identify a seizure focus in children. Pediatr Neurosurg 1995;22(4):174–180

22. Ojemann SG, Berger MS, Lettich E, Ojemann GA. Localization of language function in children: results of electrical stimulation mapping. J Neurosurg 2003;98(3):465–470

23. Sarang A, Dinsmore J. Anaesthesia for awake craniotomy—evolution of a technique that facilitates awake neurological testing. Br J Anaesth 2003;90(2):161–165

24. Soriano SG, Eldredge EA, Wang FK, et al. The effect of propofol on intraoperative electrocorticography and cortical stimulation during awake craniotomies in children. Paediatr Anaesth 2000;10(1):29–34

25. Ard J, Doyle W, Bekker A. Awake craniotomy with dexmedetomidine in pediatric patients. J Neurosurg Anesthesiol 2003;15(3):263–266

26. Keifer JC, Dentchev D, Little K, Warner DS, Friedman AH, Borel CO. A retrospective analysis of a remifentanil/propofol general anesthetic for craniotomy before awake functional brain mapping. Anesth Analg 2005;101(2):502–508, table

27. Brian JE Jr, Deshpande JK, McPherson RW. Management of cerebral hemispherectomy in children. J Clin Anesth 1990;2(2):91–95

28. Piastra M, Pietrini D, Caresta E, et al. Hemispherectomy procedures in children: haematological issues. Childs Nerv Syst 2004;20(7):453–458

29. Reid RW, Zimmerman AA, Laussen PC, Mayer JE, Gorlin JB, Burrows FA. The efficacy of tranexamic acid versus placebo in decreasing blood loss in pediatric patients undergoing repeat cardiac surgery. Anesth Analg 1997;84(5):990–996

30. Sethna NF, Zurakowski D, Brustowicz RM, Bacsik J, Sullivan LJ, Shapiro F. Tranexamic acid reduces intraoperative blood loss in pediatric patients undergoing scoliosis surgery. Anesthesiology 2005;102(4):727–732

31. Riviello JJ Jr, Holmes GL. The treatment of status epilepticus. Semin Pediatr Neurol 2004;11(2):129–138

32. Furst SR, Sullivan LJ, Soriano SG, McDermott JS, Adelson PD, Rockoff MA. Effects of ondansetron on emesis in the first 24 hours after craniotomy in children. Anesth Analg 1996;83(2):325–328

33. Wise-Faberowski L, Soriano SG, Ferrari L, et al. Perioperative management of diabetes insipidus in children. J Neurosurg Anesthesiol 2004;16(3):220–225

34. Bray RJ. Propofol infusion syndrome in children. Paediatr Anaesth 1998;8(6):491–499

15 Implantation of Strip, Grid, and Depth Electrodes for Invasive Electrophysiological Monitoring

Oğuz Çataltepe and Julie Pilitsis

The main goal of resective surgical interventions in the management of medically refractory epilepsy is the complete removal of the epileptogenic zone while preserving adjacent functionally critical cortical areas. Therefore, the precise localization of the epileptogenic zone in epilepsy surgery has critical significance for achieving postoperative seizure-free outcome.[1-3] This is especially true for the patients with extratemporal epilepsy and radiologically occult abnormalities. Although scalp electroencephalography (EEG) is very helpful in determining the location of the epileptogenic zone, it does not delineate the surgical target precisely in magnetic resonance imaging (MRI) negative cases and in many extratemporal epilepsy cases. The main contribution and value of extraoperative monitoring with intracranial electrodes in epilepsy surgery is its role in the precise determination and mapping of the epileptogenic zone and eloquent cortex. Invasive monitoring is required more frequently in children than adults because of the high frequency of extratemporal epilepsy and dysplastic cortical lesions in the pediatric age group. In these cases, preoperative data obtained with noninvasive monitoring techniques may be inconclusive with multiple foci or even unclear lateralization. Invasive monitoring is frequently required in these patients and constitutes 25 to 40% of cases in some pediatric series.[2,4-6]

■ Indication

Invasive monitoring is indicated if preoperative assessment with noninvasive tests

1. is inconclusive with unclear lateralization or localization of epileptogenic zone;
2. provide noncongruent data; or
3. reveal the following:
   - multiple epileptiform areas,
   - multiple structural lesions with ill-defined electrographic focus,
   - no clearly defined structural lesion on MRI despite electrographic evidence of epileptogenic zone in a certain cortical region,
   - electrographic evidence implying a larger epileptogenic zone than lesional zone on MRI, or
   - epileptogenic zone adjacent to eloquent cortex.

However invasive monitoring is not an exploratory procedure and is helpful only if the noninvasive workup is suggestive for certain cortical locations. In these cases, further delineation and accurate localization of the epileptogenic zone is required to be able to offer surgical resection as a management option to the patient.[2-9]

Although other indications can be defined, the most common indications for invasive monitoring in temporal lobe epilepsy (TLE) include the following:

1. Presence of noninvasive electrographic data showing bilateral temporal seizure onset
2. Semiological and electrographic difficulty in differentiating temporal lobe seizures from possible frontal lobe seizures
3. Presence of electrographic data suggestive for unilateral temporal onset in presence of bilateral imaging abnormalities
4. Ill-defined electrographic abnormalities with a unilateral structural abnormality on imaging studies
5. Dual pathologies[2-9]

Sperling defined some major and minor criteria for the role of invasive monitoring in TLE. He did not recommend invasive monitoring if the patient has concordant data fully or with either two major plus one minor or one major plus three minor criteria listed in **Table 15.1**. If tests are discordant or there are an insufficient number of concordant test results, he recommends invasive monitoring with intracranial electrodes.[6]

In extratemporal epilepsy, invasive monitoring is indicated not only to define the epileptogenic zone but also to map the eloquent cortex. Even in cases with an extratemporal lesion with well-defined borders, if it is adjacent to eloquent cortex, invasive monitoring with grid placement may still be needed for stimulation and mapping purposes. This is also true for cortical dysplasia cases that often have ill-defined borders and more extensive electrographically abnormal areas than imaging studies suggest.[2,3,5,6]

■ Invasive Monitoring Techniques

Several invasive monitoring electrodes may be used in epilepsy patients. The most commonly used electrodes are

Table 15.1 Criteria for the Role of Invasive Monitoring in Temporal Lobe Epilepsy

Major criteria	Scalp/sphenoidal EEG: temporal lobe interictal spikes
	Scalp/sphenoidal EEG: temporal lobe ictal onset
	MRI: hippocampal atrophy
	PET: temporal lobe hypometabolism
Minor criteria	Wada test: lateralized memory deficit
	EEG: interictal focal θ or δ (> 50% of time)
	SPECT: ictal temporal lobe hyperperfusion

Abbreviations: electroencephalogram, EEG; magnetic resonance imaging, MRI; positron emission tomography, PET; single photon emission computed tomography, SPECT.

subdural strip, grid, and depth electrodes (**Fig. 15.1**). Epidural peg electrodes are also available but not as widely used. Invasive monitoring electrodes can be chosen among commercially available electrodes or can be custom made based on the specific needs of the case. These can be used separately or in combination to determine the epileptogenic zone. The extent of the coverage, ideal electrode type, and configuration should be determined by the epileptologist, epilepsy surgeon, and neurophysiologist together after review of the available data for each patient. The initial step in invasive monitoring is determining the cortical area with the highest likelihood of epileptogenicity to cover with invasive electrodes. Scalp EEG data and MRI studies provide the most valuable data in defining the cortical area that needs to be covered.[5,6] Invasive electrodes are frequently placed bilaterally, but if lateralization of the seizures is clear and localization is questionable, coverage may be asymmetrical with more extensive sampling from the suspicious hemisphere.[6] Each electrode and invasive monitoring modality has certain advantages and disadvantages. Although depth

and strip electrodes are more useful to lateralize the seizure onset, grids are much more helpful to further localize the epileptogenic zone.

Depth Electrodes

Depth electrodes are most valuable in assessing deep cortical structures such as the amygdala, hippocampus, parahippocampus, cingulum, and orbitofrontal cortex.[10] Depth electrodes in pediatric epilepsy surgery are mostly used in older children, although still not as commonly as in adults. These are multicontact electrode arrays, consisting of up to 12 nickel-chromium or platinum contacts embedded in a thin, tubular, biologically inert Silastic material. They can be placed through a drill or burr hole using a stereotactic frame or frameless neuronavigation guidance. Typical indications for depth electrodes include bilateral mesial temporal epilepsy (MTS), dual pathology, differentiation between mesial and neocortical temporal epilepsy or temporal lobe and orbitofrontal seizure onset, and presence of epileptogenic lesion located in deep brain parenchyma, such as in cases of hypothalamic hamartoma or periventricular heterotopia. Depth electrodes are also useful in clarifying conflicting data such as the presence of unilateral MTS on MRI and bilateral independent or nonlocalizing interictal/ictal epileptogenic activities in noninvasive EEG monitoring. Although depth electrodes provide excellent data from deep structures, they do not have cortical surface coverage and have very limited stimulation capabilities. Therefore, depth electrodes are frequently used in combination with strip electrodes.[4] Bilateral hippocampal depth electrodes combined with bilateral temporal subdural strip electrodes provide perfect coverage for both neocortical and mesial temporal areas bilaterally. This already large coverage can be easily further extended to both

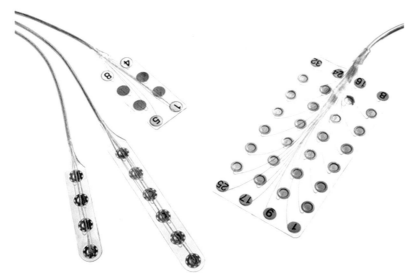

Fig. 15.1 Subdural strip and grid electrodes (courtesy of Integra Neurosciences, Plainsboro, NJ, USA).

orbitofrontal regions by adding two more subdural strip electrodes. Depth electrodes can also be placed in the cingulum and orbitofrontal cortex; for additional frontal coverage, they can be combined with strip electrodes, such as bilateral orbitofrontal depth electrodes with bilateral convexity, lateral frontal, and interhemispheric strip electrodes.[4,7,10]

Depth electrodes can be placed into the mesial temporal structures through two different approaches: occipitotemporal and temporal (**Fig. 15.2A–F**). The occipitotemporal approach provides a trajectory parallel to the long axis of hippocampus, whereas the temporal approach provides a trajectory orthogonal to hippocampus. We prefer the occipitotemporal approach because it has the advantage of placing multiple contacts throughout the amygdala and hippocampal head and body with a single-depth electrode. Because this approach would not provide any information regarding neocortical electrical activity, additional subdural strips can be easily placed to cover temporal neocortex at the same time. Conversely, the temporal orthogonal approach has an advantage of providing data both from mesial as well as neocortical structures through a single-depth electrode. However, this approach often necessitates multiple-depth electrodes (two or three) on each side and results in only

one or two contacts truly in the mesial structures whereas the other contacts are in neocortex. However, this approach provides very limited neocortical electrographic data compared with strip electrodes.

Subdural Strip and Grid Electrodes

Both subdural strip and grid electrodes are thin, biologically inert, Silastic or Teflon sheets with embedded nickel-chromium or platinum, electrically isolated electrode contacts. Each electrode contact is 2 to 4 mm in diameter, and generally the interelectrode distance is 10 mm. Subdural strips are a single row of contact electrodes with 10 mm interelectrode distances (1×4, 1×6, 1×8). Subdural grids are larger plates of rectangular arrays with several parallel rows of up to 64 electrodes (2×4, 2×6, 4×8, 8×8 . . .). Both subdural strips and grid electrodes are very thin and flexible sheets and can be contoured to the underlying cortical surface. They are also transparent and thus allow visualization of the underlying anatomical structures. There are many commercially available strip and grids with various configurations and shapes, such as curvilinear, dual-faced grid electrodes for interhemispheric coverage. Custom-made options are also

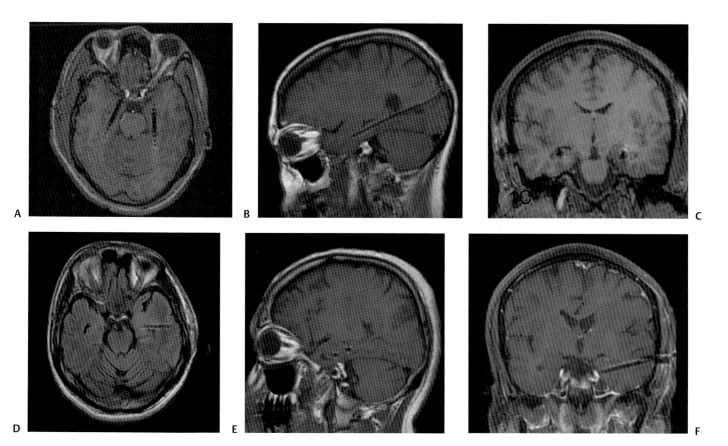

Fig. 15.2 (A–C) Postoperative magnetic resonance imaging (MRI) images of bilateral hippocampal depth electrodes through occipitotemporal approach: Axial **(A)**, sagittal **(B)**, and coronal **(C)** planes. **(D–F)** Unilateral hippocampal depth electrode placement through lateral temporal approach. Postoperative MRI images: Axial **(D)**, sagittal **(E)**, and coronal **(F)** planes.

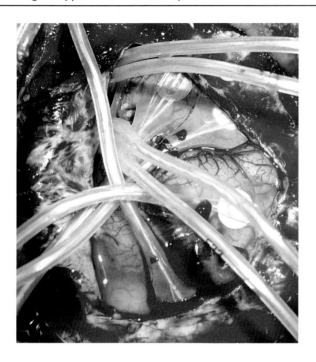

Fig. 15.3 Interhemispheric grid and frontal multiple strip electrode placement through a frontal craniotomy.

readily available. Strip electrodes are placed through burr holes or can be slid under craniotomy edges if they will be used in combination with grid electrodes (**Fig. 15.3**). Multiple subdural strip electrodes using different trajectories to sample large cortical areas can be placed through a single burr hole. Strip electrodes are ideal to lateralize and grossly localize the most suspicious cortical areas for seizure onset. This area would need further exploration by grid electrodes for more precise mapping to define the surgical resection area. Grid electrode placement is performed with a large craniotomy (**Fig. 15.4A,B**). Grid electrode recording is an ideal technique to locate the epileptogenic zone and to stimulate and map the adjacent eloquent cortex by covering large cortical surfaces more completely. Subdural grid electrodes are frequently used in pediatric epilepsy surgery to cover large extratemporal cortical areas.[4–7,11]

■ Advantages and Limitations of Invasive Monitoring Techniques

Invasive electrode recording has many advantages as well as many significant limitations. One of the main advantages of

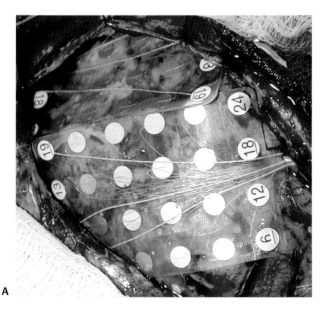

A

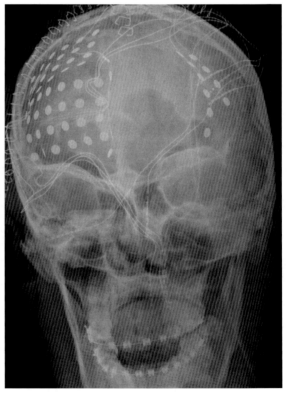

B

Fig. 15.4 (A) Intraoperative photograph of frontal multiple grid placement. Note the absence of any gap between the two grid electrode plates. **(B)** Postoperative skull x-ray showing large grid cover-

age on the right frontal convexity and interhemispheric space as well as strip sampling from the left frontal cortex.

invasive monitoring is the reliability of the electrophysiological recording, because it is directly obtained from a small number of neurons with stable impedances and higher amplitudes; and signal attenuation caused by scalp and skull, as well as muscle artifact, are eliminated.[6,7,12] Other advantages are being able to detect EEG activity from deep structures such as the amydala, hippocampus, basal frontal or temporal cortex, and interhemispheric cortical surfaces and providing an opportunity to perform extraoperative stimulation and cortical mapping that is a very helpful feature in the pediatric age group especially.[6,11,12]

It is prudent to know the advantages and limitations of each invasive monitoring technique to choose the most appropriate modality for individual patients. Depth electrodes are excellent choices for recording from deep structures. They may be placed with a small incision, through a small drill hole, and can be removed at bedside easily without going back to the operating room.[4] The most significant advantages of depth electrodes are their ability to record directly from hippocampus and the precision with which the electrodes can be placed. This is especially relevant in mesial TLE because seizure activities originating from mesial temporal structures may spread very rapidly, and thus seizure onset may not be clearly defined with surface recording alone in selected cases.[11] Conversely, the placement of depth electrodes requires sophisticated equipments such as a stereotactic frame and neuronavigation systems, surgical expertise and experience with these techniques, longer operating time, and higher cost associated with the additional perioperative imaging studies required.

The main advantage of strip electrodes is their versatility. They can be easily placed through a small burr hole without requiring any special equipment or expertise. Multiple strip electrodes can be placed in different trajectories through a single burr hole and large cortical areas including basal temporal and frontal cortex can be sampled with a low-risk procedure. Strip electrodes can even be used for mesial temporal lobe coverage; although they record from the parahippocampus rather than hippocampus, valuable information is still provided. Conversely, the placement of strip electrodes is not as precise as depth electrodes, and the location of the electrodes can easily be suboptimal because the placement is done blindly and free-handed. Injury to cortical veins and bleeding risks are also present with this technique for the same reasons. Strip electrodes are only able to provide cortical sampling data because their coverage of a large cortical area is discontinuous and somewhat limited. Thus, their ability to localize the epileptogenic zone is more limited than grid electrodes. The risk of cerebrospinal fluid (CSF) leak and infection is also much higher with strip electrodes than with depth electrodes.[7,11]

Grid electrode is an excellent choice for covering a large cortical area in its entirety to record both interictal and ictal epileptogenic activity and to perform extraoperative stimu-lation and mapping. However grids can be placed only after seizures are lateralized and grossly localized with other modalities.[11] Although extraoperative cortical stimulation and mapping ability is one of the greatest advantages of grid electrodes, its value in small children is limited. The absence of responses to cortical stimulation in children younger than 4 years old does not indicate nonfunctional cortex, and the cortical stimulation results in this age group are inconsistent, at best. Furthermore, the cortical identification of language with extraoperative cortical stimulation in children younger than 10 years old is not reliable.[4,13] Grid electrode placement is also performed with a large craniotomy and thus exposes the patient to considerable postoperative risks, including cerebral edema, mass effect, cortical injury, bleeding, and related problems.

Invasive monitoring techniques have many advantages as described previously; however, they also have an inherent bias secondary to limited cortical sampling (tunnel vision) that is prone to false localization. Because of limited spatial coverage, invasive monitoring techniques may define the epileptogenic zone incompletely if the coverage is less than perfect, and the electrographic abnormal activity detected by intracranial electrodes can easily be a propagated activity more than a true seizure onset.[7] Although a single scalp electrode can record electrical activity from a relatively large cortical area (~6 cm^2), a single subdural or depth electrode contact can cover only a few square millimeters of cortical area.[9] This limited sampling subsequently provides perfect recording at the contact area but can easily miss seizure onset from adjacent areas. Therefore, interictal spikes, especially, recorded by depth electrodes are accepted as unreliable for the determination of the epileptogenic zone. It should also be emphasized that grid and strip coverage is basically a surface sampling limited to the crown portion of the cortex. The majority of the cortex in covered areas stays buried in the sulci below the surface or under opercular surfaces such as insular cortex. Therefore, strip and grid electrodes do not have any direct contact with cortical tissues on these embedded cortical areas.

Another well-known potential technical problem of invasive monitoring techniques is an issue with signal detection problems secondary to orientation of the angle of the dipole.[1,4–6] Other disadvantages and limitations are cost, patient discomfort secondary to the surgical procedure and because of the immobility during the postoperative monitoring period, surgical risks that may cause morbidity and even mortality, and the necessity for two separate surgical interventions. It is also possible that invasive monitoring still may not provide any localizing information at the end of the monitoring period and further cortical resection to treat seizures may not be an option for the patient. This rate has been reported between 12 and 34% in some large series.[1,4,5]

■ Surgical Technique

Depth and Strip of Electrode Placement

Depth electrode placement in epilepsy patients has traditionally been performed with stereotactic frames. However, frameless stereotactic techniques using neuronavigation system guidance has been becoming increasingly more popular in recent years.[5,14] We place depth electrodes using stereotactic frames (CRW (Integra Radionics, Burlington, MA) or Leksell (Elektra, Stockholm, Sweden)) in our patients but application of a stereotactic frame in the pediatric age group is limited by age. We have not used the stereotactic frame for depth electrode placement in children younger than 13 years old. Frameless systems have many advantages in children, including their ability for use in younger patients, more freedom to choose appropriate trajectories, concurrent use in guiding precise strip electrode trajectories and grid placement in the same setting, and eliminating the need to remove or work around the frame if craniotomy is needed.[5,14] Conversely, the stereotactic frame has a very reliable track record and unsurpassed precision for depth electrode placement.

For depth electrode placement, we obtain a brain MRI with gadolinium in all patients 1 to 2 days before surgery date. Then the stereotactic frame base is attached to the patient's head in the operating room under general anesthesia, and the patient is transferred to the computed tomography (CT) scanner. A head CT scan with contrast is obtained after the stereotactic localizer is attached to the frame, and the head is secured to the scanner table. The digital data are then transferred via Ethernet to our computer workstation, and MRI and CT scan images are fused using image fusion software. The most appropriate trajectories for both depth electrodes are subsequently chosen. Image fusion enables us to combine a CT scan's precision for targeting with the enhanced neuroanatomy and multiplanar imaging capabilities of MRI.

Although depth electrodes can also be placed into orbitofrontal cortex or cingulum, hippocampal depth electrode placement is the most commonly used technique. We describe this approach here. We insert depth electrodes with 10–12 contacts via an occipitotemporal approach in TLE to maximize the number of electrode contacts in the amygdala and hippocampus. First, target and entry points are selected, and the trajectory is defined. The ideal trajectory avoids cortical vascular structures and does not pass through sulci or the ventricle. The target point of the most distal electrode contact is in amygdala, and the other contacts lay in hippocampal head and body (**Fig. 15.2A–C**). This may not be possible in some cases because of the individual anatomical variations, and some compromises may be needed while choosing the entry point and trajectory.[8] The trajectory is checked in axial, sagittal, and coronal slices carefully using the probe's eye view on the workstation, and the entry and target points are subsequently slightly altered, if necessary,

to obtain a safer trajectory. After the most appropriate trajectory is chosen, coordinates are calculated and recorded. Simultaneously, the patient's head is attached to the operating table using the Mayfield (Codman Inc., Raynham, MA) attachment for the stereotactic frame, and the patient's neck is slightly flexed. The head of the bed is elevated up to 45 degrees for a semisitting position. This position provides a perfect exposure to the parietooccipital region.

The surgical site is prepared and draped with a transparent adhesive cover. Then the appropriate coordinates are chosen on the frame and arc, and a guide cannula is inserted to the scalp to mark the entry point. A small linear scalp incision is made for the burr hole. We prefer using a burr hole, rather than a drill hole, to allow direct visualization of cortical vessels and to avoid any accidental alterations of trajectory caused by bony edges. The dura is coagulated and opened. Next, the rigid guide cannula and its obturator are placed to target; then the obturator is removed, and the depth electrode is inserted through the cannula. The cannula is then removed while holding the depth electrode and its semirigid stylet steadily. Then the stylet of the depth electrode is removed. The depth electrode is next tunneled several centimeters away from the incision using either a specially designed tunneler or a 14-gauge angiocath and is tied down to scalp with 3–0 silk. Then a purse-string suture, using 3–0 silk, passing through the galea is placed around the cable to decrease risk for CSF leak. Then the electrode cable is again sutured to scalp by making a small loop.

We almost always use depth-strip electrode combinations in TLE; frequently, three subdural strip electrodes are placed on each side to cover both temporal neocortexes. After applying sterile dressings on depth electrode incisions, a small incision is made on the temporal region for strip electrode placement. A burr hole is placed 2 cm above the zygoma, just anterior to pinna, then dura is opened carefully while protecting the underlying arachnoid. The temporal strip electrodes are gently slid into the subdural space using smooth forceps and continuous irrigation. A Penfield (Codman Inc., Raynham, MA) #3 dissector may be helpful during strip electrode placement to guide the electrodes' trajectory. We place an eight-contact electrode to cover the parahippocampus in patients older than 10 years and a six-contact electrode in patients younger than 10. This electrode is placed parallel to the sylvian fissure on a trajectory toward the medial portion of the temporal pole just lateral to the sphenoid wing so that it curves down at the tip and lies under the anterior parahippocampus. Then, a second electrode with six contacts is placed, perpendicular to the sylvian fissure/base of the middle fossa, covering the middle, inferior, and fusiform gyri with the most distal electrode under the middle-posterior portion of the parahippocampus. The third electrode (four to six contacts) is placed posteriorly to cover the posterior temporal region over the middle temporal gyrus. If a strip electrode does not slide in smoothly, it should be pulled back and reoriented to a slightly different trajectory for the second attempt.[3,12] After placement of strip electrodes, the cables are tunneled several centimeters away from incision using an angiocath or specially designed tunnelers. The burr hole is plugged with Gelfoam (Pfizer Inc, NY, USA) and covered with DuraSeal (Confluent Surgical, MA, USA). The galea and scalp layers are closed separately. Strip electrodes are also frequently used for extratemporal epilepsy cases. The burr hole location is determined in these cases individually on the basis of the suspicious area and planned coverage sites.

Grid Electrode Placement

For grid placement, the patient is in the supine position, and the head is either placed on a horseshoe head holder or secured with three-point fixation systems. The extent of skin incision and scalp flap is determined by considering the electrode coverage area as well as the projected craniotomy for possible resective surgery in the future. The surgical procedure for grid placement is a standard craniotomy and is performed under general anesthesia. The dura is opened largely, and tacking sutures are placed. At this stage, neuronavigation guidance can be used again to determine the cortical coverage area more precisely. Then the grid plate is placed over the cortex with smooth forceps. Although it is possible to slide the grid plate slightly beyond the craniotomy edges,

this type of blind advancement should be avoided as much as possible to decrease cortical injury and bleeding risk. Dual-sided grid electrodes are perfect for interhemispheric bilateral coverage, if needed. We place our craniotomy flap two thirds anterior and one third posterior to the coronal suture in these cases if the plan is to place only interhemispheric grid and a few subdural frontal strips (**Fig. 15.5A, B**). Although grid electrodes can often be slid into the interhemispheric space easily, we place interhemispheric grid electrodes after fully dissecting and exploring the interhemispheric space because of the frequent presence of adhesions and bridging veins in this area. We also prefer to expose and dissect the interhemispheric space all the way down to corpus callosum if the goal is also to cover cingulum. Both cingulate gyri are almost always tightly attached to each other, and the edge of the grid electrode would either stay above cingulum or injure them if it is placed blindly by sliding the plate without separating both gyri. After grid placement is completed, the edges of the plate should be checked carefully to avoid any compression by the edge of the grid on large cortical veins or injury to bridging veins or cortical areas with adhesions. If the cortical area covered by grid plate is a site of previous surgery or trauma or if there is an underlying mass lesion, more caution is needed while placing grid electrodes and during the closure. It is also critical to be sure that all electrodes have a firm contact with cortical surface because grid plates can be folded under the bone.

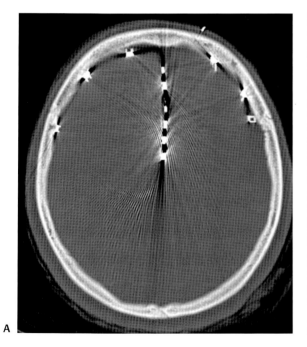
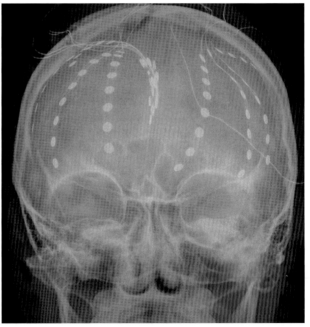

A   B

Fig. 15.5 Mesial frontal cortex coverage with interhemispheric dual-sided grid electrodes and bilateral frontal convexity coverage with multiple strip electrodes. **(A)** Head computed tomography scan shows grid electrode contacts in the interhemispheric space and multiple strip electrode contacts in different trajectories on the frontal convexities. **(B)** Skull x-ray shows interhemispheric grid plates and multiple bilateral strip electrodes covering frontal convexities.

In some cases, adjacent grid/grid or grid/strip combinations may be needed to gain more extensive coverage. In these cases, these adjacent electrodes should be placed so that no space is present between subdural electrodes to prevent herniation of brain or cortical vasculature between the edges of the two subdural electrode plates (**Fig. 15.4A**). After placement of the grid plate, cables are tunneled several centimeters away from the incision lines using an angiocath or specifically designed cable tunnelers. Then a digital photo is taken to document the grid position, and dural closure is performed. Duraplasty is almost always needed to have a comfortable closure with a watertight technique as much as possible. We also cover the suture lines with first Duragen (Integra Lifesciences, NJ, USA) and then DuraSeal (Confluent Surgical, MA, USA). Then a surface recording is performed by checking each electrode contact separately, and the bone flap is replaced with loose sutures if recording is satisfactory. At this stage, it is necessary to ensure that leads are not compressed between bone edges. We perform meticulous hemostasis before skin closure to avoid any need for subgaleal drain placement. Then the galea and skin are closed as separate layers with appropriate sutures. All cable exit points are closed with purse-string sutures, and all cables are marked and numbered separately to identify the related electrodes. A bulky head dressing is applied.

■ Postoperative Monitoring

Patients receive pre- and postoperative intravenous antibiotics. We also use small dosages of dexamethasone (Decadron) for a few days in subdural grid cases. Skull x-rays and a head CT scan are obtained to document the electrode positions, and the patient is transferred to the intensive care unit for an overnight stay. EEG monitoring starts the next day. Supplemental drawings of the electrode locations are prepared by the epilepsy surgeon after surgery, and these are placed into the patient file as well as the neurophysiology file. We also obtain a postoperative brain MRI, especially in depth electrode cases, to see the electrode contact locations more precisely. Although MRI is a concern because of potential heating/electrical injury to brain parenchyma, we have not encountered any issues to date; these results were confirmed in a large study showing that MRI is safe for invasive monitoring patients.[15] Duration of monitoring and the ideal seizure numbers necessary to complete a monitoring period are somewhat controversial. We aim to record at least three habitual seizures before removing the electrodes, and we verify the seizure types with family members to be sure these are typical seizures. If the patient does not have the sufficient number of seizures, then provocative measures such as sleep deprivation are considered, along with discontinuation of medications. Patients are closely monitored for CSF leak, and if any leak is noted, additional sutures are placed. We do not use lumbar drains to prevent CSF leak. After obtaining satisfactory electrophysiological data, the patient returns to the operating room for removal of the electrodes with or without cortical resection, and all removed electrodes are sent for culture.

■ Complications

Invasive monitoring has a relatively high rate of complications. The most common complications reported in some large series including both adult and children are subdural hematoma (SDH; 0–16%), cerebral edema (2–14%), CSF leak (19–33%), and infection (2–16%).[1,8,11,12] CSF leak was reported between 12 and 31% in three large pediatric series.[2,4,16] In these pediatric series, infection rate was reported between 0 and 8.6%, and hemorrhage rate was between 0 and 25%. Reported infections include wound infection (0.6–11%), meningitis (0.3–2%), osteomyelitis, and brain abscess.[2,4,16] One of these series reported a detailed list of complications in 35 children who underwent invasive monitoring[16]: CSF leak (20%), cerebral edema (14%), SDH (14%), intracerebral hemorrhage (9%), wound infection (9%), and osteomyelitis (3%). The same study reported associated neurological deficits as well: mild-moderate temporary hemiparesis (69%), dysphasia (51%), facial weakness (48%), and visual field defect (37%). Another large series, which included 187 adults and children, reported an overall complication rate of 26.3%.[12] Authors reported a 12.6% incidence of neurological deficit (hemiparesis 7.6%, only 1.5% permanent neurological deficit), 12.1% infection, (7.1% meningitis, 3% osteomyelitis), 3% hematoma, and 2.5% mental status change.[12] SDH is a concern especially in grid cases, and some surgeons even leave a drain in the subdural space. We do not leave any drain and do not consider any intervention for subdural thin hematoma unless they are symptomatic. We believe meticulous hemostasis with copious irrigation and checking adjacent vasculature to the grid edges is essential to decrease the risk of SDH. Intracranial bleeding risk is reportedly higher in depth electrodes compared with strip electrodes in some series, whereas other series report much lower rates of intracranial bleeding with depth electrode placement.[1–3,5,8,12,16] Cerebral edema is another significant problem; although not clinically relevant in most cases, it can also be severe with midline shift and herniation findings and necessitate urgent removal of electrodes. Cerebral edema risk is higher with grid electrodes, multiple plates, in the pediatric age group, and in the presence of mass lesion. Therefore, large duraplasty, hinging the skull flap, or craniectomy may be considered in high-risk patients. Among risk factors in invasive monitoring patients, grid electrodes, higher number of grids and strips, longer monitoring periods, presence of CSF leak, previous surgeries at the same site, and presence of mass lesions are also reported.[2,3,12]

■ Conclusion

In conclusion, invasive monitoring constitutes a significant portion of epilepsy surgery in the pediatric age group and may provide essential additional data in selected patients. Invasive monitoring techniques often include a combination of depth, strip, and grid electrodes and the precise configuration is determined by individual patient pathology. The surgeon and epilepsy team must be aware of the advantages, limitations, and potential complications of each technique and must be versatile with them in order to provide the best possible electrophysiological data to direct potential resective procedures.

References

1. Johnston JM Jr, Mangano FT, Ojemann JG, Park TS, Trevathan E, Smyth MD. Complications of invasive subdural electrode monitoring at St. Louis Children's Hospital, 1994-2005. J Neurosurg 2006; 105(5, suppl):343–347
2. Simon SL, Telfeian A, Duhaime A-C. Complications of invasive monitoring used in intractable pediatric epilepsy. Pediatr Neurosurg 2003;38(1):47–52
3. Bruce DA, Bizzi JWJ. Surgical technique for the insertion of grids and strips for invasive monitoring in children with intractable epilepsy. Childs Nerv Syst 2000;16(10-11):724–730
4. Adelson PD, O'Rourke DK, Albright AL. Chronic invasive monitoring for identifying seizure foci in children. Neurosurg Clin N Am 1995;6(3):491–504
5. Blount JP, Cormier J, Kim H, Kankirawatana P, Riley KO, Knowlton RC. Advances in intracranial monitoring. Neurosurg Focus 2008;25(3): E18
6. Sperling MR. Clinical challenges in invasive monitoring in epilepsy surgery. Epilepsia 1997;38(suppl 4):S6–S12
7. Diehl B, Lüders HO. Temporal lobe epilepsy: when are invasive recordings needed? Epilepsia 2000;41(suppl 3):S61–S74
8. Blatt DR, Roper SN, Friedman WA. Invasive monitoring of limbic epilepsy using stereotactic depth and subdural strip electrodes: surgical technique. Surg Neurol 1997;48(1):74–79
9. Dubeau F, McLachlan RS. Invasive electrographic recording techniques in temporal lobe epilepsy. Can J Neurol Sci 2000;27(suppl 1): S29–S34, discussion S50–S52
10. Mulligan L, Vives K, Spencer D. Placement of depth electrodes. In: Luders HO, ed. Textbook of Epilepsy Surgery. London, UK: Informa; 2008:938–944
11. Salazar F, Bingaman WE. Placement of subdural grids. In: Luders HO, ed. Textbook of Epilepsy Surgery. London, UK: Informa; 2008:931–937
12. Hamer HM, Morris HH, Mascha EJ, et al. Complications of invasive video-EEG monitoring with subdural grid electrodes. Neurology 2002;58(1):97–103
13. Schevon CA, Carlson C, Zaroff CM, et al. Pediatric language mapping: sensitivity of neurostimulation and Wada testing in epilepsy surgery. Epilepsia 2007;48(3):539–545
14. Chamoun RB, Nayar VV, Yoshor D. Neuronavigation applied to epilepsy monitoring with subdural electrodes. Neurosurg Focus 2008;25(3):E21
15. Davis LM, Spencer DD, Spencer SS, Bronen RA. MR imaging of implanted depth and subdural electrodes: is it safe? Epilepsy Res 1999;35(2):95–98
16. Onal C, Otsubo H, Araki T, et al. Complications of invasive subdural grid monitoring in children with epilepsy. J Neurosurg 2003;98(5):1017–1026

16 Mesial Temporal Sclerosis in Children

Mackenzie C. Cervenka and Adam L. Hartman

Temporal lobe epilepsy (TLE) is the most common partial seizure disorder in the adult population, and the most frequent cause is mesial temporal sclerosis (MTS). Seizures usually begin in late childhood or early adolescence. The prevalence of MTS among children with newly diagnosed seizure disorders is reportedly much lower: approximately 1% of those presenting with initial recurrent seizures and even lower when evaluating children younger than 12 years.[1–3] Ng et al recently studied the baseline prevalence of childhood MTS.[4] Their review of 3100 brain magnetic resonance imaging (MRI) reports from children younger than 14 years old (obtained for a variety of reasons, including seizure, head injury, brain tumor, headache, and developmental delays) showed that 24 (0.77%) had MTS. All patients with MTS in this series initially presented with seizures, so the authors concluded that although MTS is uncommon in children, it is invariably presents with seizures.

Pathophysiology

The mesial temporal structures include the hippocampus, amygdala, and parahippocampal gyrus. MTS refers to atrophy and gliosis of the hippocampus. Synonyms for MTS include Ammon's horn sclerosis and hippocampal sclerosis. MTS is the cause for TLE in 50 to 65% of patients undergoing temporal lobectomy.[5,6] Pathological variants observed in MTS include hippocampal neuronal loss and gliosis, neuronogenesis, and axonal reorganization.[7] Classic Ammon's horn sclerosis is defined as primary neuronal loss involving sectors CA1 and CA4 (the sectors most vulnerable to hypoxic damage), occurring less frequently in sectors CA2 and CA3.[8] Total Ammon horn sclerosis consists of severe neuronal loss involving all four sectors.

The molecular pathology of MTS is not completely understood. Certain types of medically refractory epilepsy may be the result of excitotoxicity secondary to excessive glutamatergic activity. Elevated extracellular glutamate levels, glutamate receptor upregulation, and loss of glutamine synthetase (a glutamate-metabolizing enzyme) have been demonstrated in affected brain tissue of patients with MTS.[9] This observation has been referred to as the "glutamate hypothesis" of MTS pathogenesis. Astrocytes, with their important role in glutamate reuptake and metabolism, probably play an important role in this process, because excessive astrocyte proliferation and accumulation and release of astrocytic glutamate has been demonstrated in MTS.[9,10]

Etiologies

There is a great deal of controversy regarding the causality between MTS and TLE (i.e., whether MTS is the cause or the result of TLE). Prolonged febrile seizures, head injury, nonfebrile status epilepticus, encephalitis, hypertensive encephalopathy, and viruses have been implicated as potential underlying causes for MTS in children.[11–14] MTS can also be a late complication of posttransplant cyclosporine-A neurotoxicity (including in children).[15,16] Dual pathology [i.e., the presence of other lesions, such as malformations of cortical development (MCD) in sites outside the hippocampus or even the temporal lobe] has been observed in approximately one third of patients who have undergone temporal lobectomy as treatment for intractable seizures.[17–22] MTS can be bilateral in up to 20% of patients.[6]

MTS and Febrile Seizures

The link between MTS and severe febrile convulsions (FCs) was suggested by Falconer et al.[23] MRI studies have suggested a causal link between prolonged and focal FCs in some patients, although some infants in that series also had evidence of pre-existing abnormalities (this has not been consistent between series).[24,25] Up to 30% of TLE patients with MTS in surgical series have a history of prolonged FCs and status epilepticus.[26] Up to 3.5% of patients with a history of febrile seizures later develop epilepsy.[27,28] Three potential hypotheses exist to explain the association with MTS and FCs (explained in ref. 29). One is that FCs cause MTS through acute hippocampal injury, which then later results in the emergence of TLE. The second hypothesis is that FCs and MTS are both a consequence of another abnormality that ultimately results in TLE. Finally, MTS may precede FCs. Other investigators believe there is no actual association between FCs and MTS. Patients with a history of complex (not simple) febrile seizures (defined in the National Collaborative Perinatal Project as those lasting greater than 15 minutes, with evidence of focal convulsions, or more than two seizures in a 24-hour period[27]) have an increased incidence of epilepsy and MTS.[22–31] The incidence of MTS after complex febrile seizures is related directly to the number of complex features.[31] However, more recent studies with long-term follow-up have questioned the strength of this association. Tarkka et al followed 24 patients with prolonged febrile seizures, 8 with an unprovoked seizure after the first event and 32 control subjects with a single simple febrile seizure over a mean of 12.3 years and found that none fit MRI criteria for MTS at the time of follow-up.[32]

Human Herpes Virus 6

Human herpes virus 6 (HHV-6) is a ubiquitous β-herpesvirus associated with roseola infantum. HHV6 has been shown to cause limbic encephalitis in immunocompromised hosts and is thought to cause seizures, meningitis, and multiple sclerosis in otherwise healthy individuals.[13,14] Theodore et al examined TLE specimens and discovered that hippocampal astrocytes contained active HHV6B in approximately two thirds of MTS patients.[14] They proposed that HHV6B may cause excitotoxicity by inhibiting transport of excitatory amino acids within astrocytes and by causing neuronal damage. A great deal of evidence also links HHV6 to febrile seizures, indicating a potential link between MTS and FC.

Dual Pathology

Postsurgical pathological evaluation of temporal lobectomy specimens in patients with MTS has often revealed not only hippocampal sclerosis, but also coexistent MCD. Mohamed et al reported mild-to-moderate MCD in 79% of specimens received from 34 children and adolescents who underwent anteromesial temporal resection.[33] Although the interictal electroencephalogram (EEG) in these patients was not as localizing as in patients with MTS alone, the finding of dual pathology did not predict a poorer postsurgical outcome. These findings are in contrast to a more recent evaluation by Kan et al showing that of 19 patients identified with MTS, only 3 had dual pathology (16%) and of those, only one third were seizure free after surgical resection.[34]

■ Presentation

Older children and adolescents with MTS often present initially with complex partial seizures that frequently secondarily generalize. The seizures can be triggered by psychological or physical stress, sleep deprivation, or hormonal fluctuations in adolescent girls. They may be preceded by a combination of auras such as a rising gastric sensation, déjà vu, psychic auras (e.g., fear, anxiety, or other strong emotions), olfactory auras, or autonomic changes (e.g., tachycardia, pallor, mydriasis). The ictal event typically lasts 1 to 2 minutes and consists

clinically of staring and automatisms such as lip smacking, puckering, chewing, or swallowing, hand picking, rubbing, or fumbling. Importantly, hand automatisms are seen more frequently ipsilateral to the MTS with contralateral dystonic posturing.[35] Patients can behave in a semipurposeful manner during these episodes but do not retain full awareness of the event. The postictal period may be of variable duration and may last up to several hours.[36] However, as in most of pediatric neurology, signs can be age dependent. Signs and symptoms are more difficult to assess when evaluating infants and toddlers with suspected MTS because assessment of subjective aura and impairment of consciousness is challenging in this age group. Bourgeois et al described the distinctive features of complex partial seizures in infants as follows: "(1) a predominance of behavioral arrest with possible impairment of consciousness, (2) no identifiable aura, (3) automatisms that are discrete and mostly orofacial, (4) more prominent convulsive activity, and (5) a longer duration (> 1 minute)."[1] Brockhaus and Elger studied 29 children with TLE and found that symmetrical limb motor signs, posturing (as expected in frontal lobe seizures), and head nodding were the most common signs.[37] Therefore, many different types of seizure semiology may indicate TLE; conversely, absence of clinical findings typical of older children and adults should not rule out the diagnosis because semiology can represent spread to extratemporal regions (i.e., rather than origin from the mesial temporal region).[38]

Adults with MTS often have memory impairment specific to the hemisphere involved (i.e., verbal memory impairment with dominant hemisphere disease and nonverbal learning impairment in nondominant MTS). However, children tend to have less-specific neuropsychological deficits with impairment in long-term memory as well as both verbal and nonverbal learning.[39] Patients with evidence of early bilateral MTS are at increased risk for more severe impairments in learning and memory.[40]

■ Evaluation

Detailed neurological examination should focus on evidence of memory and language dysfunction and additional signs of focal neurological deficits. The most frequently reported neurological abnormality in MTS patients is a mild contralateral facial paresis.[41,42] The standard of care in evaluating a patient for the cause of a first seizure is to obtain a routine 30-minute EEG.[43,44] In adults, the first routine EEG reveals epileptiform abnormalities in approximately 23% of patients.[44]

Electroencephalography and Electrocorticography

The interictal EEG in patients with suspected MTS often reveals unilateral or bilateral independent anterior temporal sharp waves and spikes (**Fig. 16.1A**).[45–47] These epileptiform discharges may be better detected with inclusion of zygomatic or sphenoidal electrodes in adults, although noninvasive cheek electrodes are just as sensitive in detecting spikes.[48] Invasive electrodes are not routinely used in the pediatric age group. Temporal intermittent rhythmic delta activity over the affected region is also highly suggestive of MTS.[49,50] The typical ictal pattern consists of θ (5–7 Hz) to low α (8–9 Hz) frequency rhythmic sharp activity originating over the anterior temporal region either at the time of ictal onset (initial focal onset) or within 30 s of ictal onset (delayed focal onset)[51,52] (**Fig. 16.1B**). In children, the initial ictal pattern is often preceded by a brief period of low voltage fast activity and can involve more diffuse generalized or bilateral activity.[33,37]

Patients with ictal and interictal patterns on scalp recording that are inconclusive or with no evidence of MTS on routine neuroimaging may require intracranial monitoring with subdural grid, strips, or depth electrodes to further differentiate MTS from a neocortical or extratemporal seizure foci. Studies reviewing these recordings have shown that patients with clear radiographic hippocampal sclerosis can

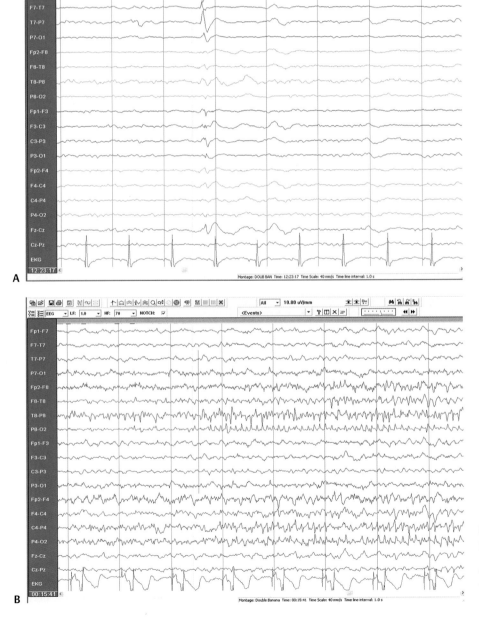

Fig. 16.1 **(A)** Interictal left anterior temporal sharp wave (longitudinal bipolar montage). **(B)** Onset of a seizure showing α frequency rhythmic spiking, maximal over the right posterior temporal head region (longitudinal bipolar montage).

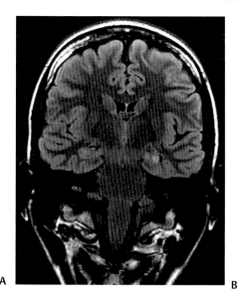
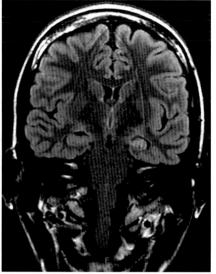
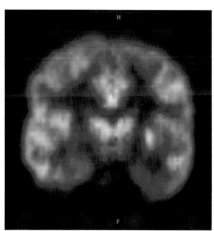

A   B   C

Fig. 16.2 **(A)** Fluid-attenuated inversion recovery (FLAIR) sequence of coronal magnetic resonance imaging (MRI) with thin cuts through the hippocampus reveals signal hyperintensity in the left hippocampus. **(B)** FLAIR sequence of coronal MRI demonstrates decreased volume of the left hippocampus. **(C)** Axial 2-deoxy-2[^{18}F]fluoro-D-glucose–positron emission tomography scan demonstrating left anterior temporal hypometabolism.

have seizure foci distant from the hippocampus, including the temporal pole,[53] amygdala,[54] or perisylvian cortex.[55]

Magnetic Resonance Imaging

A variety of neuroimaging modalities have been used to detect MTS. Routine MRI is relatively insensitive in detecting MTS.[56] MRI with thin, coronal oblique sections through the temporal lobes, hippocampi, and amygdala using high-resolution, T1-weighted images with inversion recovery and T2-weighted images with spin echo or fast spin echo is considered the gold standard in radiographically diagnosing MTS. Classic findings of MTS on MRI include decreased hippocampal volume and abnormal increased T2 signal of the mesial temporal structures (**Fig. 16.2A** and **16.2B**). T2 hyperintensity represents gliosis and increased free-water content within the hippocampus. Associated findings include atrophy of the adjacent fornix, mammillary body, or other limbic system structures.[57] Fluid-attenuated inversion recovery imaging can demonstrate abnormal signal intensity in the hippocampus, taking into account that normal limbic structures are slightly hyperintense relative to the neocortex. Hippocampal volume calculations also can be performed through volumetric thin-section T1-weighted imaging analysis (volumetric MRI) and provide significant improvement in detection of mild unilateral MTS.[21,58] The significance of these findings varies with age because children younger than 6 years old have hippocampal volumes that increase linearly with age.[59] Sensitivity of high-resolution MRI in detecting MTS is as high as 97% with a specificity of 83%.[60,61]

Magnetic resonance spectroscopy demonstrates the anatomic distribution of biologic metabolites, and N-acetylaspartate is focally reduced in MTS, indicating some degree of focal neuronal metabolic dysfunction.[62] There are regional metabolic abnormalities with maximal focal accentuation at the site of the epileptogenic focus. This technique has been useful in noninvasively localizing seizure foci and in predicting surgical outcome in bilateral TLE patients.[63]

Positron Emission Tomography and Single Proton Emission Tomography

Positron emission tomography (PET) scanning with [^{18}F]fluorodeoxyglucose (FDG) reveals hypometabolism in the mesial temporal structures during the interictal period in patients with MTS (**Fig. 16.2C**). The temporal pole and lateral temporal cortex also may be hypometabolic in MTS patients as well as extratemporal regions such as the parietal cortex, orbitofrontal cortex, and insula.[64,65] Hypometabolism in the temporopolar region predicts a favorable postoperative outcome.[66] MTS patients without imaging evidence of hippocampal sclerosis still can be identified on the basis of PET results revealing ipsilateral hippocampal hypometabolism and adjacent cortical hypometabolism.[67]

Single positron emission tomography (SPECT) scans are performed after injection of a radiotracer ictally and interictally to reveal differences in distribution of blood flow. During a seizure, there is relative hyperperfusion at the site of ictal onset and, therefore, greatest uptake of radiotracer. Interictally, there is relative hypoperfusion and hence a decrease in radiotracer uptake compared with the surrounding unaffected brain tissue. In a meta-analysis of SPECT imaging in localization of epileptic foci, Devous et al found the overall sensitivity for SPECT in seizure localization for patients with TLE was 44% interictally, 75% postictally, and 97% ictally.[68] Few studies in children have confirmed efficacy of ictal–interictal SPECT in localizing epileptic foci.[69] Ictal–interictal subtraction techniques with MRI coregistration provide more accurate lateralization and localization of ictal onset.[70]

■ Differential Diagnosis

Pathological abnormalities associated with temporal lobe seizure in infancy and childhood include MCD, migrational disorders, hamartomas, low-grade brain tumors (such as astrocytomas, gangliogliomas, and dysembryoplastic neuroepithelial tumors) and vascular malformations. These abnormalities have been identified pathologically or radiographically in 15 to 20% of children with TLE.[6,71,72] Of these, glial and neuronal neoplasms account for 10 to 15%.[6] The lesions may be subtle and not apparent even with high-resolution MRI until later in childhood and initially may be indistinguishable from MTS—only noted once a specimen has been obtained for histopathology. Electrographically, focal epilepsy of childhood (particularly benign epilepsy with centrotemporal spikes) may lead to a misdiagnosis of MTS.

■ Treatment

Antiepileptic Medications

Patients who have a single, unprovoked seizure have an approximate subsequent seizure risk of 50%.[72] Once the patient has suffered a second unprovoked seizure, the risk of further seizures within the next 4 years increases to 75%.[73] Of patients newly diagnosed with epilepsy, roughly 60% will respond to initial monotherapy, and 40% will ultimately be considered refractory to pharmacologic treatment.[74] Overall, patients with MTS appear to be more refractory to pharmacotherapy, as shown in several studies in which between 0 and 25% of MTS patients had their seizures well controlled with anticonvulsant medication only.[75,76] In these studies, many patients were treated for several years and presented for potential temporal lobectomy, thus representing a biased sample of patients with MTS. Stephen et al studied 73 patients with newly diagnosed MTS and found that 42% responded to pharmacotherapy.[74] Only 48% of these patients required more than one agent to become seizure free, suggesting an important role of anticonvulsants as initial management in the treatment of TLE in MTS.[74]

Aggressive anticonvulsant management at the time of diagnosis is important to help prevent psychosocial dysfunction and possibly limit cognitive decline and interference with school performance. Medication titration should be implemented with the goal of achieving seizure freedom with minimal side effects. If the initial medication is ineffective, it is our practice to either switch drugs or add a second agent with a different mechanism of action from the first. Overall, success in obtaining seizure freedom with multiple agents in MTS once monotherapy fails is poor.[75,76]

Previous studies support the use of sodium channel blockers (e.g., phenytoin, carbamazepine), although all commercially available anticonvulsants (with the exception of ethosuximide) have been found to be useful.[77,78] Of the newer agents, only topiramate carries a Level A recommendation as adjunctive therapy in children with refractory partial epilepsy.[79,80]

Resective Surgery

Once patients have failed optimal treatment with multiple anticonvulsants, surgical intervention becomes a consideration.[81] Delaying surgery can worsen long-term outcomes, especially in the pediatric population; intractable epilepsy has a negative impact on cognitive and behavioral issues.[9,39,74]

Presurgical evaluation varies considerably among centers performing epilepsy surgery. However, the general approach includes evaluation with continuous video-EEG monitoring, high-resolution MRI, and a preoperative neuropsychological evaluation.[72] Based on this initial result, patients may also receive an interictal PET scan, or an ictal SPECT scan to further localize the seizure focus. Functional MRI is performed in select patients to localize sensorimotor and language function, and the Wada test (intracarotid amobarbital) is used to lateralize language and memory. Patients may undergo intraoperative mapping and electrocorticography or extraoperative invasive recordings to more precisely identify an epileptogenic focus. Ideally, these measures yield concordant information regarding the localization of the epileptogenic zone. However, some studies in the pediatric population have demonstrated favorable postsurgical outcomes, even when results are discordant.[37,82] With subdural grids or strips in place, patients may undergo functional localization mapping with electrocortical stimulation. The goal of mapping is to define eloquent cortex that should be avoided during a surgical resection. Several surgical strategies have been used to treat patients with TLE.

With regard to postoperative outcome measures, most studies have defined Engel Class I as their criteria for seizure freedom. The time to last follow-up has varied between studies. Wyllie et al. reported seizure-free outcomes in 72 children ages 3 months to 12 years and adolescents 13 to 20 years who underwent all types of seizure (including temporal lobectomy, lesionectomy, and hemispherectomy) surgery to be as high as 78% postoperatively after more than

3 years of follow-up.[71] In a review of previous literature addressing seizure outcome after temporal lobe resection in children, Wyllie reported an overall 74 to 82% rate of seizure freedom.[83] Clusmann et al evaluated 89 children with TLE, ages 1 to 18 years for an average of 46 months after surgery and found that maximum seizure control was obtained with anterior mesial temporal resection (AMTR) (95%) compared with selective amygdalohippocampectomy (SAH) (75%), although this study included TLE patients with and without MTS.[84] Cohen-Gadol et al reported 2-year postoperative outcomes in unilateral MTS patients diagnosed on the basis of surgical pathology results who underwent anterior temporal lobectomy with hippocampectomy. They evaluated the percentage of patients that remained Engel

Class I and found that 86% were seizure free at 6 months, 83% at 1 year, 80% at 2 years, and 79% at 5 and 10 years.[85] Baldauf et al reported a greater than 90% remission rate in 41 patients diagnosed with unilateral MTS on the basis of four or more interictal EEG recordings and diagnostic MRI results alone, followed for more than 3 years after cortico-amygdalo-hippocampectomy.[86] In a pediatric population of carefully selected patients diagnosed with MTS on the basis of ictal semiology, EEG, and MRI findings who underwent temporal lobectomy, 73 to 100% received benefit from surgery.[6] Surgical outcomes are predictably not as favorable for patients with bilateral disease as those with clear unilateral MTS,[33] and other treatment modalities must be considered.

References

1. Bourgeois BF. Temporal lobe epilepsy in infants and children. Brain Dev 1998;20(3):135–141
2. King MA, Newton MR, Jackson GD, et al. Epileptology of the first-seizure presentation: a clinical, electroencephalographic, and magnetic resonance imaging study of 300 consecutive patients. Lancet 1998;352(9133):1007–1011
3. Berg AT, Testa FM, Levy SR, Shinnar S. Neuroimaging in children with newly diagnosed epilepsy: a community-based study. Pediatrics 2000;106(3):527–532
4. Ng YT, McGregor AL, Duane DC, Jahnke HK, Bird CR, Wheless JW. Childhood mesial temporal sclerosis. J Child Neurol 2006;21(6): 512–517
5. National Institutes of Health Consensus Conference. Surgery for epilepsy. JAMA 1990;264(6):729–733
6. Blume WT, Hwang PA. Pediatric candidates for temporal lobe epilepsy surgery. Can J Neurol Sci 2000;27(suppl 1):S14–S19, discussion S20–S21
7. Velísek L, Moshé SL. Temporal lobe epileptogenesis and epilepsy in the developing brain: bridging the gap between the laboratory and the clinic. Progression, but in what direction? Epilepsia 2003;44(suppl 12):51–59
8. Graham DI, Lantos PL, eds. Greenfield's Neuropathology. 7th ed. London, UK: Arnold; 1997:950
9. Eid T, Williamson A, Lee TS, Petroff OA, de Lanerolle NC. Glutamate and astrocytes—key players in human mesial temporal lobe epilepsy? Epilepsia 2008;49(suppl 2):42–52
10. Liu Z, Mikati M, Holmes GL. Mesial temporal sclerosis: pathogenesis and significance. Pediatr Neurol 1995;12(1):5–16
11. Scott RC, Gadian DG, Cross JH, Wood SJ, Neville BG, Connelly A. Quantitative magnetic resonance characterization of mesial temporal sclerosis in childhood. Neurology 2001;56(12):1659–1665
12. Solinas C, Briellmann RS, Harvey AS, Mitchell LA, Berkovic SF. Hypertensive encephalopathy: antecedent to hippocampal sclerosis and temporal lobe epilepsy? Neurology 2003;60(9):1534–1536
13. Donati D, Akhyani N, Fogdell-Hahn A, et al. Detection of human herpesvirus-6 in mesial temporal lobe epilepsy surgical brain resections. Neurology 2003;61(10):1405–1411
14. Theodore WH, Epstein L, Gaillard WD, Shinnar S, Wainwright MS, Jacobson S. Human herpes virus 6B: a possible role in epilepsy? Epilepsia 2008;49(11):1828–1837
15. Faraci M, Lanino E, Dallorso S, et al. Mesial temporal sclerosis—a late complication in four allogeneic pediatric recipients with persistent seizures after an acute episode of cyclosporine-A neurotoxicity. Bone Marrow Transplant 2003;31(10):919–922
16. Gaggero R, Haupt R, Paola Fondelli M, et al. Intractable epilepsy secondary to cyclosporine toxicity in children undergoing allogeneic hematopoietic bone marrow transplantation. J Child Neurol 2006;21(10):861–866
17. Lévesque MF, Nakasato N, Vinters HV, Babb TL. Surgical treatment of limbic epilepsy associated with extrahippocampal lesions: the problem of dual pathology. J Neurosurg 1991;75(3):364–370
18. Cendes F, Cook MJ, Watson C, et al. Frequency and characteristics of dual pathology in patients with lesional epilepsy. Neurology 1995;45(11):2058–2064
19. Prayson RA, Reith JD, Najm IM. Mesial temporal sclerosis. A clinicopathologic study of 27 patients, including 5 with coexistent cortical dysplasia. Arch Pathol Lab Med 1996;120(6):532–536
20. Li LM, Cendes F, Watson C, et al. Surgical treatment of patients with single and dual pathology: relevance of lesion and of hippocampal atrophy to seizure outcome. Neurology 1997;48(2):437–444
21. Ho SS, Kuzniecky RI, Gilliam F, Faught E, Morawetz R. Temporal lobe developmental malformations and epilepsy: dual pathology and bilateral hippocampal abnormalities. Neurology 1998;50(3):748–754
22. Cendes F, Li LM, Andermann F, et al. Dual pathology and its clinical relevance. Adv Neurol 1999;81:153–164
23. Falconer MA, Serafetinides EA, Corsellis JAN. Etiologies and pathogenesis of temporal lobe epilepsy. Arch Neurol 1964;10:233–248
24. Scott RC, Gadian DG, King MD, et al. Magnetic resonance imaging findings within 5 days of status epilepticus in childhood. Brain 2002;125(pt 9):1951–1959
25. VanLandingham KE, Heinz ER, Cavazos JE, Lewis DV. Magnetic resonance imaging evidence of hippocampal injury after prolonged focal febrile convulsions. Ann Neurol 1998;43(4):413–426
26. Davies KG, Hermann BP, Dohan FC Jr, Foley KT, Bush AJ, Wyler AR. Relationship of hippocampal sclerosis to duration and age of onset of epilepsy, and childhood febrile seizures in temporal lobectomy patients. Epilepsy Res 1996;24(2):119–126
27. Nelson KB, Ellenberg JH. Predictors of epilepsy in children who have experienced febrile seizures. N Engl J Med 1976;295(19): 1029–1033

28. Verity CM, Golding J. Risk of epilepsy after febrile convulsions: a national cohort study. BMJ 1991;303(6814):1373–1376

29. Arzimanoglou A, Guerrini R, Aicardi J. Aicardi's Epilepsy in Children. 3rd ed. Philadelphia, PA: Lippincott, Williams & Wilkins: 2004

30. Annegers JF, Hauser WA, Shirts SB, Kurland LT. Factors prognostic of unprovoked seizures after febrile convulsions. N Engl J Med 1987;316(9):493–498

31. Lewis DV. Febrile convulsions and mesial temporal sclerosis. Curr Opin Neurol 1999;12(2):197–201

32. Tarkka R, Pääkkö E, Pyhtinen J, Uhari M, Rantala H. Febrile seizures and mesial temporal sclerosis: No association in a long-term follow-up study. Neurology 2003;60(2):215–218

33. Mohamed A, Wyllie E, Ruggieri P, et al. Temporal lobe epilepsy due to hippocampal sclerosis in pediatric candidates for epilepsy surgery. Neurology 2001;56(12):1643–1649

34. Kan P, Van Orman C, Kestle JRW. Outcomes after surgery for focal epilepsy in children. Childs Nerv Syst 2008;24(5):587–591

35. Kotagal P, Lüders H, Morris HH, et al. Dystonic posturing in complex partial seizures of temporal lobe onset: a new lateralizing sign. Neurology 1989;39(2 pt 1):196–201

36. Engel J Jr. Mesial temporal lobe epilepsy: what have we learned? Neuroscientist 2001;7(4):340–352

37. Brockhaus A, Elger CE. Complex partial seizures of temporal lobe origin in children of different age groups. Epilepsia 1995;36(12):1173–1181

38. Cendes F, Kahane P, Brodie M, Andermann F. The mesio-temporal lobe epilepsy syndrome. In: Roger J, Bureau M, Dravet, Genton P, Tassinari CA, Wolf P, eds. Epileptic Syndromes in Infancy, Childhood, and Adolescence. 3rd ed. Eastleigh, London, England: John Libbey 2002:513–530

39. Aldenkamp AP, Alpherts WC, Dekker MJ, Overweg J. Neuropsychological aspects of learning disabilities in epilepsy. Epilepsia 1990;31(suppl 4):S9–S20

40. DeLong GR, Heinz ER. The clinical syndrome of early-life bilateral hippocampal sclerosis. Ann Neurol 1997;42(1):11–17

41. Remillard GM, Andermann F, Rhi-Sausi A, Robbins NM. Facial asymmetry in patients with temporal lobe epilepsy. A clinical sign useful in the lateralization of temporal epileptogenic foci. Neurology 1977;27(2):109–114

42. Cascino GD, Jack CR, Parisi JE, et al. Facial asymmetry, hippocampal pathology, and remote symptomatic seizures: a temporal lobe epileptic syndrome. Ann Neurol 1991;30:31–36

43. Hirtz D, Berg A, Bettis D, et al. Quality Standards Subcommittee of the American Academy of Neurology; Practice Committee of the Child Neurology Society. Practice parameter: treatment of the child with a first unprovoked seizure: Report of the Quality Standards Subcommittee of the American Academy of Neurology and the Practice Committee of the Child Neurology Society. Neurology 2003;60(2):166–175

44. Krumholz A, Wiebe S, Gronseth G, et al. Quality Standards Subcommittee of the American Academy of Neurology; American Epilepsy Society. Practice Parameter: evaluating an apparent unprovoked first seizure in adults (an evidence-based review): report of the Quality Standards Subcommittee of the American Academy of Neurology and the American Epilepsy Society. Neurology 2007;69(21):1996–2007

45. Gambardella A, Gotman J, Cendes F, Andermann F. The relation of spike foci and of clinical seizure characteristics to different patterns of mesial temporal atrophy. Arch Neurol 1995;52(3):287–293

46. Cascino GD, Trenerry MR, So EL, et al. Routine EEG and temporal lobe epilepsy: relation to long-term EEG monitoring, quantitative MRI, and operative outcome. Epilepsia 1996;37(7):651–656

47. Gilliam F, Bowling S, Bilir E, et al. Association of combined MRI, interictal EEG, and ictal EEG results with outcome and pathology after temporal lobectomy. Epilepsia 1997;38(12):1315–1320

48. Krauss GL, Lesser RP, Fisher RS, Arroyo S. Anterior "cheek" electrodes are comparable to sphenoidal electrodes for the identification of ictal activity. Electroencephalogr Clin Neurophysiol 1992;83(6):333–338

49. Gambardella A, Gotman J, Cendes F, Andermann F. Focal intermittent delta activity in patients with mesiotemporal atrophy: a reliable marker of the epileptogenic focus. Epilepsia 1995;36(2):122–129

50. Sharbrough FW. Nonspecific abnormal EEG patterns. In: Niedermeyer E, Lopes da Silva F, eds. Electroencephalography: Basic Principles, Clinical Applications, and Related Fields. 5th ed. Baltimore, MD: Lippincott Williams and Wilkins; 2005:235–254

51. Ebersole JS, Pacia SV. Localization of temporal lobe foci by ictal EEG patterns. Epilepsia 1996;37(4):386–399

52. Assaf BA, Ebersole JS. Visual and quantitative ictal EEG predictors of outcome after temporal lobectomy. Epilepsia 1999;40(1):52–61

53. Kahane P, Chabardès S, Minotti L, Hoffmann D, Benabid AL, Munari C. The role of the temporal pole in the genesis of temporal lobe seizures. Epileptic Disord 2002;4(suppl 1):S51–S58

54. Spanedda F, Cendes F, Gotman J. Relations between EEG seizure morphology, interhemispheric spread, and mesial temporal atrophy in bitemporal epilepsy. Epilepsia 1997;38(12):1300–1314

55. Kahane P, Huot JC, Hoffman D, et al. Perisylvian cortex involvement in seizures affecting the temporal lobe. In: Avanzini G, Beaumanoir A, Munari C, eds. Limbic Seizures in Children. London, UK: John Libbey; 2001:115–127

56. McBride MC, Bronstein KS, Bennett B, Erba G, Pilcher W, Berg MJ. Failure of standard magnetic resonance imaging in patients with refractory temporal lobe epilepsy. Arch Neurol 1998;55(3):346–348

57. Chan S, Erickson JK, Yoon SS. Limbic system abnormalities associated with mesial temporal sclerosis: a model of chronic cerebral changes due to seizures. Radiographics 1997;17(5):1095–1110

58. Free SL, Li LM, Fish DR, Shorvon SD, Stevens JM. Bilateral hippocampal volume loss in patients with a history of encephalitis or meningitis. Epilepsia 1996;37(4):400–405

59. Szabó CA, Wyllie E, Siavalas EL, et al. Hippocampal volumetry in children 6 years or younger: assessment of children with and without complex febrile seizures. Epilepsy Res 1999;33(1):1–9

60. Berkovic SF, McIntosh AM, Kalnins RM, et al. Preoperative MRI predicts outcome of temporal lobectomy: an actuarial analysis. Neurology 1995;45(7):1358–1363

61. Jack CR Jr, Rydberg CH, Krecke KN, et al. Mesial temporal sclerosis: diagnosis with fluid-attenuated inversion-recovery versus spin-echo MR imaging. Radiology 1996;199(2):367–373

62. Capizzano AA, Vermathen P, Laxer KD, et al. Temporal lobe epilepsy: qualitative reading of 1H MR spectroscopic images for presurgical evaluation. Radiology 2001;218(1):144–151

63. Li LM, Cendes F, Antel SB, et al. Prognostic value of proton magnetic resonance spectroscopic imaging for surgical outcome in patients with intractable temporal lobe epilepsy and bilateral hippocampal atrophy. Ann Neurol 2000;47(2):195–200

64. Semah F, Baulac M, Hasboun D, et al. Is interictal temporal hypometabolism related to mesial temporal sclerosis? A positron emission

tomography/magnetic resonance imaging confrontation. Epilepsia 1995;36(5):447–456

65. Arnold S, Schlaug G, Niemann H, et al. Topography of interictal glucose hypometabolism in unilateral mesiotemporal epilepsy. Neurology 1996;46(5):1422–1430

66. Dupont S, Semah F, Clémenceau S, Adam C, Baulac M, Samson Y. Accurate prediction of postoperative outcome in mesial temporal lobe epilepsy: a study using positron emission tomography with 18fluorodeoxyglucose. Arch Neurol 2000;57(9):1331–1336

67. Carne RP, O'Brien TJ, Kilpatrick CJ, et al. 'MRI-negative PET-positive' temporal lobe epilepsy (TLE) and mesial TLE differ with quantitative MRI and PET: a case control study. BMC Neurol 2007;7:16

68. Devous MD Sr, Thisted RA, Morgan GF, Leroy RF, Rowe CC. SPECT brain imaging in epilepsy: a meta-analysis. J Nucl Med 1998;39(2):285–293

69. Harvey AS, Bowe JM, Hopkins IJ, Shield LK, Cook DJ, Berkovic SF. Ictal 99mTc-HMPAO single photon emission computed tomography in children with temporal lobe epilepsy. Epilepsia 1993;34(5):869–877

70. O'Brien TJ, So EL, Mullan BP, et al. Subtraction ictal SPECT co-registered to MRI improves clinical usefulness of SPECT in localizing the surgical seizure focus. Neurology 1998;50(2):445–454

71. Wyllie E, Comair YG, Kotagal P, Bulacio J, Bingaman W, Ruggieri P. Seizure outcome after epilepsy surgery in children and adolescents. Ann Neurol 1998;44(5):740–748

72. Ray A, Wyllie E. Treatment options and paradigms in childhood temporal lobe epilepsy. Expert Rev Neurother 2005;5(6):785–801

73. Hauser WA, Rich SS, Lee JR, Annegers JF, Anderson VE. Risk of recurrent seizures after two unprovoked seizures. N Engl J Med 1998;338(7):429–434

74. Stephen LJ, Kwan P, Brodie MJ. Does the cause of localisation-related epilepsy influence the response to antiepileptic drug treatment? Epilepsia 2001;42(3):357–362

75. Semah F, Picot MC, Adam C, et al. Is the underlying cause of epilepsy a major prognostic factor for recurrence? Neurology 1998;51(5):1256–1262

76. Kim WJ, Park SC, Lee SJ, et al. The prognosis for control of seizures with medications in patients with MRI evidence for mesial temporal sclerosis. Epilepsia 1999;40(3):290–293

77. Brodie MJ, Dichter MA. Antiepileptic drugs. N Engl J Med 1996;334(3):168–175

78. Brodie MJ. Management strategies for refractory localization-related seizures. Epilepsia 2001;42(suppl 3):27–30

79. French JA, Kanner AM, Bautista J, et al; Therapeutics and Technology Assessment Subcommittee of the American Academy of Neurology; Quality Standards Subcommittee of the American Academy of Neurology; American Epilepsy Society. Efficacy and tolerability of the new antiepileptic drugs I: treatment of new onset epilepsy: report of the Therapeutics and Technology Assessment Subcommittee and Quality Standards Subcommittee of the American Academy of Neurology and the American Epilepsy Society. Neurology 2004;62(8):1252–1260

80. French JA, Kanner AM, Bautista J, et al; Therapeutics and Technology Assessment Subcommittee of the American Academy of Neurology; Quality Standards Subcommittee of the American Academy of Neurology; American Epilepsy Society. Efficacy and tolerability of the new antiepileptic drugs II: treatment of refractory epilepsy: report of the Therapeutics and Technology Assessment Subcommittee and Quality Standards Subcommittee of the American Academy of Neurology and the American Epilepsy Society. Neurology 2004;62(8):1261–1273

81. Brodie MJ, French JA. Management of epilepsy in adolescents and adults. Lancet 2000;356(9226):323–329

82. Castro LH, Serpa MH, Valério RM, et al. Good surgical outcome in discordant ictal EEG-MRI unilateral mesial temporal sclerosis patients. Epilepsia 2008;49(8):1324–1332

83. Wyllie E. Surgical treatment of epilepsy in children. Pediatr Neurol 1998;19(3):179–188

84. Clusmann H, Kral T, Gleissner U, et al. Analysis of different types of resection for pediatric patients with temporal lobe epilepsy. Neurosurgery 2004;54(4):847–859, discussion 859–860

85. Cohen-Gadol AA, Wilhelmi BG, Collignon F, et al. Long-term outcome of epilepsy surgery among 399 patients with nonlesional seizure foci including mesial temporal lobe sclerosis. J Neurosurg 2006;104(4):513–524

86. Baldauf CM, Cukiert A, Argentoni M, et al. Surgical outcome in patients with refractory epilepsy associated to MRI-defined unilateral mesial temporal sclerosis. Arq Neuropsiquiatr 2006; 64(2B, 2-B) 363–368

17 Anteromesial Temporal Lobectomy

Oğuz Çataltepe and John Weaver

Anteromesial temporal lobectomy (AMTL) is the most commonly performed surgical procedure for the treatment of patients with medically refractory epilepsy. Although temporal lobe epilepsy (TLE) is more common in adults, AMTL is still a frequently performed procedure in surgical treatment of children with epilepsy. AMTL constitutes 30 to 44% of all surgical resections in published pediatric epilepsy series compared with reported rates of 62 to 73% of cases in adult epilepsy surgery series.[1-5]

The main reason for this discrepancy is related to the differences in neuropathological substrates causing epilepsy in children and adults. Mesial temporal sclerosis (MTS) is the most common substrate in adult epilepsy patients, and it occurs with a greater frequency compared with low-grade neoplasms and developmental lesions such as cortical dysplasia, which are more commonly seen in the pediatric age group. AMTL is a very effective surgical intervention in controlling medically refractory seizures in well-selected pediatric patients, and its efficiency in the treatment of children with intractable TLE has been demonstrated in many surgical series.[1,2,6-11]

This chapter gives a step-by-step description of the surgical technique we use for AMTL. The surgical technique may change based on the underlying lesion and extent of the epileptogenic zone, especially in patients with cortical dysplasia. Briefly, all patients undergo a comprehensive presurgical assessment by our pediatric epilepsy service including a detailed clinical examination, magnetic resonance imaging (MRI) with epilepsy protocol, electroencephalography (EEG), and long-term EEG-video monitoring to obtain ictal and interictal electrophysiological data. Positron emission tomography/single photon emission computed tomography, neuropsychological assessment, and intracarotid amobarbital procedure (Wada test) are among other commonly used diagnostic modalities and tests. Despite all of these tests, locating the epileptogenic zone remains problematic in a significant number of children with TLE, and these patients frequently are candidates for invasive monitoring. Further details on patient selection criteria/preoperative workup as well as surgical techniques for other pathologies can be found in related chapters in this book.

■ Historical Evolution of the Surgical Technique

Temporal lobe resection in epilepsy surgery is not a standard technique.[12,13] Because temporal lobectomy suggests removal of the whole temporal lobe, *anterior* or *anteromesial temporal lobectomy* are the more appropriate terms for the technique commonly used by epilepsy surgeons. Early variations of the surgical technique we use today were developed in the 1950s. The first application of the technique was a temporal neocortical resection without removing mesial temporal structures. Then, Wilder Penfield and colleagues reported better results by resecting the hippocampus and uncus along the temporal neocortex.[14-16] After the initial studies regarding the role of hippocampus in memory function, the surgical technique evolved toward electrophysiologically tailored temporal lobectomy with significant preservation of the hippocampus.[12,13,17,18] Also in the mid 1950s, Niemeyer described selective transcortical amygdalohippocampectomy.[19] Later, Yasargil and colleagues developed a selective amygdalohippocampectomy technique through the transsylvian approach and reported impressive seizure control rates without removing temporal neocortex.[20] The details of this approach are discussed in the next chapter.

At the Montreal Neurological Institute (MNI), Rasmussen performed anterior temporal lobectomy by including uncus and amygdala and used electrocorticography to determine the extent of hippocampal resection. His approach was to remove the anterior 1 to 1.5 cm of the hippocampus.[21-25] Conversely, Feindel and colleagues, in the same institution (MNI), routinely avoided the removal of hippocampus to preserve memory functions but aggressively resected the amygdala.[26-28] Then Goldring and colleagues described an anterior temporal lobectomy technique that spares the amygdala.[29] Today, the most commonly used technique is the resection of anterior temporal neocortex and mesial temporal structures, including amygdala and hippocampus. Even this technique has some variations, including en bloc resection of both neocortex and mesial temporal structures that was described by Falconer and later applied by Polkey and Crandal.[30] Another modification of the technique was described by Spencer and colleagues at Yale.[31] Spencer's technique is the most commonly used technique today, although many differences among epilepsy surgeons of the application of this surgical technique still exist. One of the main differences is resection length of anterior temporal lobe. The majority of epilepsy surgeons do not exceed a 4-cm neocortical resection length (from the tip of anterior temporal lobe) in the dominant hemisphere, whereas the length of resection may increase up to 5.5 to 6 cm in the nondominant hemisphere. Another difference among surgeons is the intent to spare the superior temporal gyrus during lateral temporal neocortical resection. Many epilepsy surgeons spare the superior temporal gyrus partially or fully to decrease the risk of postoperative complications. The extent of the hippocampal resection is also controversial. Although some find it sufficient to remove the anterior 1.5 cm of the hippocampus, others extend their hippocampal resection up to 3 cm by reaching back to the posterior part of the tail. The current trend is limiting anterior temporal neocortical resection while being more aggressive with the resection of mesial temporal structures.[12,13] The size of the resection is also related to the patient's age; therefore, it probably is more reasonable, especially in pediatric epilepsy surgery, to describe the extent of temporal neocortical and hippocampal resections based on anatomical landmarks, such as sylvian end of the central sulcus and the quadrigeminal plate.

■ Surgical Technique

Here we will describe the anteromesial temporal lobectomy technique we use at the University of Massachusetts Medical Center. In general, our temporal lobe resection includes the anterior 3.5 cm of the temporal neocortex in the dominant hemisphere with most of the superior temporal gyrus spared, as described by Spencer et al.[31] Our resection also includes the uncus, a large part of the amygdala, and an approximately 3-cm length of the hippocampus/parahippocampus excised en bloc. The neocortical resection is extended to 5 cm in the nondominant hemisphere. Mesial structures are resected in the same manner in both dominant and nondominant hemispheres if neuropsychological assessment and Wada test results are reassuring. This technique may be modified depending on the patient's age, imaging, and electrophysiological characteristics. If there is radiologically defined dysplastic cortex or an electrophysiologically more extensive abnormality, our neocortical resection borders are redefined and may be extended further. If the epileptogenic zone is limited to a certain part of the temporal neocortex based on the invasive monitoring data, the resection may be tailored based on these data. In these cases, mesial structures may be spared, especially in some lesional epilepsy cases. Alternatively, if the radiological findings of hippocampal sclerosis are more pronounced at the hippocampal tail, then we extend our resection of the hippocampal tail much fur-

ther than our standard limits. The surgical plan is extensively discussed in advance with the pediatric epilepsy team in a multidisciplinary epilepsy surgery conference, and the extent of resection is predetermined based on the aforementioned considerations. All patients receive their regular antiseizure medications on the day of surgery. We also give an age-appropriate dosage of dexamethasone after induction of anesthesia and prophylactic antibiotics before incision and for 24 hours postoperatively. We do not use mannitolours routinely.

Positioning the Patient

The patient is placed in supine position, and the head is placed in the pin head holder if the patient is older than 3 years. The horseshoe head holder is used for younger patients. A gel roll is placed under the ipsilateral shoulder, and the head is turned to the contralateral side approximately 60 degrees. The neck is slightly extended by lowering the vertex approximately 15 degrees downward, just enough to bring the zygoma to the surgeon's eyeline and to make the zygoma the most prominent point on the midline. Lastly, the occiput is tilted slightly toward the ipsilateral shoulder (**Fig. 17.1**). This head position places the base of the temporal fossa perpendicular to the horizontal plane. The surface of the lateral temporal lobe will be in a horizontal position, and the long axis of the hippocampus will be oriented vertically relative to the surgeon with this approach. Thus, the head position will create a good alignment of the mesial structures to the surgeon's eyeline and will provide an excellent exposure to the uncus–amygdala complex, the whole length of hippocampus, and the lateral–basal temporal neocortex.

Scalp Incision

A smoothly curved, question mark–shaped scalp incision is drawn starting just above the zygoma and approximately 10 mm anterior to tragus, based on the location of palpated superficial temporal artery. Then the incision is extended upward such that it makes a smooth anterior turn at the upper point of the pinna by following the superior temporal line toward the keyhole. It ends approximately 3 to 4 cm behind the keyhole, depending on the patient's hairline (**Fig. 17.1**). Then the incision is infiltrated with 0.5% bupivacaine hydrochloride (Marcaine) diluted in 1:200.000 epinephrine solution. The superficial temporal artery is palpated and protected during the scalp incision. Some small branches of superficial temporal artery may be occasionally sacrificed, but generally the main body can be protected by dissecting and mobilizing it during the incision. Then the incision of the temporal fascia, muscle, and periosteum is also completed sharply by cutting these layers parallel to the scalp incision. Scalp, temporal fascia, muscle, and underlying periosteum are dissected subperiosteally to create a single musculocutaneous

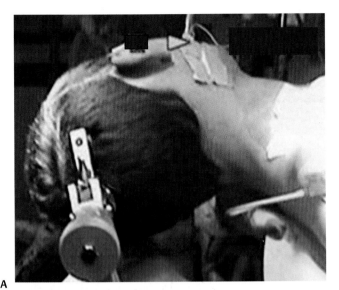

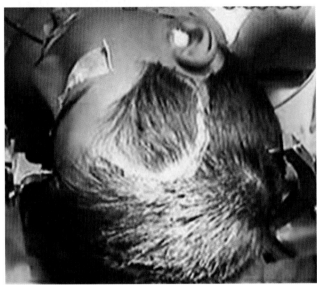

Fig. 17.1 Head positioning of the patient. **(A)** Neck is extended by lowering the vertex approximately 15 degrees downward with a slight occipital tilt toward the ipsilateral shoulder and making the zygoma the most prominent point on the midline. **(B)** Head is turned to the contralateral side approximately 60 degrees. A question mark–shaped incision starts just above the zygoma and extends anteriorly toward the keyhole by ending just behind the hairline.

flap. The lower part of the incision is extended down to the zygoma. Having an exposure down to the zygomatic root is critical for satisfactory access to the base of the temporal fossa during the neocortical resection. The other critical point at this stage is exposure of the orbital-zygomatic ridge or the keyhole. It should be palpated, and the temporal muscle should be cut and dissected from the keyhole by retracting the scalp further and working beneath it. Then the temporal muscle is subperiosteally dissected using sharp

periosteal elevators by keeping the periosteum attached to the temporal muscle as much as possible to preserve muscle innervation and vascular supply. Monopolar cautery should not be used during this dissection for the same reason. Strict adherence to this technique is critical to prevent future temporal muscle atrophy. Although application of this technique may be difficult in elderly patients, it is much easier to have an excellent subperiosteal dissection that keeps the whole periosteum intact and attached to temporal muscle in the pediatric age group. Fish hooks are then placed to reflect the musculocutaneous flap anterolaterally to expose the temporal bone widely.

Craniotomy

Three burr holes are placed with locations at the keyhole, just above the zygoma and on the superior temporal line and approximately 4 to 5 cm posterior to the burr hole on the keyhole. A free bone flap is removed after dissecting the dura with Penfield dissectors. The sphenoid ridge is removed with rongeurs to create a smooth anterior-medial bony wall. This maneuver has critical significance to have a good exposure for uncus/amygdala resection. Further bone removal is needed along the floor of the temporal fossa down to the root of the zygoma and toward the temporal tip. This will provide a comfortable access to the inferobasal neocortical region and temporal pole during the resection. Dural tack-up sutures are placed at this stage, and the epidural space at bone edges is filled with an injectable hemostatic agent, such as Surgifoam (Johnson & Johnson, Gateway, NJ, USA). Then the dura is opened C-shaped, starting from the keyhole site on frontal region and ending at temporal pole by following the craniotomy edges. The dura is folded and tacked up with 4–0 Nurolon sutures to the muscle flap over the sphenoid wing. At this stage, the exposed area in the surgical field includes the full extent of the sylvian fissure/vein, superior and middle temporal gyri, and the upper part of the inferior temporal gyrus (**Fig. 17.2**).

Neocortical Resection

The previously planned resection length of the lateral temporal neocortex is measured and marked on the cortex at this stage. The tip of the temporal pole can be seen easily seen with the help of a cortical ribbon placed on a Cottonoid over the middle temporal gyrus. A predetermined 3.5- or 5-cm resection length (depends on being on the dominant or nondominant side) from the tip of the temporal lobe is measured along the middle temporal gyrus and marked on the cortex with bipolar coagulation. The resection line starts at the medial edge of the temporal pole and turns toward the middle temporal gyrus approximately 2 cm behind the temporal tip (**Fig. 17.2**). The remaining part of the incision continues along the upper border of the middle temporal

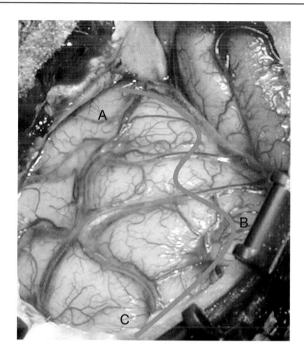

Fig. 17.2 Exposed surgical field includes anterior part of the inferior frontal gyrus, sylvian vein, and superior and middle temporal gyri. The blue line marks the surgical incision lines. First incision line (A–B) stays parallel to the sylvian fissure and second incision line (B–C) stays perpendicular to the first incision line. The first incision line starts from the most anteromedial part of the temporal pole and extends posteriorly approximately 2 cm by following the sylvian vein and staying just a few millimeters below the vein. Then the incision makes a smooth curve toward the superior temporal sulcus to preserve the superior temporal gyrus and follows the sulcus until the posterior resection line. The second incision line starts from the most posterior point of the first incision line and extends toward the floor of the temporal fossa by traversing the middle and inferior temporal gyri.

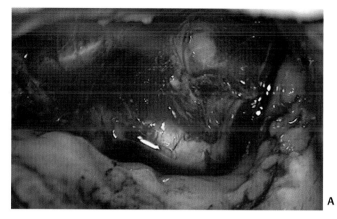

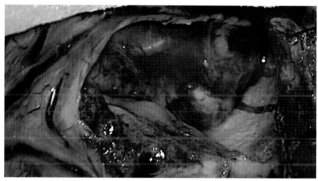

Fig. 17.3 (A) Temporal neocortex is subpially dissected from the sylvian fissure by keeping the pia intact to avoid any risk of injury to the middle cerebral artery (MCA) branches. **(B)** The entire temporal neocortex is removed en bloc by exposing the tentorium and mesial temporal structures.

gyrus to spare most of the superior temporal gyrus posteriorly. This resection line is marked on the pia-arachnoid of the superior and middle temporal gyri with a fine-tip bipolar coagulator staying parallel and 5 to 6 mm below the sylvian vein or superior temporal sulcus. After coagulation of the pia-arachnoid over the gyri, it is incised with microscissors throughout the length of the marked incision line. After completing the incision, the pia-arachnoid adjacent to sylvian vein is coagulated thoroughly to create an appropriate handle to hold during the subpial dissection of superior and middle temporal gyri. Then cortex is subpially dissected from pia of the sylvian fissure anteriorly and from the superior temporal sulcus posteriorly. Meticulous subpial dissection technique is used to avoid injury to the middle cerebral artery (MCA) branches in the sylvian fissure (**Fig. 17.3A**) and to protect the vascular supply of the unresected part superior temporal gyrus by leaving both pial layers of the superior temporal sulcus undisrupted on the lower bank

of the superior temporal gyrus. Some bleeding is generally encountered while peeling the cortex from pia that can be easily controlled by placing Surgifoam and Cottonoid patties. We would like to remind the reader that subpial dissection is much more challenging in pediatric patients than adults because of the very thin and fragile nature of the pia at this age. Appropriate application of this technique may not be feasible in very young children.

The next critical step is finding the temporal horn. There are several approaches for this and a close review of the patient's MRI, especially coronal spoiled gradient recalled (SPGR) cuts, will be helpful to determine the best approach. The temporal horn starts approximately 3 cm behind the temporal tip, and the average distance between the surface of superior temporal gyrus and the ventricle is approximately 31 to 34 mm.[32,33] We prefer to perform our dissection to reach the temporal horn at a point on the superior temporal sulcus approximately 3.5 cm behind the tip of the temporal pole. Frequently, the T1 sulcus (superior temporal sulcus) directly brings the surgeon into the temporal horn. This can be done through an intrasulcal approach or by remaining subpial and following either the inferior wall of the superior temporal gyrus or superior wall of the middle temporal gyrus, which we prefer. The bottom of the sulcus can be easily recognized by visualizing the end of the pial bank at first. Then the ependyma can be appreciated after deepening the same incision approximately 11 to 12 mm further.[33] This distance can be measured case by case on MRI coronal cuts easily. The ependyma can be opened with Penfield #4 dissector (Codman, MA) and cerebrospinal fluid will verify the intraventricular location. If the surgeon passes the estimated distance and the temporal horn is not in sight, the best strategy is to redirect the dissection. The most common two reasons for not being able to find the ventricle are either placing the entry point of the dissection too anteriorly or directing the dissection either too medially or too laterally. At this stage, the appropriate strategy is to redirect the dissection toward the floor of the middle fossa but not medially. The dissection is then deepened toward the floor of the middle fossa until gray matter is encountered on the adjacent occipitotemporal (or fusiform) gyrus. Then the dissection is redirected again, this time medially into the white matter until temporal horn is entered. Deepening the dissection medially to search the temporal horn without taking the aforementioned strategies may easily lead the surgeon into the temporal stem and basal ganglia and may cause significant complications. Therefore redirecting the dissection intentionally too laterally initially is a much safer approach, as defined very clearly by Wen et al.[32] When we enter into the ventricle, we place a tiny cottonoid patty in it to prevent blood contamination and then subpially dissect first the superior wall of the medial temporal gyrus and then sylvian pia anteriorly to the temporal pole using microsuction in a low setting and a Penfield dissector. This subpial dissection is performed down to the ependymal level throughout the sulcus. Then the ependyma is easily opened using a bipolar coagulator, the temporal horn is unroofed all the way to its tip, and a small cotton ball is placed into the temporal horn toward the atrium to avoid intraventricular dissemination of blood products.

Several other approaches to the temporal horn exist. One is to follow the collateral sulcus. This approach is only feasible after completing the second cortical incision, which will be described in the following paragraphs. Alternatively, the temporal horn can be found after completing the resection of the anterolateral temporal lobe without locating the temporal horn. In this case, the uncus is located first by following the tentorial edge anteromedially. When removal of the uncus is completed, its posterior segment will open and expose the tip of the temporal horn automatically. Lastly, the use of a neuronavigation system to assist the localization of the temporal horn is an option.

The second cortical incision line starts from the most posterior extent of the first incision and is directed perpendicularly toward the floor of temporal fossa (**Fig. 17.2**). The

posterior line of the neocortical resection extends inferiorly traversing the superior, middle, inferior temporal, and fusiform gyri, respectively, and ends at the collateral sulcus. The temporal horn is located generally just dorsal to the base of the collateral sulcus and can be found by following the collateral sulcus pia as described previously. The average distance from the depth of the collateral sulcus to the temporal horn is 3 to 6 mm.[33] Thus, the posterior end of the first incision and superior end of the second incision lines intersect at the temporal horn. A third incision is directed to the collateral sulcus by cutting across the temporal stem and the white matter of the basal temporal lobe. This third incision disconnects the temporal neocortex from parahippocampus/hippocampus and completes the lateral neocortical temporal resection by dividing the collateral sulcus from its posterior end to the tip of the temporal horn at rhinal sulcus level. The entire lateral neocortex is removed as an en bloc specimen (**Fig. 17.3A,B**).

Mesial Temporal Resection

For the next step, it is important to locate several anatomical landmarks and structures before proceeding to resect the mesial temporal structures. Hippocampus, fimbria, lateral ventricular sulcus, collateral eminence, choroid plexus, choroidal fissure, inferior choroidal point, and amygdala need to be fully exposed and can be distinctly recognized at this stage. The hippocampus sits over the parahippocampal gyrus

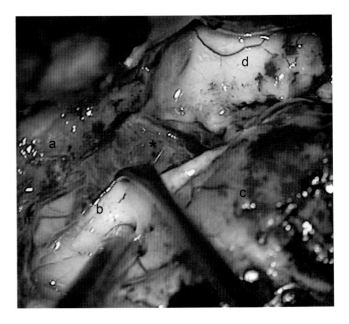

Fig. 17.4 Choroidal point (*) and anterior part of the choroidal fissure is exposed by peeling the fimbria. Note surrounding structures including choroidal plexus (a), fimbria (b), hippocampus (c), and posteromedial part of uncus (d).

and has a short, wide head that continues with a gradually narrowing body and tail. The tail makes a backward–upward turn at the trigone level around the posterior cerebral peduncle. The anterior portion of the hippocampal head blends into the posterior uncus and amygdala (**Fig. 17.4**). The hippocampus can be easily recognized between the collateral eminence and choroidal fissure. The lateral ventricular sulcus lies between the hippocampus proper and the collateral eminence, extending anteriorly toward the amygdala–hippocampal junction. The medial border of the hippocampus is lined by the choroid plexus over the choroidal fissure and the choroidal point at the most anterior part. If the choroidal plexus is lifted gently upward and medially, the choroidal fissure and fimbria would be fully exposed (**Fig. 17.4**). Retraction

of the choroid plexus laterally over the hippocampus would expose stria terminalis. When the anterior end of the choroid plexus is pulled backward, the velum terminale and the choroidal point at the tip of the posterior uncus can be visualized (**Fig. 17.5**). The anterior choroidal artery (AChA) runs across the ambient and crural cisterns near the choroid plexus. It pierces the arachnoid plane to supply the choroid plexus at the inferior choroidal point by giving rise to numerous branches. The anterior fimbria and stria terminalis join to form the velum terminale and create the anterior border of the choroidal fissure where the inferior choroidal point is also located (**Fig. 17.5**). The fimbria is a narrow, flat band covering the mesial border of the hippocampus. It is located just above the dentate gyrus and continues as fimbria fornix posteriorly. The temporal horn is fully unroofed to expose the most anterior part of the temporal horn that includes the bulging amygdala, posterior uncus, amygdala–hippocampal junction, and posteriorly the head and body of the hippocampus. The uncal recess is a distinct landmark that separates the head of the hippocampus from the amygdala. Better exposure of the hippocampal tail can be provided with the help of a tapering retractor ribbon (**Fig. 17.6A**).

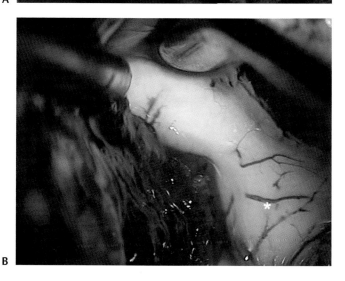

A

B

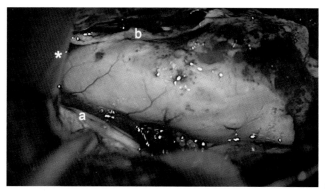

A

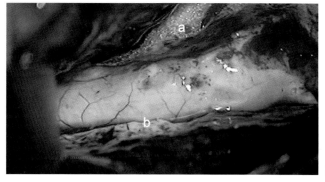

B

Fig. 17.5 **(A)** Choroidal point (*) is seen surrounded by anterior tip of choroidal plexus (a), fimbria (b), velum terminale (c), stria terminalis (d), head of hippocampus (e), and posteromedial part of uncus (f). **(B)** The anterior part of the fimbria and stria terminalis joins to form velum terminale (*).

Fig. 17.6 **(A)** Head and body of the hippocampus are exposed, and a retractor (*) is placed to elevate the temporal roof for further exposure of the hippocampal tail. Note choroidal sulcus (a) and surgical resection line on collateral eminence (b). **(B)** Entire hippocampus is subpially dissected as an en bloc specimen between collateral eminence (a) and fimbria (b).

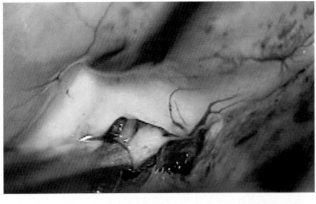

A

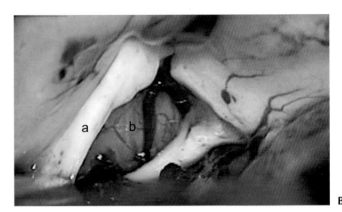

B

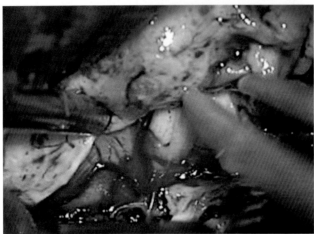

C

Fig. 17.7 **(A)** Fimbria is lifted with a dissector to expose the hippocampal sulcus and hippocampal arteries. **(B)** Further dissection and elevation of fimbria (a) exposes subiculum (b) and hippocampal arteries extending into hippocampal sulcus. **(C)** Subiculum and hippocampal sulcus are fully exposed, and hippocampal arteries have been coagulated.

The ribbon is placed on the most posterior end of the unroofed part of the temporal horn and the remaining part of the roof is gently elevated laterally for this purpose. The hippocampal tail can be exposed with this maneuver back to the point where it makes a medial and upward turn. Obtaining this exposure is very critical for a satisfactory resection of mesial temporal structures.

After locating the intraventricular landmarks, resection of mesial temporal structures starts with an incision on the lateral ventricular sulcus that is the demarcation line between the collateral eminence and hippocampus. The ependyma of the lateral ventricular sulcus is coagulated posteroanteriorly as an entry point to the parahippocampal gyrus. The medial pial bank of the collateral sulcus is exposed by suctioning parahippocampus intragyrally. Intragyral removal of parahippocampus is completed along the collateral eminence, starting from hippocampus proper to the amygdala–hippocampal junction. Then the lateral wall of the parahippocampus–hippocampus complex is subpially dissected by peeling it from the collateral sulcus pia using the Penfield dissectors **(Fig. 17.6B)**. Then the dissection continues mesially toward the tentorial edge until the pia along the mesial border of the parahippocampus and hippocampal sulcus is

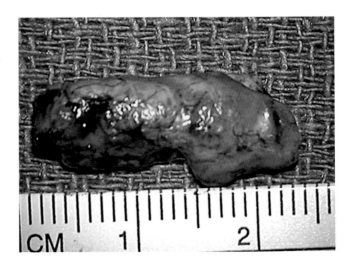

Fig. 17.8 Hippocampus proper is removed en bloc for histological examination. Further resection of the hippocampal tail is performed with the ultrasonic aspirator.

encountered. At this stage, the subiculum of the hippocampus is peeled off toward the hippocampal sulcus. The parahippocampal gyrus lateral to this line is emptied further by suctioning it anteriorly toward the entorhinal area and uncus. At this stage, the hippocampus proper can easily be retracted laterally into the cavity created by intragyral aspiration of the parahippocampus. This maneuver provides an excellent view of the anterior end of the hippocampal sulcus. The hippocampal sulcus fans out at this junction between pes hippocampi, uncus, and anterior end of the parahippocampus **(Fig. 17.5A)**. This anatomy provides the surgeon with

an excellent starting point for the dissection of hippocampal sulcus between fimbria, inferior choroidal point, and choroidal fissure. The most anterior end of the fimbria can be easily opened and peeled away from the pia of the choroidal fissure just lateral to tela choroidea. Then the fimbria can be lifted with Rhoton microdissectors (Codman, MA) at the inferior choroidal point level and underlying pia and vasculature can be exposed **(Fig. 17.4)**. The fimbria is further opened with Rhoton dissectors along its length all the way to the hippocampal tail. At this stage, the hippocampus is further retracted laterally with the suction, and the hippocampal

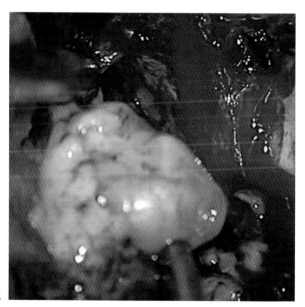

A

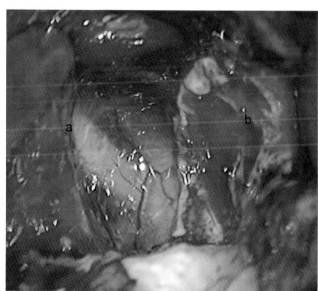

B

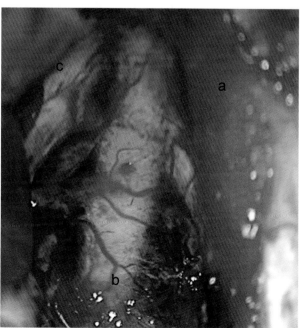

C

Fig. 17.9 (A) Uncus and amygdala are peeled from the pia are with dissectors or low-power suction. **(B)** Uncus is emptied subpially. Third nerve (a) under the pia is visible along with some residual part of amygdala (b). **(C)** After subpial removal of amygdala and uncus, edge of tentorium (a), third nerve (b), and posterior cerebral artery (PCA) (c) are visible under intact pia.

sulcus is exposed as a two-layered pial folding with several tiny arteries running between pial layers. The hippocampal sulcus is a very critical landmark in this procedure and should be fully visualized. It separates the hippocampus proper and the subiculum. The subiculum constitutes the most medial part of the parahippocampus bulging into the middle incisural space. The hippocampal arteries and arising arterioles (Uchimura arteries) are located within the hippocampal sulcus (**Fig. 17.7**). These thin hippocampal arteries mostly form a group of 2–6 thin vessels from the AChA and medial P2 segment of posterior cerebral artery close to the free edge of the tentorium. After having a satisfactory exposure of the hippocampal sulcus, hippocampal arterioles are coagulated with fine-tipped bipolar forceps and cut with microscissors one by one (**Fig. 17.7C**). Again, it should be noted that these arteries in young pediatric patients are extremely thin and can rupture easily with manipulation. Further, the distances between the hippocampal arteries and the AChA and P2 segment are very short in pediatric patients. Therefore coagulation of hippocampal arteries should be performed carefully using very fine-tipped bipolars by staying close to hippocampus proper. Then the head of the hippocampus is fully dissected subpially from the underling pia and lifted upward and posteriorly. This maneuver provides a very nice subpial plane at the base of the whole hippocampus–parahippocampus complex. Then the hippocampal head is mobilized and lifted upward and posteriorly and the remaining parahippocampal attachments are dissected subpially using a Penfield # 4 dissector. This way the whole hippocampus and underlying part of the parahippocampus are dissected back to the hippocampal tail. Then the tail is resected with bipolar coagulation at its upward turn behind the quadrigeminal plate and the hippocampus is removed en bloc (**Fig. 17.8**).

The final step of the procedure is the resection of the amygdala while emptying the content of the anterior uncus. During this stage of the procedure, using strictly subpial dissection and showing the utmost respect to pial barriers are critical to protect the underlying vasculature, third nerve, and cerebral peduncle. The anterior amygdala blends into the uncus, and we use a microsuction with the suction regulator at the low-suction setting and Penfield dissectors to peel the uncal content from the pia below the incisura (**Fig. 17.9A**). Ultrasonic aspirator in a low setting is also a very useful tool to empty the uncal content. After completing the resection of uncus and anterior basal amygdala, the cerebral peduncle and third nerve can be seen under the intact pia (**Fig. 17.9B**). Although the anterior and basal borders of the amygdala are very well defined, there are no dorsomedial anatomical boundaries of the amygdala. Therefore, it is more challenging to define the dorsomedial resection borders of the amygdala. The M1 segment of the MCA, which can be seen subpially, corresponds to the anterior–superior border of the amygdala. The line extending from the anterior tip of the temporal horn to the angle of the MCA at the limen in-

sula makes the anterior–superior border of the resection line of amygdala. The dissection at the anterior–superior border should be done very carefully because of the presence of the small MCA branches supplying the basal ganglia here. After completing the amygdala resection, the surgical cavity is re-explored and all devascularized residual cortical tissues are removed with the ultrasonic aspirator without violating the pia. At this stage, the tentorial edge, third nerve, internal cerebral artery (ICA), posterior cerebral artery (PCA), lateral edge of the midbrain between cerebral peduncle, and tectum can be seen under the pia in the ambient and crural cisterns. After hemostasis, the surgical cavity is filled with warm saline irrigation, and the dura is closed in a watertight fashion with 4–0 Nurolon sutures. The bone flap is replaced with microplates, and the temporal muscle, fascia, and galea are closed as two separate layers using 3–0 and 4–0 Vicryl sutures. The skin is closed with 4–0 Prolene sutures.

■ Complications

The complication rates in temporal lobe surgery series in children have been reported to be between 2 and 8%.[2,6,8] Mortality is a rare occurrence and is reported as lower than 0.5%.[34] Postoperative complications, although rare, may be devastating; using appropriate surgical techniques and extreme caution at critical stages of the surgery are essential to avoid complications. The most commonly reported complications are visual field defects, infection, stroke, manipulation or retraction hemiparesis, third nerve palsy, and language disturbances. The most common visual field defect is superior quadrantanopsia, with a reported incidence of 9% in a Benifla et al series of 126 children with TLE.[6] Benifla et al also reported a 4% incidence of homonymous hemianopia. The overall complication rate was 14.9% in Clusmann and colleagues' series, but only 2.2% had permanent deficits.[7] The incomplete or complete quadrantanopsia incidences were 28.2% and 3.8%, respectively. In a separate study by Kim et al, the rate of postoperative visual field defect was 22%.[3]

Another common complication is dysphasia, which is mostly transient. Transient dysphasia can be seen in approximately half of the dominant site temporal resections and frequently resolves within a few weeks.[35] A possible reason for this finding is the disconnection of the mesial and neocortical temporal lobe and retraction related to physiological disruption. Although rare, third and fourth nerve palsies can be seen after AMTL. Using strict subpial technique and avoiding cautery around the tentorium or high-power suction application during the uncus resection may help to avoid these complications. Partial seventh nerve palsy is another well-known complication and occurs secondary to injury of the facial nerve branches located within the temporalis fascia. This injury can be easily avoided with the technique we described here by avoiding dissection of the temporalis fascia. However, traction and monopolar cauterization in close proximity to the facial nerve may also cause facial palsy and should be taken into consideration during the craniotomy. One of the most devastating, although rare, complications in temporal lobe resection is hemiplegia. It is a well-recognized complication, with an incidence of 1 to 2%.[5] It has also been termed *manipulation hemiplegia* and frequently is related to injuries of the AChA and PCA during the resection of the mesial temporal structures. Maintaining the utmost respect to subpial technique, meticulous protection of the pia throughout the surgery, coagulation and cutting of the hippocampal arterioles strictly in hippocampal sulcus, and staying away from the main arteries (AChA or PCA) decreases the risk of injury to these vessels. MCA-related hemiplegia secondary to compression with retractors may cause this problem as well.

◼ Outcome

The seizure control rate of temporal resections in children is different than it is in adults; the main reason is the heterogeneity of underlying pathologies. The most common neuropathological substrates in children are cortical dysplasia and neoplasms followed by gliosis and MTS.[1,6,36] Temporal lobe resection is a safe and effective surgical technique in the management of TLE with reported seizure control rates between 60 and 80%.[1,2,6-11,37,38] Seizure-free outcome rate was reported as 78% by Sinclair et al[8] in their series of 42 patients. Benifla et al[6] reported 74%, and Clusmann et al[7] reported 87% good seizure control rates (Engel Class I and II) with temporal lobe resection in 126 and 89 children, respectively. The best outcome was seen in the patients with temporal lobe neoplasms (88–92%) followed by the patients with gliosis (86%) and MTS (70%) in Benifla's series.[6] The lowest seizure control rate was seen in the patients with cortical dysplasia. Mittal et al reviewed their experience with 109 children at the Montreal Neurological Institute and reported Engel Class I and II outcomes in 86.3% of patients at more than 5 years of follow-up.[39] Jarrar et al found that the seizure-free rate in their series was 82% 5 years after surgery but decreased to 53% after 10 years.[40] Maton et al reported their experience with temporal lobe resection during early life in 20 children younger than 5 years old.[11] Sixty-five percent of the children were seizure free, and an additional 15% had more than 90% seizure reduction at a mean follow-up of 5.5 years. Smyth et al[41] reported 63.3% overall good seizure control rate (Engel I and II) in the preadolescent age group. MTS patients had a 76.9% seizure control rate, which compared favorably to cortical dysplasia and gliosis groups in this study. The Great Orman Street Hospital series reported seizure-free rates as 73% in lesional, 58% in MTS, and 33% in dual pathology groups.[5] Kim et al reported 88% seizure-free outcome in the temporal resection group of their epilepsy surgery series in children.[3]

References

1. Wyllie E, Comair YG, Kotagal P, Bulacio J, Bingaman W, Ruggieri P. Seizure outcome after epilepsy surgery in children and adolescents. Ann Neurol 1998;44(5):740–748

2. Adelson PD, Peacock WJ, Chugani HT, et al. Temporal and extended temporal resections for the treatment of intractable seizures in early childhood. Pediatr Neurosurg 1992;18(4):169–178

3. Kim SK, Wang KC, Hwang YS, et al. Epilepsy surgery in children: outcomes and complications. J Neurosurg Pediatr 2008;1(4):277–283

4. Cossu M, Lo Russo G, Francione S, et al. Epilepsy surgery in children: results and predictors of outcome on seizures. Epilepsia 2008;49(1):65–72

5. Harkness W. Temporal lobe resections. Childs Nerv Syst 2006;22(8):936–944

6. Benifla M, Otsubo H, Ochi A, et al. Temporal lobe surgery for intractable epilepsy in children: an analysis of outcomes in 126 children. Neurosurgery 2006;59(6):1203–1213, discussion 1213–1214

7. Clusmann H, Kral T, Gleissner U, et al. Analysis of different types of resection for pediatric patients with temporal lobe epilepsy. Neurosurgery 2004;54(4):847–859, discussion 859–860

8. Sinclair DB, Aronyk K, Snyder T, et al. Pediatric temporal lobectomy for epilepsy. Pediatr Neurosurg 2003;38(4):195–205

9. Duchowny M, Levin B, Jayakar P, et al. Temporal lobectomy in early childhood. Epilepsia 1992;33(2):298–303

10. Mohamed A, Wyllie E, Ruggieri P, et al. Temporal lobe epilepsy due to hippocampal sclerosis in pediatric candidates for epilepsy surgery. Neurology 2001;56(12):1643–1649

11. Maton B, Jayakar P, Resnick T, Morrison G, Ragheb J, Duchowny M. Surgery for medically intractable temporal lobe epilepsy during early life. Epilepsia 2008;49(1):80–87

12. Schramm J. Temporal lobe epilepsy surgery and the quest for optimal extent of resection: A review. Epilepsia 2008;49(8):1296–1307

13. de Almeida AN, Teixeira MJ, Feindel WH. From lateral to mesial: the quest for a surgical cure for temporal lobe epilepsy. Epilepsia 2008;49(1):98–107

14. Penfield W, Flanigin H. Surgical therapy of temporal lobe seizures. AMA Arch Neurol Psychiatry 1950;64(4):491–500

15. Penfield W, Baldwin M. Temporal lobe seizures and the technique of subtemporal lobectomy. Ann Surg 1952;134:625 634

16. Penfield W, Jasper H. Epilepsy and Functional Anatomy of the Human Brain. Boston, Ma.: Little Brown; 1954:815–816

17. Penfield W, Milner B. Memory deficit produced by bilateral lesions in the hippocampal zone. Arch Neurol Psychiatry 1958;79:475–497

18. Scoville WB, Milner B. Loss of recent memory after bilateral hippocampal lesions. J Neurol Neurosurg Psychiatry 1957;20(1):11–21

19. Niemeyer P. The transventricular amygdalo-hippocampectomy in temporal lobe epilepsy. In: Baldwin M, Bailey P, eds. Temporal Lobe Epilepsy. Springfield, IL: CC Thomas; 1958:461–482

20. Yasargil MG, Teddy PJ, Roth P. Selective amygdalohippocampectomy: operative anatomy and surgical technique. In: Symon L et al., eds. Advances and Technical Standards in Neurosurgery. Vol 12. New York, NY: Springler-Wien; 1985:93–123

21. Rasmussen T, Jasper H. Temporal lobe epilepsy: indication for operation and surgical technique. In: Baldwin M, Bailey P, eds. Temporal Lobe Epilepsy. Springfield, IL: CC Thomas; 1958:440–460

22. Rasmussen T, Branch C. Temporal lobe epilepsy: indication for and results of surgical therapy. Postgrad Med J 1962;31:9–14

23. Rasmussen T. Surgical treatment of patients with complex partial seizures. In: Penry JK, Daly DD, eds. Advances in Neurology. Vol 11, Complex Partial Seizures and Their Treatment. New York, NY: Raven Press; 1975:415–449

24. Rasmussen T. Surgical aspects of temporal lobe epilepsy: results and problems. In: Gillingham J, Gybels J, Hitchcock ER, & Szikla G, eds. Advances in Stereotactic and Functional Neurosurgery Acta Neurochirurgica, Supp 30. Vienna: Springer-Verlag; 1980:13–24

25. Rasmussen TB. Surgical treatment of complex partial seizures: results, lessons, and problems. Epilepsia 1983;24(suppl 1):S65–S76

26. Feindel W, Penfield W, Jasper H. Localization of epileptic discharges in temporal lobe automatism. Transactions of the American Neurological Association. American Neurological Association; New York: Springer; 1952:14–17

27. Feindel W, Penfield W. Localization of discharge in temporal lobe automatism. AMA Arch Neurol Psychiatry 1954;72(5):603–630

28. Feindel W, Rasmussen T. Temporal lobectomy with amygdalectomy and minimal hippocampal resection: review of 100 cases. Can J Neurol Sci 1991; 18(4, suppl):603–605

29. Goldring S, Edwards I, Harding GW, Bernardo KL. Results of anterior temporal lobectomy that spares the amygdala in patients with complex partial seizures. J Neurosurg 1992;77(2):185–193

30. Olivier A. Transcortical selective amygdalohippocampectomy in temporal lobe epilepsy. Can J Neurol Sci 2000;27(suppl 1):S68–S76, discussion S92–S96

31. Spencer DD, Spencer SS, Mattson RH, Williamson PD, Novelly RA. Access to the posterior medial temporal lobe structures in the surgical treatment of temporal lobe epilepsy. Neurosurgery 1984;15(5):667–671

32. Wen HT, Rhoton AL Jr, Marino R Jr. Gray matter overlying anterior basal temporal sulci as an intraoperative landmark for locating the temporal horn in amygdalohippocampectomies. Neurosurgery 2006; 59(4, suppl 2):ONS221–ONS227, discussion ONS227

33. Campero A, Tróccoli G, Martins C, Fernandez-Miranda JC, Yasuda A, Rhoton AL Jr. Microsurgical approaches to the medial temporal region: an anatomical study. Neurosurgery 2006; 59(4, suppl 2): ONS279–ONS307, discussion ONS307–ONS308

34. Adelson PD. Temporal lobectomy in children with intractable seizures. Pediatr Neurosurg 2001;34(5):268–277

35. Kraemer DL, Spencer DD. Temporal lobectomy under general anesthesia. Tech Neurosurg 1995;1:32–39

36. Spencer S, Huh L. Outcomes of epilepsy surgery in adults and children. Lancet Neurol 2008;7(6):525–537

37. Arruda F, Cendes F, Andermann F, et al. Mesial atrophy and outcome after amygdalohippocampectomy or temporal lobe removal. Ann Neurol 1996;40(3):446–450

38. Clusmann H, Schramm J, Kral T, et al. Prognostic factors and outcome after different types of resection for temporal lobe epilepsy. J Neurosurg 2002;97(5):1131–1141

39. Mittal S, Montes JL, Farmer JP, et al. Long-term outcome after surgical treatment of temporal lobe epilepsy in children. J Neurosurg 2005; 103(5, suppl):401–412

40. Jarrar RG, Buchhalter JR, Meyer FB, Sharbrough FW, Laws E. Long-term follow-up of temporal lobectomy in children. Neurology 2002;59(10):1635–1637

41. Smyth MD, Limbrick DD Jr, Ojemann JG, et al. Outcome following surgery for temporal lobe epilepsy with hippocampal involvement in preadolescent children: emphasis on mesial temporal sclerosis. J Neurosurg 2007; 106(3, suppl):205–210

18 Transsylvian Selective Amygdalohippocampectomy

Uğur Türe, Ahmet Hilmi Kaya, and Canan Aykut Bingöl

With the introduction of microneurosurgical techniques and extensive experience with mediobasal temporal tumors and arteriovenous malformations, Yaşargil developed the modern form of selective amygdalohippocampectomy by using the pterional–transsylvian route.[1–3] This technique is the preferred surgical approach in our epilepsy unit and is the focus of this chapter.

The soul of selective amygdalohippocampectomy is the selective resection of the amygdala (except medial and central nuclei), the piriform cortex, which includes the uncus, the anterior two thirds of the hippocampus, and the parahippocampal gyrus through the pterional–transsylvian approach.[1–6] A profound knowledge of the vascular supply of this area and its possible variations, and a full understanding of the surgical anatomy of the limbic system, are the "sine qua non" of this approach.

Recently, developments in neuroimaging, especially magnetic resonance imaging (MRI) with high resolution, have enabled clear visualization of abnormalities in the mediobasal temporal structures.[7–9] In turn, this development has facilitated surgical decision making. The availability of fiber tractography, especially with 3-Tesla MRI, and an interest in the white matter anatomy, especially information gained from fiber dissection, have also contributed to our experience with this technique.[9–12]

The efficacy of surgery in the management of drug-resistant temporal lobe epilepsy has been demonstrated in a prospective randomized trial.[13] However, controversy remains regarding which resection method yields the best results for seizure freedom and neuropsychological function. Temporal neocortical resection by leaving the hippocampus or amygdala behind can result in seizure-free rates of approximately 50%.[14] Conversely, seizure control rates with selective amygdalohippocampectomy are similar to those of anteromesial temporal lobectomy, and there is considerable evidence that the neuropsychological outcome is better in patients undergoing selective amygdalohippocampectomy.[13–17] Although, class I evidence for seizure outcome based on the type and extent of resection of mediobasal temporal lobe structures is rare, selective amygdalohippocampectomy appears to provide a similar seizure outcome and a better cognitive outcome than temporal lobe resection based on the available data.[14,17] Still, it remains unclear whether larger mediobasal resection leads to a better seizure outcome. In children, seizure outcome and functional recovery are better.[15]

■ Patient Evaluation before Selective Amygdalohippocampectomy

Patient selection for selective amygdalohippocampectomy is important in terms of cognitive outcome and freedom from seizures. Patients with mediobasal temporal lobe epilepsy with hippocampal sclerosis and intractable seizures should be clearly identified through a defined underlying hippocampal pathology shown on MRI, clinical seizure types, and electrophysiological and functional imaging techniques. Initial precipitating incidents, including febrile seizures, trauma, hypoxia, and intracranial infections before the age of 5 and before the onset of habitual nonfebrile seizures are very common.[18] Habitual seizures begin earlier for mediobasal temporal lobe epilepsy with hippocampal sclerosis, with the majority occurring in patients between the ages of 4 and 16 years; however, these seizures can begin earlier or much later, and the patient can still show the same pathological changes and excellent response to surgery. Focal seizures occur in more than 90% of patients but secondary generalized seizures are rare and may correlate with the extent of the lesion. Auras and automotor seizures, sometimes with impaired consciousness, are characteristics of mediobasal temporal lobe epilepsy with hippocampal sclerosis. Auras are mainly characterized by an ascending epigastric sensation, gradual impairment of consciousness, and are typically associated with oroalimentary automatism in approximately 70% of patients.[18] Dystonic posturing occurs in 20 to 30% of patients and is contralateral to the side of seizure onset. Specific baseline and follow-up neuropsychological testing is important. MRI is the most important investigational tool. Improvements in MRI techniques, especially 3-Tesla MRI scanners, contributes to diagnosis of hippocampal sclerosis significantly. MRI volumetric investigations and spectroscopy give more information on T1, T2 and fluid attenuation inversion recovery (FLAIR) findings. 18F-deoxyglucose positron emission tomography (FDG-PET) demonstrates ipsilateral hypometabolism interictally. However, 11C flumazenil PET is more sensitive than FDG-PET. Ictal

147

and postictal single photon emission computed tomography (SPECT) are preferred over interictal SPECT. In one third of patients, interictal epileptiform anomalies are lateralized and localized to the lesion. In the other two thirds, bilateral dependent or independent (or both) epileptic activity is detected. Sphenoid electrode recordings also disclose more information about lateralization. The ictal onset is not always detected by scalp electroencephalography (EEG) video recording, and seizures are lateralized in 80% of patients.[18] Invasive EEG recordings with depth and subdural electrodes are needed in patients with discordant findings on MRI, semiology, functional imaging exams, and electrophysiology.

■ Surgical Technique

An exact knowledge of the topographical, white matter, and arteriovenous anatomy of the region is crucial for a successful outcome after selective amygdalohippocampectomy (**Figs. 18.1** and **18.2**).[10–12,19–29]

A pterional craniotomy is performed in the usual way, and the posterior ridge of the greater wing of the sphenoid bone is removed with a high-speed electric drill down to the level of the superior orbital fissure.[1,3,4,6] The dura is opened in a semicircular fashion above the sylvian fissure, and the incision is arched toward the sphenoid ridge and orbit.

Chiasmatic and carotid cisterns must be explored through the fronto-orbital aspect of the frontal lobe before opening the sylvian fissure. The arachnoid between the optic nerve and the internal carotid artery (ICA) must then be opened. These procedures release large amounts of cerebrospinal fluid, which relaxes the brain and facilitates further dissection. Next, the proximal part of the sylvian fissure is opened medially or laterally to the superficial sylvian veins, depending on the variations in the venous anatomy. A simple spreading action with fine bipolar forceps is usually adequate to dissect the fissure. As the sylvian fissure is dissected more deeply, longer fine-tipped forceps are needed. The thickened arachnoid bands must be divided with microscissors where necessary, and dissection continues with a fine suc-

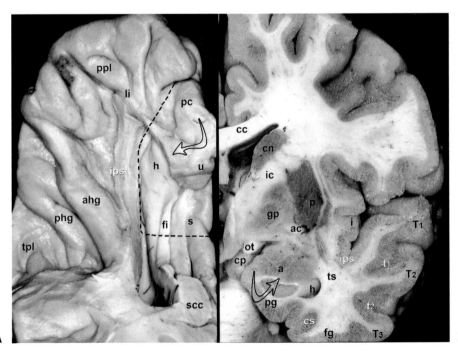

Fig. 18.1 (A) Medial surface of the left temporal operculum and mediobasal temporal region in a cadaver brain, superomedial view. The dotted line indicates the incision through the collateral eminence to the collateral sulcus and the incision through the posterior limit of the hippocampus and parahippocampal gyrus via the transsylvian–transamygdalar approach. The *arrow* indicates the angle of the surgical approach. **(B)** Coronal section of the left cerebral hemisphere in a cadaver through the amygdala, anterior view. The hippocampus (h) is shown at the tip of the temporal horn, and the amygdala (a) is located at the antero-superomedial side of the hippocampus. The *arrow* indicates the angle of the surgical approach. a = amygdala; ac = anterior commissure; ahg = anterior Heschl gyrus; cc = corpus callosum; cn = caudate nucleus; cp = cerebral peduncle; cs = collateral sulcus; fg = fusiform gyrus; fi = fimbria; gp = globus pallidus; h = hippocampus; i = insula; ic = internal capsule; ips = inferior peri-insular sulcus; li = limen insula; ot = optic tract; p = putamen; pc = piriform cortex; pg = parahippocampal gyrus; phg = posterior Heschl gyrus; ppl = polar planum; s = subiculum; scc = splenium of corpus callosum; T1 = superior temporal gyrus; T2 = middle temporal gyrus; T3 = inferior temporal gyrus; t1 = superior temporal sulcus; t2 = inferior temporal sulcus; tp = temporal pole; tpl = temporal planum; ts = temporal stem; u = uncus. White letters denote the sulci and fissures.

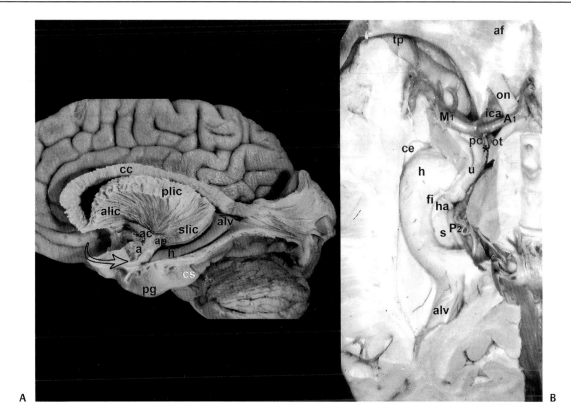

Fig. 18.2 (A) Superolateral view of the left mediobasal temporal structures and internal capsule after fiber dissection in a cadaver brain. The *arrow* indicates the angle of the surgical approach for the transsylvian selective amygdalohippocampectomy. **(B)** Superior view of the left mediobasal temporal region with arterial vascularization in a cadaver brain. A1 = first segment of the anterior cerebral artery; a = amygdala; ac = anterior commissure; af = anterior fossa; alic = anterior limb of internal capsule; alv = atrial portion of lateral ventricle; ap = ansa peduncularis; ce = collateral eminence; cc = corpus callosum; cp = cerebral peduncle; cs = collateral sulcus; fi = fimbria; h = hippocampus; ha = hippocampal arteries; ica = internal carotid artery; M1 = first segment of the middle cerebral artery; on = optic nerve; ot = optic tract; P2 = second segment of the posterior cerebral artery; pc = piriform cortex; pg = parahippocampal gyrus; plic = posterior limb of the internal capsule; s = subiculum; slic = sublentiform portion of the internal capsule; tp = temporal pole; u = uncus. The *asterisk* indicates the anterior choroidal artery.

tion tip on a moist Cottonoid sponge. Dissection continues to expose the area from the bifurcation of the ICA to 10 to 15 mm beyond the bifurcation of the middle cerebral artery. It also encompasses the anterior third of the insula and the M2 segment of the middle cerebral artery. At this point, the arachnoid fibers between the temporal and fronto-orbital areas are well separated, as are the vessels along the proximal sylvian fissure down to the ICA and its branches. These structures, as well as the position of the oculomotor nerve, the tentorial edge, and the medial basal areas of the temporal pole, may be inspected. The lateral branches of the internal carotid artery (ICA) (posterior communicating artery [PCoA], anterior choroidal artery [AChA] and striocapsular arteries) and the cortical branches of the M1 segment (temporopolar, anterior, and middle temporal arteries) and its variations are identified, as are the number, position, variation, and courses of the lenticulostriate arteries. The limen insula and the inferior trunk of the M2 segment are observed. The M2 segment curves slightly laterally in the

inferior peri-insular sulcus and lies just over the inferior insular vein.

As in many procedures using the pterional approach, the dissection is performed medial to the sylvian vein (on the frontal lobe side) while the surgeon opens the sylvian fissure. However, anatomical variations, such as a large fronto-orbital vein and too many major branches of this vessel, make sacrifice necessary to carry out medial dissection. In such cases, dissection must proceed in an epipial plane, lateral to the sylvian vein along the medial surface of the superior temporal gyrus, until the inferior peri-insular sulcus and the inferior insular vein are reached. Variations of the M1 segment and its lateral branches are also frequently encountered.[1] In such cases, the surgeon must find sufficient space to make an incision in the piriform cortex between the temporal arteries by mobilizing them if needed. Significant variations exist among patients regarding the major vascular supply to the amygdala, uncus, hippocampus, and parahippocampal gyrus.[1,4,19,20,24,25,27]

The resection of the piriform cortex just anterolateral to the M1 segment and anteroinferior to the limen insula enables the surgeon to reach the amygdala. The superior part of the amygdala is identified a few millimeters under the incision line by its hazelnut color in the white matter. The amygdala must first be removed piecemeal with both a tumor forceps (to gain histological specimens) and gentle suction. During the removal of amygdala, the temporal horn of the lateral ventricle must be entered, allowing a clearer orientation of the hippocampus and the extent of the superior, posterior, and lateral aspects of the amygdala. Removing the amygdala is not usually a bloody procedure. While approaching the ventricular wall, however, particularly in the medial plane, the surgeon must keep in mind the presence of subependymal veins returning from the amygdala. These vessels run subependymally to the atrial vein of the temporal horn, which runs through the choroidal fissure to the basal vein of Rosenthal. Any damage to these veins and their branches may cause torrential, retrograde venous hemorrhage from the basal vein and the vein of Galen. The surgeon should also note that the basal vein may not run in a semicircular fashion around the cerebral peduncle to drain into the vein of Galen but instead may course diagonally over the cerebral peduncle from anteromedial to posterolateral in the direction of the tentorial incisura, draining into the superior petrosal sinus or tentorial veins. The variations in the venous drainage of the insular mediobasal temporal structures, cerebral peduncle, optic tract, and thalamus to the basal vein have been described comprehensively elsewhere.[22,29]

At this stage of the operation, it is of utmost importance that the optic tract is clearly identified. Thus, great caution must be used when removing the lateral, basal, and cortical nuclei of the amygdala. Care must also be taken not to resect the most medial parts of the amygdala (especially medial and central nuclei) lying superolateral to the optic tract and projecting to the claustrum, putamen, and globus pallidus. After these sections of the amygdala are taken out, the rest of the piriform cortex and the anterior part of the parahippocampal gyrus are removed subpially. The transparent curtain of pial and arachnoidal membranes near the lateral part of the carotid cistern and the anterior part of the crural and ambient cisterns may be identified readily anteroinferiorly, after subpial resection. After the pia is opened, important anatomical details can be identified, such as the entrance of the AChA to the choroidal fissure along the crural cistern and the optic tract and the basal vein of Rosenthal, which lie medial to the AChA, the cerebral peduncle, the P2 segment of the posterior cerebral artery, and the oculomotor nerve.

To remove the uncus, hippocampus, and parahippocampal gyrus, the surgical microscope must be angled posteroinferiorly. This avenue provides access from the tip of the temporal horn to the trigone and supplies an excellent view of the choroid plexus and of the pes hippocampus. The tela

choroidea, the transparent membrane from which the choroid plexus arises, can be isolated by displacing the choroid plexus medially over the choroidal fissure. Through the tela choroidea, important structures such as the AChA, the hippocampal vein, and ventricular tributaries of the basal vein of Rosenthal can be identified. Subsequently, fine forceps are used to reflect the choroid plexus medially and open the tela choroidea between the choroid plexus and the tenia fimbria. At this point, the hippocampal and uncal branches of the AChA must be coagulated and divided. However, great care must be taken not to injure the main stem of the AChA and its medial branches to the peduncle, optic tract, pallidum, internal capsule, thalamus, lateral geniculate body, and choroid plexus. The surgeon may encounter anatomical variations of the branches to the uncus and amygdala, which may arise separately and proximally from the AChA or even separately from the lateral wall of the ICA or from the M1 segment. Occasionally, these variations arise from the temporal and anterior temporal arteries.[4,19,20,24,25,27]

As the choroidal fissure along the tenia fimbria is opened, the medial part of the parahippocampal gyrus (subiculum) within the lateral wing of the transverse fissure can be identified. Hippocampal and parahippocampal veins, which run over the subiculum direction, exit the hippocampal sulcus and drain into the basal vein of Rosenthal. They should be isolated from the arachnoidal membranes and meticulously preserved. The hippocampus is supplied by the hippocampal arteries, which lie beneath the veins described previously and enter the hippocampus most often by penetrating the hippocampal sulcus. They usually originate from the P2 segment just proximal to the P2-P3 junction, or from the P3 segment itself, or from branches of the P3 segment and occasionally from the AChA.[4,19,20,24,25,27] At this stage of the operation, the hippocampal arteries are coagulated and divided.

The head of the hippocampus–parahippocampal gyrus is transected at the level of the proximal portion of the fimbria and en bloc resection is done. The middle and posterior portions of the hippocampus and parahippocampal gyrus are removed with suction or the ultrasonic aspirator. We prefer this technique instead of en bloc resection of the whole hippocampus–parahippocampal gyrus because it preserves the anterior temporal stem **(Figs. 18.3, 18.4,** and **18.5)**. The posterior limit of the resection of the hippocampal tail is just at the level of the posterior rim of the cerebral peduncle, some 10 to 15 mm before and inferior to the isthmus cinguli. The resection is performed inferolaterally through the posterior part of the hippocampus–parahippocampal gyrus, in the direction of the collateral sulcus and tentorial edge. Resection continues with forceps and suction along the sulcus in a semicircular fashion within the temporal horn lateral to the hippocampus, then enters the collateral and rhinal sulci. This semicircular resection, 4 to 5 cm long and 5 to 10 mm deep, extends down to the free edge of the tentorium, leaving the fusiform gyrus untouched laterally.

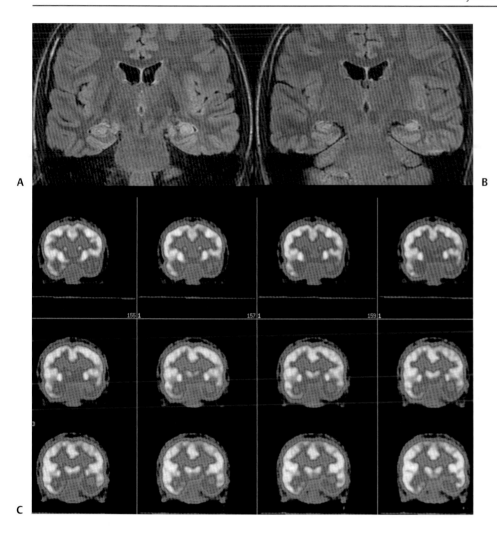

Fig. 18.3 Coronal sections of the fluid attenuation inversion recovery magnetic resonance images show left-sided hippocampal sclerosis in a 12-year-old child with mediobasal temporal epilepsy (**A** and **B**). A preoperative 2-deoxy-2[18F]fluoro-D-glucose positron emission tomography scan show left-sided temporal hypoactivity (**C**).

The loops and branches of the temporooccipital trunk arising from the P2–P3 junction can be identified within the collateral sulcus. The branches that supply the parahippocampal gyrus are coagulated and divided. As the limbic areas are resected, the hippocampal veins are again exposed and coagulated and divided at a proper distance from the basal vein of Rosenthal. Occasionally, bleeding may occur from the pial bed of the resected limbic structures in the cavity; these areas require coagulation with bipolar forceps. Generally, opening the extension of the collateral sulcus provides access to the tentorium some 2.5 cm from its free edge and in its anterior half. In patients with herniation of the mediobasal temporal structures, the mediobasal dissection must be done meticulously because of the potential for damage to the underlying structures. In such cases, staying in the subpial plane allows removal of the parahippocampal gyrus, whereas the P2 segment with its branches, the superior cerebellar artery, third nerve, and fourth nerve (lying below the tentorial edge) are protected by the pia and a double layer of arachnoid.

During this procedure, retractors should never be placed in the small entrance and the tip of the suction tube, covered with a moist Cottonoid sponge, can be used as a gentle temporary retractor. After careful hemostasis is achieved in the resection cavity and around the middle cerebral artery, the ICA, the AChA, the PCoA, and their branches, the dura is closed with a running suture and the bone flap is replaced in the usual fashion.

After the amygdala and uncus–hippocampus–parahippocampal gyrus are removed, the neighboring structures, including the superior, middle, and inferior temporal gyri, and the fusiform (lateral temporooccipital) and lingual (medial temporooccipital) gyri remain undamaged. Furthermore, removal of the anterior one third of the hippocampus–parahippocampal gyrus enables the pathologist to carry out scientific studies on resected structures. Because it is less complex and allows the surgeon to preserve the anterior temporal stem, piecemeal removal or subpial suction of the rest of the hippocampus–parahippocampal gyrus is a preferable approach compared with en bloc resection.

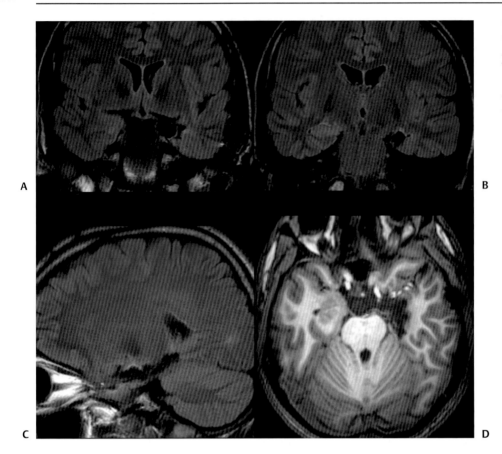

Fig. 18.4 Postoperative coronal **(A** and **B)** and sagittal **(C)** sections of the fluid attenuation inversion recovery and T1-weighted **(D)** magnetic resonance images show a left-sided selective amygdalohippocampectomy in a 12-year-old child with mediobasal temporal epilepsy. Please note the preserved temporal stem.

■ Surgical Considerations

The mediobasal temporal structures, such as the amygdala, uncus, hippocampus, and parahippocampal gyrus, can vary considerably in size and form.[19,26] In some cases, these structures are seen to bend only gently around the cerebral peduncle parallel to the optic tract, whereas in others they may resemble a coiled shrimp. Advances in neuroradiology, particularly in MRI technology, have provided considerable help in studying the extension, variations, and exact preoperative and postoperative morphology of the mediobasal temporal area.[8,9] The MRI findings that suggest mediobasal temporal sclerosis include the loss of hippocampal volume on coronal thin-slice FLAIR and T2-weighted images with associated ex vacuo enlargement of the temporal horn of the lateral ventricle and the loss of gray/white matter differentiation within the temporal tip.[8] The presence of small vascular malformations or gliomas is also readily identified. Concomitant MRI angiography has established itself as a noninvasive, standard procedure to diagnose vascular pathologies and has supplanted formal angiography in all but exceptional cases. It is imperative that the surgeon review the MRI images in detail to appreciate the mesiotemporal anatomy of the patient before proceeding the surgical intervention.

The term *selective amygdalohippocampectomy* is misleading for several reasons. Approximately 10 to 20% of the most medial part of the amygdala, where it abuts the basal ganglia, anterior commissure, and tail of the caudate nucleus, remains intact. Thus, the amygdala is not totally removed. Furthermore, posterior transection of the hippocampus–parahippocampal gyrus is generally done at the level of the posterior margin of the cerebral peduncle, where the P2–P3 segment junction is located, at the level of the ascending tail of the hippocampus and 10 to 15 mm before the isthmus cinguli, where the anterior portion of the lingual gyrus lies. If this dissection is carried too far posteromedially, there is a risk of damaging the lateral geniculate body or Meyer's loop.[5,12]

Selective amygdalohippocampectomy can be regarded as safe because it does not damage the neocortical part of the temporal lobe (apart from the piriform cortex, amygdala, uncus, hippocampus, and parahippocampal gyrus). After selective amygdalohippocampectomy, the remaining structures of the temporal lobe, namely the superior, middle, and inferior temporal gyri, and the fusiform and lingual gyri remain surgically untouched. Although subpial resection of the amygdala and the anterior portion of the parahippocampal gyrus compromise the connecting areas of

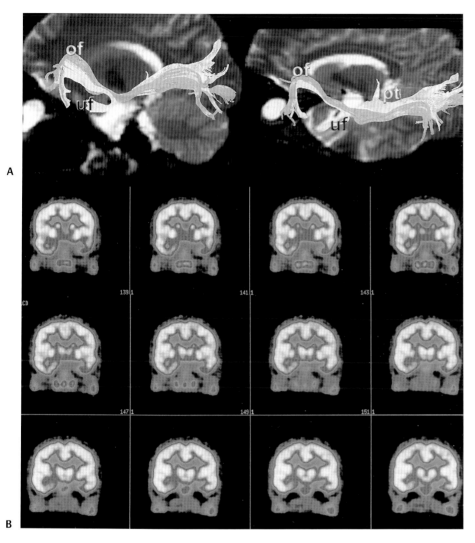

Fig. 18.5 Postoperative fiber tractography shows the preserved uncinate fasciculus (uf), occipitofrontal fasciculus (of), and posterior thalamic peduncle (pt), which includes the optic radiation **(A and B).** The postoperative 2-deoxy-2[18F]fluoro-D-glucose positron emission tomograph scan show ametabolic activity in the left mediobasal temporal region.

the superior, middle, and inferior temporal gyri within the mediobasal temporal pole, postoperative imaging does little to show such damage. In addition, because the adjacent preserved basal gyri, such as the fusiform and lingual gyri, migrate and occupy the surgically created space, postoperative volumetric studies may reveal conflicting results. This situation necessitates careful examination of the postoperative triplane MRIs.[8,30] Our results suggest that the transsylvian–transamygdalar approach prevents injury to the temporal stem compared with a standard temporal lobectomy. This is demonstrated by postoperative fiber tractography **(Fig. 18.5)**. Available data imply that preserving more functional temporal lobe tissue is critical for improved preservation of a patient's neurocognitive function postoperatively, particularly in high-functioning patients with dominant temporal lobe epilepsy.

Possible complications such as hemiparesis and homonymous field defects can be minimized if care is taken to prevent damage to the branches of the AChA and branches of the P2 segment. Visual field defects seen in this approach are more likely to result from injury or vasospasm of vessels supplying the optic tract than from direct damage to Meyer's loop. Because of their close anatomical relationship, iatrogenic injury to the optic tract while attempting to radically resect the medial and central nuclei of the amygdala is another possible cause of postoperative visual field defects.

■ Outcome

We believe it is most helpful to review the outcome data gathered by the medical/surgical team of the institute where this technique was developed.[4,16] They assessed postoperative seizure outcome in their series using the criteria recommended by the International League Against

Epilepsy Commission for Neurosurgery for Epilepsy as follows: I, seizure free; II, rare seizures (not more than one or two per year); III, worthwhile improvement, that is, more than 90% reduction in seizure frequency and improvement in quality of life; IV, unchanged; and V, worse. According to this classification, the seizure outcome at 1-year follow-up in more than 100 patients was as follows: 59% of the patients were in category I, 13% in II, 12% in III, and 16% in IV, and none of the patients' seizure patterns were worse than the preoperative pattern. The histopathological assessment of the surgical specimens obtained from the patients who had no neoplastic or vascular pathology revealed, in decreasing order of frequency, gliosis, sclerosis, hamartoma, scar, dysplasia, and microinfarct. Gliosis was present in half of patients. Selective amygdalohippocampectomy resulted in a much better neuropsychological and psychosocial outcome compared with the standard anterior temporal lobe resection. Furthermore, verbal learning scores, verbal memory at 30 minutes, visual learning, and visual memory at 30 minutes were all statistically significantly better in postoperative assessment of the patients who had a selective procedure compared with the dominant temporal lobectomy group. Although not statistically significant, the percentage of seizure-free patients was also greater in the group having undergone selective amygdalohippocampectomy compared with standard temporal lobectomy.

■ Conclusion

The comparison of the most commonly used surgical techniques in the management of temporal lobe epilepsy (selective amygdalohippocampectomy and anteromesial temporal lobectomy) is still an unresolved issue.[14] According to a recently published review, "selective amygdalohippocampectomy appears to have similar seizure outcome and possibly a better cognitive outcome than temporal lobectomy." If the patient data that are obtained using appropriate preoperative tests strictly show that the origin of the

seizures is the unilateral mediobasal temporal region, and again, if detailed MRI studies shows that mediobasal temporal structures are structurally abnormal but lateral cortical structures are normal, then selective amygdalohippocampectomy provides an opportunity to reach and to remove the pathological region (mediobasal temporal) without disturbing overlying healthy tissue (lateral temporal). In addition, for patients with dominant temporal lobe epilepsy who are highly functional or for those whose preoperative Wada results suggest that they are at risk of significant verbal memory loss with temporal neocortical resection, the selective procedure is the preferred operation. However, if preoperative evaluation data show discordant findings, the epilepsy team should carry out additional tests, such as invasive EEG monitoring with depth electrodes, stimulation with invasive monitoring for better evaluation of functional areas, and intraoperative mapping/recording to determine the extent of resection.

There is an increasing tendency for recommending surgical interventions to pediatric epilepsy patients in earlier ages.[31] This recommendation is based on previous observations that chronic epilepsy in children inhibits the development of personality and is frequently associated with debilitating behavioral and psychiatric problems, including tamper tantrums, aggressiveness, attention deficit disorders, and hyperactivity.[32-35] Although the number of appropriate candidates for selective amygdalohippocampectomy in the pediatric age group is much more limited than adults, this surgical approach is a viable approach in some carefully selected pediatric epilepsy patients.

To perform selective amygdalohippocampectomy safely and effectively, an exact knowledge of the vascular supply and of the surgical anatomy is essential along with skillful microsurgical techniques. Selective amygdalohippocampectomy is a safe microneurosurgical procedure with a favorable chance of success in relieving medically refractory seizures originating in the mediobasal temporal region. Postoperative neuropsychological performance also appears to be better with selective resection of mesial temporal structures.

References

1. Yaşargil MG. Microneurosurgery. Vol I. Stuttgart, Germany: Georg Thieme; 1984
2. Wieser HG, Yaşargil MG. Selective amygdalohippocampectomy as a surgical treatment of mesiobasal limbic epilepsy. Surg Neurol 1982;17(6):445–457
3. Yaşargil MG, Teddy PJ, Roth P. Selective amygdalohippocampectomy: operative anatomy and surgical technique. In: Symon L, Brihaye J, Guidetti B, et al., eds. Advances and Technical Standards in Neurosurgery. Vienna, Austria: Springer; 1985:93–123
4. Yaşargil MG, Wieser HG, Valavanis A, von Ammon K, Roth P. Surgery and results of selective amygdala-hippocampectomy in one hundred patients with nonlesional limbic epilepsy. Neurosurg Clin N Am 1993;4(2):243–261
5. Yaşargil MG. Experiences and reflections about selective amygdalohippocampectomy (AHE). Epileptologie 2005;22:74–80
6. Yaşargil MG, Türe U, Boop FA. Selective amygdalohippocampectomy. In: Kaye AH, Black PM, eds. Operative Neurosurgery. Vol 2. London, UK: Harcourt Publishers Limited; 2000:1275–1283

7. Briellmann RS, Berkovic SF, Syngeniotis A, King MA, Jackson GD. Seizure-associated hippocampal volume loss: a longitudinal magnetic resonance study of temporal lobe epilepsy. Ann Neurol 2002;51(5):641–644

8. Jack CR Jr, Rydberg CH, Krecke KN, et al. Mesial temporal sclerosis: diagnosis with fluid-attenuated inversion-recovery versus spin-echo MR imaging. Radiology 1996;199(2):367–373

9. Widjaja E, Raybaud C. Advances in neuroimaging in patients with epilepsy. Neurosurg Focus 2008;25(3):E3

10. Türe U, Yaşargil DCH, Al-Mefty O, Yaşargil MG. Topographic anatomy of the insular region. J Neurosurg 1999;90(4):720–733

11. Türe U, Yaşargil MG, Friedman AH, Al-Mefty O. Fiber dissection technique: lateral aspect of the brain. Neurosurgery 2000;47(2):417–426, discussion 426–427

12. Yaşargil MG, Türe U, Yaşargil DCH. Impact of temporal lobe surgery. J Neurosurg 2004;101(5):725–738

13. Tanriverdi T, Olivier A, Poulin N, Andermann F, Dubeau F. Long-term seizure outcome after mesial temporal lobe epilepsy surgery: corticalamygdalohippocampectomy versus selective amygdalohippocampectomy. J Neurosurg 2008;108(3):517–524

14. Schramm J. Temporal lobe epilepsy surgery and the quest for optimal extent of resection: a review. Epilepsia 2008;49(8):1305–1307

15. Gleissner U, Sassen R, Schramm J, Elger CE, Helmstaedter C. Greater functional recovery after temporal lobe epilepsy surgery in children. Brain 2005;128(pt 12):2822–2829

16. Khan N, Wieser HG. Psychosocial outcome of patients with amygdalohippocampectomy. J Epilepsy 1992;5:128–134

17. Paglioli E, Palmini A, Portuguez M, et al. Seizure and memory outcome following temporal lobe surgery: selective compared with nonselective approaches for hippocampal sclerosis. J Neurosurg 2006;104(1):70–78

18. Wieser HG; ILAE Commission on Neurosurgery of Epilepsy. ILAE Commission Report. Mesial temporal lobe epilepsy with hippocampal sclerosis. Epilepsia 2004;45(6):695–714

19. Duvernoy H. The Human Hippocampus. 3rd ed. Berlin, Germany: Springer-Verlag; 2005

20. Erdem A, Yaşargil G, Roth P. Microsurgical anatomy of the hippocampal arteries. J Neurosurg 1993;79(2):256–265

21. Gloor P. The Temporal Lobe and Limbic System. New York, NY: Oxford University Press; 1997

22. Huang YP, Wolf BS. The basal cerebral vein and its tributaries. In: Newton TH, Potts DG, eds. Radiology of the Skull and Brain. St Louis, MO: CV Mosby; 1974:2111 2154

23. Klingler J, Gloor P. The connections of the amygdala and of the anterior temporal cortex in the human brain. J Comp Neurol 1960;115:333–369

24. Marinković S, Milisavljević M, Puskas L. Microvascular anatomy of the hippocampal formation. Surg Neurol 1992;37(5):339–349

25. Marinković SV, Milisavljević MM, Vucković VD. Microvascular anatomy of the uncus and the parahippocampal gyrus. Neurosurgery 1991;29(6):805–814

26. Nieuwenhuys R, Voogd J, van Huijzen C. The human central nervous system. Berlin, Germany: Springer; 1991

27. Rhoton AL Jr. The supratentorial arteries. Neurosurgery 2002; 51(4, suppl):S53–S120

28. Rhoton AL Jr. The cerebral veins. Neurosurgery 2002; 51(4, suppl): S159–S205

29. Wolf BS, Huang YP. The insula and deep middle cerebral venous drainage system: Normal anatomy and angiography. Am J Roentgenol Radium Ther Nucl Med 1963;90:472–489

30. Siegel AM, Wieser HG, Wichmann W, Yasargil GM. Relationships between MR-imaged total amount of tissue removed, resection scores of specific mediobasal limbic subcompartments and clinical outcome following selective amygdalohippocampectomy. Epilepsy Res 1990;6(1):56–65

31. Mittal S, Montes JL, Farmer JP, et al. Long-term outcome after surgical treatment of temporal lobe epilepsy in children. J Neurosurg 2005;103(5, suppl):401–412

32. Harbord MG, Manson JI. Temporal lobe epilepsy in childhood: reappraisal of etiology and outcome. Pediatr Neurol 1987;3(5):263–268

33. Kotagal P, Rothner AD, Erenberg G, Cruse RP, Wyllie E. Complex partial seizures of childhood onset. A five-year follow-up study. Arch Neurol 1987;44(11):1177–1180

34. Lindsay J, Ounsted C, Richards P. Long-term outcome in children with temporal lobe seizures. I: Social outcome and childhood factors. Dev Med Child Neurol 1979;21(3):285–298

35. Wyllie E. Surgical treatment of epilepsy in pediatric patients. Can J Neurol Sci 2000;27(2):106–110

19 Tailored Temporal Lobectomy Techniques

Jeffrey G. Ojemann

Temporal lobe epilepsy is a common cause of intractable epilepsy. In adults, temporal lobectomy is the most common surgery and has been proven effective with class I evidence for its efficacy.[1] The disease in children has some features different from adults. In particular, the finding of mesial temporal (hippocampal) sclerosis is less common in children than in adults.[2,3] Further, even when present in histopathology, sclerosis is evident on magnetic resonance imaging (MRI) in only approximately half the instances.[4] The increased incidence of dual pathology[5,6] and dysplasia, which can involve medial, anterolateral, or basal temporal structures, argues for an electrophysiological approach to temporal lobectomy that combines anatomical boundaries with electrophysiological information. Thus, a wide range of temporal lobectomy may be indicated—from highly selective hippocampal/basal temporal resections to full temporal lobectomy[7] (**Fig. 19.1**).

A *tailored resection* can refer to modification of the resection (larger, smaller, or different location from a standard anterior temporal lobectomy or amygdalohippocampectomy) based on interictal measurements or modification based on functional information, in particular language mapping.[8-11]

In adults with mesial temporal abnormalities, intraoperative electrocorticography (ECoG) has been used to guide the extent of hippocampal resection,[12,13] and the presence or absence of residual epileptiform activity (e.g., spikes) has been associated with postoperative seizure control.[13] Postoperative spikes outside the medial temporal lobe may be of less value,[12] although some reports have found better outcome when neocortical spikes are eliminated with resection.[14,15]

Tailoring occurs de facto when invasive monitoring is used. The prolonged observation of interictal abnormalities and ictal onset will determine the resective strategy. This information can be augmented by intraoperative recordings. In this chapter, the strategies for using intraoperative ECoG are discussed, methods for hippocampal recordings are described, and approaches to functional considerations are reviewed.

■ Strategies

The advantages to tailoring a resection are seen in several circumstances. First, in the case of a clear lesion, intraoperative ECoG can identify particularly epileptogenic areas

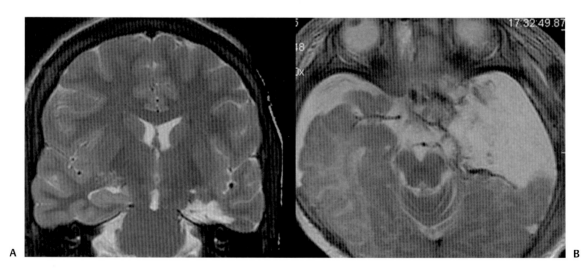

Fig. 19.1 Two different temporal lobectomies. **(A)** A selective resection through very inferior approach was used for selective pathology. This may minimize cognitive deficits, especially on the dominant side.[7] **(B)** A more aggressive temporal lobectomy was appropriate for a younger patient with more diffuse temporal lobe pathology (cortical dysplasia).

156

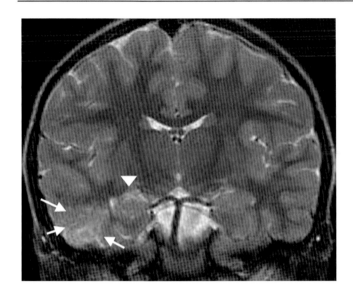

Fig. 19.2 Coronal magnetic resonance imaging (T2 weighted) of a 6-year-old with intractable seizures. The basal temporal abnormality (*arrows*) and the abnormal architecture of the right hippocampus (*arrowhead*) are both possible foci. Scalp electroencephalography findings were concordant with right temporal onset. Intraoperatively, the extent of the interictal abnormality included medial and basal temporal cortex. Histopathology of the lesion in basal temporal lobe and of the hippocampus was consistent with cortical dysplasia.

covering both the suspected or evident lesion and other electrodes covering the medial temporal lesion. Either subtemporal electrodes placed medially or depth electrodes into the hippocampus should give similar results.[22] Alternatively, if the lesions are in the same functional-anatomical region (e.g., basal and medial temporal lobes or anterior temporal lobe), intraoperative recordings can guide the relevant extents. Areas outside the hippocampus have been implicated in the genesis of anterior temporal lobe seizures,[23] and their interictal abnormalities can be identified during intraoperative recordings (**Fig. 19.2**).

■ Functional Considerations

Another role for tailoring is in the setting of minimizing resection to avoid postoperative deficits. In lateral temporal cortex, this may involve mapping language and avoiding, by at least 1 cm, areas where stimulation disrupts naming tasks.[24] In dominant temporal lobe, this may involve mapping language[8] and even memory,[25] because lateral temporal cortex resection has been associated with memory difficulties,[25] although the presence of a normal hippocampus on MRI and good preoperative memory are very strong risk factors for postoperative memory decline[26] that may be impossible to escape.

of cortex surrounding the lesion, and such an approach has been associated with excellent outcomes.[15–19] A lesion can co-exist with functional cortex, even if grossly abnormal,[20,21] and adjacent brain is, of course, vulnerable to functional loss; therefore, particularly in suspected language areas, a functional map is needed as well.

Other situations in which tailoring is useful are cases of suspected dual pathology. Two approaches can be taken. One option is to perform invasive monitoring, with electrodes

Functional information can often be determined without direct cortical mapping. The location of language areas is similar in adults and children, although younger children may have a more limited distribution of language sites than adults.[27] Thus, a preoperative assessment of the risk to language can be judged. Functional MRI (fMRI) continues to hold promise as a method to determine language sites noninvasively, but it remains a challenging tool.[28,29] We have found language fMRI can be, with practice, performed to as young as age 6. Silent action generation from both pictures

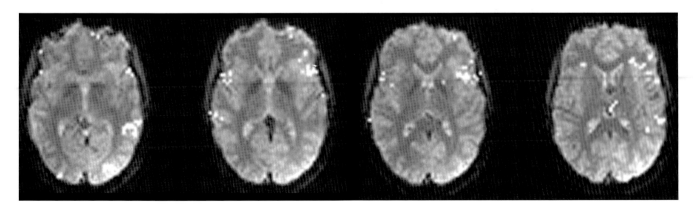

Fig. 19.3 Language functional magnetic resonance imaging. A 12-year-old girl with temporal lobe epilepsy performed a silent verb generation task to visually presented words. The left inferior frontal and posterior superior temporal gyri were strongly activated (*white pixels*) compared with a fixation point control.

and words can be effective (**Fig. 19.3**). The cerebral amytal (Wada) test may be necessary when features are present such as left-handedness, seizure semiology, or incongruent neuropsychological testing or when a proposed resection would be more radical if atypical dominance were confirmed. The Wada test is difficult in younger patients, and only very skilled teams are likely to be successful with children younger than age 12.

When direct cortical mapping is desired intraoperatively, preoperative practice is all the more critical in younger children. Below age 12 in the operating room may be impractical, but the use of dexmedetomidine has been described in very young children[30] and appears to have minimal effect on the ECoG.[31] Any anesthetic agent will influence the ECoG; benzodiazepines in particular should be avoided, if possible. Propofol is extensively used because of its effects on the depth of suppression of cortical activity, potentially masking epileptiform activity in the ECoG, can usually be titrated rapidly.[32]

■ Technique

In the case of a cortical lesion, ECoG can often be obtained simply with surface electrodes. These can be conventional arrays of platinum/iridium electrodes as commonly used for long-term monitoring, or an electrode array of carbon-tipped electrodes distributed around areas of concern can monitor and be used to guide electrical stimulation threshold for functional mapping.[11] The array is held in place by a skull clamp, which can be modified to allow for frameless stereotaxy without placing the patient in pins.[33]

For involvement of the hippocampus and medial temporal structures, the first step is to identify the temporal horn, thus visualizing the hippocampus, amygdala, and roof of the ventricle. The roof of the lateral ventricle, the anterior aspect of the choroidal fissure (found by following the choroid plexus anteriorly), and the lateral amygdala (that portion of the amygdala visible from the temporal horn, are several key landmarks (**Figs. 19.4A** and **19.4B**). Resecting tissue anterior to the choroidal point can be safely performed in a subpial manner, leaving the pial membrane over the carotid, third nerve, and brainstem and thus keeping these structures safe. Above the roof of the ventricle, there is no such pial plane, and a resection in this direction will soon come on descending motor fibers with significant potential consequences.

ECoG in the basal and medial temporal lobe is primarily performed with strip electrode arrays. These may be placed over inferior, fusiform, and parahippocampal regions in a lateral to medial direction and another can be placed over the tip of the temporal lobe. Once the ventricle is open, a very useful method is to place a four-contact (1-cm interelectrode distance) array over the ependyma of the hippocampus

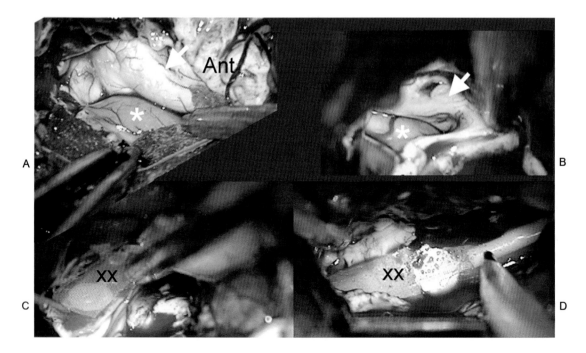

Fig. 19.4 Electrocorticography of the hippocampus. All frames are from a left medial temporal lobectomy, with anterior to the right and inferior to the top of each image. **(A)** The hippocampus is opened widely, demonstrating its extent within the lateral ventricle. The head of the hippocampus (*arrow*) is found opposite the amygdala (*asterisk*) at the anterior aspect of the temporal horn. **(B)** With a much more limited opening of the lateral ventricle, the hippocampal head (*arrowhead*) is exposed and the amygdala visualized (*asterisk*). **(C)** The electrode array (xx) is directed over the hippocampus, aimed posteriorly, without significant medial direction until **(D)** the hippocampus is covered by the electrodes (xx) allowing for an assessment of the epileptic properties, if any, of the medial temporal complex.

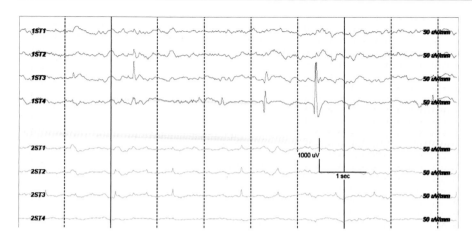

Fig. 19.5 Intraoperative electrocorticography tracing showing large (nearly 1mV) spikes from electrodes placed over the hippocampus. Note that only the most proximal electrodes (1ST3 and 1ST4) were involved, thus guiding a less extensive dominant hippocampal resection. The patient remains seizure free 1 year postoperatively.

(**Figs. 19.4C** and **19.4D**). This requires placing the tip of the array into the ventricle, which will run more superior-posteriorly than might be expected. The array should be roughly parasagittal in direction because the lateral geniculate and rest of the thalamus will be vulnerable if the electrode array is forced medially.

The hippocampus may look irregular. In the setting of hydrocephalus, choroidal cysts, or severe hippocampal atrophy, landmarks may be distorted. In some cases, the basal temporal gyri may be irregular,[34] and, anecdotally, a very prominent sulcus just lateral to the head of the hippocampus can create a confusing view from the lateral approach.

When hippocampal electrodes are in place, the interictal activity can be quite robust (**Fig. 19.5**). When the abnormal physiology is more focal, a limited hippocampal resection can be performed and the electrodes reapplied over the surgical margins. Typically, resection is taken back to the limits of hippocampal epileptiform activity. The parahippocampus is included with the resection, although posterior to the brainstem, this is no longer taken all the way to the medial pia because this dives well medial toward occipital lobe, whereas the hippocampus remains more lateral as it travels superior-posterior. At the very posterior aspect of a residual recording, the recording electrodes may be into the occipital horn. Occasionally, fast activity can be seen in these electrodes, which, contrary to the polymorphic fast activity seen over dysplasia, does not appear to be pathological and certainly should not be pursued without other evidence for more posterior temporal-occipital pathology.

Although a highly active, epileptogenic region is likely to be the location of ictal onset as well, not all interictal abnormalities will indicate the epileptopenic zone. Occasional spikes on the resection margin do not have to be chased, and certainly not at the expense of additional functional deficit. Fast activity can be seen over the posterior temporal horn electrodes within the occipital horn. This should not be confused with the continuous spiking and bursts of spikes suggestive of an area of dysplasia.[35] The occipital changes do not have to be pursued. The bursting activity often seen with dysplasia can be a very useful marker.

■ Conclusion

Most neurosurgical resections are tailored in some sense because a surgery is adjusted to the particulars of individual anatomy, pathology, patient and family concepts of risk–benefit trade-offs, presurgical workup (such as positron emission tomography [PET], single photon emission computed tomography [SPECT], EEG, neuropsychological testing), and direct cortical electrophysiology. The varied nature of epilepsy makes direct proof of the validity of any of these steps difficult, however the ambiguities inherent in many cases of pediatric temporal lobe epilepsy may particularly benefit from the additional information gained from ECoG and a physiological assessment of function and disease.

References

1. Wiebe S, Blume WT, Girvin JP, Eliasziw M; Effectiveness and Efficiency of Surgery for Temporal Lobe Epilepsy Study Group. A randomized, controlled trial of surgery for temporal-lobe epilepsy. N Engl J Med 2001;345(5):311–318
2. Mohamed A, Wyllie E, Ruggieri P, et al. Temporal lobe epilepsy due to hippocampal sclerosis in pediatric candidates for epilepsy surgery. Neurology 2001;56(12):1643–1649
3. Harvey AS, Cross JH, Shinnar S, Mathern BW; ILAE Pediatric Epilepsy Surgery Survey Taskforce. Defining the spectrum of international practice in pediatric epilepsy surgery patients. Epilepsia 2008;49(1):146–155
4. Smyth MD, Limbrick DD Jr, Ojemann JG, et al. Outcome following surgery for temporal lobe epilepsy with hippocampal involvement in preadolescent children: emphasis on

mesial temporal sclerosis. J Neurosurg 2007; 106(3, suppl):205–210

5. Lévesque MF, Nakasato N, Vinters HV, Babb TL. Surgical treatment of limbic epilepsy associated with extrahippocampal lesions: the problem of dual pathology. J Neurosurg 1991;75(3):364–370

6. Li LM, Cendes F, Watson C, et al. Surgical treatment of patients with single and dual pathology: relevance of lesion and of hippocampal atrophy to seizure outcome. Neurology 1997;48(2):437–444

7. Robinson S, Park TS, Blackburn LB, Bourgeois BFD, Arnold ST, Dodson WE. Transparahippocampal selective amygdalohippocampectomy in children and adolescents: efficacy of the procedure and cognitive morbidity in patients. J Neurosurg 2000;93(3):402–409

8. Ojemann GA, Ojemann JG, Lettich E, Berger M. Cortical language localization in left, dominant hemisphere. An electrical stimulation mapping investigation in 117 patients. J Neurosurg 1989;71(3):316–326

9. Ojemann JG. Managing epilepsy III: surgery for intractable epilepsy. Nep J Neuroscience 2004;1:92–97

10. Ojemann JG. Surgical treatment of pediatric epilepsy. Semin Neurosurg 2002;13:71–80

11. Silbergeld DL, Ojemann GA. The tailored temporal lobectomy. Neurosurg Clin N Am 1993;4(2):273–281

12. Schwartz TH, Bazil CW, Walczak TS, Chan S, Pedley TA, Goodman RR. The predictive value of intraoperative electrocorticography in resections for limbic epilepsy associated with mesial temporal sclerosis. Neurosurgery 1997;40(2):302–309, discussion 309–311

13. McKhann GM II, Schoenfeld-McNeill J, Born DE, Haglund MM, Ojemann GA. Intraoperative hippocampal electrocorticography to predict the extent of hippocampal resection in temporal lobe epilepsy surgery. J Neurosurg 2000;93(1):44–52

14. Fiol ME, Gates JR, Torres F, Maxwell RE. The prognostic value of residual spikes in the postexcision electrocorticogram after temporal lobectomy. Neurology 1991;41(4):512–516

15. Sugano H, Shimizu H, Sunaga S. Efficacy of intraoperative electrocorticography for assessing seizure outcomes in intractable epilepsy patients with temporal-lobe-mass lesions. Seizure 2007;16(2):120–127

16. Weber JP, Silbergeld DL, Winn HR. Surgical resection of epileptogenic cortex associated with structural lesions. Neurosurg Clin N Am 1993;4(2):327–336

17. Berger MS. Functional mapping-guided resection of low-grade gliomas. Clin Neurosurg 1995;42:437–452

18. Jooma R, Yeh HS, Privitera MD, Gartner M. Lesionectomy versus electrophysiologically guided resection for temporal lobe tumors manifesting with complex partial seizures. J Neurosurg 1995;83(2):231–236

19. Tran TA, Spencer SS, Javidan M, Pacia S, Marks D, Spencer DD. Significance of spikes recorded on intraoperative electrocorticography in patients with brain tumor and epilepsy. Epilepsia 1997;38(10):1132–1139

20. Ojemann JG, Miller JW, Silbergeld DL. Preserved function in brain invaded by tumor. Neurosurgery 1996;39(2):253–258, discussion 258–259

21. Skirboll SS, Ojemann GA, Berger MS, Lettich E, Winn HR. Functional cortex and subcortical white matter located within gliomas. Neurosurgery 1996;38(4):678–684, discussion 684–685

22. Vossler DG, Kraemer DL, Haltiner AM, et al. Intracranial EEG in temporal lobe epilepsy: location of seizure onset relates to degree of hippocampal pathology. Epilepsia 2004;45(5):497–503

23. Wennberg R, Arruda F, Quesney LF, Olivier A. Preeminence of extrahippocampal structures in the generation of mesial temporal seizures: evidence from human depth electrode recordings. Epilepsia 2002;43(7):716–726

24. Haglund MM, Berger MS, Shamseldin M, Lettich E, Ojemann GA. Cortical localization of temporal lobe language sites in patients with gliomas. Neurosurgery 1994;34(4):567–576, discussion 576

25. Ojemann GA, Dodrill CB. Verbal memory deficits after left temporal lobectomy for epilepsy. Mechanism and intraoperative prediction. J Neurosurg 1985;62(1):101–107

26. Stroup E, Langfitt J, Berg M, McDermott M, Pilcher W, Como P. Predicting verbal memory decline following anterior temporal lobectomy (ATL). Neurology 2003;60(8):1266–1273

27. Ojemann SG, Berger MS, Lettich E, Ojemann GA. Localization of language function in children: results of electrical stimulation mapping. J Neurosurg 2003;98(3):465–470

28. Rutten GJ, Ramsey NF, van Rijen PC, Noordmans HJ, van Veelen CW. Development of a functional magnetic resonance imaging protocol for intraoperative localization of critical temporoparietal language areas. Ann Neurol 2002;51(3):350–360

29. Ojemann JG. Preoperative assessment of temporal lobe function with fMRI. In: Miller JW, Silbergeld DL, eds. Epilepsy Surgery: Principles and Controversies. New York: Taylor & Francis; 2006:336–341

30. Everett LL, van Rooyen IF, Warner MH, Shurtleff HA, Saneto RP, Ojemann JG. Use of dexmedetomidine in awake craniotomy in adolescents: report of two cases. Paediatr Anaesth 2006;16(3):338–342

31. Souter MJ, Rozet I, Ojemann JG, et al. Dexmedetomidine sedation during awake craniotomy for seizure resection: effects on electrocorticography. J Neurosurg Anesthesiol 2007;19(1):38–44

32. Silbergeld DL, Mueller WM, Colley PS, Ojemann GA, Lettich E. Use of propofol (Diprivan) for awake craniotomies: technical note. Surg Neurol 1992;38(4):271–272

33. Leuthardt EC, Fox DJ, Ojemann GA, et al. Frameless stereotaxy without rigid pin fixation during awake craniotomies. Stereotact Funct Neurosurg 2002;79(3-4):256–261

34. Kim H, Bernasconi N, Bernhardt B, Colliot O, Bernasconi A. Basal temporal sulcal morphology in healthy controls and patients with temporal lobe epilepsy. Neurology 2008;70(22 pt 2):2159–2165

35. Ferrier CH, Aronica E, Leijten FS, et al. Electrocorticographic discharge patterns in glioneuronal tumors and focal cortical dysplasia. Epilepsia 2006;47(9):1477–1486

20 Surgical Management of Lesional Temporal Lobe Epilepsy

Oğuz Çataltepe and G. Rees Cosgrove

Temporal lobe lesions constitute 30 to 70% of surgical specimens obtained from children with intractable temporal lobe epilepsy (TLE).[1–8] Developmental brain tumors and low-grade neoplasms are the most common causes of TLE in children. Although hippocampal sclerosis is the most common lesion in adults with TLE, it is much less frequent in the pediatric patient population. In this chapter, we will discuss the surgical strategies in children with lesional temporal epilepsy, mainly focusing on tumors and vascular malformations, because they are the most common neuropathological substrates in children after cortical dysplasia and mesial temporal sclerosis (MTS).

The goal in neuro-oncological surgery is always total resection of the tumor when it is feasible. This is also relevant for tumor-related epilepsy cases with one significant difference: there is an equally important additional surgical target—the epileptogenic zone. Therefore, surgical interventions for lesional TLE in children have dual therapeutic goals: stopping the seizures and removing the lesion while preserving cortical function. These dual therapeutic goals can be achieved by determining both the causative relationship between the lesion and the seizures and the spatial relationship between the lesion and the epileptogenic zone. Although the epileptogenic zone frequently corresponds to the cortex immediately adjacent to the lesion, it may also stretch far beyond the anatomical boundaries of the lesion. Therefore, determining the extent of resection in lesional epilepsy patients is critical to optimizing surgical outcome but also quite challenging at times. Furthermore, reaching these goals may not always be feasible, and certain compromises may be required in some cases.

Here we will discuss the surgical management of lesional TLE patients based on published data and our own clinical experience. There is very limited published data specifically obtained from children with TLE, and there are even smaller numbers of reports addressing lesional TLE in children. The real frequency of lesional TLE cases is not clear, and reported rates show wide variations in large surgical series (**Table 20.1**).[1–8]

■ Pathological Substrate

The most common pathological substrates in medically refractory epilepsy patients are MTS, tumors, vascular abnormalities, gliosis, and developmental disorders.[9] We will review lesional TLE in childhood by focusing on neoplasms and vascular abnormalities and refer the reader to related chapters in this book for details regarding the surgical management of MTS and cortical dysplasia. Published series describing pathological substrates in TLE patients mostly include mixed patient populations, both adults and children. Only a few reports exclusively cover the pediatric age group.[1–8] As we can see in **Table 20.1**, published data are heterogeneous and most likely heavily biased by referral pat-

Table 20.1 Pathological Substrates in Pediatric Lesional TLE Series

	Number	Tumor	MTS	CD	Vasc.	Dual Pathology
Sinclair[1]	42	33%	19%	9%	—	11%
Clusmann[2]	89	46%	31%	1%	—	—
Mittal et al[3]	109	35%	45%	35%	5%	25%
Benifla et al[4,54]	126	52%	13%	7%	3%	8%
Kan et al[5]	33	28%	28%	22%	9%	5%
Kim et al[6]	59	54%	23%	18%	—	—
Maton et al[7]	20	40%	20%	30%	—	—

Sources: Mittal S, Montes JL, Farmer JP, et al. Long-term outcome after surgical treatment of temporal lobe epilepsy in children. J Neurosurg 2005; 103 (5, suppl)401–412; Benifla M, Otsubo H, Ochi A, et al. Temporal lobe surgery for intractable epilepsy in children: an analysis of outcomes in 126 children. Neurosurgery 2006;59(6):1203–1213, discussion 1213–1214; Kan P, Van Orman C, Kestle JRW. Outcomes after surgery for focal epilepsy in children. Childs Nerv Syst 2008;24(5):587–591; Kim SK, Wang KC, Hwang YS, et al. Epilepsy surgery in children: outcomes and complications. J Neurosurg Pediatr 2008;1(4):277–283; Maton B, Jayakar P, Resnick T, Morrison G, Ragheb J, Duchowny M. Surgery for medically intractable temporal lobe epilepsy during early life. Epilepsia 2008;49(1):80–87.

Abbreviations: TLE, temporal lobe epilepsy, MTS, mesial temporal sclerosis; CD, cortical displasia; Vasc., vascular lesion.

Table 20.2 Tumor Types in Pediatric TLE Series

	Number	DNET	GG	LGA	Oligo
Sinclair[1]	14	14%	57%	21%	—
Clusmann[2]	41	17%	56%	7%	7%
Mittal et al[3]	38	13%	55%	13%	7%
Çataltepe et al[10]	29	52%	13%	21%	10%
Benifla et al[4,54]	65	15%	24%	24%	—
Kim et al[6]	32	37%	40%	—	9%
Maton et al[7]	8	25%	25%	50%	—

Abbreviations: TLE, temporal lobe epilepsy, DNET, dysembryoplastic neuroepithelial tumors; GG, ganglioplioma; LGA, low grade astrocytoma; Oligo, oligodendroglioma.

terns to the related epilepsy centers. However, it is still fair to state that neoplasms are the most common pathological substrates seen in children with lesional TLE followed by MTS, cortical dysplasia, and vascular lesions. MTS constitutes, at least in some series, a substantial percentage of the cases, but the true frequency of MTS in children with TLE is still not clear.

Tumors

The exact frequency of tumors in children with intractable TLE is not well established yet because of the limited number of studies focusing exclusively on the pediatric population. Çataltepe et al[10] reported that temporal-tumor–related epilepsy patients constituted 40% of pediatric epilepsy surgery cases in their series. Published data imply that the most common neoplasms in TLE patients are developmental tumors, such as dysembryoneuroepithelial tumor (DNET), or slowly growing low-grade glial tumors and oligodendrogliomas.[1,3–5,13] However, the frequencies of the neoplasms seen in epilepsy patients are quite different among published series. Although ganglioglioma is the most common neoplasm in some series, low-grade astrocytoma or DNET is the most common neoplasm in other studies (**Table 20.2**). The vast majority of the patients with temporal lobe tumor–related epilepsy have some common distinctive characteristics, and some authors even define them as a distinct clinico-pathological group. These characteristics include a well-differentiated histological pattern, cortical localization of the tumors (69–91%), frequent involvement of mesial structures (48%), indolent biological nature, young age, seizures frequently as the only symptom, long-standing history of seizure disorder, normal neurological exam, and favorable outcome after surgery.[10,12,13]

Vascular Malformations

Most common vascular malformations causing epilepsy are arteriovenous malformations (AVM) and cavernous hemangiomas. The most common presenting symptoms of AVM are hemorrhage and seizures. Hemorrhage is by far the commonest initial manifestation of AVM in children, whereas 10 to 25% of the patients present with seizures.[14–17] Seizures in

AVM patients most likely originate from gliotic, nonfunctional brain parenchyma interspersed in and around the AVM nidus. These gliotic changes develop secondary to focal ischemia induced by "steal" phenomena and possibly constitute the main reason for seizures in AVM patients. In Yasargil's series of 414 operated cerebral AVM patients that included both children and adults, initial manifestations were hemorrhage and seizures in 77.8% and 14.7% of the patients, respectively.[18] Yasargil's series includes 74 children (17.8%) younger then 15 years old, and approximately 11% of them had temporal lobe AVMs (6.8% extramesial and 4.1% hippocampal AVM). In the same series, seizure as an initial manifestation was found in 40% of the patients when the AVM was located in the temporal lobe and in 10.6% of the children overall in this series.

Cavernous hemangiomas are relatively common congenital lesions that occur in 0.4 to 0.5% of the general population and constitute 5 to 13% of all intracerebral vascular malformations.[19–21] Cavernous hemangiomas occur mostly in the supratentorial region, 15 to 20% of them being in temporal lobe.[20–23] In a large series, temporal lobe location in cavernous hemangioma patients was found to be significantly higher (48%), and 40% were located in mesiobasal structures.[24] Epilepsy incidence in symptomatic patients with cavernous hemangioma has been reported between 35 and 79%.[19,21,22,25–27] Cavernous hemangiomas that are located in the temporal lobe have a much higher tendency to be associated with intractable epilepsy, and they are far more likely than AVM to be medically refractory.[19,27,28] In children, seizures are the most common manifestation of cavernous malformations (45–54%).[23,25,29,30] The estimated risk for seizure development was reported as 1.5%/year/patient in single lesions and 2.5%/lesion/year in patients with multiple lesions.[24,29]

■ Mechanism of Seizures

The epileptogenic mechanisms involved in lesion-related epilepsy are not clear. Several mechanisms, including direct pressure and irritation of the cortical tissue, gliotic changes and disruption of vascular structures of the surrounding cortex, morphological alterations at the cellular level, changes in inhibitory and excitatory neurotransmitter levels, and denervation hypersensitivity have been proposed to play a role.[11,31,32] Chronic changes in surrounding brain tissue either by mechanical or vascular mechanisms can also be responsible for seizures induced by slowly growing low-grade tumors. Developmental tumors may even have intrinsic epileptogenicity because they are frequently associated with cortical dysplasia and contain cells with a rich array of neurochemical properties, including altered inhibitory and excitatory local circuits.[11,31] The location of the lesion is also a critical factor. Brain tumors associated with epilepsy are often located in the cortex or in gray–white matter junction. When the lesion is located in the temporal lobe, its direct or indirect effects on hippocampus may cause seizures. The lesion location may interfere with cortical afferents and efferents and lead to relative deafferentation of a certain cortical area that has intrinsic epileptogenicity. Small hemorrhages in and around the tumors also cause hemosiderin deposits, which are highly epileptogenic.[11] Secondary epileptogenesis might also be responsible for seizures in some patients. It has been shown with intracranial electroencephalography (EEG) recording that approximately one half of the patients with neocortical temporal tumors have independent epileptogenic areas in ipsilateral mesial structures.[33] The proposed mechanisms for seizures in patients with AVMs include vascular steal phenomenon, focal ischemia of the adjacent cortex secondary to A-V shunting, progressive intralesional and perilesional gliosis, demyelination, hemosiderin lining in AVM bed, and secondary epileptogenesis in the temporal lobe.[14,16,28] It has also been suggested that mass effect on the surrounding brain, cortical irritation, presence of calcification, gliosis in the surrounding brain tissue, and accumulation of iron-containing substances in hemosiderin fringe are responsible for the seizures in cavernous hemangioma patients.[19-22]

■ Surgical Strategy

Although the histological subtype of the lesion is always the major factor influencing clinical outcome in any given patient, the determinants of the seizure-related outcome in lesional epilepsy are more complicated. The factors effecting good outcome in epilepsy patients are not only dependent on the type of the lesion but also related to the location of the lesion as well as the extent of the epileptogenic zone and the area of resection.[32-34] Therefore, the surgical strategy in lesional epilepsy patients is a multifaceted topic. It should be defined based on the location, extent of both the lesion and the epileptogenic zone, as well as the histopathological diagnosis. Determining the optimal surgical strategy in these cases is a challenging task and still involves some controversy. Lesionectomy alone, lesionectomy with resection of the epileptogenic zone, or lesionectomy with resection

of the ipsilateral mesial structures all have their advocates in discussions about the appropriate surgical approaches in these cases. However, there is limited clinical evidence to support specific resective strategies in lesional-TLE cases.[32] Therefore, until more data are available, the surgical strategy for each patient should be determined on an individual basis by considering histological type and location of the lesion, extent of the epileptogenic zone, and the spatial relation between the lesion and the epileptogenic zone.

Extent of Resection

The spatial relationship between the epileptogenic zone and the lesion is the most critical factor to determine the extent of surgical resection in lesional epilepsy patients. There are several conditions for optimizing seizure control in children with lesional epilepsy. First, the lesion should be completely identified and resected. Second, the epileptogenic zone should be contained within the resected area, and finally the remaining cortical and subcortical areas should not develop independent seizures after surgery. Unsuccessful results in lesional epilepsy surgery are frequently related to incomplete resection of the lesion/epileptogenic zone or the presence of additional or secondary epileptogenic foci.[35] Another reason may be having an extensive epileptogenic zone beyond the boundaries of the lesion. Some well-known examples of this include the presence of surrounding gliosis in AVM, hemosiderosis rim associated with cavernous hemangioma, dysplastic areas associated with developmental tumors, and dual pathology.

Lesion

Lesionectomy alone is probably the most commonly used surgical approach in lesional epilepsy cases. Although there is wide consensus regarding the significance of total tumor resection for good seizure control, the results of this surgical approach in the published epilepsy series are quite different. Khajavi et al[36] reported that seizure-free outcome was only correlated with the extent of tumor resection but not with additional resection of the surrounding cortex. Conversely, Jooma et al[37] reported that epilepsy patients who underwent lesionectomy procedure alone had a significantly lower seizure-free outcome rate compared with patients who had additional cortical resections of the adjacent epileptogenic zone. Sugano et al[38] reported that after complete resection of mass lesions, they still found residual spikes in the mesial structures in up to 86% of the patients and recommended additional resection in these areas for better seizure control.

Epileptogenic Zone

The first step in the planning lesional epilepsy surgery is to define the relationship between the localization of the

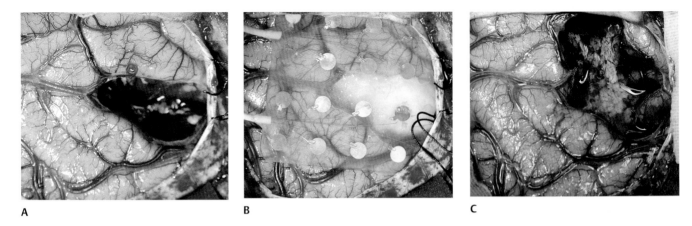

A   B   C

Fig. 20.1 Intraoperative pictures from a 14-year-old patient with a cortical lesion (dysembryoplastic neuroepithelial tumor) associated with focal cortical dysplasia in posterior temporal region. **(A)** Surgical cavity after resection of the tumor by completely emptying the involved gyrus. **(B)** Intraoperative electrocorticography after resection of the lesion to map the adjacent dysplastic epileptogenic cortex. **(C)** Further resection of the adjacent dysplastic cortex based on electrocorticographic mapping.

seizures and the location of the lesion. If the clinical and electrophysiological characteristics of the seizures are fully correlated with the location of the lesion, then the next step would be to determine whether the epileptogenic zone exceeds the anatomical boundaries of the lesion. The surgeon needs to work closely with the epilepsy/neurophysiology team to map the epileptogenic zone and to determine its spatial relationships with the structural lesion **(Fig. 20.1)**. The surgical resection strategy is then designed based on lesion location, the extent of the epileptogenic zone, and the relative position of adjacent eloquent cortex. Anterior temporal lobectomy (ATL) including the lesion **(Fig. 20.2)** or tailored lesionectomy including the surrounding epileptogenic cortex are the two commonly used surgical approaches in lesional TLE. Clussmann et al[2] describe their "preoperative tailoring" technique as aiming for complete resection of the lesion demonstrated on magnetic resonance imaging (MRI) and extending the resection further whenever clinical or electrophysiological data suggest a seizure onset in the respective distant areas, such as the hippocam-

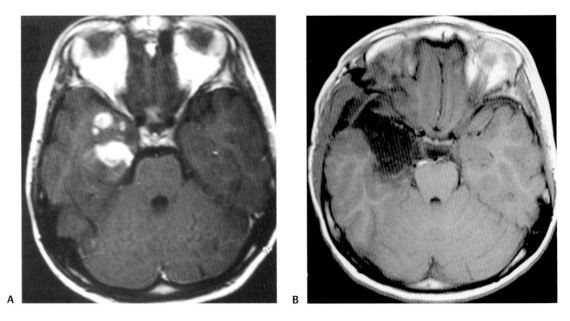

A   B

Fig. 20.2 Preoperative **(A)** and postoperative **(B)** axial magnetic resonance images of a 10-year-old patient with ganglioglioma located in the right parahippocampus. The tumor was resected along with anterior temporal lobe and mesiotemporal structures.

pus. Imaging techniques such as functional imaging studies, magnetoencephalography, diffusion tensor imaging (DTI), intraoperative electrocorticography (ECoG), and invasive monitoring data obtained with depth/subdural electrodes are among the recommended techniques to determine the extent of the neocortical and hippocampal resections.

Mesial Temporal Structures

It has been generally assumed that the primary epileptogenic activity arises in the vicinity of the lesion. However, the situation may be more complicated if the lesion is located in the temporal lobe because secondary involvement of the mesial temporal structures in seizure generation is not rare with temporal lobe lesions. It is well known that the hippocampus is a very epileptogenic structure and may even generate a focus for secondary epileptogenesis. Therefore, much attention is given to the mesial structures in TLE patients even if the lesion is located in temporal neocortex. This is a legitimate concern because it is possible that epileptogenic zone may not be limited to cortex adjacent to the lesion itself but may also include the mesial temporal structures. If that is the case, then resection of the mesial temporal structures along with the lesion may be needed to obtain a seizure-free outcome. However, indications for resection of the adjacent mesial temporal structures in lesional TLE cases are highly controversial. If the tumor directly involves mesial temporal structures, then the surgical decision is relatively straightforward. Conversely, if mesial temporal structures are not directly in the lesional zone, then the risks and benefits of the resection of mesial temporal structures should be assessed carefully. Well-defined histological and electrophysiological changes in the hippocampus are very important to determine the most appropriate surgical approach in these cases. Unfortunately, imaging findings of hippocampal neuronal loss are quite subtle in lesional TLE patients, unlike MTS patients. Therefore it may be very difficult to appreciate pathological changes, such as neuronal loss, in the hippocampus of the patients with temporal neocortical lesions using available imaging techniques. Similarly, even if the hippocampus demonstrates epileptogenic properties by intracranial monitoring techniques, imaging studies may not be grossly abnormal.[33] Usui et al[33] reviewed 15 TLE patients who had structural lesions in temporal lobe but normal appearing mesial temporal structures on MRI. They reviewed intracranial EEG data obtained through bilateral temporal subdural and depth electrodes and documented independent ictal discharges arising from ipsilateral mesial structures in 47% of the patients. They concluded that these findings support the presence of independent epileptogenicity of mesial structures in lesional temporal lobe epilepsy. In this series, clinical semiology, scalp EEG, and MRI images were not found predictive for mesial onset of the seizures. Furthermore, the presence of mesial temporal onset of sei-

zures was not associated with hippocampal neuronal loss in histological exam. In another study, Mathern et al[39] showed, using depth electrodes, that ictal onset EEG activity either started from mesial temporal structures or first propagated in the mesial contacts of depth electrodes in 94% of the patients with temporal lobe lesions. Mihara and Baba[40] identified independent ictal discharges arising from ipsilateral mesial structures in 47% of the patients with neocortical temporal lesions and concluded that there is independent epileptogenicity of both neocortical lesions and ipsilateral mesial structures in this subgroup of patients. The potential complexity of accurately localizing the epileptogenic zone in lesional TLE patients causes difficulties in determining the correct surgical approach for all cases.

Clusmann et al classified their surgical approach toward mesial structures of lesional TLE cases in five groups as complete amygdalohippocampectomy, partial (anterior) hippocampectomy, resection of temporal pole plus amygdalohippocampectomy, basal temporal resection plus amygdalohippocampectomy, and removal of a mesial lesion that extends into the lateral temporal lobe.[2] They reported comparable rates of seizure relief with all these approaches. Similarly, Fried et al published their results of 41 temporal tumors and stated that seizure-free outcome rate was 87% without any correlation with the extent of hippocampal resection.[12] Another report showed similar (81%) seizure-free outcome with hippocampal-sparing resections in lesional TLE cases.[41] Morris et al also published a high rate of seizure-free outcome in their temporal lobe tumor series using a surgical approach that spared hippocampus.[42] Therefore, they recommended that hippocampus not be resected unless it is structurally abnormal. Two other series showed similar seizure control rates without resecting hippocampus of the epilepsy patients with occult vascular malformations in temporal lobe.[43,44] In summary, it is still not clear whether resection of mesial structures along the lesion is needed for good seizure control in lesional TLE cases. Currently there is no clear-cut evidence in relevant literature to devise an optimal strategy regarding resection of the mesial structures along the temporal lobe lesions.

The presence of radiologically normal-appearing mesial structures along with a temporal lobe lesion presents an additional challenge because even if the mesial structures are radiologically normal appearing, they may still be histologically abnormal and capable of generating independent seizures. This may be related to abnormal synaptic reorganization of hippocampus that may be induced by seizures propagating from temporal neocortical lesions. The critical question is whether the epileptogenic capacity of the ipsilateral radiologically normal-appearing hippocampus would still continue after resection of the temporal tumor. Unfortunately, little data exist to answer this question. Another avenue to assess the ipsilateral radiologically normal-appearing hippocampus is its functional status. Impaired performance on the Wada test correlates well with the extent of hippo-campal neuronal loss according to Morioka et al.[45] Therefore, if PET, neuropsychological, and Wada test results are sugges-tive of dysfunction of the ipsilateral mesial temporal struc-tures, then these should be considered when determining the extent of the mesial temporal resection. Conversely, if these test results show well-functioning mesial structures, then they should be preserved.[33]

Dual Pathology

Dual pathology in TLE cases is the co-existence of hippo-campal sclerosis with another epileptogenic lesion, such as a tumor or cavernoma and is not a rare occurrence in epi-lepsy patients. Although its incidence in the literature var-ies, Drake et al reported a 56% dual pathology rate in their series of pediatric TLE secondary to pediatric temporal lobe tumors.[46] Otsubo et al reported dual pathology in 54% of pa-tients with epileptogenic ganglioglioma.[47] Conversely, we found a dual pathology rate of 8% in our pediatric tempo-ral lobe tumor series.[10] The presence of dual pathology cre-ates a challenge in surgical strategy of lesional TLE patients similar to the one that we discussed previously. Few studies address this issue. Li et al demonstrated that seizure-free outcome rate was significantly low if only one of the lesions was removed in dual-pathology patients, but it was quite high (73%) when both sclerotic hippocampus and the lesion were removed.[48] Morris et al also recommend resection of sclerotic hippocampus along with the temporal tumor if im-aging studies are correlated with hippocampal sclerosis.[49] In another study, Cascino et al reported that lesionectomy alone yielded unsatisfactory results in TLE with a dual path-ological entity and recommended resection of hippocampus along with the tumors in these cases.[50] These reports all em-phasize the significance of careful evaluation of lesional TLE patients with dual pathology to determine the necessity of

amygdalohippocampectomy along with lesion removal. This decision needs to be tailored case by case based on the elec-trophysiological findings and functional status of the mesial temporal structures.

Location

The surgical approaches in lesional TLE cases are closely re-lated to the location of the lesion within temporal lobe and its proximity to mesial temporal structures (**Fig. 20.3**). The accessibility of the lesion, its relationship to eloquent cortex, and mesial structures are all critical components in deter-mining the surgical approach and extent of the resection. There is no well-defined, localization-based classification of temporal lobe lesions to describe and to discuss surgical ap-proaches in TLE patients. We prefer to classify temporal lobe lesions, mainly tumors, in three groups based on their loca-tion within the temporal lobe as we described previously.[10] Here we will summarize our surgical approaches in these cases based on this classification:

- Mesial temporal lobe tumors: parahippocampus, amygdala, and hippocampus
- Basal temporal lobe tumors: inferior temporal and fusiform gyri
- Lateral temporal lobe tumors: superior and middle temporal gyri

It is our observation that mesial temporal tumors generally respect pial boundaries of the collateral sulcus and very com-monly remain restricted to the mesial temporal region (**Figs. 20.4** and **20.5**). The only exception to this is the high-grade, malignant tumor. Therefore, mesial temporal lobe tumors can be classified separately from temporal neocortical tu-mors. Conversely, separation between basal and lateral tem-poral tumors is less precise and tumors extending to both sides are not rare. However, surgical access to basal tempo-

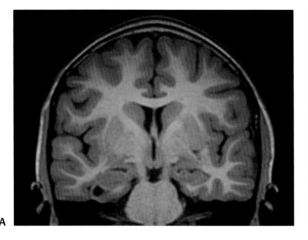
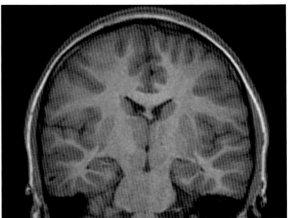

Fig. 20.3 Dysembryoplastic neuroepithelial tumors located in **(A)** mesial temporal and **(B)** lateral temporal regions.

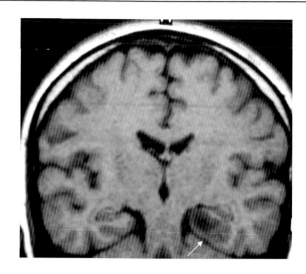

Fig. 20.4 Magnetic resonance image of a mesiotemporal tumor that is entirely confined in the parahippocampus. Note that collateral sulcus (*arrow*) is well-preserved without any tumor involvement in the fusiform gyrus.

a case-by-case basis by considering many factors, including age, availability of detailed electrophysiological data, and feasibility of Wada and neuropsychological tests. The critical part of the decision-making process in these cases is defining the spatial relationship between the epileptogenic zone and the lesion itself. Invasive monitoring techniques may be needed in some cases to define the epileptogenic zone more clearly. This way, the surgical resection area can be carefully mapped using invasive monitoring, stimulation studies, and functional imaging.

Mesial Temporal Tumors

Tumors in the Nondominant Mesial Temporal Region

Total removal of the tumor along with the mesial temporal structures is the goal (**Fig. 20.5**). If the tumor does not involve adjacent mesial structures, such as an amygdala tumor with radiologically normal-appearing hippocampus, we still consider hippocampectomy unless neuropsychological tests suggest a high risk for memory dysfunction.

ral tumors has its unique challenges, and it is still helpful to use this classification to define the surgical approach and its rationale more clearly. We define our approach based not only on the tumor location in the temporal lobe but also on being in the dominant or nondominant hemisphere to provide a framework to discussion. It should be emphasized that the location-based description of our surgical approach is defined simply to provide a general perspective to our discussion and certainly should not be considered as a strict guideline. In practicality, we define our surgical approach on

Tumors in the Dominant Mesial Temporal Region

Total removal of the tumor is the goal if the adjacent mesial structures are radiologically and electrophysiologically normal and the neuropsychological tests are normal. If the adjacent mesial structures are not radiologically and electrophysiologically normal, then Wada and neuropsychological test results become critical in determining the extent of the resection. If the potential risks are acceptable, then resection of the tumor along with the mesial temporal structures is performed.

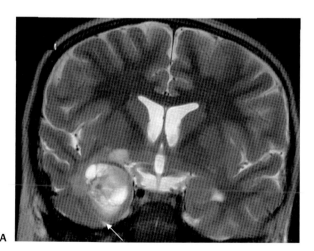
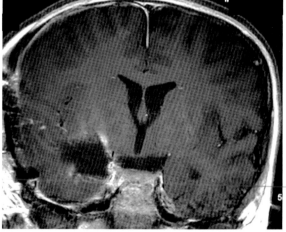

Fig. 20.5 Preoperative **(A)** and postoperative **(B)** magnetic resonance images (MRIs) of a dysembryoplastic neuroepithelial tumor located in mesiotemporal region, invading both the parahippocampus and hippocampus. The tumor was resected along with mesial temporal structures. Note that the preoperative MRI shows no tumor involvement in the fusiform gyrus despite the large size of tumor and significant enlargement of the parahippocampus. Although displaced, the collateral sulcus (*arrow*) remains intact and well-preserved.

Basal Temporal Tumors

Tumors in the Nondominant Basal Temporal Region

If the epileptogenic zone does not extend to the mesial temporal region, then we perform lesionectomy only. If the epileptogenic zone extends to the mesial temporal region, then we resect mesial structures as well.

Tumors in the Dominant Basal Temporal Region

If the epileptogenic zone does not extend to the mesial temporal region, we perform lesionectomy only. If the epileptogenic zone extends to the mesial temporal region as well, then we resect mesial structures only if the potential risks are acceptable based on the Wada and neuropsychological test results.

Lateral Temporal Tumors

Tumors in the Dominant or Nondominant Lateral Temporal Region

If the epileptogenic zone does not extend beyond the anatomical boundaries of the lesion, we perform lesionectomy only. If the epileptogenic zone extends to the surrounding cortical tissue, then tailored resection is performed by including both the lesion and the epileptogenic area.

There are certainly lesions that cannot be classified strictly within these three anatomical subgroups, such as dual pathologies, AVMs, and lesions covering very large areas in the temporal lobe. These are challenging cases, and the surgical approach should be tailored carefully in these patients by considering the histological, radiological, functional, and electrophysiological characteristics of each case. When the neurophysiological and clinical semiological findings are not co-localized with the lesion, further investigation including invasive monitoring should be considered.

■ Special Considerations in Vascular Malformations

Cavernous Hemangioma

Adequate seizure control rate with medical management is approximately 60% in cavernous hemangioma-related epilepsy, and the surgical indications and approaches in TLE patients with cavernous hemangioma remain controversial.[19–22] If the patient has rare seizures, medical management can be considered as a first-line treatment. However, the location of the lesion and the risk of bleeding should also be considered to decide whether surgical management is preferable. If the seizures are medically intractable or associated with recurrent bleeding and functional impair-

ment, then surgery should be strongly considered.[27] The extent of resection and the timing of the surgical intervention are the main controversial topics in these patients. Some authors discuss that early operation in patients with shorter duration of seizures provides better seizure control and helps to avoid creating secondary epileptogenic foci in hippocampus.[27] However limited data exist to support this approach. Surgical approaches include lesionectomy limited to the cavernous hemangioma itself, extended lesionectomy (cavernoma and additional removal of perilesional tissue), and tailored temporal lobectomy (cavernoma resection and anteromesial temporal lobectomy).[19] Simple lesionectomy provides seizure-free outcome in 70 to 80% of the patients.[19] Complete resection of the cavernoma along with surrounding hemosiderin fringe is the most commonly recommended technique. It is suggested that hemosiderin fringe is responsible for the epileptogenic activity because of the iron content of hemosiderin and the induced gliotic changes in the surrounding tissues. Therefore, resection of these tissues is critical for good seizure control, according to some authors.[24,28] However, this approach remains controversial, and some study results could not verify this assumption. Although it is not well established, there are data suggesting that the extended resection based on the ECoG provides better seizure control in this patient group.[27]

Another topic of discussion is the timing of the surgery. Early surgical intervention for seizure control in cavernous hemangioma patients was correlated with a better postoperative outcome according to some authors. Stefan and Hammen[27] reported 91.7% seizure-free outcome in patients who were operated on within 2 years of seizure onset. Cappabianca et al stated that lesionectomy was the treatment of choice for patients with a short history of seizures (<1 year).[22] However for longer seizure histories, they recommend tailored surgery with neurophysiological investigations to detect possible secondary seizure foci. Another critical issue in surgical strategy is determining whether the patient has dual pathology (i.e., cavernous hemangioma with hippocampal sclerosis). Hammen et al[25] found that it is critical to remove both cavernoma and sclerotic hippocampus in dual-pathology cases. Stefan and Hammen[27] also emphasized the importance of assessment for dual pathology.

If there is no discordance between location of the lesion and clinical and electrophysiological features of the seizures, then simple lesionectomy might be a reasonable approach in cavernomas located in the temporal lobe. We prefer lesionectomy with removal of the surrounding hemosiderin fringe as the first step in cavernous hemangioma patients **(Fig. 20.6)**. If the seizures persist, then more rigorous investigations including invasive monitoring can be performed as a second step. Again, invasive monitoring before removal of cavernoma should be considered if there is poor concordance between the location of the cavernoma and the electrophysiological and clinical semiology data. We also believe

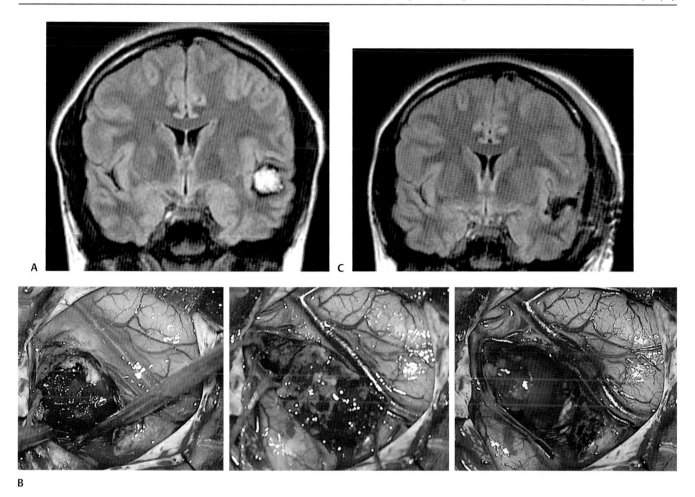

Fig. 20.6 **(A)** Preoperative coronal magnetic resonance image (MRI) of a 12-year-old patient shows a cavernous hemangioma located in superior temporal gyrus. **(B)** Intraoperative pictures of the same patient: surgical exposure, dissection, and removal of cavernous hemangioma and surgical field after resection of the hemosiderin fringe on the cavity walls. **(C)** Postoperative coronal MRI shows residual surgical cavity.

that removal of the ipsilateral mesial structures is the correct approach if the cavernoma is located in the mesial temporal lobe.

Arteriovenous Malformations

AVM-related seizures are frequently well controlled with medical management.[28] Radiosurgery is also very effective for seizure control in many AVM patients.[17,51] Therefore, the surgical treatment decision for AVMs is usually related to intracerebral bleeding or the risk of future hemorrhage. Conversely, data in the literature are limited regarding the natural course of seizures in AVM patients because the main focus of AVM literature is mostly vascular events and their surgical management. The main goal in cerebral AVM surgery is removal of the AVM nidus without disruption or damage to the surrounding brain tissue. There are some data in the literature suggesting that AVM resection not only provides

protection from potentially catastrophic hemorrhage but also helps to control the seizures.[16] Yeh et al have published two studies on the surgical management of seizures in AVM patients.[52,53] They recommend intraoperative ECoG covering temporal neocortex and mesial structures if the seizures involve temporal lobe in AVM patients. Using this technique, they performed additional cortical excisions, based on the ECoG data, including resection of mesial temporal structures in 9 of 17 patients with temporal lobe AVMs with good seizure control rates. In another study, Turjman et al identified several characteristics of AVMs that correlate with a high risk of epilepsy as the initial presentation.[16] These features are a superficial nidus in close proximity to the cortex, temporoparietal location, and feeders from the middle cerebral artery. The main questions regarding AVM-related epilepsy are whether the surrounding brain tissue and gliotic areas around the AVM have independent epileptogenic properties, the rate of secondary epileptogenesis of mesial temporal structures in temporal lobe AVMs, the appropriate diagnostic techniques to determine independent epileptogenic activities, and the right approach to improve postoperative seizure control in AVM patients. Unfortunately, little data exist in the literature to answer these questions. There are not even satisfactory data to determine whether the extent of resection beyond the gliotic margins of an AVM has any influence over postoperative seizure control.[28] We believe these are critical questions on AVM-related seizures that deserve more detailed investigation.

■ Outcome

Tumors

Surgical outcome in tumor-related pediatric TLE cases are much better than some other lesional epilepsy cases, such as cortical dysplasia. In a large study, the best seizure control rate was seen in children with TLE secondary to neoplasm: 88 to 92% Engel Class I and II outcome. This rate was 70% in the MTS group and 50% in the patients with cortical dysplasia in the same series.[54] Choi et al reported Class I seizure-free outcome in 77% of the patients with tumor-related TLE.[55] They noted that complete resection of the tumor was the most significant factor in obtaining a seizure-free outcome. Other authors have reported seizure-free outcomes in 75 to 95% of patients with tumor-related epilepsy.[3,5,56]

The main predictor of seizure-free outcome is complete resection of the tumor according to some studies.[13,36] Another predictor is histological type of the tumor. Luyken et al noted that seizure-free outcome was the highest in patients with ganglioglioma and oligodendroglioma (> 90%) compared with those with pilocytic and grade II astrocytomas (61% and 66%, respectively).[57] The same study revealed clinical and radiological predictors for poorer seizure control as having a longer history of seizures, additional EEG focus, dual pathology, and incomplete tumor resection. Clusmann et al reported on 89 children with TLE and 46.6% of the patients had neoplastic lesions.[2] They reported a good outcome (Engel Class I and II) in 83.3% of ganglioglioma and DNET patients.

The location of the tumor within the temporal lobe also appears to have a significant effect on the outcome. Giulioni et al reported the results of 21 tumor-related (ganglioglioma) TLE patients who all underwent lesionectomy only.[58] In this series, 66.6% and 33.3% of the patients had Engel Class I and Class II outcomes, respectively. Although the seizure-free outcome rate was 100% in temporal neocortical tumors, this rate was only 5/11 (60%) in temporomesial tumors in this series. This was despite of gross total tumor resection in 80% of patients with temporomesial tumor. Therefore, Giulioni et al suggested that further neurophysiological assessment should be performed to define and resect the additional epileptogenic zone in patients with temporomesial ganglio-

glioma. Again, Giulioni et al[59] reported their experience with glioneuronal tumors associated with epilepsy in children. In their series of 15 children, 9 had temporal tumors. Seizure-free outcome rate was 86.6%. Interestingly, they did not find any difference between lateral temporal and mesial temporal tumors in terms of the postoperative outcomes. They also did not observe an effect of the duration of seizure history on the postoperative seizure outcomes. They also reported a high rate (40%) of associated dysplastic cortex among these patients.

Surgical approach is another factor that might potentially affect clinical outcome. Unfortunately, the data comparing the results of different surgical techniques are very limited. Chan et al compared the results of two different surgical approaches in patients with DNET.[60] They performed tumor resection with temporal lobectomy in 12 patients and only lesionectomy in 6 patients. Although all patients with temporal lobectomy had seizure-free outcomes, this rate was only 33% in patients who underwent lesionectomy alone. Chan et al explained this difference with the presence of dysplastic cortex around DNET lesions.[60] In another study, Minkin et al reported on 24 children with DNETs. A total of 15 lesions were located in the temporal lobe, 10 were in the lateral temporal, and 5 were in the mesial temporal lobe.[61] Overall, 83.3% of the patients had seizure-free outcome. Minkin et al performed lesionectomy alone in 73% of the patients, whereas the remaining 4 patients had incomplete seizure control. They performed lesionectomy and amygdalohippocampectomy in the remaining 4 patients, and all of these patients had seizure-free outcomes. Therefore, Minkin et al stressed the significance of amygdalohippocampectomy in the treatment of temporal DNETs and recommended extensive presurgical evaluation in this patient group. However, all these studies are retrospective assessments, most include a relatively small number of patients, and none is specifically designed to compare the effect of different surgical approaches on outcome.

Cavernous Hemangioma

Postoperative seizure control rates are greater than 70% in most of the surgical cavernous hemangioma series.[23] Baumann et al[24,62] reported Engel Class I outcome in 70% of cavernous hemangioma patients in a series that included both adults and children. In contrast to other studies, Baumann et al[24,62] did not find that longer seizure duration is a predictor for poorer outcome in cavernous hemangioma patients. They reported favorable outcome predictors as mesiotemporal location, removing hemosiderin-stained brain tissue along the cavernous hemangioma, older than 30 years of age, no additional seizure foci, and no secondarily generalized seizures. In another study, Fortuna et al reviewed 56 pediatric cavernous hemangioma patients and reported seizure-free outcome in 73.2% of them and significant improvement in an additional 19.6% of the patients.[65] Two other studies, reported respectively 82.9% and 84% seizure-free outcome postoperatively in cavernous hemangioma patients.[21,22]

Arteriovenous Malformation

As mentioned previously, the goal in the surgical management of AVMs is the complete removal of the AVM nidus. Whether this is sufficient to have good postoperative seizure control is not clear. Again the benefit of resecting the surrounding brain parenchyma and gliotic tissue or ipsilateral mesial temporal structures is not clear from a seizure-control standpoint. Data to answer these questions are simply very limited. In one of the studies addressing this question, Yeh et al[52,53] documented remote seizure foci in mesial temporal region using depth electrodes in temporal AVM patients. They then resected mesial structures in addition to AVM nidus in 67% of the patients to control seizures. They reported excellent seizure control in 78% of the patients. Another large series was published by Hoh et al.[63] They reported 141 patients with brain AVMs who had multimodality treatment. In this series, 33% of the patients had seizures before the treatment. They found that large size (> 3cm) of the AVM and temporal location was associated with seizures more frequently. The seizure-free (Engel Class I) outcome rate was 66% and Class II outcome was 10% after surgical treatment. Yasargil[18] reported a postoperative seizure-free outcome without any medication in all patients (*n* = 12) with hippocampal AVMs. This rate was 18% in extramesial temporal AVM patients,

with an additional 56% with good seizure control with medications. Gerszten et al[64] reported 72 children with AVM who were treated with Gamma knife radiosurgery. Twenty-one percent had seizures, and 85% became seizure-free after the Gamma knife treatment.

■ Conclusion

Low-grade tumors are one of the most common pathological substrates in TLE during childhood. No consensus in the surgical management of lesion-related TLE has been established to date. Although there is consensus that complete lesion resection is essential, the importance of additional resection of adjacent cortex or the mesial temporal structures remains controversial. There are strong implications in the published series on dual pathology lesions that lesionectomy alone without removal of the sclerotic hippocampus may not yield good seizure-control rates. Further investigation is needed in these patients to determine whether the resection of both the lesion and sclerotic hippocampus is indicated for better outcomes. Data are very limited regarding AVM-related TLE and the most effective surgical approach in its management. Lesionectomy is the most commonly used technique in the surgical management of intractable TLE in cavernous hemangioma patients, and a significant number of studies suggest that removal of surrounding hemosiderin fringe in addition to lesionectomy would further increase seizure control rates in these patients.

References

1. Sinclair DB, Wheatley M, Aronyk K, et al. Pathology and neuroimaging in pediatric temporal lobectomy for intractable epilepsy. Pediatr Neurosurg 2001;35(5):239–246
2. Clusmann H, Kral T, Fackeldey E, et al. Lesional mesial temporal lobe epilepsy and limited resections: prognostic factors and outcome. J Neurol Neurosurg Psychiatry 2004;75(11):1589–1596
3. Mittal S, Montes JL, Farmer JP, et al. Long-term outcome after surgical treatment of temporal lobe epilepsy in children. J Neurosurg 2005; 103(5, suppl)401–412
4. Benifla M, Otsubo H, Ochi A, et al. Temporal lobe surgery for intractable epilepsy in children: an analysis of outcomes in 126 children. Neurosurgery 2006;59(6):1203–1213, discussion 1213–1214
5. Kan P, Van Orman C, Kestle JRW. Outcomes after surgery for focal epilepsy in children. Childs Nerv Syst 2008;24(5):587–591
6. Kim SK, Wang KC, Hwang YS, et al. Epilepsy surgery in children: outcomes and complications. J Neurosurg Pediatr 2008;1(4):277–283
7. Maton B, Jayakar P, Resnick T, Morrison G, Ragheb J, Duchowny M. Surgery for medically intractable temporal lobe epilepsy during early life. Epilepsia 2008;49(1):80–87
8. Hennessy MJ, Elwes RDC, Honavar M, Rabe-Hesketh S, Binnie CD, Polkey CE. Predictors of outcome and pathological considerations in

the surgical treatment of intractable epilepsy associated with temporal lobe lesions. J Neurol Neurosurg Psychiatry 2001;70(4):450–458
9. Bronen RA, Fulbright RK, Spencer DD, Spencer SS, Kim JH, Lange RC. MR characteristics of neoplasms and vascular malformations associated with epilepsy. Magn Reson Imaging 1995;13(8):1153–1162
10. Çataltepe O, Turanli G, Yalnizoglu D, Topçu M, Akalan N. Surgical management of temporal lobe tumor-related epilepsy in children. J Neurosurg 2005; 102(3, suppl)280–287
11. Fish DR. How do tumors cause epilepsy? In: Kotagal P, Luders HO, eds. The Epilepsies: Etiologies and Prevention. San Diego, CA: Academic Press; 1999:301–314
12. Fried I, Kim JH, Spencer DD. Limbic and neocortical gliomas associated with intractable seizures: a distinct clinicopathological group. Neurosurgery 1994;34(5):815–823, discussion 823–824
13. Zaatreh MM, Firlik KS, Spencer DD, Spencer SS. Temporal lobe tumoral epilepsy: characteristics and predictors of surgical outcome. Neurology 2003;61(5):636–641
14. Horgan MA, Florman J, Spetzler RF. Surgical management of AVM in children. In: Alexander MJ, Spetzler RF, eds. Pediatric Neurovascular Disease. New York, NY: Thieme;2006:104–115

15. Menovsky T, van Overbeeke JJ. Cerebral arteriovenous malformations in childhood: state of the art with special reference to treatment. Eur J Pediatr 1997;156(10):741–746
16. Turjman F, Massoud TF, Sayre JW, Viñuela F, Guglielmi G, Duckwiler G. Epilepsy associated with cerebral arteriovenous malformations: a multivariate analysis of angioarchitectural characteristics. AJNR Am J Neuroradiol 1995;16(2):345–350
17. Schäuble B, Cascino GD, Pollock BE, et al. Seizure outcomes after stereotactic radiosurgery for cerebral arteriovenous malformations. Neurology 2004;63(4).683–687
18. Yasargil MG. Microneurosurgery. New York, NY: Thieme Medical Publishers; 1988:13–23, 11–136, 393–396
19. Cosgrove GR. Occult vascular malformations and seizures. Neurosurg Clin N Am 1999;10(3):527–535
20. Mottolese C, Hermier M, Stan H, et al. Central nervous system cavernomas in the pediatric age group. Neurosurg Rev 2001;24(2-3):55–71, discussion 72–73
21. Moran NF, Fish DR, Kitchen N, Shorvon S, Kendall BE, Stevens JM. Supratentorial cavernous haemangiomas and epilepsy: a review of the literature and case series. J Neurol Neurosurg Psychiatry 1999;66(5):561–568
22. Cappabianca P, Alfieri A, Maiuri F, Mariniello G, Cirillo S, de Divitiis E. Supratentorial cavernous malformations and epilepsy: seizure outcome after lesionectomy on a series of 35 patients. Clin Neurol Neurosurg 1997;99(3):179–183
23. Yeh D, Crone KR. Cavernous malformations in children. In: Alexander MJ, Spetzler RF, eds. Pediatric Neurovascular Disease. New York, NY: Thieme;2006:65–71
24. Baumann CR, Acciarri N, Bertalanffy H, et al. Seizure outcome after resection of supratentorial cavernous malformations: a study of 168 patients. Epilepsia 2007;48(3):559–563
25. Hammen T, Romstöck J, Dörfler A, Kerling F, Buchfelder M, Stefan H. Prediction of postoperative outcome with special respect to removal of hemosiderin fringe: a study in patients with cavernous haemangiomas associated with symptomatic epilepsy. Seizure 2007;16(3):248–253
26. Requena I, Arias M, López-Ibor L, et al. Cavernomas of the central nervous system: clinical and neuroimaging manifestations in 47 patients. J Neurol Neurosurg Psychiatry 1991;54(7):590–594
27. Stefan H, Hammen T. Cavernous haemangiomas, epilepsy and treatment strategies. Acta Neurol Scand 2004;110(6):393–397
28. Kraemer DL, Awad IA. Vascular malformations and epilepsy: clinical considerations and basic mechanisms. Epilepsia 1994;35(suppl 6): S30–S43
29. Giulioni M, Acciarri N, Padovani R, Galassi E. Results of surgery in children with cerebral cavernous angiomas causing epilepsy. Br J Neurosurg 1995;9(2):135–141
30. Di Rocco C, Iannelli A, Tamburrini G. Cavernomas of the CNS in children. A report of 22 cases. Acta Neurochir (Wien) 2006;138:1267–1274
31. Bartolomei JC, Christopher S, Vives K, Spencer DD, Piepmeier JM. Low-grade gliomas of chronic epilepsy: a distinct clinical and pathological entity. J Neurooncol 1997;34(1):79–84
32. Çataltepe O, Comair YG. Strategies in operating on patients with tumor-related epilepsy. In: Kotagal P, Luders HO, eds. The Epilepsies: Etiologies and Prevention. San Diego, CA: Academic Press;1999:365–370
33. Usui N, Mihara T, Baba K, et al. Intracranial EEG findings in patients with lesional lateral temporal lobe epilepsy. Epilepsy Res 2008;78(1):82–91
34. Awad IA, Rosenfeld J, Ahl J, Hahn JF, Lüders H. Intractable epilepsy and structural lesions of the brain: mapping, resection strategies, and seizure outcome. Epilepsia 1991;32(2):179–186
35. Van Ness PC. Pros and cons of lesionectomy as treatment for partial epilepsy. In : Kotagal P, Luders HO, eds. The Epilepsies: Etiologies and Prevention. San Diego, CA: Academic Press;1999:391–397
36. Khajavi K, Comair YG, Wyllie E, Palmer J, Morris HH, Hahn JF. Surgical management of pediatric tumor-associated epilepsy. J Child Neurol 1999;14(1):15–25
37. Jooma R, Yeh HS, Privitera MD, Gartner M. Lesionectomy versus electrophysiologically guided resection for temporal lobe tumors manifesting with complex partial seizures. J Neurosurg 1995;83(2):231–236
38. Sugano H, Shimizu H, Sunaga S. Efficacy of intraoperative electrocorticography for assessing seizure outcomes in intractable epilepsy patients with temporal-lobe-mass lesions. Seizure 2007;16(2):120–127
39. Mathern GW, Babb TL, Pretorius JK, Melendez M, Lévesque MF. The pathophysiologic relationships between lesion pathology, intracranial ictal EEG onsets, and hippocampal neuron losses in temporal lobe epilepsy. Epilepsy Res 1995;21(2):133–147
40. Mihara T, Baba MK. Combined use of subdural and depth electrodes. In: Luders H, Comair Y, eds. Epilepsy Surgery. 2nd ed. Philadelphia, PA: Lippincott Williams & Wilkins; 2001
41. Lee SK, Lee SY, Kim KK, Hong KS, Lee DS, Chung CK. Surgical outcome and prognostic factors of cryptogenic neocortical epilepsy. Ann Neurol 2005;58(4):525–532
42. Morris HH, Estes ML, Gilmore R, Van Ness PC, Barnett GH, Turnbull J. Chronic intractable epilepsy as the only symptom of primary brain tumor. Epilepsia 1993;34(6):1038–1043
43. Cohen DS, Zubay GP, Goodman RR. Seizure outcome after lesionectomy for cavernous malformations. J Neurosurg 1995;83(2):237–242
44. Kraemer DL, Griebel ML, Lee N, Friedman AH, Radtke RA. Surgical outcome in patients with epilepsy with occult vascular malformations treated with lesionectomy. Epilepsia 1998;39(6):600–607
45. Morioka T, Hashiguchi K, Nagata S, et al. Additional hippocampectomy in the surgical management of intractable temporal lobe epilepsy associated with glioneuronal tumor. Neurol Res 2007;29(8):807–815
46. Drake J, Hoffman HJ, Kobayashi J, Hwang P, Becker LE. Surgical management of children with temporal lobe epilepsy and mass lesions. Neurosurgery 1987;21(6):792–797
47. Otsubo H, Hoffman HJ, Humphreys RP, et al. Detection and management of gangliogliomas in children. Surg Neurol 1992;38(5):371–378
48. Li LM, Cendes F, Andermann F, et al. Surgical outcome in patients with epilepsy and dual pathology. Brain 1999;122(Pt 5):799–805
49. Morris HH, Matkovic Z, Estes ML, et al. Ganglioglioma and intractable epilepsy: clinical and neurophysiologic features and predictors of outcome after surgery. Epilepsia 1998;39(3):307–313
50. Cascino GD, Jack CR Jr, Parisi JE, et al. Operative strategy in patients with MRI-identified dual pathology and temporal lobe epilepsy. Epilepsy Res 1993;14(2):175–182
51. Trussart V, Berry I, Manelfe C, Arrue P, Castan P. Epileptogenic cerebral vascular malformations and MRI. J Neuroradiol 1989;16(4):273–284
52. Yeh HS, Kashiwagi S, Tew JM Jr, Berger TS. Surgical management of epilepsy associated with cerebral arteriovenous malformations. J Neurosurg 1990;72(2):216–223

53. Yeh HS, Tew JM Jr, Gartner M. Seizure control after surgery on cerebral arteriovenous malformations. J Neurosurg 1993;78(1):12–18

54. Benifla M, Otsubo H, Ochi A, et al. Temporal lobe surgery for intractable epilepsy in children: an analysis of outcomes in 126 children. Neurosurgery 2006;59(6):1203–1213, discussion 1213–1214

55. Choi JY, Chang JW, Park YG, Kim TS, Lee BI, Chung SS. A retrospective study of the clinical outcomes and significant variables in the surgical treatment of temporal lobe tumor associated with intractable seizures. Stereotact Funct Neurosurg 2004;82(1):35–42

56. Kim SK, Wang KC, Hwang YS, Kim KJ, Cho BK. Intractable epilepsy associated with brain tumors in children: surgical modality and outcome. Childs Nerv Syst 2001;17(8):445–452

57. Luyken C, Blümcke I, Fimmers R, et al. The spectrum of long-term epilepsy-associated tumors: long-term seizure and tumor outcome and neurosurgical aspects. Epilepsia 2003;44(6):822–830

58. Giulioni M, Gardella E, Rubboli G, et al. Lesionectomy in epileptogenic gangliogliomas: seizure outcome and surgical results. J Clin Neurosci 2006;13(5):529–535

59. Giulioni M, Galassi E, Zucchelli M, Volpi L. Seizure outcome of lesionectomy in ganglioneuronal tumors associated with epilepsy in children. J Neurosurg Pediatr 2005;102:288–293

60. Chan CH, Bittar RG, Davis GA, Kalnins RM, Fabinyi GCA. Long-term seizure outcome following surgery for dysembryoplastic neuroepithelial tumor. J Neurosurg 2006;104(1):62–69

61. Minkin K, Klein O, Mancini J, Lena G. Surgical strategies and seizure control in pediatric patients with dysembryoplastic neuroepithelial tumors: a single-institution experience. J Neurosurg Pediatr 2008;1:206–210

62. Baumann CR, Schuknecht B, Lo Russo G, et al. Seizure outcome after resection of cavernous malformations is better when surrounding hemosiderin-stained brain also is removed. Epilepsia 2006;47(3):563–566

63. Hoh BL, Chapman PH, Loeffler JS, Carter BS, Ogilvy CS. Results of multimodality treatment for 141 patients with brain arteriovenous malformations and seizures: factors associated with seizure incidence and seizure outcomes. Neurosurgery 2002;51(2):303–309, discussion 309–311

64. Gerszten PC, Adelson PD, Kondziolka D, Flickinger JC, Lunsford LD. Seizure outcome in children treated for arteriovenous malformations using gamma knife radiosurgery. Pediatr Neurosurg 1996;24(3):139–144

65. Fortuna A, Ferrante L, Mastronardi L, Acqui M, d'Addetta R. Cerebral cavernous angioma in children. Child's Nerv Syst 1989;5:201–207

21 Extratemporal Resection

Erich G. Anderer, Robert J. Bollo, and Howard L. Weiner

The safety and efficacy of surgery for temporal lobe epilepsy has been well established and represents the paradigm for resective epilepsy surgery.[1–5] By contrast, surgery for epilepsy of extratemporal origin poses several unique challenges, which require the team of treating physicians to engage in a rigorous preoperative workup often culminating in a technically demanding operative procedure, with traditionally less successful outcomes regarding seizure freedom. Surgery for medically refractory partial extratemporal epilepsy involves cortical resection of the areas of ictal onset and seizure propagation anywhere outside of the temporal lobe. It is the more common type of epilepsy surgery performed in children. Although anteromesial temporal lobectomy for temporal lobe epilepsy is known to carry a reasonably low morbidity, the resections necessary for extratemporal seizure foci typically involve larger areas of cortex, which often may either encompass or abut functionally significant regions of the brain.

Although much of the literature pertaining to extratemporal epilepsy surgery describes treatment of frontal lobe epilepsy, all cortical areas outside of the temporal lobe have the potential to be involved. The ultimate surgical plan, which should ideally be devised by a multidisciplinary team in the setting of a comprehensive epilepsy center, is based on a multitude of factors and includes a consideration of pathological substrate, neuroimaging data, electroencephalography (EEG)/neurophysiological information, functional mapping data, and the specific risk–benefit profile of the individual patient. Published rates of seizure freedom after surgery for extratemporal epilepsy vary between 30 and 80%, compared with more than 80% for temporal lobe epilepsy.[6–13] However, the treatment goals are the same: the reduction or elimination of seizures with minimal morbidity, as well as the preservation or improvement neurocognitive function. Several published studies have demonstrated both the safety and efficacy of epilepsy surgery in children.[6–9]

■ Unique Considerations in Pediatric Extratemporal Epilepsy Surgery

There is a growing body of literature on extratemporal epilepsy surgery in children. This patient population warrants special consideration for several reasons. First, the pathological substrate differs in the adult and pediatric populations. The most common cause of intractable partial epilepsy in adults is hippocampal sclerosis, classically treated surgically by anterior temporal lobectomy with amygdalohippocampectomy. In children, however, the predominance of epilepsy of extratemporal origin is related to developmental brain abnormalities (e.g., cortical dysplasia, tuberous sclerosis complex, Sturge-Weber syndrome) and low-grade cortical tumors (e.g., gangliogliomas, desmoplastic infantile gangliogliomas, oligodendrogliomas, astrocytomas).[14,15] Cortical dysplasia is especially prominent in the pathological specimens of children who undergo resections for extratemporal epilepsy.[15] By contrast, adults who undergo extratemporal resections are typically found to harbor a different pathological profile than children, often including such variable entities as gliosis and focal cell loss. Although good outcomes have been reported for adults after extratemporal epilepsy surgery, they appear not to fare as well after surgical intervention as children do.[16–22]

Second, the treating physician must take into account the developmental implications of intervention on an affected child with a still-developing nervous system. Although the developing brain is very sensitive to the detrimental effects of recurrent seizures, with potentially permanent neuropsychological and cognitive sequelae, the plasticity of the developing brain also lends itself to better functional recovery after cortical resections that may involve eloquent cortex.[23–25] Nevertheless, it is now increasingly appreciated that uncontrolled epilepsy in childhood can have a detrimental effect on a child's intelligence and cognitive abilities and, moreover, that epilepsy surgery performed in childhood may play a critical role in enhancing development and overall quality of life.[26] Finally, because medically refractory partial seizures are unlikely to remit when an adequate response is not achieved with the first two major antiepileptic medications administered, early surgery is now often advocated for both adult and pediatric populations at many centers.[1,14,16,25,27]

■ Evaluation

Because of the pathological complexity of extratemporal epilepsy, patients who are being considered for surgery are best evaluated in a comprehensive epilepsy center by a multidisciplinary team of epilepsy neurologists, epilepsy surgeons, neuropsychologists, psychiatrists, and social workers. Typically, the preoperative evaluation consists of a comprehensive battery of tests all designed to localize the epileptogenic zone. A thorough understanding of the potential strengths and limitations of each of these techniques is critical for appropriate patient selection and satisfactory surgical outcomes.

Noninvasive Modalities

Routine structural imaging with magnetic resonance imaging (MRI) together with scalp video-EEG (VEEG) comprise the most basic requirements of any preoperative epilepsy evaluation. However, other noninvasive techniques are now commonly used to localize the ictal onset zone and map functionally eloquent cortex. These include magnetoencephalography (MEG), single photon emission computed tomography (SPECT), and positron emission tomography (PET).

Although invasive video-EEG (iVEEG) with subdural electrodes is felt to be superior in localizing extratemporal ictal onset zones in children undergoing resective surgery for refractory epilepsy, other studies have shown the promise of MEG as a technique for localizing the epileptogenic zone.[28-33] This may partially be explained by a differential sensitivity to radial compared with tangential pacemakers, making these techniques complementary.[32-34] The resection of remote ictal zones identified by MEG and electrocorticography (ECoG) does not contribute to epilepsy outcome in patients with tumors. However, in patients with cortical dysplasia, the resection of remote ictal regions may be critical to seizure outcome.[29]

SPECT has become a common tool in the evaluation of refractory epilepsy in children.[35] Subtraction ictal SPECT scanning coregistered to MRI imaging (SISCOM) improves the sensitivity of ictal SPECT for localization of the ictal onset zone and has demonstrated clinical utility in guiding placement of intracranial electrodes.[36-38] Ictal SPECT and SISCOM may be especially useful in providing preoperative guidance for intracranial electrode placement in children with frontal lobe epilepsy, because rapid seizure spread often renders false-localizing clinical and electrophysiological data.[39,40]

PET uses radiolabeled tracers to image cerebral perfusion, glucose and protein metabolism, and γ-aminobutyric acid (GABA) and serotonin receptor density.[41] Interictal 2-deoxy-2[^{18}F]fluoro-D-glucose (FDG)-PET has a reported sensitivity of 60–80% for identification of foci of hypometabolism among patients with chronic, refractory extratemporal epilepsy and a normal MRI; this sensitivity is similar to that reported for similar patients with ictal SPECT.[42,43] However, the clinical utility of FDG-PET in presurgical seizure focus localization is limited by low specificity relative to iVEEG. Studies in children with tuberous sclerosis complex suffering from chronic, refractory epilepsy have shown that FDG-PET may complement MRI with diffusion-weighted imaging in

differentiating epileptogenic from clinically silent tubers.[44] In addition, α-[^{11}C]-methyl-L-tryptophan (AMT), which images tryptophan metabolism, has shown promising results in preliminary clinical studies aimed at distinguishing between epileptogenic and electrically silent lesions in children with multifocal pathology.[45]

Functional Mapping

Precisely identifying eloquent cortex essential for sensorimotor, language, and memory function, as well as defining the anatomical relationship between ictal foci and functional centers, is critical for surgical risk assessment and decision making in extratemporal epilepsy. Several noninvasive imaging techniques, including functional MRI, MEG, and FDG-PET, provide accurate maps of primary sensorimotor cortex in children. Functional mapping may also be performed intraoperatively via direct cortical stimulation or extraoperatively via implanted subdural electrodes. Wada testing (intracarotid amobarbital test) is useful for establishing the laterality of language and memory function in cooperative children. In addition, a thorough neuropsychological evaluation is essential not only for providing a preoperative baseline but also for potentially providing corroborative data to a suspected ictal focus. Comparison of preoperative and postoperative neuropsychiatric tests may help determine whether ictal behavior has been altered.[46,47]

■ Surgery

The major factors that potentially complicate the surgical intervention in extratemporal epilepsy include the multifocality of seizure foci, the higher incidence of nonlesional MRI-negative epilepsy, and the frequent proximity of the epileptogenic zone to eloquent cortex. As a result, surgical strategies should consider a wide array of therapeutic options, which must be tailored to the individual patient's risk–benefit profile.

When the preoperative comprehensive evaluation does not reveal an apparent localized seizure focus that can be approached surgically, the treating team of specialists is left with a dilemma regarding how to proceed. The options include either no surgery or the use of a palliative procedure, such as vagal nerve stimulation or corpus callosotomy, in the appropriate clinical setting. At our institution, we have offered selected patients, in whom we highly suspect partial seizures, but in whom we have nonetheless found nonlocalizing data, bilateral strip electrode survey studies to lateralize and localize their seizures. This is accomplished in a two-stage fashion, in which either a vertex craniotomy of bilateral craniotomies are performed to insert subdural strip electrodes in a survey fashion over the cortical surface (**Fig. 21.1**). This technique has been useful in both lesional

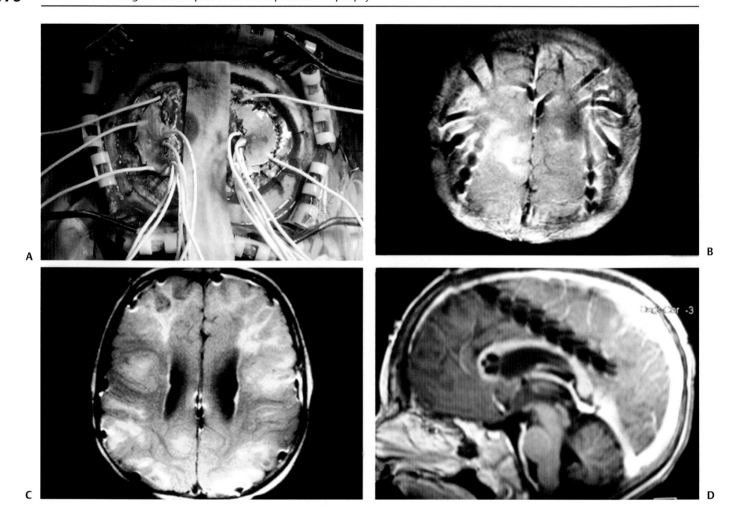

Fig. 21.1 Bilateral strip electrode survey via vertex craniotomy. **(A)** A midline craniotomy is performed, and the dura is opened on either side of the superior sagittal sinus. Strip electrodes containing between four and eight electrodes are carefully passed over both the mesial and lateral surfaces of both hemispheres. Postoperative T1-weighted axial **(B, C)** and postcontrast T1-weighted midsagittal **(D)** magnetic resonance imaging demonstrating strip electrodes.

and nonlesional cases, in our experience, and has led several patients to successful resections once the ictal onset zone can be localized. For example, in our extratemporal tuberous sclerosis complex patients, we have performed this technique successfully in patients not considered to be classic epilepsy surgery patients based on their nonlocalizing preoperative evaluations. If the bilateral strip study reveals a unilateral focus, this is then approached at a later date, with a classic two-stage procedure consisting of initial grid placement, followed by resection of the ictal focus.

Traditionally, the goal of surgical management of patients suffering from medically refractory partial epilepsy has been cortical resection of the defined epileptogenic zone. This may be accomplished in one of several ways, from a surgical standpoint: single-, two-, or multistage approach. Patients harboring a radiographic lesion, which is identified as the clear source of seizures by the comprehensive preoperative evaluation, can be treated with a single-stage lesionectomy.

If concerns exist that the epileptogenic zone extends beyond the boundaries of the radiographic lesion, then one can identify the extent of ictal zone by either using intraoperative ECoG or by placing a subdural grid over the lesion to define this extraoperatively. Intraoperatively, ECoG may assist in the identification of the epileptogenic zone. Limitations of this technique include analysis of interictal data only and significantly diminished interictal spike frequency under general anesthesia. Technically, this procedure is similar in adults and children: electrodes are placed over the putative epileptogenic zone and interictal electrical spike activity is characterized. It is generally reliable if an interictal spike frequency reaches at least one spike per minute. This technique is widely applied in children with brain tumors and refractory epilepsy, where the ictal onset zone is frequently localized to cortex adjacent to the tumor and the resection of perilesional cortex with abnormal interictal spike activity correlates with long-term seizure freedom.[48,49]

Although there are clearly limitations to performing intraoperative ECoG in awake pediatric patients, chronic implanted subdural electrodes not only appear to be well tolerated in this population but may also yield more useful data with the longer sampling times.[25,50] With the two-stage approach, the epilepsy team is able to develop a map of the ictal zone and the associated epileptogenic network that would need to be addressed surgically (**Fig. 21.2**). Extraoperative ictal focus mapping via stimulation across subdural electrodes (arrays of 2.5-mm platinum electrodes either 5 mm or 10 mm apart, mounted on Silastic strips, implanted

under general anesthesia) is a well-established technique.[51,52] Reports in children with extratemporal epilepsy indicate a sensitivity of approximately 90%.[53] A significant advantage is the ability to capture ictal and interictal events over several days of monitoring. Conversely, a disadvantage is the need for an additional operation for electrode implantation.[51] Most centers report an overall complication rate of 10 to 15% among patients with chronic intracranial electrodes.[54–59]

The reported complications include cerebrospinal fluid (CSF) leak or positive CSF cultures, usually in the absence of clinically evident meningitis.[50,55,56,58] Other reported

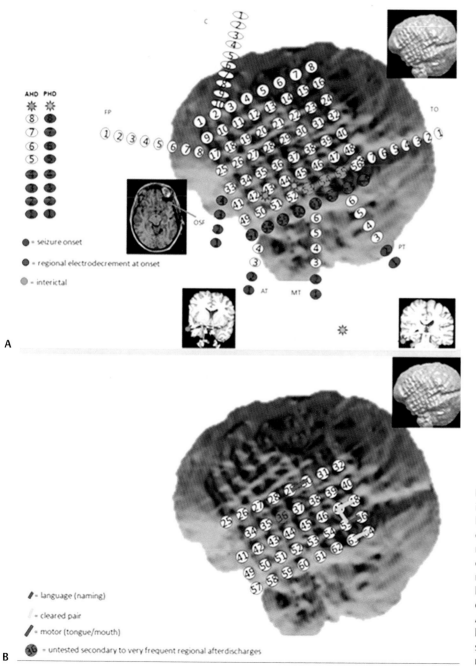

A

B

Fig. 21.2 Ictal and functional mapping via intracranial electrodes. **(A)** Ictal focus map based on accumulated ictal and interictal data demonstrates regions of seizure onset, regional electrodecrements, and interictal discharges in multilobar epilepsy. **(B)** Corresponding functional map demonstrating language function at the posterior border of electrophysiologically abnormal cortex. All electrodes shown were tested against at least one adjacent electrode. Functional results and clinically relevant electrodes with no evident function are shown.

complications include transient neurological deficit, epidural or subdural hematoma, and stroke. A reduction in complication rate with increasing surgical experience and lower complication rates in children have been reported.[54,57] Class 2 data indicate that dexamethasone may reduce cerebral swelling in children with implanted subdural grid electrode arrays. However, it also decreases the seizure frequency, which may lead to longer extraoperative monitoring periods to capture sufficient data to localize the ictal focus.[60] Studies of the pathological changes seen in cortex underlying subdural arrays have revealed focal, transient aseptic meningitis in all patients. However, the severity of this reaction does not correlate with the incidence of infection or long-term surgical outcome.[61]

In addition to the seizure information, functional data can be obtained using the same grid with extraoperative functional mapping. In many of these patients, the extent of resection of the seizure focus may be limited by its extent of involvement of eloquent cortex. Because awake cortical mapping may not be possible in younger pediatric patients, other modalities such as extraoperative grid mapping, MEG, or functional MRI may be necessary to define eloquent cortex. Once these regions have been satisfactorily mapped, the surgeon can discuss the various treatment options with the patient's family in light of the specific risk–benefit considerations: resection, multiple subpial transections, or no resection. The refinement of neuronavigational techniques over the last several years has also aided the epilepsy surgeon. Both frameless and frame-based systems have been used in placing monitoring electrodes, particularly depth electrodes, and to aid in resection. Three-dimensional MRI reconstructions, functional imaging data, and MR angiography have all been used effectively to help delineating the extent of resection.[62]

For a select group of patients with the most complex manifestations of extratemporal epilepsy, we have advocated the use of a multistage surgical approach.[50] This typically consists of electrode implantation, an extraoperative monitoring period, resection and electrode reimplantation, a second monitoring period, and a third operation for electrode removal and further resection if necessary (**Fig. 21.3**). The additional monitoring period often reveals secondary ictal foci that only become apparent after removal of the primary seizure focus. Criticisms of this philosophy include the additional risk of further invasive monitoring and an additional surgery. In our experience, a second intraoperative monitoring period followed by a third surgical stage is simpler than a return to the operating room several months later. In this select group of pediatric patients with poor surgical prognostic factors (i.e., multifocal ictal onset, ictal overlap with eloquent cortex, or previous surgical failure), we believe that this additional stage has the potential to improve surgical outcomes. We have postulated that it is difficult to assess adequately the potential of secondary seizure foci to become independent

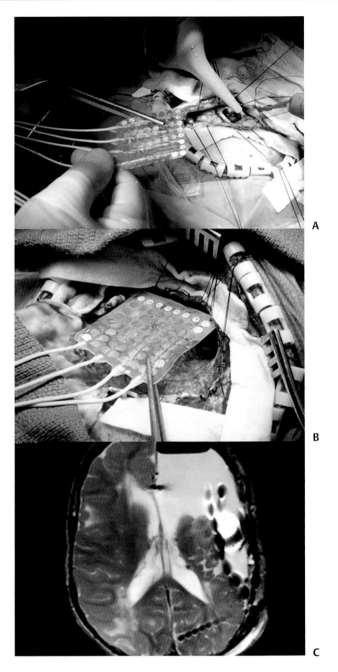

Fig. 21.3 Multistage approach. Replacement of 64-contact subdural grid array (5-mm electrode spacing) after extratemporal ictal focus resection. **(A)** The grid is contoured and **(B)** laid over the resection cavity. **(C)** Postoperative T2-weighted axial magnetic resonance imaging demonstrating grid overlying resection cavity and also depth electrode after the second stage of a three-stage procedure.

ictal generators once the primary focus has been resected. Multifocal epilepsy involving purely extratemporal or temporal and extratemporal regions of seizure onset is common in the pediatric population. In addition, acute seizures after ictal focus resection reflect a poor prognosis.[63-65] This supports the strategy of multistage procedures, in which

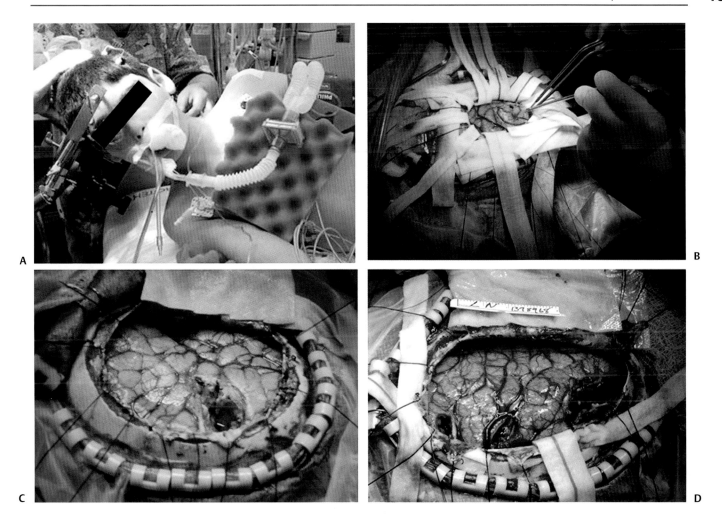

A

B

C

D

Fig. 21.6 Craniotomy for extratemporal seizure focus resection. **(A)** The lateral decubitus position allows the neck to remain in line with the body, preventing jugular venous compression. **(B)** Bipolar coagulation of the cortical surface over the area to be resected. **(C)** Right parietal ictal focus resection. After pial coagulation, ultrasonic aspiration is used to empty all gray matter from gyri containing the mapped ictal focus as permitted by functional anatomy. **(D)** Multifocal resection.

ture. A Jackson Pratt drain is always left in the subgaleal space. In fact, during the last several years, we have had the practice of keeping the Jackson–Pratt (Cardinal Health, IL) drain in place for the entire period of monitoring, which has essentially eliminated all instances of CSF leakage from the wire exit sites. In our practice, intravenous antibiotics are given at induction of anesthesia and for the duration of monitoring. We have also used frameless stereotactic image guidance for insertion of depth electrodes. In our experience, the depth electrodes have been particularly useful for monitoring deep lesions, such as tubers, and more remote cortex, such as the mesial frontal and parietal areas. Culture swabs of the epi- and subdural spaces are taken at the second and third operative stages. MRI scans are performed postoperatively to document electrode position. Whereas some surgeons choose to freeze the bone flap during the period of invasive monitoring, it has been our practice to leave the bone flap in

situ. We use irrigation very liberally at each stage of surgery, and surgical gloves are changed at least twice during an epilepsy operation.

Resection Technique

The surgical resection techniques used in epilepsy surgery are unique and critical for its success. Epileptogenic cortex typically involves specific gyri of the brain, and its safe removal therefore requires absolute preservation of arteries and veins in the subarachnoid space, as well as the underlying subcortical white matter. To accomplish the safe resection of this cortical tissue, we have found the Cavitron Ultrasonic Surgical Aspirator (CUSA) (Integra Neuro Sciences, Plainsboro, NJ) to be an indispensable tool. The initial cortical incision is performed using bipolar cautery and straight microscissors. On a low setting, the CUSA can then be used to resect safely the gray matter tissue filling any gyrus in a subpial fashion, with total preservation of the underlying pia and blood vessels. Bleeding from the raw edge of exposed pia after resection is easily managed by placing small square strips of surgical gauze.

When performing extratemporal resections, it is critical to ensure that the resection is completed all the way to the pial surface and that the gyrus in question has been emptied of all gray matter. This is especially true when the surgery calls for resecting the mesial frontal, parietal, or occipital cortex, in which case the surgeon must be sure to visualize the mesial pia to be confident that the resection is complete (**Fig. 21.6B–D**).

■ Results

Although seizure freedom rates as high as 80% have been reported in some published pediatric extratemporal epilepsy surgery series, these usually include a large proportion of lesional cases, which are biased toward a more favorable outcome.[10] In general, the success rate for pediatric extratemporal epilepsy surgery has been consistently inferior to that for temporal lobe epilepsy. Two long-term follow-up studies in pediatric populations reported Engel Class I outcomes of 78% and 74% versus 54% and 60% for temporal and extratemporal resections, respectively.[11,14] Similarly, pediatric patients with nonlesional epilepsy who undergo surgery do not achieve surgical outcomes comparable to those with lesions noted on MRI.[3,12] However, most reports describe a retrospective analysis of a small group of patients treated at a single institution. Meta-analyses indicate that a more extensive surgical resection, structural pathology on MRI, and concordant imaging and electrophysiologic data predict long-term seizure freedom. Acute postoperative seizures consistently predict a poor long-term outcome.[65-68]

In our subset of patients who underwent multistaged surgery, we observed an Engel Class I outcome in 60% of children, with 87% of the group demonstrating worthwhile improvement (Engel Class III or higher).[50] In addition, retrospective data suggest similar improvements in quality of life among patients undergoing temporal and extratemporal resections.[69] Other data in children have suggested similar long-term outcome compared with adults, despite a much higher frequency of extratemporal seizures in this population.[70] Most authors recommend early surgical intervention in children with refractory seizures.[65,67,68,70]

■ Conclusion

Despite significant technological advances that have been made in functional neuroimaging, neuronavigation, and neuromonitoring, the epileptogenic zone in pediatric extratemporal epilepsy often remains elusive. With enhanced surgical innovation however, we remain optimistic that more effective treatment algorithms are forthcoming that will render patients seizure free with the lowest possible surgical morbidity.

References

1. Wiebe S, Blume WT, Girvin JP, Eliasziw M; Effectiveness and Efficiency of Surgery for Temporal Lobe Epilepsy Study Group. A randomized, controlled trial of surgery for temporal-lobe epilepsy. N Engl J Med 2001;345(5):311–318

2. Yasuda CL, Tedeschi H, Oliveira EL, et al. Comparison of short-term outcome between surgical and clinical treatment in temporal lobe epilepsy: a prospective study. Seizure 2006;15(1):35–40

3. Engel J Jr, van Ness PC, Rasmussen TB, et al. Outcome with respect to epileptic seizures. In: Engel J Jr, ed. Surgical Treatment of the Epilepsies, 2nd ed. New York, NY: Raven Press; 1993:609–621

4. Kellett MW, Smith DF, Baker GA, Chadwick DW. Quality of life after epilepsy surgery. J Neurol Neurosurg Psychiatry 1997;63(1):52–58

5. Birbeck GL, Hays RD, Cui X, Vickrey BG. Seizure reduction and quality of life improvements in people with epilepsy. Epilepsia 2002;43(5):535–538

6. Wyllie E, Lüders H, Morris HH III, et al. Subdural electrodes in the evaluation for epilepsy surgery in children and adults. Neuropediatrics 1988;19(2):80–86

7. Morrison G, Duchowny M, Resnick T, et al. Epilepsy surgery in childhood. A report of 79 patients. Pediatr Neurosurg 1992;18(5-6):291–297

8. Rossi GF. Epilepsy in the pediatric age and its surgical treatment. Childs Nerv Syst 1995;11(1):23–28

9. Adelson PD, Black PM, Madsen JR, et al. Use of subdural grids and strip electrodes to identify a seizure focus in children. Pediatr Neurosurg 1995;22(4):174–180

10. Pomata HB, González R, Bartuluchi M, et al. Extratemporal epilepsy in children: candidate selection and surgical treatment. Childs Nerv Syst 2000;16(12):842–850

11. Van Oijen M, De Waal H, Van Rijen PC, Jennekens-Schinkel A, van Huffelen AC, Van Nieuwenhuizen O; Dutch Collaborative Epilepsy Surgery Program. Resective epilepsy surgery in childhood: the Dutch experience 1992-2002. Eur J Paediatr Neurol 2006;10(3):114–123

12. Sinclair DB, Aronyk K, Snyder T, et al. Extratemporal resection for childhood epilepsy. Pediatr Neurol 2004;30(3):177–185

13. Quesney LF. Extratemporal epilepsy: clinical presentation, preoperative EEG localization and surgical outcome. Acta Neurol Scand Suppl 1992;140:81–94

14. Wyllie E, Comair YG, Kotagal P, Bulacio J, Bingaman W, Ruggieri P. Seizure outcome after epilepsy surgery in children and adolescents. Ann Neurol 1998;44(5):740–748

15. Paolicchi JM, Jayakar P, Dean P, et al. Predictors of outcome in pediatric epilepsy surgery. Neurology 2000;54(3):642–647

16. Cascino GD. Surgical treatment for extratemporal epilepsy. Curr Treat Options Neurol 2004;6(3):257–262

17. Zentner J, Hufnagel A, Ostertun B, et al. Surgical treatment of extratemporal epilepsy: clinical, radiologic, and histopathologic findings in 60 patients. Epilepsia 1996;37(11):1072–1080

18. Cascino GD, Jack CR Jr, Parisi JE, et al. MRI in the presurgical evaluation of patients with frontal lobe epilepsy and children with temporal lobe epilepsy: pathologic correlation and prognostic importance. Epilepsy Res 1992;11(1):51–59

19. Kim DW, Lee SK, Yun CH, et al. Parietal lobe epilepsy: the semiology, yield of diagnostic workup, and surgical outcome. Epilepsia 2004;45(6):641–649

20. Lee JJ, Lee SK, Lee SY, et al. Frontal lobe epilepsy: clinical characteristics, surgical outcomes and diagnostic modalities. Seizure 2008;17(6):514–523

21. Olivier A. Surgery of frontal lobe epilepsy. Adv Neurol 1995;66:321–348, discussion 348–352

22. Jobst BC, Siegel AM, Thadani VM, Roberts DW, Rhodes HC, Williamson PD. Intractable seizures of frontal lobe origin: clinical characteristics, localizing signs, and results of surgery. Epilepsia 2000;41(9):1139–1152

23. Mizrahi EM, Kellaway P, Grossman RG, et al. Anterior temporal lobectomy and medically refractory temporal lobe epilepsy of childhood. Epilepsia 1990;31(3):302–312

24. Wyllie E, Comair YG, Kotagal P, Bulacio J, Bingaman W, Ruggieri P. Seizure outcome after epilepsy surgery in children and adolescents. Ann Neurol 1998;44(5):740–748

25. Centeno RS, Yacubian EM, Sakamoto AC, Ferraz AF, Junior HC, Cavalheiro S. Pre-surgical evaluation and surgical treatment in children with extratemporal epilepsy. Childs Nerv Syst 2006;22(8):945–959

26. Loddenkemper T, Holland KD, Stanford LD, Kotagal P, Bingaman W, Wyllie E. Developmental outcome after epilepsy surgery in infancy. Pediatrics 2007;119(5):930–935

27. Kwan P, Brodie MJ. Early identification of refractory epilepsy. N Engl J Med 2000;342(5):314–319

28. Oishi M, Kameyama S, Masuda H, et al. Single and multiple clusters of magnetoencephalographic dipoles in neocortical epilepsy: significance in characterizing the epileptogenic zone. Epilepsia 2006;47(2):355–364

29. Otsubo H, Ochi A, Elliott I, et al. MEG predicts epileptic zone in lesional extrahippocampal epilepsy: 12 pediatric surgery cases. Epilepsia 2001;42(12):1523–1530

30. Knowlton RC, Laxer KD, Aminoff MJ, Roberts TP, Wong ST, Rowley HA. Magnetoencephalography in partial epilepsy: clinical yield and localization accuracy. Ann Neurol 1997;42(4):622–631

31. Minassian BA, Otsubo H, Weiss S, Elliott I, Rutka JT, Snead OC III. Magnetoencephalographic localization in pediatric epilepsy surgery: comparison with invasive intracranial electroencephalography. Ann Neurol 1999;46(4):627–633

32. Wheless JW, Willmore LJ, Breier JI, et al. A comparison of magnetoencephalography, MRI, and V-EEG in patients evaluated for epilepsy surgery. Epilepsia 1999;40(7):931–941

33. Papanicolaou AC, Pataraia E, Billingsley-Marshall R, et al. Toward the substitution of invasive electroencephalography in epilepsy surgery. J Clin Neurophysiol 2005;22(4):231–237

34. Jansen FE, Huiskamp G, van Huffelen AC, et al. Identification of the epileptogenic tuber in patients with tuberous sclerosis: a comparison of high-resolution EEG and MEG. Epilepsia 2006;47(1):108–114

35. Pirotte B, Goldman S, Salzberg S, et al. Combined positron emission tomography and magnetic resonance imaging for the planning of stereotactic brain biopsies in children: experience in 9 cases. Pediatr Neurosurg 2003;38(3):146–155

36. Buchhalter JR, So EL. Advances in computer-assisted single-photon emission computed tomography (SPECT) for epilepsy surgery in children. Acta Paediatr Suppl 2004;93(445):32–35, discussion 36–37

37. Van Paesschen W. Ictal SPECT. Epilepsia 2004;45(suppl 4):35–40

38. Ahnlide JA, Rosén I, Lindén-Mickelsson Tech P, Källén K. Does SISCOM contribute to favorable seizure outcome after epilepsy surgery? Epilepsia 2007;48(3):579–588

39. Lee SK, Lee SY, Yun CH, Lee HY, Lee JS, Lee DS. Ictal SPECT in neocortical epilepsies: clinical usefulness and factors affecting the pattern of hyperperfusion. Neuroradiology 2006;48(9):678–684

40. Fukuda M, Masuda H, Honma J, Kameyama S, Tanaka R. Ictal SPECT analyzed by three-dimensional stereotactic surface projection in frontal lobe epilepsy patients. Epilepsy Res 2006;68(2):95–102

41. Duncan JD, Moss SD, Bandy DJ, et al. Use of positron emission tomography for presurgical localization of eloquent brain areas in children with seizures. Pediatr Neurosurg 1997;26(3):144–156

42. Juhász C, Chugani HT. Imaging the epileptic brain with positron emission tomography. Neuroimaging Clin N Am 2003;13(4):705–716, viii

43. Sood S, Chugani HT. Functional neuroimaging in the preoperative evaluation of children with drug-resistant epilepsy. Childs Nerv Syst 2006;22(8):810–820

44. Chandra PS, Salamon N, Huang J, et al. FDG-PET/MRI coregistration and diffusion-tensor imaging distinguish epileptogenic tubers and cortex in patients with tuberous sclerosis complex: a preliminary report. Epilepsia 2006;47(9):1543–1549

45. Chugani DC, Chugani HT, Muzik O, et al. Imaging epileptogenic tubers in children with tuberous sclerosis complex using alpha-[11C]methyl-L-tryptophan positron emission tomography. Ann Neurol 1998;44(6):858–866

46. Jones-Gotman M, Smith ML, Zatorre RJ. Neuropsychological testing for localizing and lateralizing the epileptogenic region. In: Engel J Jr., ed. Surgical Treatment of the Epilepsies. 2nd ed. New York, NY: Raven Press; 1993:245–261

47. Bernstein JH, Prather PA, Rey-Casserly C. Neuropsychological assessment in preoperative and postoperative evaluation. Neurosurg Clin N Am 1995;6(3):443–454

48. Pilcher WH, Silbergeld DL, Berger MS, Ojemann GA. Intraoperative electrocorticography during tumor resection: impact on seizure outcome in patients with gangliogliomas. J Neurosurg 1993;78(6):891–902

49. Ojemann SG, Berger MS, Lettich E, Ojemann GA. Localization of language function in children: results of electrical stimulation mapping. J Neurosurg 2003;98(3):465–470

50. Bauman JA, Feoli E, Romanelli P, Doyle WK, Devinsky O, Weiner HL. Multistage epilepsy surgery: safety, efficacy, and utility of a novel approach in pediatric extratemporal epilepsy. Neurosurgery 2005;56(2):318–334

51. Tharin S, Golby A. Functional brain mapping and its applications to neurosurgery. Neurosurgery 2007;60(4, suppl 2):185–201, discussion 201–202

52. Duffau H. Lessons from brain mapping in surgery for low-grade glioma: insights into associations between tumour and brain plasticity. Lancet Neurol 2005;4(8):476–486

53. Bruce DA, Bizzi JWJ. Surgical technique for the insertion of grids and strips for invasive monitoring in children with intractable epilepsy. Childs Nerv Syst 2000;16(10-11):724–730

54. Hamer HM, Morris HH, Mascha EJ, et al. Complications of invasive video-EEG monitoring with subdural grid electrodes. Neurology 2002; 58(1):97–103

55. Johnston JM Jr, Mangano FT, Ojemann JG, Park TS, Trevathan E, Smyth MD. Complications of invasive subdural electrode monitoring at St. Louis Children's Hospital, 1994-2005. J Neurosurg 2006; 105(5, suppl):343–347

56. Onal C, Otsubo H, Araki T, et al. Complications of invasive subdural grid monitoring in children with epilepsy. J Neurosurg 2003; 98(5):1017–1026

57. Rydenhag B, Silander HC. Complications of epilepsy surgery after 654 procedures in Sweden, September 1990-1995: a multicenter study based on the Swedish National Epilepsy Surgery Register. Neurosurgery 2001;49(1):51–56, discussion 56–57

58. Simon SL, Telfeian A, Duhaime AC. Complications of invasive monitoring used in intractable pediatric epilepsy. Pediatr Neurosurg 2003;38(1):47–52

59. Swartz BE, Rich JR, Dwan PS, et al. The safety and efficacy of chronically implanted subdural electrodes: a prospective study. Surg Neurol 1996;46(1):87–93

60. Araki T, Otsubo H, Makino Y, et al. Efficacy of dexamethasone on cerebral swelling and seizures during subdural grid EEG recording in children. Epilepsia 2006;47(1):176–180

61. Stephan CL, Kepes JJ, SantaCruz K, Wilkinson SB, Fegley B, Osorio I. Spectrum of clinical and histopathologic responses to intracranial electrodes: from multifocal aseptic meningitis to multifocal hypersensitivity-type meningovasculitis. Epilepsia 2001;42(7):895–901

62. Maciunas RJ. Computer-assisted neurosurgery. Clin Neurosurg 2006;53:267–271

63. Garcia PA, Barbaro NM, Laxer KD. The prognostic value of postoperative seizures following epilepsy surgery. Neurology 1991; 41(9):1511–1512

64. Lüders H, Murphy D, Awad I, et al. Quantitative analysis of seizure frequency 1 week and 6, 12, and 24 months after surgery of epilepsy. Epilepsia 1994;35(6):1174–1178

65. Mani J, Gupta A, Mascha E, et al. Postoperative seizures after extratemporal resections and hemispherectomy in pediatric epilepsy. Neurology 2006;66(7):1038–1043

66. Tanriverdi T, Olivier NP, Olivier A. Quality of life after extratemporal epilepsy surgery: a prospective clinical study. Clin Neurol Neurosurg 2008;110(1):30–37

67. Tonini C, Beghi E, Berg AT, et al. Predictors of epilepsy surgery outcome: a meta-analysis. Epilepsy Res 2004;62(1):75–87

68. Beghi E, Tonini C. Surgery for epilepsy: assessing evidence from observational studies. Epilepsy Res 2006;70(2-3):97–102

69. Gilliam F, Wyllie E, Kashden J, et al. Epilepsy surgery outcome: comprehensive assessment in children. Neurology 1997;48(5):1368–1374

70. Terra-Bustamante VC, Fernandes RM, Inuzuka LM, et al. Surgically amenable epilepsies in children and adolescents: clinical, imaging, electrophysiological, and post-surgical outcome data. Childs Nerv Syst 2005;21(7):546–551

22 Surgical Approaches in Cortical Dysplasia

Lorie D. Hamiwka, Ronald T. Grondin, and Joseph R. Madsen

Cortical dysplasias are malformations of cortical development initially identified as a pathological substrate in individuals with intractable epilepsy by Taylor and colleagues in 1971.[1] They are characterized by a disruption of the normal lamination of the cortex that can vary in severity, ranging from mild disruption of lamination and normal-appearing neurons to significant loss of laminar organization with neuronal clustering, dysmorphic abnormally oriented neurons, cytomegalic neurons, and balloon cells[2-4] (see **Figs. 22.1**, showing a lesion at the base of a right frontal sulcus, and **22.2**, showing left occipital cortical dysplasia). In addition, there is gliosis of the white matter with heterotopic neurons.[2-4] Cortical dysplasias are reported as the most common underlying pathology in children undergoing surgical resection for medically resistant partial epilepsy.[5,6] Advances in structural neuroimaging and the increased use of multimodal imaging have improved the ability to recognize cortical dysplasia resulting in the development of classification systems and increased interest in the epileptogenic

mechanisms of these lesions.[3,5-9] Despite these advances, long-term surgical outcomes remain poor, with significant challenges regarding the localization of the epileptogenic zone and the extent of the surgical margin allowing for a complete resection.[10-13]

■ Epidemiology of Cortical Dysplasia in Intractable Epilepsy

The clinical presentation of cortical dysplasias is variable and depends on the function of the involved region. Children may exhibit epilepsy, developmental delay, and, often, motor impairment. Epilepsy is usually chronic and consists of partial or generalized seizures, depending on the lesion. Not all individuals with cortical dysplasias will have seizures, and their response to antiepileptic medications is variable.

The Pediatric Epilepsy Surgery Subcommission of the International League Against Epilepsy conducted a survey of 20 programs in the United States, Europe, and Australia. The study found that in 42% of children undergoing surgical resection, the pathological diagnosis was cortical dysplasia, representing the most common underlying etiology in this cohort.[14] This diagnosis was more common in younger children and in those with extratemporal or multilobar seizures.[14] These findings are similar to those previously reported in the literature.[6,15,16]

■ Classification of Cortical Dysplasia

Advances in neuroimaging, improved understanding of pathogenetic mechanisms, the development of animal models, descriptions of clinical–electrographic correlations, and the delineation of surgical strategies have resulted in the proposal classification schemes.

In 1996, a classification system was proposed for malformations of cortical development based on the timing at which the developmental process was disturbed.[17] In 2001, this classification was revised as a result of increased knowledge of biologic mechanisms and the discovery of new malformations.[18] A subsequent revision was undertaken in 2005, with revision made predominantly related

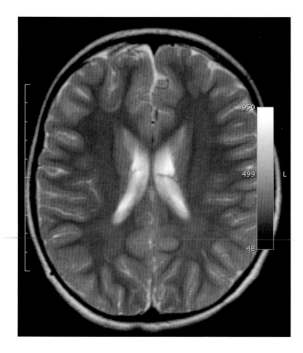

Fig. 22.1 Frontal lobe bottom of sulcus cortical dysplasia.

185

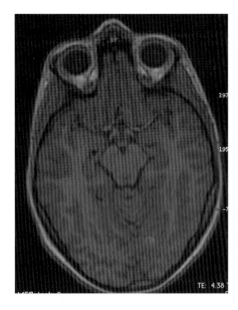 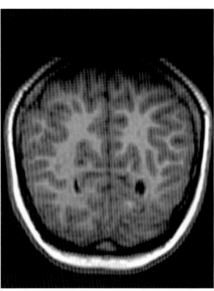

Fig. 22.2 Cortical dysplasia located in left occipital lobe (*left*).

to advances in genetics and neuroimaging.[19] In this classification, cortical dysplasias are categorized as malformations of cortical development associated with abnormal neuronal and glial proliferation or apoptosis and as malformations caused by abnormal late neuronal migration and cortical organization, depending on the timing in development. This classification, however, does not focus on focal cortical dysplasias increasingly recognized in individuals with medically resistant epilepsy undergoing surgical resection.

In 2004, Palmini and colleagues suggested that cortical dysplasias should be applied only to the subtype of malformations of cortical development in which the abnormality was, for the most part, intracortical.[3] They proposed a detailed classification system for focal cortical dysplasia using predominantly histopathological features. This classification is outlined in **Table 22.1**.

■ Why Do Malformations of Cortical Development Cause Epilepsy?

Studies on the epileptogenesis of cortical dysplasia have been performed both on resected human tissue and in animal models. Animal models of cortical dysplasia include in utero manipulation (methylazoxymethanol [MAM] injection, γ irradiation), manipulations in the newborn (ibotenate cortical injection, cortical freeze lesions), spontaneously epileptic animals with cortical malformations (Ihara's genetically epileptic rat, telencephalic internal structure heterotopia [TISH] rat) and knockouts (PAFAH β subunit knockouts, tuberous

sclerosis complex 2 knockouts). Although these models may help in determining why dysplastic cortex is hyperexcitable, it is less clear how well they can be related to the human condition, because phenotypes in animal models are often much milder and many, although showing enhanced sensitivity to seizure-inducing agents, are not associated with spontaneous seizures.

Abnormal cells or abnormal neuronal circuitry may explain the epileptogenicity in cortical dysplasia. In general, more focal malformations of cortical developments (MCDs) often have abnormal cells that may act as pacemakers of epileptiform discharges.[20] By contrast, more diffuse MCDs have normal-appearing cells but abnormal connectivity of the cellular aggregate.[20]

Abnormal Neurons

Epileptiform discharge in a large group of neurons can be triggered by a small group of abnormal cells that generate bursting behavior. The most dramatic examples of abnormal neurons in cortical dysplasia are the balloon cell, which stains positively for markers of both neurons and glia, and has multiple dendritic trees that show little orientation specificity, and the giant cell, which is often found together with balloon cells in Taylor-type focal dysplasia.

These neurons have been known to display intrinsic hyperexcitability,[21] possibly because of modification of N-methyl-D-aspartate (NMDA) receptors predisposing to hyperexcitability. NR1 and NR2 are the two subunits of the NMDA receptor. In vitro studies have shown that NR2 alone is nonfunctional, whereas NR1 alone produces only

Table 22.1   Palmini Classification of the Cortical Dysplasias

Mild malformations of cortical development	*Type 1:* with ectopically placed neurons in or adjacent to layer 1 *Type 2:* with microscopic neuronal heterotopia outside layer 1 *Structural imaging:* not detectable by current MRI techniques *Histopathology:* architectural disorganization, clusters of misplaced neurons *Clinical manifestations:* some individuals have epilepsy and those who do may have learning disabilities and cognitive impairments

Focal cortical dysplasias	*Type I:* no dysmorphic neurons or balloon cells
	   Type IA: isolated architectural abnormalities (dyslamination, accompanied or not by other abnormalities of mild MCD)
	   Type IB: architectural abnormalities, plus giant or "immature," but not dysmorphic, neurons
	Structural imaging: currently no specific findings
	Histopathology: dyslamination and other mild abnormalities (architectural abnormalities), immature neurons, giant neurons
	Clinical manifestations: commonly have medically resistant seizures, often temporal in origin
	Type II: Taylor-type FCD (dysmorphic neurons without or with balloon cells)
	   Type IIA: architectural abnormalities with dysmorphic neurons but without balloon cells
	   Type IIB: architectural abnormalities with dysmorphic neurons and balloon cells
	Structural imaging: focal lesions commonly identified on MRI
	Histopathology: in addition to Type I, the presence of dysmorphic neurons and balloon cells
	Clinical manifestations: commonly have medically resistant seizures, often extratemporal in origin with motor manifestations or secondary generalization

Dysplastic tumors	*DNETs, gangliogliomas:* may represent an extreme end of FCD spectrum, may be associated with abnormal cortex including dyslamination, large dysmorphic neurons and glial cells with subcortical heterotopic neurons *Structural imaging:* cortically based lesions with cystic and calcified areas, irregular and poorly delineated with no perilesional edema or mass effect *Clinical manifestations:* oncologically benign, often medically refractory with seizures beginning before 20 years of age

Source: Data from Palmini A, Najm I, Avanzini G, et al. Terminology and classification of the cortical dysplasias. Neurology 2004; 62(6 suppl 3):S2–S8.
Abbreviations: magnetic resonance imaging, MRI; malformations of cortical development, MCD; focal cortical dysplasia, FCD; dysembryoplastic neuroepithelial tumor, DNET.

weak currents to glutamate. Heteromeric co-assembly of NR1 and NR2 subunits, however, leads to marked increases in the NMDA channel current.[22] In studies on human surgical specimens, Ying et al noted that dysplastic neurons have increased NMDA receptor subunits NR1 and NR2A/B.[23] Furthermore, in human epileptic focal cortical dysplasia, NR1 co-assembled with NR2,[24] and NR1-NR2A/B were co-expressed in single dysplastic neurons,[25] leading to neurons that are hyperexcitable to glutamate.

MAM-treated rats showed an increased number of bursting neurons in regions of heterotopia and dysplastic cortex,[26] which supports the concept that epileptogenesis may result from a few abnormal cells. Evidence of decreased binding to γ-aminobutyric acid (GABA) receptors using autoradiography[27] and decreased sensitivity of GABA$_A$ receptors to zolpidem, a benzodiazepine agonist,[28] in the freeze lesion cortical dysplasia model, also suggests a role for decreased inhibition in dysplasia.

Altered Synaptic Connectivity

Cortical dysplasias are associated with reorganization of cortical circuitry. Abnormal connectivity has been best studied in the freeze lesion model of cortical dysplasia. In this model, the epileptogenic zone is actually adjacent to the microgyrus of the lesion, and the cells in this adjacent region appear normal.

Jacobs and Prince have shown that the pyramidal neurons adjacent to the dysplastic microgyrus receive more excitatory input, perhaps because of hyperinnervation by excitatory cortical afferents that were originally destined for the microgyrus.[29] Furthermore, axons that would normally project out of the epileptic zone may also be interrupted and instead make excitatory synapses locally. In addition, in the MAM model of cortical dysplasia, aberrant connections have been shown between the heterotopic cell regions and other, more distant brain regions, facilitating spread of abnormal epileptiform activity.[30] Decreased numbers of inhibitory neurons have also been noted in and around dysplastic lesions, which would contribute to the overall hyperexcitability.[31,32]

■ Do Uncontrolled Seizures Worsen Long-Term Outcome in Children with Cortical Dysplasias?

Single electroencephalography (EEG) discharges have been shown to cause transient cognitive impairment.[33,34] If single spikes can cause cognitive impairment, frequent multifocal discharges might be expected to more profoundly affect cognition. Frequent epileptiform discharges during sleep may have a particularly disruptive effect on memory consolidation by interfering with storage of memory in the neocortex.[35]

Epilepsy may be progressive, with resulting cognitive decline. Oki and colleagues reported on two children with focal cortical dysplasia in their dominant hemispheres who experienced significant decline in verbal IQ with recurrence of frequent seizures in mid to late childhood.[36] An adult study tested cognitive function on two occasions separated by at least 10 years.[37] The onset of epilepsy was in childhood (median of 8 years of age). The study showed severe cognitive decline that occurred across a wide range of cognitive functions. Generalized tonic–clonic seizure frequency was the strongest predictor of decline. Complex partial seizure frequency correlated with a decline in memory and executive skills but not in IQ. Seizure-related head injuries and advancing age were associated with a poor prognosis, and periods of remission were associated with a better cognitive outcome.

There is further clinical evidence that in certain patients, particularly those with recurrent, generalized seizures or status epilepticus, epilepsy may be a progressive disease, with cognitive deterioration, progressive brain atrophy, and potential development of intractable seizures. In a study of temporal lobe epilepsy, Hermann et al found that patients with childhood onset (younger than 14 years) had significantly reduced intellectual status and memory function compared with those with onset later in life, and the longer the epilepsy duration was, the worse the cognitive problems were.[38] They also found reduced total brain tissue on volumetric magnetic resonance imaging (MRI) in the childhood onset group. There is ongoing debate as to whether seizures beget seizures, with this argument being predominantly refuted by large epidemiological studies and supported by experimental animal models of epilepsy.[39,40]

■ Structural Neuroimaging in Children with Cortical Dysplasia

Although the presence of an abnormality on MR neuroimaging has not been a predictor for successful long-term seizure

freedom in children with cortical dysplasia after surgery,[11,12] it is a critical tool in the evaluation of for surgical candidacy (**Figs. 22.1** and **Fig. 22.2**). Over the past decade, there have been significant advances in structural neuroimaging in an attempt to improve the signal-to-noise ratio (SNR) and therefore optimize the quality of such studies. The use of high field strength (>1.5 T) and, more importantly, phased array head coils, have enhanced spatial and contrast resolution compared with routine quadrature head coils.[41] At 1.5 T using an eight-channel phased array coil, the SNR is increased by approximately fourfold. In a study of 13 children in which 9 had normal neuroimaging on 1.5 T MRI, 4 were found to have a cortical abnormality on subsequent imaging using phased array head coils.[41] Phased array coils have also been used at 3 T with approximately a twofold increase in SNR. A prospective study of 40 patients with epilepsy, using phased array coils at 3 T, yielded additional diagnostic information in 19 cases compared with clinical read at 1.5 T.[42] In 14 of these cases, the information resulted in a change in clinical management. Further advances involving the application of 7-T phased array technology has the potential to allow visualization of structure at or below the 100-µm level.[43]

Quantitation of cerebral structures is still, for the most part, a research tool.[44,45] Reports of cortical segmentation and thickness in patients with cortical dysplasia are emerging.[46–48] This may be a useful tool in the future in patients for whom the MRI is negative. As both structural and quantitative neuroimaging continue to evolve with ongoing improvements SNR, standardized use of high-resolution MRI in the clinical setting, the clinical application of segmentation, and improved recognition of cortical dysplasias in children may lead to improved outcomes in this group.

■ Surgical Management

Defining Epileptogenic Zone Boundaries

The surgical boundary is typically determined by some combination of the presurgical evaluation techniques, including intracranial monitoring and intraoperative electrocorticography (ECoG). The presurgical evaluation begins with a detailed history of the semiology of the seizures. A careful history will usually allow for lateralization of the seizure onset zone and will often provide useful localizing information. Further evaluation includes ictal as well as interictal EEG and video-EEG recordings. These are done in combination with primary imaging modalities, such as MRI and computed tomography (CT), and secondary imaging modalities, such as single photon emission computed tomography (SPECT) and position emission tomography (PET).

Occasionally, the dysplastic cortex may be visualized on MRI with a variety of patterns, including heterotopic gray matter, or abnormal cortical thickness. These abnormalities may be focal or diffuse. When present, they do not necessarily delineate the full extent of neuronal disorganization and may not correlate to the area of seizure onset. Therefore, other imaging modalities pointing to abnormal electrical activity, such as increased blood flow, are needed.

PET delineates regional or focal central activity according to the degree of uptake of radioactive agents in the interictal state related to blood flow. A wide variety of radioactive ligands are available with PET for investigating pathophysiological mechanisms underlying the epileptic process.

SPECT provides similar blood flow information; however, it can also be used successfully during the ictal phase. The principle of ictal SPECT in localizing seizure onset is based on the phenomenon of increased cerebral blood flow in the regions affected by seizure activity. When the radiotracer is injected soon after seizure onset, it is distributed and bound by cerebral tissues in proportion to the amount of local cerebral perfusion. The distribution and uptake of radiotracer is usually completed within 1 minute and provides information on brain perfusion at seizure onset. Thus, SPECT is functionally correlated to the ictal metabolism of the seizure onset zone.

When data from the clinical history and all imaging studies agree with a similar location, they are said to be *convergent* and are associated with the best likelihood that resection of that area will result in a favorable outcome, namely reduction or elimination of seizures. Occasionally, some data will be nonconvergent, and the challenge then arises about how to appropriately weigh all data.

Defining Eloquent Cortex

When the epileptogenic zone has been identified, the next task is to identify areas of eloquent cortex so that these areas may be preserved during surgery. Recent advances in neuroimaging and the development of functional paradigms for functional MRI (fMRI) and magnetoencephalography (MEG) have led to improvements in identification of eloquent cortex. fMRI involves dynamic visualization of change in cerebral blood flow (more specifically balance between oxy- and deoxyhemoglobin in the microvascular bed) as a consequence of stimulation or task performance. It has also been used with EEG for source localization and an entity coined spike-triggered MRI. Clinical studies have suggested the utility of fMRI for mapping sensorimotor cortex and centers involved in language processing and production.[49]

MEG is a technology that measures magnetic fields formed by flow of electrical current and has been used in the investigation of children with both lesional[50,51] and nonlesional epilepsy being considered for surgical treatment. It is valuable as a diagnostic tool in lesional cases involving MCD because it has been shown that removal of MEG cluster spike sources extending from the lesion are necessary for favorable outcome.[13,50] However, for lesional cases involving

tumors (excluding developmental tumors), lesionectomy alone yields a favorable outcome despite extramarginal MEG spikes.[50] MEG has also been reported as a useful tool in the presurgical evaluation of nonlesional extratemporal epilepsy in children with good convergence of intracranial video-EEG and interictal MEG data.[52]

Resection

Often the data obtained from the presurgical assessment will be enough to compose a surgical plan. When the epileptogenic zone is far away from any eloquent cortex, then a single-stage resection can be performed with the goal being complete resection of abnormal tissue. Although intraoperative ECoG has been widely used to try to improve surgical outcomes by achieving a complete surgical resection, the clinical utility remains controversial. Variability in the location of the interictal discharges, multifocal discharges in chronic epilepsy, secondary propagation, intraoperative time constraints leading to brief recording periods, and decreased spike frequency associated with anesthetic can lead to inaccurate assumptions. Currently, there are no individual features of the preoperative ECoG that are clearly indicative of the site of origin of a child's seizures or the extent of the epileptogenic zone, although preresection spike distribution and postresection spike presence or absence may have prognostic significance.

Currently, the gold standard for identification of areas of seizure onset and areas of eloquent cortex is invasive EEG monitoring with implanted subdural or depth electrodes. This procedure allows for both ictal and interictal data to be obtained with the greater accuracy of having closely spaced electrodes directly on the surface of the brain. Functional mapping can also be performed by electrical stimulation through the electrodes.

A focal cortical resection is undertaken when data show a well-localized epileptogenic focus, whereas lobectomy or multilobar resections are considered when the ictal area is large. Subcortical white matter pathways should be preserved in cases of focal cortical resection.

Abnormally appearing gyral and sulcal patterns, arterial supply, and venous drainage are common in cortical dysplasia and need to be considered in the surgical planning. Frequently, anatomical considerations such as proximity to functional eloquent cortex and vascular structures, have a significant effect on the size and extent of the resected area.

Case Scenario

A 3-year-old boy presented to the hospital with a 1-week history of staring episodes, decreased responsiveness, and posturing of the right arm. In retrospect, the parents noted that he also had similar, but less frequent, episodes several

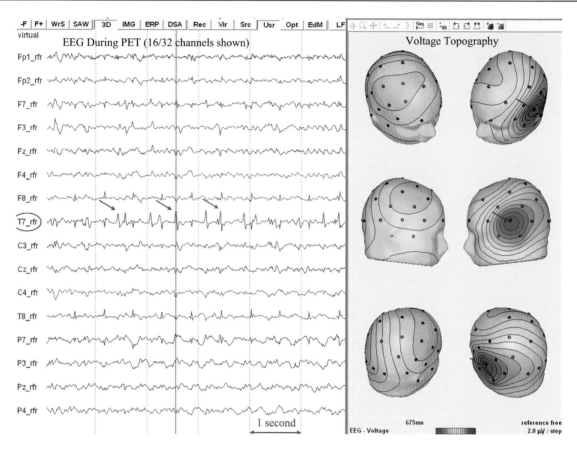

Fig. 22.3 Brain electrical source analysis of ictal spikes with decrease in isoflurane. Source analysis identified a dipole originating in the left mid temporal lobe.

months earlier. Ictal and interictal EEG studies demonstrated left temporal slowing with left frontotemporal seizure onset and rapid spread to temporal and central areas. This was associated with leftward eye deviation and right hand posturing. Initial MRI studies did not demonstrate any structural abnormalities. The seizures became progressively more frequent, and the patient went into status epilepticus, necessitating intubation for airway control and medical control of seizures. These were ultimately controlled with isoflurane anesthesia for burst suppression. A tissue biopsy was obtained from the left temporal lobe, which demonstrated focal cortical dysplasia type IIA.

It was noted that a reduction in the amount of isoflurane resulted in the appearance of left mid temporal interictal spikes. Brain electrical source analysis localized this to the mid temporal lobe (**Fig. 22.3**) near the T7 electrode. A PET scan was obtained at the same time that also demonstrated increased signal in the left mid temporal lobe (**Fig. 22.4**). Based on these findings, surgeons elected to proceed with a single-stage left temporal cortical resection using intraoperative ECoG.

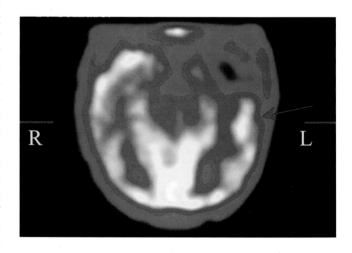

Fig. 22.4 Ictal positron emission tomography. Note the asymmetrically increased left mid temporal activity with decrease in isoflurane.

The patient was brought to the operative theater and underwent a left temporal craniotomy (**Fig. 22.5**). Preresection ECoG demonstrated spikes centered over the left mid and anterior temporal lobe (corresponding to electrodes 10, 11, and 12 in **Fig. 22.5**, box 2; focus A in **Fig. 22.5**, box 3). A cortical resection of the inferior and middle temporal gyri anterior to the vein of Labbé was performed. Further ECoG then demonstrated continued activity just deep to the vein of Labbé, and, therefore, further resection was performed deep to the vein. Subsequent ECoG then revealed a new area of activity in the inferior temporal gyrus posterior to the vein of Labbé (focus B in **Fig. 22.5**, box 3). After resection of this focus of activity, ECoG was again performed, which did not demonstrate any further epileptiform activity. The final area of resection is demonstrated in **Fig. 22.5** (green area in box 3

and box 4). Histological analysis demonstrated focal cortical dysplasia with balloon cells, modifying the final diagnosis to focal cortical dysplasia type IIB. Postoperatively, the patient did not have any further seizures.

■ Surgical Challenges in Children with Cortical Dysplasias

Although there has been an increase in the number of children with medically resistant epilepsy who are considered for surgery, even in the most ideal candidates, there is a considerable delay between onset of the epilepsy and time to surgery. The reasons for this may be related to the

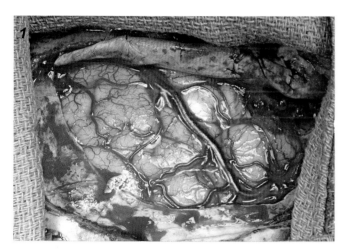

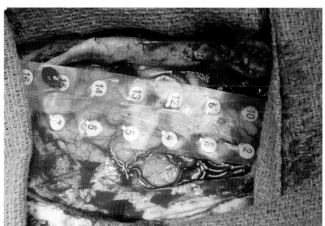

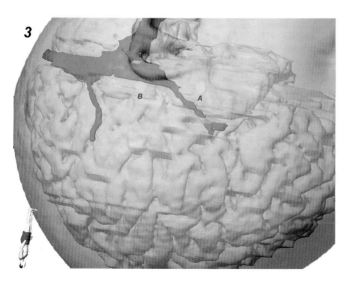

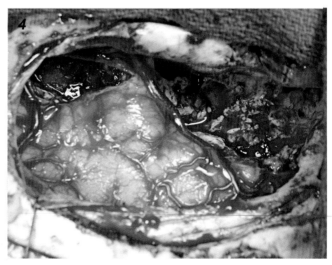

Fig. 22.5 Left temporal craniotomy for focal cortical resection with intraoperative electrocorticography (ECoG). Exposure of the left temporal lobe is shown in box 1. The vein of Labbé can be seen crossing the temporal lobe, and the anterior temporal biopsy is demonstrated to the upper right of the photo. Intraoperative ECoG (box 2) demonstrated ictal spikes in two areas (A and B in box 3). The resected areas are demonstrated in box 3 (shaded in green). Final cortical resection is shown in box 4.

definition of intractability for children and concerns about operating in a child in whom the natural history might be self-limited. There is also the concern regarding the risk of surgery in young children. Both of these are especially important in cortical dysplasias, because these lesions are more common in younger children.[7,14] In terms of defining candidacy for epilepsy surgery, medically resistant epilepsy may be defined as seizures that continue despite a trial of at least two first-line drugs at maximally tolerated serum levels for 2 years.[53] If two medications are ineffective, the chance of responding to a third is less than 5%.[54] Children referred to comprehensive epilepsy centers for consideration of surgical treatment typically have tried multiple medications and other therapies before referral.

A successful outcome from epilepsy surgery is generally defined as a seizure-free state with no imposition of neurological deficit. Achieving this state requires precise localization of the epileptogenic zone and the determination of the anatomical regions of eloquent cortex. Predictors of successful surgical outcome in cortical dysplasias are completeness of the resection and proximity to eloquent cortex.[11,12,55] Advances in neuroimaging have improved recognition of small cortical abnormalities. Despite these advances, nearly one half of children undergoing surgery remain MRI negative[41] and approximately 25% of pathologically confirmed focal cortical dysplasia were a lesion not seen on neuroimaging.[56,57] Even when the MRI does show an abnormality, the full extent of the lesion may not be visible. For example, the prognosis for seizure freedom in children presenting with dysembryoplastic neuroepithelial tumors was initially felt to be very good with short-term follow-up studies documenting seizure freedom at 80%.[58] Long-term follow-up studies showed a significant recurrence of intractable seizures and pathological evidence of

Table 22.2 Surgical Outcome in Children with Cortical Dysplasia

	Sample Size (N)	Age	Location of the Resection (T = temporal, E = extratemporal, M = multilobar)	Abnormal MRI (Y = yes/ N = no)	Follow-up (years)	Outcome (Engel Classification)	Predictors for Good Outcome	Complications
Kloss et al 2002[64]	68	< 18 years	T = 8 E = 47 M = 13	Y = 47 N = 21	2	I–34 (50%) II–7 III–22 IV–5	Completeness of the resection	Increased motor deficit, 2; Subdural, 1
Francione et al[65]	10	20 months– 11 years	T = 3 E = 4 M = 3	Y = 8 N = 2	25 months	I–7 (70%) II–1 III–0 IV–2	Completeness of the resection Location in the temporal lobe	Homonymous hemianopia, 1
Hader et al 2004[11]	39	2 months– 18 years	T = 11 E = 17 M = 11	Y = 32 N = 7	18 months	I /II–28 (72%)	Completeness of the resection	No comments
Hamiwka et al 2005[12]	38	6 months– 18 years	T = 13 E = 20 M = 5	Y = 18 N = 20	10 years	I–15 (40%) II–10 III/IV–13	Completeness of the resection	No comments
Hudgins et al 2005[55]	15	3 months– 14 years	T = 7 E = 6 M = 2	Y = 11 N = 4	4 years	I–10 (66%) II–2	Completeness of the resection	None
Park et al 2006[63]	30	1.5–18 years	T = 16 E = 13 M = 1	Y = 22 N = 8	3.2 years	I–20 (66%) II–6 III–1 IV–3	Presence of a lesion Location in the temporal lobe	Transient hemiparesis–3 Subdural–1

Source: Kloss S, Pieper T, Pannek H, et al. Epilepsy surgery I children with focal cortical dysplasia: Results of longterm outcome. Neuropediatrics 2002;33(1): 21–26; Francione S, Viplano P, Tassi L et al. Surgery for drup resistant partial epilepsy in children with focal cortical dysplasia: Anatoomical-clinical correlations and neurophysiological data in 10 patient. J Neurol Neurosurg Pyschiatry 74(11):1493–1501; Hader WJ, Mackay M, Otsubo H, et al. Cortical dysplastic lesions in children with intractable epilepsy: role of complete resection. J Neurosurg 2004;100(2, suppl Pediatrics):110–117; Hamiwka L, Jayakar P, Resnick T, et al. Surgery for epilepsy because of cortical malformations: ten-year follow-up. Epilepsia 2005;46(4):556–560; Hudgins RJ, Flamini JR, Palasis S, Cheng R, Burns TG, Gilreath CL. Surgical treatment of epilepsy in children caused by focal cortical dysplasia. Pediatr Neurosurg 2005;41(2):70–76; Park CK, Kim SK, Wang KC, et al. Surgical outcome and prognostic factors of pediatric epilepsy caused by cortical dysplasia. Childs Nerv Syst 2006;22(6):586–592.

cortical dysplasia adjacent to the resection margin.[13] Thus, the presence of an MRI lesion has not been shown to be a predictor of seizure freedom,[12,59] and seizure recurrence is thought to be a result of extension of the dysplastic cortex beyond the visible abnormality.

Cortical dysplasias are more commonly seen in extratemporal resections and eloquent cortex.[5] Proximity to critical function can limit the resection margin in an attempt to avoid postoperative neurological disability and has, at least in part, resulted in poorer surgical outcomes.[6] This is particularly true if there is a normal neurological examination before surgery. In an effort to treat lesions in surgically unresectable or eloquent cortex, the technique of multiple subpial transections was developed.[60] Vertical cuts through the cortex are believed to disrupt spread of epileptic activity in a horizontal direction while allowing preservation of functional vertical columns.[60] Although this technique has been found to be safe with few complications,[61] it has not improved surgical success.[11] Surgically, the dilemma remains in determining the extent of the surgical resection to maximize the potential for seizure freedom and minimize the possibility of neurologic impairment.

■ Surgical Outcomes in Children with Cortical Dysplasias

The most widely used system for classifying seizure outcome in epilepsy surgery is that described by Engel et al in 1993.[62] This method classifies postoperative seizure frequency and only considers quality-of-life issues when surgery does not result in a dramatic reduction in seizures. A good surgical outcome is considered to be Engel Class 1 or 2 (seizure free or only rare disabling seizures).

Six studies have published outcome data specifically for cortical resections in children with cortical dysplasia (**Table 22.2**). One study also evaluated mesial temporal sclerosis (MTS) and did not find any benefit when used in combination with cortical resection.[11] All studies focused primarily on seizure freedom. Only one commented on the effect of surgery on learning and social adaptation and found that 43% of children had improved school performance and 77% had good social adaptation.[63] Both, however, were related to successful surgical outcomes.

The follow-up period varies between from 18 months to 10 years. Seizure-free reported outcomes are from 40 to 70% and are inversely proportional to the length of follow-up. Completeness of the resection and, in some cases, the presence of an MRI lesion were predictors of good surgical outcome.[55,63]

■ Future Directions

The primary goal of surgical treatment is to stop seizures in children with epilepsy refractory to other therapies including medication. Early surgery has been advocated because of the suggestion that refractory, ongoing, daily, and repetitive seizures are potential negative effects on learning, psychosocial development, and neurobiological mechanisms. Further research is necessary to better understand the possible relationship between surgical treatment and improvements in cognition, behavior, and other neuropsychiatric co-morbidities associated with medically resistant epilepsy. These questions are likely of significant importance in cortical dysplasia because they affect very young children when learning and neurobehavioral pathways are developing.

References

1. Taylor DC, Falconer MA, Bruton CJ, Corsellis JA. Focal dysplasia of the cerebral cortex in epilepsy. J Neurol Neurosurg Psychiatry 1971;34(4):369–387
2. Mischel PS, Nguyen LP, Vinters HV. Cerebral cortical dysplasia associated with pediatric epilepsy. Review of neuropathologic features and proposal for a grading system. J Neuropathol Exp Neurol 1995;54(2):137–153
3. Palmini A, Najm I, Avanzini G, et al. Terminology and classification of the cortical dysplasias. Neurology 2004; 62(6, suppl 3):S2–S8
4. Prayson RA, Frater JL. Cortical dysplasia in extratemporal lobe intractable epilepsy: a study of 52 cases. Ann Diagn Pathol 2003;7(3):139–146
5. Cepeda C, André VM, Flores-Hernández J, et al. Pediatric cortical dysplasia: correlations between neuroimaging, electrophysiology and location of cytomegalic neurons and balloon cells and glutamate/GABA synaptic circuits. Dev Neurosci 2005;27(1):59–76
6. Wyllie E, Comair YG, Kotagal P, Bulacio J, Bingaman W, Ruggieri P. Seizure outcome after epilepsy surgery in children and adolescents. Ann Neurol 1998;44(5):740–748
7. Cepeda C, Hurst RS, Flores-Hernández J, et al. Morphological and electrophysiological characterization of abnormal cell types in pediatric cortical dysplasia. J Neurosci Res 2003;72(4):472–486
8. Kuzniecky RI. Malformations of cortical development and epilepsy, part 1: diagnosis and classification scheme. Rev Neurol Dis 2006;3(4):151–162
9. Zhang W, Simos PG, Ishibashi H, et al. Multimodality neuroimaging evaluation improves the detection of subtle cortical dysplasia in seizure patients. Neurol Res 2003;25(1):53–57
10. Fauser S, Bast T, Altenmüller DM, et al. Factors influencing surgical outcome in patients with focal cortical dysplasia. J Neurol Neurosurg Psychiatry 2008;79(1):103–105

11. Hader WJ, Mackay M, Otsubo H, et al. Cortical dysplastic lesions in children with intractable epilepsy: role of complete resection. J Neurosurg 2004;100(2, suppl Pediatrics):110–117

12. Hamiwka L, Jayakar P, Resnick T, et al. Surgery for epilepsy because of cortical malformations: ten-year follow-up. Epilepsia 2005;46(4):556–560

13. Sakuta R, Otsubo H, Nolan MA, et al. Recurrent intractable seizures in children with cortical dysplasia adjacent to dysembryoplastic neuroepithelial tumor. J Child Neurol 2005;20(4):377–384

14. Harvey AS, Cross JH, Shinnar S, Mathern BW; ILAE Pediatric Epilepsy Surgery Survey Taskforce. Defining the spectrum of international practice in pediatric epilepsy surgery patients. Epilepsia 2008;49(1):146–155

15. Mathern GW, Giza CC, Yudovin S, et al. Postoperative seizure control and antiepileptic drug use in pediatric epilepsy surgery patients: the UCLA experience, 1986–1997. Epilepsia 1999;40(12):1740–1749

16. Nordborg C, Eriksson S, Rydenhag B, Uvebrant P, Malmgren K. Microdysgenesis in surgical specimens from patients with epilepsy: occurrence and clinical correlations. J Neurol Neurosurg Psychiatry 1999;67(4):521–524

17. Barkovich AJ, Kuzniecky RI, Dobyns WB, Jackson GD, Becker LE, Evrard P. A classification scheme for malformations of cortical development. Neuropediatrics 1996;27(2):59–63

18. Barkovich AJ, Kuzniecky RI, Jackson GD, Guerrini R, Dobyns WB. Classification system for malformations of cortical development: update 2001. Neurology 2001;57(12):2168–2178

19. Barkovich AJ, Kuzniecky RI, Jackson GD, Guerrini R, Dobyns WB. A developmental and genetic classification for malformations of cortical development. Neurology 2005;65(12):1873–1887

20. Schwartzkroin PA, Walsh CA. Cortical malformations and epilepsy. Ment Retard Dev Disabil Res Rev 2000;6(4):268–280

21. Mathern GW, Cepeda C, Hurst RS, Flores-Hernandez J, Mendoza D, Levine MS. Neurons recorded from pediatric epilepsy surgery patients with cortical dysplasia. Epilepsia 2000;41(suppl 6):S162–S167

22. Monyer H, Sprengel R, Schoepfer R, et al. Heteromeric NMDA receptors: molecular and functional distinction of subtypes. Science 1992;256(5060):1217–1221

23. Ying Z, Babb TL, Comair YG, Bingaman W, Bushey M, Touhalisky K. Induced expression of NMDAR2 proteins and differential expression of NMDAR1 splice variants in dysplastic neurons of human epileptic neocortex. J Neuropathol Exp Neurol 1998;57(1):47–62

24. Mikuni N, Babb TL, Ying Z, et al. NMDA-receptors 1 and 2A/B coassembly increased in human epileptic focal cortical dysplasia. Epilepsia 1999;40(12):1683–1687

25. Ying Z, Babb TL, Mikuni N, Najm I, Drazba J, Bingaman W. Selective coexpression of NMDAR2A/B and NMDAR1 subunit proteins in dysplastic neurons of human epileptic cortex. Exp Neurol 1999;159(2):409–418

26. Baraban SC, Schwartzkroin PA. Flurothyl seizure susceptibility in rats following prenatal methylazoxymethanol treatment. Epilepsy Res 1996;23(3):189–194

27. Zilles K, Qü M, Schleicher A, Luhmann HJ. Characterization of neuronal migration disorders in neocortical structures: quantitative receptor autoradiography of ionotropic glutamate, GABA(A) and GABA(B) receptors. Eur J Neurosci 1998;10(10):3095–3106

28. Hablitz JJ, DeFazio RA. Altered receptor subunit expression in rat neocortical malformations. Epilepsia 2000;41(suppl 6):S82–S85

29. Jacobs KM, Prince DA. Excitatory and inhibitory postsynaptic currents in a rat model of epileptogenic microgyria. J Neurophysiol 2005;93(2):687–696

30. Colacitti C, Sancini G, Franceschetti S, et al. Altered connections between neocortical and heterotopic areas in methylazoxymethanol-treated rat. Epilepsy Res 1998;32(1–2):49–62

31. Roper SN, Eisenschenk S, King MA. Reduced density of parvalbumin- and calbindin D28-immunoreactive neurons in experimental cortical dysplasia. Epilepsy Res 1999;37(1):63–71

32. Spreafico R, Battaglia G, Arcelli P, et al. Cortical dysplasia: an immunocytochemical study of three patients. Neurology 1998;50(1):27–36

33. Aarts JH, Binnie CD, Smit AM, Wilkins AJ. Selective cognitive impairment during focal and generalized epileptiform EEG activity. Brain 1984;107(pt 1):293–308

34. Binnie CD. Cognitive impairment during epileptiform discharges: is it ever justifiable to treat the EEG? Lancet Neurol 2003;2(12):725–730

35. Káli S, Dayan P. Off-line replay maintains declarative memories in a model of hippocampal-neocortical interactions. Nat Neurosci 2004;7(3):286–294

36. Oki J, Miyamoto A, Takahashi S. [Longitudinal study of cognitive function in two patients with focal cortical dysplasia]. No To Hattatsu 2000;32(5):408–414

37. Thompson PJ, Duncan JS. Cognitive decline in severe intractable epilepsy. Epilepsia 2005;46(11):1780–1787

38. Hermann BP, Seidenberg M, Bell B. The neurodevelopmental impact of childhood onset temporal lobe epilepsy on brain structure and function and the risk of progressive cognitive effects. Prog Brain Res 2002;135:429–438

39. Berg AT, Shinnar S. Do seizures beget seizures? An assessment of the clinical evidence in humans. J Clin Neurophysiol 1997;14(2):102–110

40. Sutula TP. Mechanisms of epilepsy progression: current theories and perspectives from neuroplasticity in adulthood and development. Epilepsy Res 2004;60(2–3):161–171

41. Goyal M, Bangert BA, Lewin JS, Cohen ML, Robinson S. High-resolution MRI enhances identification of lesions amenable to surgical therapy in children with intractable epilepsy. Epilepsia 2004;45(8):954–959

42. Knake S, Triantafyllou C, Wald LL, et al. 3T phased array MRI improves the presurgical evaluation in focal epilepsies: a prospective study. Neurology 2005;65(7):1026–1031

43. Grant PE. Imaging the developing epileptic brain. Epilepsia 2005;46(suppl 7):7–14

44. Dale AM, Fischl B, Sereno MI. Cortical surface-based analysis. I. Segmentation and surface reconstruction. Neuroimage 1999;9(2):179–194

45. Fischl B, Sereno MI, Dale AM. Cortical surface-based analysis. II: Inflation, flattening, and a surface-based coordinate system. Neuroimage 1999;9(2):195–207

46. Bernasconi A. Quantitative MR imaging of the neocortex. Neuroimaging Clin N Am 2004;14(3):425–436, viii

47. Colliot O, Mansi T, Bernasconi N, Naessens V, Klironomos D, Bernasconi A. Segmentation of focal cortical dysplasia lesions using a feature-based level set. Med Image Comput Comput Assist Interv Int Conf Med Image Comput Comput Assist Interv 2005;8(pt 1):375–382

48. Colliot O, Mansi T, Bernasconi N, Naessens V, Klironomos D, Bernasconi A. Segmentation of focal cortical dysplasia lesions on MRI using level set evolution. Neuroimage 2006;32(4):1621–1630

49. Binder J. Functional magnetic resonance imaging. Language mapping. Neurosurg Clin N Am 1997;8(3):383–392

50. Otsubo H, Ochi A, Elliott I, et al. MEG predicts epileptic zone in lesional extrahippocampal epilepsy: 12 pediatric surgery cases. Epilepsia 2001;42(12):1523–1530

51. Bast T, Oezkan O, Rona S, et al. EEG and MEG source analysis of single and averaged interictal spikes reveals intrinsic epileptogenicity in focal cortical dysplasia. Epilepsia 2004;45(6):621–631

52. Minassian BA, Otsubo H, Weiss S, Elliott I, Rutka JT, Snead OC III. Magnetoencephalographic localization in pediatric epilepsy surgery: comparison with invasive intracranial electroencephalography. Ann Neurol 1999;46(4):627–633

53. Bourgeois B. General concepts of medical intractability. In: HO L, ed. Epilepsy Surgery. New York, NY: Raven Press; 1992:77–81

54. Kwan P, Brodie MJ. Early identification of refractory epilepsy. N Engl J Med 2000;342(5):314–319

55. Hudgins RJ, Flamini JR, Palasis S, Cheng R, Burns TG, Gilreath CL. Surgical treatment of epilepsy in children caused by focal cortical dysplasia. Pediatr Neurosurg 2005;41(2):70–76

56. Widdess-Walsh P, Diehl B, Najm I. Neuroimaging of focal cortical dysplasia. J Neuroimaging 2006;16(3):185–196

57. Ruggieri PM, Najm I, Bronen R, et al. Neuroimaging of the cortical dysplasias. Neurology 2004;62(6, suppl 3);S27–S29

58. Nolan MA, Sakuta R, Chuang N, et al. Dysembryoplastic neuroepithelial tumors in childhood: long-term outcome and prognostic features. Neurology 2004;62(12):2270–2276

59. Alarcón G, Valentín A, Watt C, et al. Is it worth pursuing surgery for epilepsy in patients with normal neuroimaging? J Neurol Neurosurg Psychiatry 2006;77(4):474–480

60. Morrell F, Whisler WW, Bleck TP. Multiple subpial transection: a new approach to the surgical treatment of focal epilepsy. J Neurosurg 1989;70(2):231–239

61. Blount JP, Langburt W, Otsubo H, et al. Multiple subpial transections in the treatment of pediatric epilepsy. J Neurosurg 2004; 100(2, suppl Pediatrics)118–124

62. Engel J Jr, Ness PV, Rasmussen T, Ojemann L. Outcome with respect to epileptic seizures. In: Engel J. Jr., ed. Surgical Treatment of the Epilepsies. 2nd ed. New York, NY: Raven Press; 1993:609–621

63. Park CK, Kim SK, Wang KC, et al. Surgical outcome and prognostic factors of pediatric epilepsy caused by cortical dysplasia. Childs Nerv Syst 2006;22(6):586–592

64. Kloss S, Pieper T, Pannek H, et al. Epilepsy surgery I children with focal cortical dysplasia: Results of longterm outcome. Neuropediatrics 2002;33(1):21–26

65. Francione S, Viplano P, Tassi L et al. Surgery for drup resistant partial epilepsy in children with focal cortical dysplasia: Anatoomical-clinical correlations and neurophysiological data in 10 patient. J Neurol Neurosurg Pyschiatry 74(11):1493–1501

23 Posterior Quadrantic Resection and Disconnection

Roy Thomas Daniel, K. Srinivasa Babu, Rebecca Jacob, and Jean-Guy Villemure

Surgery is often contemplated when patients with medical intractability suffer from widespread areas of hemispheric epileptogenicity. When the whole hemisphere is involved with accompanying hemiplegia, hemispherectomy is the treatment of choice. In subhemispheric epilepsy (epilepsy involving two or more lobes), where there is residual motor neurological function (finger opposition and foot tapping) secondary to a condition that is static, multilobar surgery sparing the functional cortices is an option that needs to be considered. Intractable multilobar epilepsy has traditionally been treated by resective surgery, which involves the removal of large parts of the hemisphere, classically, either the frontal and temporal lobes, or the temporal, parietal, and occipital lobes (posterior quadrant resection), leaving behind a large operative cavity. Akin to the evolution of disconnective techniques in hemispherectomy, the surgical approach for posterior quadrantic epilepsy has evolved progressively toward more disconnection and less resection. These techniques, while maintaining similar seizure outcomes to resective surgery, are aimed at reducing perioperative morbidity and long-term complications.

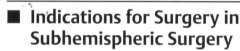 Indications for Surgery in Subhemispheric Surgery

The surgical treatment of posterior quadrantic subhemispheric epilepsy has been increasingly used in the last decade, but the frequency of these surgeries accounts for less than 5% of all epilepsy surgeries.[1,2] The increased use of these techniques has been due to advances in neuroimaging, increased awareness, advances in pediatric anesthesia, and introduction of disconnective techniques in epilepsy surgery. Posterior quadrantic epilepsy surgery is indicated when the epileptogenic zone encompasses large areas of the temporal, parietal, and occipital lobes (posterior quadrant) and spares the central and frontal areas. The indication rests on a good concordance between the imaging (magnetic resonance imaging [MRI], computed tomography, nuclear) studies, electroencephalography (EEG), and clinical and neuropsychological evaluations that localize the lesion to the posterior quadrant unilaterally. The etiologies for posterior quadrantic epilepsy in our series were cortical dysplasia,

Sturge-Weber syndrome, ischemic prenatal lesion, and sequela of ruptured arteriovenous malformations.

■ Preoperative Assessment

The examination of the neurological status generally confirms the presence of homonymous hemianopsia. Patients will demonstrate the ability to perform fine finger movements and foot tapping, although some may have parietocortical sensory loss. The preoperative investigations include MRI and prolonged EEG recordings with telemetry. MRI should reveal the presence of an extensive radiological abnormality of the temporo-parieto-occipital lobes, with imaging characteristics of the causative pathology (**Fig. 23.1**). The interictal EEG and prolonged EEG telemetry confirm the origin of the epileptiform activity arising from the large radiological abnormality with propagation of activity to anterior cortices or contralaterally in ictal recordings. The concordance achieved with presurgical investigations (that aim at localizing the epileptogenic zone) generally obviates the need for chronic invasive recording. Invasive recording is reserved for difficult cases in which phase I presurgical evaluation results in discordant findings. The pathological substrate responsible for the seizure disorder should be static and should necessarily not be a progressive one like Rasmussen encephalitis. The presence of residual voluntary motor function of the contralateral distal musculature, that is, finger opposition and foot tapping, contraindicates a hemispherectomy but forms the indication for posterior quadrant resection or disconnection. The presence of a visual field defect imparts greater confidence to the surgeon in his or her decision to carry out this extensive surgery. However, the possibility of creation or aggravation of a homonymous field deficit is not an absolute contraindication to this surgery in cases in which the risk–benefit ratio is favorable. In dominant posterior quadrantic surgery, speech is a significant concern. In our experience, all patients who underwent surgery for dominant quadrantic lesions had congenital lesions and consequently had language functions residing in the right hemisphere. This hypothesis was made on the basis of the seizure semiology, neuropsychological examination, and more so on the basis of the nature and location of the

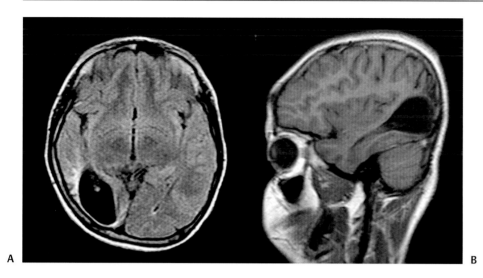

Fig. 23.1 Preoperative magnetic resonance imaging (MRI) scan of an 11-year-old boy who presented with left focal motor seizures with secondary generalization of 9 years duration. He had no neurological deficits except for a left homonymous hemianopsia. Despite treatment with multiple anticonvulsants, he had three to four episodes of seizures every week. Axial fluid attenuated inversion recovery (FLAIR) MRI **(A)** shows atrophy of the temporo-occipital lobes with a porencephalic cyst. **(B)** Sagittal T1-weight MRI shows atrophy of the right posterior parietal and occipital lobes and a porencephalic cyst.

A

B

radiological abnormalities. This precluded the need for a Wada test. Our presurgical hypothesis was validated by the absence of postoperative language dysfunction.

■ Evolution of Surgery for Subhemispheric Epilepsy

We have recently described the evolution of procedures for subhemispheric epilepsy.[3] Over the past 15 years, the surgical procedure has evolved from anatomical multilobar resection to the introduction of disconnective techniques similar to the development of functional hemispherectomy techniques in hemispheric epilepsy. In the early years, the surgical procedure for this disease was anatomical posterior quadrantectomy, which entails the removal of the temporal, parietal, and occipital lobes. The next step in the evolution was the description of functional posterior quadrantectomy. In this procedure, an extended temporal lobectomy is performed, then the parietooccipital lobe is disconnected. The latest progress in the surgical treatment of subhemispheric epilepsy has been the introduction of peri-insular posterior quadrantectomy (PIPQ). In this surgery, no lobe is resected, and the entire posterior quadrant (temporo-parieto-occipital cortex) is disconnected but remains viable because of the preservation of vessels supplying or draining the disconnected lobes.[3]

■ Anesthetic Considerations

Most patients with intractable subhemispheric epilepsy are children; some are infants.[4] Anesthesia in these situations poses a formidable challenge. Some important consider-

ations are therefore mandatory. Many of these children are often developmentally delayed and uncooperative. They may have carious or loose teeth, gum hypertrophy, enlarged adenoids or tonsils, or cardiac involvement, and all of them will be on one or more seizure medications. Chronic carbamazepine and phenytoin usage is associated with resistance to muscle relaxants and narcotics. Posterior quadrantic surgery is a major, complex, long-duration procedure that can have massive blood loss and fluid shifts. Because the skull of a child is larger in proportion to the body than that of the adult. The scalp and skull are very vascular; massive bleeding may be expected. Therefore, venous access with at least two large bore cannulae should be assured, and meticulous monitoring of oximetry, invasive arterial pressure, central venous pressure, temperature, expired carbon dioxide and anesthetic gases, urine output (indwelling catheter), serial hematocrit, arterial blood gases, electrolytes, and coagulation parameters is required. Continuous intra-arterial blood pressure and central venous pressure monitoring is mandatory because these monitors help in optimizing volume replacement. A depth-of-anesthesia monitor is helpful to measure the level of anesthesia, prevent awareness, and prevent overdose of inhalational or narcotic agents. An ideal anesthetic regime would rapidly induce sleep without interfering with the EEG, provide analgesia when required, provide cerebral protection with a stable ICP, provide hemodynamic stability, and end with a rapid awakening to a safe state when the procedure is finished. The smaller the patient is and the more complex the surgery is, the more difficult it is to manage the blood loss, hemodynamics, and temperature. Isoflurane and sevoflurane with mild hyperventilation may be used. Propofol will produce a consistent reduction in cerebral blood volume and intracronial pressure (ICP). Neuroprotection is best done by ensuring adequate cerebral perfusion. The target for fluid therapy is normovolemia. Normal saline is the commonly used crystalloid, although large volumes of normal saline will cause acidosis. Colloids such as Voluven are an option. The child may tolerate low hematocrit, but, if necessary, transfusion may be started to maintain normal volume. There is also a need to check coagulation profile and get specific blood products like fresh frozen plasma (FFP) and cryoprecipitate, if required, as in cases of massive transfusion. The ambient temperature needs to be kept up with a body warmer, warm intravenous fluids, and airway heat-moisture exchangers.

■ Intraoperative Functional Mapping

Intraoperative electrophysiological monitoring assumes major importance in posterior quadrantic epilepsy surgery because the motor areas need to be identified and preserved, and the area of the brain that is epileptogenic needs to be defined for disconnection or resection.

Electrocorticogram (ECoG) is used mainly to delineate the extent of the epileptogenic foci or to confirm the success of the predetermined resection or disconnection. This is performed using electrodes placed on the surface of the cortex, usually in strip or grid format. The choice of electrodes will depend on the size of the craniotomy (exposed cortex). Localization of the epileptogenic foci will need grid electrodes that are either rectangle or square format; their number can vary between 4 and 64 electrodes. Dedicated intraoperative monitoring machines enable one to do either monopolar or bipolar recording through software control. In posterior quadrantic surgery, ECoG helps in identifying the limits of the epileptogenic zone. However, the practitioner must be cautious when choosing the extent of excision. Primary consideration for excision should be based on clinical factors, MRI, and EEG recordings done in the laboratory preoperatively. The ECoG would only reinforce one's preoperative hypothesis as far as localization of the epileptogenic zone is concerned.

Functional mapping of the cortex assumes great importance in posterior quadrantic epilepsy surgery because of the risk of damaging functional cortices. Although the relationship of the epileptogenic lesion to the central sulcus (CS) can be determined with MRI, the location of the CS during surgery is difficult because of its wide variability and brain shifts. Lesions (atrophic or mass) may shift the CS thus rendering standard surface markings of the CS erroneous. The relationship of the sensorimotor cortex to the superficial venous system is, at best, inconsistent. Based on our earlier study localizing the CS in patients with perirolandic tumors, we have noted that in 13% of cases, large veins were absent in relation to the motor strip and a predominant vein was present over the CS in only 68% of the cases.[5] Despite numerous technological advances in localization of functional cortex such as functional MRI, magnetic encephalography, Wada testing, surgical navigation systems, and intraoperative MRI, electrophysiological methods are still very much in use in the operation theater and in most cases considered the gold standard.

SSEP Localization of CS

The recording of somatosensory evoked potentials (SSEPs) in the operation room is relatively easy. SSEPs are obtained almost independent of anesthetic agents and are not influenced by muscle relaxants.[6] The median nerve contralateral to the lesion is stimulated percutaneously at the wrist, each stimulus being a constant electric square pulse of 200 microseconds at a rate of 4.7/second. Stimulus strength is set above a moderate thumb twitch. Filters are set to 10 Hz and 1000 Hz with notch filter (50 Hz) turned off. Each recording is an average of 100 to 200 responses. Simultaneous recordings are obtained from an array of silver/silver chloride plate electrodes (SLE Ltd., South Croydon, UK). The reference electrode is placed at Fpz (International 10–20 system) and the ground electrode at Erb's point. The electrode array is placed over the exposed cortex, and contact of the electrodes is ensured. The electrode plate is moved in different directions over the probable hand area to get the maximal response at approximately 20-millisecond latency. Studies have suggested that these 20-millisecond potentials originate from area 3b of Brodmann, which is located in the posterior wall of the CS.[7] Of the 20 channel recordings, the 2 channels that show a maximum negative (N20) and a positive (P20) response are chosen. To further confirm the location of the maximum response, the grid electrodes are replaced with two individual disc electrodes. The amplitudes are measured from peak to peak N20/P25 and P20/N25. The gyrus from which the maximum N20 response is recorded is identified as the post central gyrus (primary sensory cortex), and the gyrus just anterior to it is identified as the precentral gyrus (primary motor cortex) from where the P20 response is usually obtained. We have earlier shown that even when patients have mild sensorimotor deficits preoperatively, it is still possible to record a phase reversal, but it is usually of a smaller amplitude.[8] Conversely, if patients have gross sensorimotor deficits, they failed to record a phase reversal. However, in posterior quadrantic epilepsy, this is not of much concern, because no gross motor or sensory deficits exist.

Cortical Stimulation

Conventionally, direct cortical stimulation of motor cortex is used in awake craniotomies, under local anesthesia to localize functional areas. Cortical stimulation can now also be reliably performed under light general anesthesia. We prefer to have the patients induced with pentothal and maintained with 50 to 60% nitrous oxide and 0.4 to 0.5% isoflurane or halothane in oxygen and an infusion of short-acting muscle relaxants. Recently, we have begun using air instead of nitrous oxide because the latter can affect the central conduction and may require a higher current strength to elicit a response. At the time of cortical stimulation, a train-of-four stimuli is delivered to the posterior tibial nerve to assess the extent of neuromuscular blockade, ensuring that at least two twitches are obtained. This is to make sure that motor responses are elicited when the cortex is directly stimulated electrically. Usually, bipolar electrodes are used for cortical stimulation. Biphasic square pulses are delivered at 60 Hz. Taniguchi et al used anodal rectangular pulses at a higher rate of stimuli to deliver a lesser amount of current for eliciting cortical responses.[9] They showed that increasing the stimulating intensity increased the number of pulses per train or the duration of each pulse, thus increasing the amplitude of the muscle responses. The optimal frequency for stimulation to elicit a large response was 500 Hz. In our practice, monopolar, monophasic anodal stimulations are delivered at 50 Hz. Each square pulse is of 200 microseconds. A maximum current of 15 mA is used. The majority of motor responses to cortical stimulation could be elicited within 12 mA of current. Because of the large representation of hand area, more often, one encounters movements of the fingers compared with other body parts. Primary motor areas are characterized by fractionated movement of the digits, whereas multiple joint movements are characteristic feature of supplementary motor areas. The common reasons for not being able to identify the CS, besides the reasons mentioned previously, are (a) the craniotomy exposes only the primary motor gyrus or sensory gyrus but not both; (b) the craniotomy does not include the hand area for SSEPs, hence no phase reversal is seen; (c) high levels of anesthetic agents suppress central conduction; (d) muscle relaxant causes neuromuscular blockage; and (e) patient has gross sensory motor deficits. Our experience has shown that in two thirds of cases, it is possible to elicit motor responses and when used in conjunction with SSEP, localization of the CS would be possible in nearly 100% of cases.

■ Operative Technique of Peri-Insular Posterior Quadrantectomy (PIPQ) and Its Functional Neuroanatomy

The surgery is performed under general anesthesia. The patient is placed in the supine position with the head fixed on the Mayfield (Integra, Plainsboro, NJ) three-pin fixation system and is turned to the opposite side and minimally extended. In small children and infants, the head rests on a soft headrest and is taped. The ipsilateral shoulder is elevated using a cushion. The incision is a "barn-door" incision with the anterior and posterior limbs ending at the zygoma and transverse sinus, respectively. The medial part of the incision extends to approximately 1.5 cm from the midline. After elevation of the bone flap, the dura can be opened based either superiorly or inferiorly. A good exposure of the opercular cortices and the central area (perirolandic) is essential for the surgery. The surgery is tailored to encompass the whole epileptogenic lesion and to avoid the central region, which is still functional **(Fig. 23.2)**. The primary motor and sensory cortices are identified and recognized from scrupulous study of the MRI and correlation with intraoperative surface anatomy, based on gyral pattern, arteries, and veins. The identification of the functional cortex is also aided by electrophysiological means under

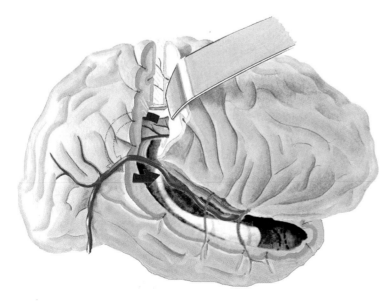

Fig. 23.2 Diagrammatic representation of peri-insular posterior quadrantectomy. The infra-insular window and the intraparietal disconnection have been demonstrated with the preservation of arteries and veins supplying/draining the disconnected cortices. The curved (*solid black and dotted*) arrow depicts the posterior callosotomy and hippocampotomy (section of fornix). The *dotted areas* in the temporal horn anteriorly depict the excision of the anterior hippocampus and amygdala.

general anesthesia before the resection or disconnection. This identification maximizes both the extent of resection or disconnection and the safety of surgery. This in turn provides the best chance of complete seizure relief, a fact that is well supported by several reports in literature.[10-15]

Stage I: Infra-Insular Window and Mesial Temporal Resection

The pia mater over the superior temporal gyrus (T1) is coagulated approximately 5 to 8 mm from the sylvian fissure. This is continued from its most anterior aspect to posterior. The temporal opercular cortex is then removed subpially. The resection of this cortex and white matter is continued until the whole inferior half of the insula can be seen through the pia. Care should be taken to preserve as many of the arteries and veins while the pial incision on T1 is made, and therefore the infra-insular window may be broken at many places by these vessels vascularizing the lateral temporal lobe. This resection would provide access to the whole length of the inferior circular cistern. At this point, the white matter is incised along the length of the circular cistern with bipolar coagulation and suction in a plane slightly oblique to the sulcus, heading toward the temporal horn of the lateral ventricle **(Fig. 23.3A)**. Once the ventricle is entered at one point, it becomes easier to open the whole temporal horn of the ventricle, extending it anteriorly and posteriorly. The amygdala is identified in the anteromedial part of the opened ventricle and is then resected along with the subpial removal of the uncus. The superior extent of the amygdalar resection is stopped at the level corresponding to the roof of the temporal horn. The anterior part of the hippocampus extending up to the choroid fissure is excised subpially.

Functional Neuroanatomy

Incision of the whole length of the inferior limb of the internal capsule (thus exposing the ventricle from the tip of the temporal horn to the atrium of the lateral ventricle) disconnects the ascending and descending fibers proceeding to the sublentiform and retrolentiform parts of the internal capsule along with the connection of these lobes to the basal ganglia and the insula. At this stage of the surgery, there remain some epileptogenic structures that need to be addressed: (1) the hippocampus through its connections proceeding along the fimbria-fornix that form the main output of the temporal lobe; (2) the amygdalar complex through its connections via the stria terminalis and projections to the basal ganglia, thalamus, hypothalamus, and brainstem; (3) the anterior temporal and paralimbic cortex through the posterior limb of the anterior commissure; and (4) the insular cortex with its projections to the basal ganglia, thalamus, hypothalamus, and brainstem. The outflow from the hippocampus passes through the fornix and is interrupted during the hippocampotomy (fornix section) at the junction of the tail of the hippocampus and fornix; this step is usually performed after the splenial callosotomy is done **(Fig. 23.2)**. Because of the degree of anatomical and functional relationship of the anterior hippocampus and amygdalar complex, anterior hippocampectomy and amygdalectomy are performed to eliminate all possible influence from the residual medial temporal structures through the anterior commissure. The insula could be resected when clearly indicated, which entails facing an increased risk of motor-sensory deficit. We believe that when there are no clear indications that the insula is contributory to the epilepsy, it is better left intact.

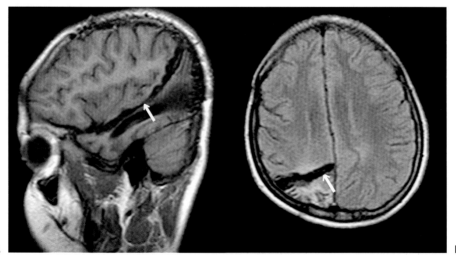

A   B

Fig. 23.3 Postoperative magnetic resonance imaging (MRI) of the patient shown in **Fig. 23.1**. Sagittal T1-weighted MRI **(A)** shows the site of the disconnection of the temporal, parietal and occipital lobes (*solid white arrow*). Axial fluid attenuated inversion recovery (FLAIR) MRI **(B)** shows the intraparietal disconnection (*solid white arrow*).

Stage II: Parietooccipital Disconnection

This stage of the surgery that deals with the disconnection of the posterior temporal, parietal, and occipital lobes and is subdivided into four distinct steps **(Fig. 23.3B)**:

- Step 1 (posterior perisylvian window): Incision in the T1 gyrus is continued posteriorly taking care to preserve the vein of Labbé and the M4 branches supplying the lobes. Reference to ventricular anatomy as the temporal horn joins the atrium makes it possible to identify the parietal opercular cortex. The opercular cortex here is aspirated, the circular cistern exposed, and the white matter is incised to reach the atrium and the posterior part of the body of the ventricle.
- Step 2 (intraparietal disconnection): The cortical incision in the parietal operculum is taken diagonally superiorly just posterior to the postcentral gyrus. The white matter along the whole length of the incision is deepened to reach the tissue along the falx, and the disconnection is done up to the pia along the falx to reach the sagittal sinus superiorly and the level of the corpus callosum inferiorly.
- Step 3 (posterior callosotomy): The incision that has reached the corpus callosum and opened the ventricle is curved posteriorly in an intraventricular parasagittal plane, and all fibers entering the posterior corpus callosum are interrupted. This would interrupt all the parietooccipital commissural fibers as they reach the corpus callosum.
- Step 4 (posterior hippocampotomy): From the limit of the splenial disconnection, the tissue in the medial ventricular wall is incised anteriorly to reach the fornix, which is found anteroinferior to the splenium. The fornix is then incised here to disconnect the hippocampus. The incision exposing the medial pia has to reach the choroidal fissure to ensure complete hippocampotomy.

Functional Neuroanatomy

Extension of the infra-insular window by removing a small part of the parietal operculum and incising the circular cistern onto its superior limb interrupts the white matter fibers connecting the posterior parietal lobe going to the posterior limb of the internal capsule. At the end of the creation of the peri-insular window, the temporal, posterior parietal, and occipital lobes have the following anatomical connections that persist: (1) cortico-cortico connections from the posterior parietal and occipital lobes via the long and short arcuate fibers to anterior cortices; (2) connections from the temporal lobe to frontal lobe through the arcuate fasciculus; (3) anatomical continuity through the cingulum; and (4) commissural fibers linking the temporal, posterior

parietal, and occipital lobes through the corpus callosum to homologous cortices in the normal hemisphere. The intraparietal disconnection at the convexity and parasagittal levels interrupts connections 1, 2, and 3 (listed previously) and functionally isolates the temporal, posterior parietal, and occipital lobes from the central and frontal regions. The intraventricular parasagittal callosotomy disconnects the commissural connections of these lobes via the posterior part of corpus callosum. At the end of both stages of the surgery, the temporo-parieto-occipital cortices are completely isolated from the ipsilateral frontal and central cortices, projection fiber systems, and basal ganglia. They are also disconnected from the contra lateral structures **(Fig. 23.4)**.

The mesial temporal resection cavity and the rest of the ventricle are irrigated, and all debris is flushed out. A drain is inserted into the opened ventricle. After careful hemostasis, the dura is completely closed and the wound is closed in layers over a subgaleal drain. The average duration of this surgical procedure in our series was 6 hours, and the average blood loss was 400 mL. Anticonvulsants are continued at the same dosages as the preoperative state. The subgaleal drain is usually removed the day after the surgery, whereas the intraventricular drain is kept for 3 to 4 days until the cerebrospinal fluid draining from the

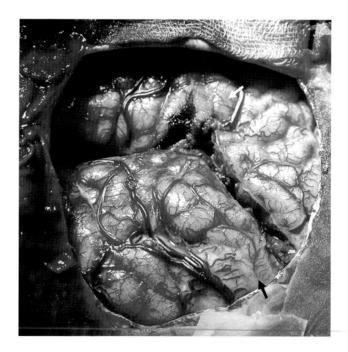

Fig. 23.4 Intraoperative photograph shows the exposed cortices along with the infra-insular window and intraparietal disconnection. The lobes marked with a *solid white arrow* have been completely disconnected functionally but remain anatomically intact and viable by preservation of vessels. The *solid black arrow* depicts the site of the central sulcus and the preserved perirolandic cortices.

ventricle becomes clear. Mild fever can be expected in the postoperative period, and antibiotic therapy is not usually necessary.

Operative Technique of Anatomical Posterior Quadrantectomy

This surgery was the procedure of choice in the past. The craniotomy needs to be larger than that described for PIPQ, because this surgery requires the removal of a massive amount of brain inclusive of the entire epileptogenic lesion. This surgery is performed in two major stages, which are subdivided into different steps.

Stage I: Extended Temporal Lobectomy

This stage consists of an extended anterior temporal lobectomy, including resection of the mesial temporal structures, and is subdivided into the following steps:

- Step 1: A cortical incision is made in the T1 gyrus extending to 5 cm from the temporal tip or up to the vein of Labbé. The T1 gyrus is then excised subpially, which exposes the inferior half of the circular cistern and the insula.
- Step 2: A posterior diagonal incision is made from the posterior end of the incision of Step 1 across T2 and T3 gyrii up to the collateral sulcus. This incision is made diagonally so that approximately 7 cm of the T3 gyrus is included in the excision. This incision is deepened through the white matter with reference to both the collateral sulcus inferiorly and the circular cistern superiorly, so that the incision reaches up to the ependyma of the temporal horn.
- Step 3 (neocortical resection): There are two parts to this step: the opening of the temporal horn and the neocortical resection.
  - The ventricle is entered posteriorly at the junction of incisions in Step 1 and 2. The ventricle is then opened from back to front up to the tip of the temporal horn by incision of the white matter between the temporal horn and the inferior aspect of the insula. This can either be done with aspiration or the bipolar, transecting the tissue.
  - An incision is made into the ventricular wall directed toward the collateral sulcus, which is visualized on the basal temporal surface. This incision is deepened through the white matter up to the pia on the basal temporal lobe, lateral to the parahippocampal gyrus. This pia is then coagulated and incised. The lateral temporal neocortex is then removed en bloc.

- Step 4 (mesial temporal resection)
  - The amygdala is identified in the anteromedial part of the opened ventricle and is then resected along with the subpial removal of the uncus. The superior extent of the amygdalar resection is stopped at the level corresponding to the roof of the temporal horn, making sure that pia is preserved and present on its medial side.
  - The hippocampus and the parahippocampal gyrus are excised subpially to the fimbria-fornix at the level of the trigone.

Stage II: Parietooccipital Lobectomy

En bloc resection of the parietal and occipital lobes is done after the temporal lobectomy. Anatomical landmarks and electrophysiological mapping (as described with PIPQ technique) guide the identification of the anterior limit of the parietal incision. The opercular cortices in the posterior parietal and posterior temporal regions are excised and the posterosuperior aspect of the circular cistern is exposed. An incision is made in the cortex just behind the post central gyrus, aiming at the lateral ventricle, taking into consideration the location of the posterior part of the temporal horn or trigone. This will correspond to a plane behind the thalamus. The ventricle is opened up to its roof, and the dissection on the medial wall-roof of the ventricle is extended to the midline, and the white matter is deepened to reach the tissue along the falx. The pia along the falx is exposed from the lateral approach, up to the sagittal sinus. The bridging veins from these lobes are coagulated and divided. The corpus callosum is identified, and the fibers entering it from the posterior aspects are interrupted, ensuring complete section of the splenium. This completes the resection of the parietal and occipital lobes, and the specimen is removed.

Complication Avoidance in Posterior Quadrantic Surgery

Surgery for posterior quadrantic epilepsy can have various complications. Most complications associated with hemispherotomy can occur in this procedure as well. In general, the risk of occurrence of these complications are less with disconnective procedures than with resective posterior quadrantic surgery. In the pediatric population, great care relative to blood loss and replacement is mandatory to avoid complications related to hypovolemia and coagulopathy. As opposed to resective surgery, disconnective posterior quadrantic surgery leaves behind a large volume of vascularized brain. It is thus essential that as many arteries and veins be preserved to lower the risk of hemorrhagic infarct and brain swelling, which have been reported earlier with hemispherotomy especially in cases with no or minimal atrophy. This may lead to increased intracranial pressure and its consequences in the postoperative period.[16] Excessive ventricular drainage of cerebrospinal fluid may also lead to hemorrhages that are distant from the operative site.[16] This can be avoided by meticulous measurement of cerebrospinal fluid drainage in the postoperative period. The incidence of early and late hydrocephalus should be lowered by reducing spillage of blood in the ventricles, using cottons to fill the ventricles as soon as possible; copious irrigation of the ventricular cavities and operative field will also contribute to prevent hydrocephalus. When the ventricular size is small, as in Sturge-Weber syndrome and dysplasias, a clear understanding of the surgical anatomy of disconnective procedures is mandatory to avoid complications and assure complete disconnection.

■ Outcome of Posterior Quadrantic Epilepsy Surgery

Surgical results for subhemispheric epilepsy (and especially for posterior quadrant epilepsy) in literature are difficult to interpret because there are few studies that focus on this subgroup of epilepsy surgery. Most centers have included the results of these surgeries along with lobar resections. Leiphart et al reported on a cohort of 111 pediatric patients after lobar or multilobar surgery that also included

tumors.[17] This group also included 24 patients with large posterior quadrantic lesions. The exact seizure outcome of this group has not been quantified, but the authors found that the results for multilobar resections were inferior to single lobar resections. However, this effect was not significant when the temporal resections were removed from the single lobe resection group. Koszewski et al obtained Engel's Class I results (seizure free or rare seizures) in 53% patients among a group of 93 patients with multilobar resections (all locations with two or more lobes).[18] The factors associated with a better outcome were radical removal, age older than 18, focal EEG abnormalities, and single seizure type. The perioperative mortality in this series was 3%. In our series of posterior quadrantic epilepsy surgery, Engel's Class I outcome was obtained in 92% of patients.[3] There was no mortality or significant morbidity in this series. Consequent to seizure freedom, the quality of life markedly improved, and antiepileptic medication could be stopped in the majority of patients. All children in this series showed "catch up" of cognitive measures and returned to full-time schooling. The hyperactive and aggressive behavior seen in many of these children stopped with the seizure control achieved after surgery. Although clear explanations do not exist, some patients show superior cognitive improvement to others. Even if cognition does not markedly improve, the progressive cognitive deterioration seen in children (before surgery) is arrested with good seizure control, and the brain is given an optimal environment for achieving its entire psychosocial development potential.

References

1. D'Agostino MD, Bastos A, Piras C, et al. Posterior quadrantic dysplasia or hemi-hemimegalencephaly: a characteristic brain malformation. Neurology 2004;62(12):2214–2220
2. Villemure JG, Peacock W. Multilobar resections and hemispherectomy. In: Engel J Jr, Pedley TA, eds. Epilepsy: A Comprehensive Textbook. Philadelphia, PA: Lippincott-Raven; 1997:1829–1839
3. Daniel RT, Meagher-Villemure K, Farmer JP, Andermann F, Villemure JG. Posterior quadrantic epilepsy surgery: technical variants, surgical anatomy, and case series. Epilepsia 2007;48(8):1429–1437
4. Daniel RT, Meagher-Villemure K, Roulet E, Villemure JG. Surgical treatment of temporoparietooccipital cortical dysplasia in infants: report of two cases. Epilepsia 2004;45(7):872–876
5. Chandy MJ, Babu KS. Surgery of perirolandic mass lesions with central sulcus mapping. Neurol India 1997;45:14–19
6. Broughton R, Rasmussen T, Branch C. Scalp and direct cortical recordings of somatosensory evoked potentials in man (circa 1967). Can J Psychol 1981;35(2):136–158
7. Allison T, McCarthy G, Wood CC, Jones SJ. Potentials evoked in human and monkey cerebral cortex by stimulation of the median nerve. A review of scalp and intracranial recordings. Brain 1991; 114(Pt 6):2465–2503

8. Babu KS, Chandy MJ. Reliability of somatosensory evoked potentials in intraoperative localization of the central sulcus in patients with perirolandic mass lesions. Br J Neurosurg 1997;11(5):411–417
9. Taniguchi M, Cedzich C, Schramm J. Modification of cortical stimulation for motor evoked potentials under general anesthesia: technical description. Neurosurgery 1993;32(2):219–226
10. Fried I, Cascino GD. Lesional surgery. In: Engel J Jr, ed. Surgical Treatment of the Epilepsies. 2nd ed. New York, NY: Raven Press; 1993:154–164
11. Ojemann GA. Intraoperative tailoring of temporal lobe resections. In: Engel J Jr, ed. Surgical Treatment of the Epilepsies. 2nd ed. New York, NY: Raven Press; 1993:481–488
12. Palmini A, Andermann F, Olivier A, Tampieri D, Robitaille Y. Focal neuronal migration disorders and intractable partial epilepsy: results of surgical treatment. Ann Neurol 1991;30(6):750–757
13. Palmini A, Gambardella A, Andermann F, et al. Operative strategies for patients with cortical dysplastic lesions and intractable epilepsy. Epilepsia 1994;35:S57–S71
14. Polkey CE. Preoperative tailoring of temporal lobe resection. In: Engel J Jr, ed. Surgical Treatment of the Epilepsies. 2nd ed. New York, NY: Raven Press; 1993:473–480

15. Rasmussen TB. Commentary: extratemporal cortical excisions and hemispherectomy. In: Engel J Jr, ed. Surgical Treatment of the Epilepsies. 2nd ed. New York, NY: Raven Press; 1993:417–424

16. Daniel RT, Villemure JG. Peri-insular hemispherotomy: potential pitfalls and avoidance of complications. Stereotact Funct Neurosurg 2003;80(1-4):22–27

17. Leiphart JW, Peacock WJ, Mathern GW. Lobar and multilobar resections for medically intractable pediatric epilepsy. Pediatr Neurosurg 2001;34(6):311–318

18. Koszewski W, Czarkwiani L, Bidziński J. Multilobar resections in surgical treatment of medically intractable epilepsy. Neurol Neurochir Pol 1998;32(suppl 2):81–94

24 Hemispherectomy and Hemispherotomy Techniques in Pediatric Epilepsy Surgery: An Overview

Oğuz Çataltepe

Hemispherectomy is the most effective surgical intervention in the management of children with unilateral hemispheric epilepsy. Since Krynauw's successful application of this technique for children with infantile hemiplegia in 1950,[1] hemispherectomy has been used in the surgical management of hemispheric epilepsy, with remarkably high cure rates. This surgical technique was originally called *anatomical hemispherectomy* and involved the removal of the entire abnormal hemisphere.[2] Since then, there have been many variations and modifications of the hemispherectomy procedure, all characterized by the gradual reduction of the volume of resected brain tissue while still achieving complete disconnection of the entire hemisphere. The first effective application of this concept was defined by Rasmussen[3] in the 1970s and called *functional hemispherectomy*. Rasmussen's functional hemispherectomy technique was further developed by the next generation of neurosurgeons, whose modifications further reduced the resection volume. In the 1990s, *hemispherotomy* techniques were developed to disconnect all neuronal fibers and to functionally isolate the damaged hemisphere without much cortical resection.[4–7]

The evolution of hemispheric surgical interventions from anatomic hemispherectomy to hemispherotomy is a fascinating chapter of pediatric epilepsy surgery. Here, we will summarize the development of these techniques and review their indications and applications in pediatric epilepsy surgery. Subsequent chapters will provide additional information about and in-depth descriptions of the main variations of hemispherectomy and hemispherotomy techniques.

■ Hemispheric Epilepsy Surgery: From Resection to Disconnection

Hemispherectomy, or resection of an entire hemisphere, was first performed by Dandy[2] in 1928 in a hemispheric glioma patient. In 1938, Canadian neurosurgeon McKenzie[8,9] used the hemispherectomy technique for the first time in the treatment of epilepsy in a patient with infantile hemiplegia. A report on the first hemispherectomy series in epilepsy patients (12 children with infantile hemiplegia) was published by Krynauw[1] in 1950. Krynauw's report popularized the procedure for the next two decades.

However, several reports regarding delayed, life-threatening complications in hemispherectomy patients were published in the late 1960s. After the publication of Oppenheimer and Griffith's report[10] in 1966 and subsequent descriptions of superficial cerebral hemosiderosis in postmortem studies,[3,5] anatomic hemispherectomy was almost completely abandoned. These reports motivated neurosurgeons to develop new strategies, some of which were effective, some of which were unsuccessful. Several new techniques to modify or replace anatomical hemispherectomy were described, including hemidecortication, modified anatomical hemispherectomy, and functional hemispherectomy.

According to Villemure and Daniel,[11] this search led to the development of the hemispherotomy techniques in use today. These techniques represent the latest stage in the conceptual and technical evolution of functional hemispherectomy. Further details regarding the historical evolution of hemispherectomy can be found in Chapter 25.

■ Epilepsy Syndromes Associated with Hemispheric Lesions

Hemispherectomy is an effective surgical procedure in hemispheric epilepsy syndromes. The typical candidate for hemispherectomy is a patient with hemiplegia secondary to a unilaterally damaged hemisphere that is the result of a congenital or acquired lesion. The most common conditions causing hemispheric epilepsy are generally seen in infants with catastrophic epilepsy, such as infantile spasms, hemiconvulsion-hemiplegia-epilepsy (HHE) syndrome, Sturge-Weber syndrome, hemimegalencephaly, multilobar cortical dysplasia, and congenital hemiplegia from a perinatal infarction. In addition, some acquired conditions may cause intractable hemispheric epilepsy, such as Rasmussen syndrome, late ischemic events, and trauma-related hemispheric injuries.

Infantile Spasms

Infantile spasms are almost entirely seen in the first year of life and are associated with developmental delay, regression, and medically refractory seizures. They present with a typical electroencephalographic (EEG) pattern: hypsarrhythmia. Seizures in infantile spasms are seen in clusters, occur even during sleep, and cause exhaustion and lethargy. Various types of myoclonic seizures, such as flexor and extensor spasms with a cry, are seen and are followed by a brief episode of akinesia. The seizures generally disappear within 5 years—50% before 3 years of age, 90% before 5 years of age. Many conditions can cause infantile spasms, such as neurocutaneous syndromes, congenital brain malformations, metabolic and degenerative diseases, and hypoxicischemic insults.[12]

Hemiconvulsion-Hemiplegia-Epilepsy Syndrome

HHE syndrome is most frequently seen within the first 2 years of life. The initial phase of the syndrome presents with unilateral, prolonged hemiconvulsive seizures that involve the face, arms, and legs. The second phase is characterized by hemiplegia, and the third phase is characterized by partial epileptic seizures. The syndrome progresses to chronic epilepsy within 1 to 2 years. Although there are many possible causes for HHE syndrome, including meningitis, subdural effusions, trauma, and hemispheric lesions, in many cases, no cause can be determined. The etiology of this condition is still poorly understood. In the course of the disease, hemiatrophia cerebri develops gradually after hemiconvulsive seizures and hemiplegia.[12,13]

Sturge-Weber Syndrome

Sturge-Weber syndrome is a progressive neurocutaneous disorder associated with pial angiomatosis involving the cerebral cortex, along with a cutaneous angioma in the trigeminal nerve territory on the face and scalp. Facial angioma (port wine stain) is seen in 90% of cases. Facial and leptomeningeal angiomas occur mostly uni- and ipsilaterally but can also be seen bilaterally in up to 20% of patients. Pial angiomatosis mostly involves the parietooccipital region, but it can be extensive and may involve the entire hemisphere in some cases.

Sturge-Weber patients have a very peculiar leptomeningeal vascular bed, with hypertrophic pial vessels and frequently absent major venous sinuses and cortical bridging veins. This peculiar vascular anatomy creates a strong retrograde venous flow into the ventricle. This abnormal hemodynamic induces hypoxia in the surrounding brain tissue because of the diversion of cerebral blood flow away from the parenchyma and associated venous stasis. This abnormal blood circulation eventually causes cellular damage in the brain parenchyma and secondary seizures.

The most common symptoms in Sturge-Weber patients are seizure (75–90%), developmental delay, hemiparesis, and various ophthalmologic problems, such as glaucoma and optic atrophy. Seizures are usually the earliest symptoms in Sturge-Weber patients, with 70% of patients experiencing seizures in the first year of life. Seizures may even occur during the newborn period. If the seizures start in infancy, the prognosis is guarded. Most seizures are simple/complex partial seizures, with frequent secondary generalization, and are often unresponsive to medications (only 10% respond well to medications). Patients may develop hemiplegia after an episode of serial seizures in the first year of life. Therefore, vigorous treatment is essential to prevent postconvulsive damage during infancy. Although hemispherectomy is the main treatment modality in Sturge-Weber patients with severe epilepsy and should be considered after diagnosis, but waiting until a child is 1 year old before proceeding to surgery may be also a reasonable approach in some cases to prove the intractability of the seizures.[12–15]

Hemimegalencephaly

Hemimegalencephaly is an extensive neuronal migrational disorder involving the entire hemisphere. This abnormal, unilaterally enlarged hemisphere generally has no cortical lamination; a wide, thickened, and flattened cortex; and shallow gyri. Other abnormal histological and radiological findings include reduced number of sulci, reduced white matter volume, subcortical heterotopia, calcifications, poor gray–white matter differentiation, hypoplastic corpus callosum, and an ipsilaterally enlarged or shrunken ventricle. The frontal and occipital lobes in an abnormal hemisphere are frequently hyperplastic, unlike the hypoplastic temporal lobe.

Hemimegalencephaly can be seen as an isolated entity or may be associated with Klippel-Trenaunay syndrome, hypomelanosis of Ito, linear nervous sebaceous of Jadassohn, or Proteus syndrome. Medically intractable seizures are the most common finding and generally start during infancy. Severe epileptic encephalopathy and developmental delay are common in these patients. If the seizures are not well controlled, patients may develop hemiparesis, hemianopia, and mental retardation. High mortality rates in the first months of life are seen in these patients because of the continuous seizures.[12,13,16]

Cortical Dysplasia

Unilateral multilobar or extensive cortical dysplasia is another congenital condition associated with medically refractory epilepsy in early childhood. Hemispherectomy or multilobar resections are frequently the best treatment options for these patients. Further information about this condition can be found in Chapter 22.

Rasmussen Syndrome

Rasmussen syndrome is a chronic encephalitis that is characterized by intractable epilepsy and progressive atrophy in one hemisphere. The syndrome was first described by Rasmussen in 1958. Although seizures in Rasmussen syndrome frequently start with a generalized tonic–clonic seizure, they usually continue as partial epilepsy.

Rasmussen syndrome is a progressive disease that causes hemiplegia in the majority of cases. The results of initial imaging studies are normal, but follow-up imaging studies reveal unilateral ventricular enlargement, followed by hyperintense changes and, finally, focal atrophy in the primary sensorimotor cortex and insula. Mesial temporal involvement in these cases is frequently seen very late, and occipital involvement is seen even later.[13,17,18] Further information about Rasmussen syndrome can be found in Chapter 26.

Porencephalic Cyst

Perinatal vascular insults, such as internal cerebral artery and middle cerebral artery infarcts, intracerebral hemorrhage secondary to arteriovenous malformations and congenital coagulopathies, and traumatic brain injuries can cause large, hemispheric porencephalic cysts.[14,17] These patients frequently have unilaterally enlarged ventricles and severe brain atrophy secondary to extensive tissue loss, with large porencephalic cystic areas. Medically intractable seizures and hemiplegia are frequent findings in these patients, who are ideal candidates for hemispherectomy and, especially, hemispherotomy procedures.

■ Preoperative Assessment

Hemispherectomy is a very extensive surgical intervention with dramatic and gratifying results. However, it is associated with significant morbidity and mortality risks. Therefore, preoperative assessment of patients to select ideal candidates is of utmost importance.

Preoperative assessment of hemispherectomy candidates should include the following questions: Is the patient's condition medically intractable? Does the patient's clinical status justify such an extensive procedure? Are the patient's electrophysiological findings strongly suggestive of a unilat-

eral hemispheric origin of seizures? Do structural and functional imaging studies show unilateral hemispheric damage? Is the contralateral hemisphere structurally, functionally, and electrographically healthy? Do the patient and family fully understand the extent of the intervention, the associated risks, and potential results? Does the patient have reliable family support?

The epilepsy surgery team should determine the answers of these questions using available preoperative assessment tools, tests, and techniques. If the answers are affirmative, then the patient is deemed an acceptable surgical candidate for hemispherectomy.

Medical Intractability

As in all epilepsy surgery cases, the first step in preoperative assessment is determining the intractability of the seizures. Although some patients may require extensive trials to prove that the seizures are intractable, children who have seizures secondary to hemispheric lesions rarely need exhaustive trials to prove medical intractability. Determining the intractability of seizures to major antiepileptic drugs (AEDs) may be relatively easy in patients with hemispheric lesions, such as Rasmussen syndrome, Sturge-Weber syndrome, and cortical dysplasia because of the very nature of these conditions. Conversely, patients with other conditions may require more time and effort to document the intractability of their seizures.

Clinical Status

The ideal candidate for hemispherectomy is a medically intractable epilepsy patient with hemiplegia and hemianopsia secondary to unilateral hemispheric damage. However, if the patient has no motor weakness or has only mild hemiparesis and partial hemianopsia, surgery will provide good seizure control, with the price being impairment of the patient's neurological status. The decision for surgery in these patients is not straightforward, and opinions about the suitability of these patients are frequently controversial. Nevertheless, some of these patients may be selected as surgical candidates for hemispherectomy because of the severity of their seizures and the debilitating effect of these seizures on the functional status of these patients.

Certain progressive conditions, such as Rasmussen syndrome, have a well-known natural course that eventually results in motor and cognitive worsening. Patients with catastrophic infantile epilepsy syndromes may present with hundreds of daily seizures, resulting in no functional life; these seizures pose a very high risk of damage to the developing brain. Even if these patients do not have hemiplegia, they may still be considered candidates for hemispherectomy procedure because early surgery may prevent an eventual decline in cognitive function and psychomotor development.[5,15–19]

■ Physical Examination

Patients with unilateral hemispheric damage generally have significant distal extremity weakness but relatively good proximal strength. Upper extremity weakness is also more pronounced than lower extremity weakness in these patients. Shoulder function is generally good, with a normal range of elbow movements; patients can lift their arms up to shoulder level horizontally. However, wrist function is typically minimal, and fine finger movements are absent.

In the lower extremities, these patients have good proximal strength, with good major joint movements but no toe movements. The vast majority of these patients have a variable degree of spasticity, but they walk quite comfortably, either independently or with help.[5,13] The most likely reason for differences in proximal and distal function in the extremities is the respective locations in the brain controlling these functions. Although fine finger movements and repeated alternating movements, such as finger–thumb oppositions and foot tapping, are mainly cortical functions, gross motor movements, such as major joint movements, originate from subcortical structures, with ipsilateral motor participation as well.[11] Therefore, distal impairment in these patients is much more pronounced than proximal impairment.

Another major neurological deficit in these patients is hemianopsia. Detailed ophthalmologic examination of these patients is important, both to assess the baseline status of vision and to counsel the parents preoperatively. In addition, some of the syndromes causing unilateral hemispheric damage may also be associated with other ophthalmologic findings, such as retinal damage, extraocular muscle weakness, and optic pathway damage. It is also very important in these patients to verify preoperatively that the visual field deficit is not bilateral.[13] However, ophthalmologic examination may not be feasible in many children because of their age or developmental status.

Electroencephalographic Assessment

Preoperative ictal and interictal EEG studies help to verify the unilaterality and determine the extent of the epileptogenic zone. Determining the extent of the epileptogenic zone is especially important for deciding whether a hemispherectomy is needed or whether a limited cortical resection will suffice. Most important, it should be preoperatively proven that a patient's seizures are unilateral and the epileptogenic zone is contained within the damaged hemisphere.

Predictors of a good outcome in these patients are the presence of ipsilateral suppression of electrical activity associated with multifocal epileptogenic abnormalities confined to the damaged hemisphere, bilateral synchronous discharges spreading from the abnormal hemisphere without contralateral slowing, and the absence of generalized discharges, bilateral independent spiking, and abnormal

background activity in the "good" hemisphere. Sporadic epileptiform activities, some abnormal secondary or independent EEG findings, and nonepileptiform abnormalities in the "good" hemisphere that are seen in some patients do not exclude those patients as candidates for hemispherectomy but may imply an unfavorable outcome, especially if independent interictal sharp wave activity in the "good" hemisphere is present.[13,14,17,20]

Structural Imaging

Anatomical imaging, mainly magnetic resonance imaging (MRI), provides detailed structural information about the damaged hemisphere to help the neurosurgeon determine the etiology and extent of the lesion, assess the integrity of the "good" hemisphere, and visualize the anatomical details of the damaged hemisphere before deciding on the most appropriate surgical technique for the patient. Anatomical details, such as ventricle size; the shape and depth of the sylvian fissure; displacement and distortion of anatomical landmarks; the thickness of the corpus callosum; surface anatomy, including cortical thickness and sulcal depth; and the severity of parenchymal atrophy are of utmost significance for the neurosurgeon. Knowledge of these details helps the neurosurgeon to visualize the patient's anatomy in three dimensions and preoperatively design the best surgical strategy.

Some findings, such as the presence of atrophy in the ipsilateral cerebral peduncle and medulla, are also helpful to predict a lower risk for postoperative worsening.[11] Conversely, other abnormal MRI findings, such as hyperintense areas in the deep gray nuclei in the "good" hemisphere, may imply mitochondrial or metabolic disease; surgical determinations in these cases should be made very carefully. Positron emission tomography (PET) scans may also be helpful for further assessment of these cases. Magnetic resonance venography is a valuable tool, especially in Sturge-Weber patients, enhancing understanding of venous drainage patterns. If needed, cerebral angiography also should be performed in these patients.[5,11,13,14,16]

Functional Imaging

Functional imaging provides information about the extent and location of functionally damaged areas, shifted locations of some cortical functions, metabolic status of the "good" hemisphere, and expected postoperative outcome. The most commonly used techniques to assess the functional status of the brain are functional MRI, PET, and single photon emission computed tomography (SPECT) scans. If the hypometabolic areas and epileptogenic zones are contained within the damaged hemisphere, this is interpreted as a good predictor. If hypometabolism is also seen in the "good" hemisphere, this is interpreted as a warning for more extensive involvement. Further details regarding these studies and their application in the preoperative assessment of patients can be found elsewhere in this book.[13,14,16]

Wada Test

The Wada test is important for verifying that the "good" hemisphere can carry on speech and memory functions satisfactorily after surgical disconnection of the damaged hemisphere is performed. However, the Wada test is not always feasible in children because of their age and developmental status. It should be emphasized that the Wada test should be performed only on the damaged hemisphere, not on the "good" hemisphere, to avoid any risk of ischemic injury to the latter.[13,14,16] Further information regarding the Wada test and its application can be found in Chapter 12.

Neuropsychological Evaluation

Neuropsychological evaluation is a routine part of the preoperative assessment of epilepsy surgical candidates. It is especially helpful in hemispherectomy candidates because one hemisphere in these patients is already severely damaged, and determining the function level of the "good" hemisphere provides critical information.

Neuropsychological assessment is performed to determine the baseline level of cognitive function status to locate certain cortical functions, to describe the extent and location of functional impairment, and to counsel parents regarding postoperative expectations. Early shift of language function is frequently seen in patients with early severe hemispheric damage. Complete lateralization of speech is acquired by the age of 5 years; thereafter, a complete shift of the speech function is very difficult. Therefore, the age of the patient at the time of hemispheric insult is critical for postoperative recovery of the speech function. In addition to age, other factors, such as the site of damage, the extent and severity of epileptogenic activities, and progression of the disease, are critical in the shifting of the speech function. A finding of severe cognitive impairment on neuropsychological assessment may imply diffuse, bilateral hemispheric involvement or structural or electrophysiological abnormality and may suggest a poor prognosis.[5,11,14,15,17]

■ Surgical Planning

If the preoperative assessment verifies that the patient is a good candidate for hemispherectomy, the following new questions will need to be addressed: What is the goal of surgery? What is the best time for surgery? What is the best hemispheric surgical approach? What is the expected seizure outcome and neurological status? And, finally, do the patient and family accept the associated risks?

The goal of surgery in pediatric epilepsy surgery is not only controlling seizures but also protecting the immature brain from the deleterious effects of seizures and AEDs during its most vulnerable period. The impact of ictal and interictal epileptogenic activities on the immature brain has become a growing concern in the last two decades, and earlier surgical intervention in pediatric epilepsy patients with hemispheric damage has increasingly become an acceptable approach. Increasing support for earlier surgery in catastrophic pediatric epilepsy patients arises not only from concerns about the burden of epilepsy on the immature brain but also from increased awareness of the plasticity window of the developing brain, during which time the young brain has the best opportunity for functional recovery from insults.[15,17]

A primary concern in hemispherectomy cases is whether the patient will have any additional neurological deficit after surgery, and, if so, whether this deficit will be permanent or temporary. If the child is younger than 3 years, no additional neurological deficit is generally expected. However, in late-onset cases, such as Rasmussen syndrome, the timing of surgery may not be straightforward. Several factors should be considered in these cases to determine the best timing for hemispherectomy: the severity of seizures and their current effect on the patient's functional status, the potential effects of seizures on the cognitive and neuropsychological development of the child, the availability of adequate AED trials, and the natural course of the disease.

It is also important to remember that the shorter the time interval between seizure onset and surgery is, the higher the success rate will be. This is especially true in patients with Rasmussen syndrome.[11] Again, it is critical to remember that earlier seizure control in children provides the best psychosocial environment with the least seizure burden, resulting in optimal psychosocial development.[11,14–17,19,20]

■ Surgical Approaches

Once surgical intervention for hemispheric epilepsy has been decided, the last step is choosing the most appropriate surgical technique. As mentioned previously, surgical intervention for hemispheric pathologies has evolved from anatomical hemispherectomy to hemispherotomy. Currently, a variety of hemispherectomy techniques are being practiced. A brief overview of these techniques appears in the following sections. In-depth information about each of these techniques can be found in other chapters.

Anatomical Hemispherectomy

Anatomical hemispherectomy was first performed by Dandy in 1928.[2] The history and details of the technique can be found in Chapter 25. In the last decade, anatomical hemispherectomy has enjoyed a revival. A recent anatomical hemispherectomy series with long-term follow-up reported much smaller complication rates than did earlier series. It has been claimed that delayed complication rates reported in earlier studies were most likely overestimated.[10,17,19,21,22]

Hemidecortication

Hemidecortication was described by Ignelzi and Bucy[9] in 1968 as an alternative to anatomical hemispherectomy. The procedure starts with sylvian cistern dissection and middle cerebral artery occlusion, followed by occlusion of the anterior and posterior cerebral arteries. The entire cerebral cortex is then removed en bloc, leaving the basal ganglia and thalamus intact with white matter coverage over the anterior horn and body of the lateral ventricle.

Hoffman used a similar technique in a series of patients with Sturge-Weber syndrome in 1979.[18] Then two other modifications of this technique were described in the 1990s. Winston et al[23] described their technique of hemidecortication in 1992 as the "de-gloving" of the entire cerebral cortex by dissecting it around the lateral ventricle, leaving only a layer of white matter around the ventricular system after developing a plane of dissection from the edges of the insula by opening the sylvian fissure. De-gloving is first performed on the frontal, parietal, and occipital lobes and then on the temporal fossa by removing the entire cortical mantle. In 1996, Carson et al[18] published a Johns Hopkins series, with some modifications. The details of this technique can be found in Chapter 26.

The main problems with hemidecortication are excessive blood loss, a heightened risk of infection, and, most especially, the technical difficulty of performing a complete cortical resection in the medial and basal sides of the lobes.

Functional Hemispherectomy

Functional hemispherectomy was developed by Rasmussen; the details were published in 1983.[3] It can be best defined as partial anatomical resection and full disconnection of the damaged hemisphere. After its introduction, this technique has become the most widely used hemispherectomy technique. It preserves the anterior frontal, posterior parietal, and occipital lobes while resecting the paracentral lobule and the anterior two thirds of the temporal lobe, including mesial structures; disconnecting all commissural and projection fibers with a complete callosotomy; and severing the connection with the brainstem and thalamus through frontobasal and occipitoparietal cuts. The rationale for this technique was to perform a functionally complete but anatomically incomplete hemispherectomy by leaving a large part of the brain intact to avoid the well-known complications associated with anatomical hemispherectomy secondary to an enormous postsurgical cavity.

Rasmussen reported seizure-free outcomes and low complication rates in 75% of patients. Other modifications of the functional hemispherectomy technique have been described, including Comair's transsylvian functional hemispherectomy technique.[13] Further details of functional hemispherectomy technique can be found in Chapter 27.

Hemispherotomy

The main goal of anatomical hemispherectomy in epilepsy surgery is the functional disconnection of the damaged hemisphere. Hemispheric resection is usually performed to achieve this goal; tissue resection is not the main objective of this procedure, as it is in neuro-oncological surgery. Rasmussen came up with the hemispheric disconnection concept by describing his functional hemispherectomy technique and showing that full functional disconnection with comparable seizure-free outcome rates is still feasible without resecting the entire hemisphere.

The next generation of neurosurgeons continued to develop new, creative surgical techniques based on this line of thought by further decreasing the amount of resected brain volume while still performing full disconnection of the hemisphere. In 1992, Delalande et al[4,5] introduced the term *hemispherotomy* to describe the evolving hemispheric surgery techniques designed to minimize resection volume while still fully disconnecting the hemisphere. Since 1992, several other neurosurgeons have developed different hemispherotomy techniques, with each technique characterized by further decreases in the resected brain volume and by smaller cortical incisions.[4,5,24–28]

Hemispherotomy is the latest step in the natural evolution of hemispheric surgery techniques. The main differences between the various hemispherotomy techniques pertain to the volume of resected brain tissue, the access route to the lateral ventricle, resecting or not resecting the insular cortex, resecting or disconnecting the hippocampus, and preserving or sacrificing the vascular structures in the peri-insular area. Although the following chapters include detailed descriptions of each technique, we will briefly summarize these approaches here to emphasize their common characteristics as well as their differences. Whether hemispherotomy or functional hemispherectomy is the correct term to describe these new techniques is debatable. Regardless, these techniques can be organized into two main groups: techniques using a vertical approach and techniques using lateral approaches.

Vertical Approach

Transventricular Vertical Hemispherotomy

Transventricular vertical hemispherotomy, the most commonly used vertical approach technique, was described by Delalande et al[4,5] in 1992. This surgical technique, like oth-

foci in the oppo
might be relate
cal tissue to the
basal ganglia an

■ Conclus

Hemispherector
factory seizure
rate, in a very d

References

1. Krynauw RA. In
hemisphere. J N
2. Dandy WE. Rem
with hemiplegi
3. Rasmussen T. H
Sci 1983;10(2):
4. Delalande O, Bul
spherotomy: su
in a population
ONS19–ONS32,
5. De Ribaupierre
nective techniqu
6. Villemure JG, N
principles and a
7. Schramm J, Be
tion: an alterna
1995;36(3):509-
8. Daniel RT, Ville
pitfalls and avoi
2003;80(1–4):2:
9. Ignelzi RJ, Bucy
of infantile cere
14–30
10. Oppenheimer D
complication of
1966;29(3):229-
11. Villemure JG, Da
epilepsy. Childs
12. Arzimanoglou A.
corresponding e
Aicardi J, eds. A
PA: Lippincott W
308–310
13. Comair YG. Tran
lection and resul
2nd ed. Philadel
699–704
14. Montes JL, Farme
Wyllie E, ed. The
ed. Philadelphia,
1159

ers, has evolved, with several changes made to it since the initial description.[5] In its current form, the surgery starts with a small linear, paramedian incision parallel to the sagittal suture. A small (3 × 5 cm) frontoparietal craniotomy is performed 1 to 2 cm lateral to midline by staying one third anterior and two thirds posterior to the coronal suture. A small (3 × 2 cm) cortical resection is then performed, by staying away from the midline, to enter the ipsilateral lateral ventricle. The body and splenium of the corpus callosum are divided intraventricularly, followed by a cut in the posterior column of the fornix at the level of the trigone by reaching the choroidal fissure behind the pulvinar. A vertical incision lateral to the thalamus is then made, guided by the choroid plexus in the temporal horn. This incision extends from the trigone to the most anterior part of the temporal horn by completely unroofing the ventricle. The callosotomy is then completed by dividing the genu and the rostrum of the corpus callosum until just above the anterior commissure. The posterior part of the gyrus rectus is resected subpially to expose the anterior cerebral artery (ACA) and optic nerve. The final step to complete the hemispheric disconnection is a straight incision anterolaterally through the caudate nucleus from the rectus gyrus to the anterior temporal horn by following the ACA.[4]

Delalande et al[4] reported 83 patients who underwent this procedure, including 30 patients (36%) with multilobar cortical dysplasia (hemimegalencephaly), 25 patients (30%) with Rasmussen syndrome, 10 patients (12%) with Sturge-Weber syndrome, and 18 patients (22%) with ischemic-vascular sequelae. The postoperative seizure-free outcome rate was 74%. The best results, a 92% seizure-free outcome, were achieved in patients with Rasmussen syndrome and Sturge-Weber syndrome. The postoperative hydrocephalus rate was 16%, and the mortality rate was 3.6%.

Another vertical approach through the interhemispheric fissure was described by Danielpour et al[29] in 2001 and used in only two patients.

Lateral Approaches

Perisylvian Transcortical Transventricular Hemispherical Deafferentation

The Perisylvian transcortical transventricular hemispherical deafferentation technique was described by Schramm et al[7] in 1995. The goal of the procedure was described as deafferenting nearly all of the cortical structures of the damaged hemisphere from its connections to the basal ganglia and the contralateral hemisphere. The first step is a classic anteromesial temporal lobectomy, followed by a circular transcortical incision starting from the temporal horn and ending at the tip of the frontal horn. Major superficial veins and some of the middle cerebral artery branches are preserved. The next step of the procedure is a posterior basal disconnec-

tion. The posterior end of the hippocampal resection at the choroidal fissure is carried through the white matter subpially, crossing the calcarine sulcus and reaching the splenium. Then, a complete corpus callosotomy is performed intraventricularly. The last step to complete the deafferentation of the hemisphere is a frontobasal disconnection between the sphenoid wing and the rostral end of the callosotomy by staying subpial and anterior to the A1 segment. Schramm et al[7] reported on 13 patients operated on with this technique. Eleven patients had perinatal brain damage or atrophy; two had Rasmussen syndrome and Sturge-Weber syndrome. After surgery, 11 patient were seizure free, and 1 patient had more than 75% reduction in seizure frequency. No mortality was reported, and only one patient needed a shunt.

Transsylvian Keyhole Functional Hemispherectomy

This technique was reported on by Schramm et al[24] in 2001 as a modification of the original technique, described previously. In this new modification, anteromesial temporal lobectomy is replaced with selective amygdalohippocampectomy. More information about this technique can be found in Chapter 28.

Peri-insular Hemispherotomy

Peri-insular hemispherotomy was described by Villemure and Mascott[6] in 1995. It was defined as a conceptual and technical evolution of the functional hemispherectomy described by Rasmussen and represented the latest stage in its development.[11,18,25,30] More information about this technique can be found in Chapter 29.

Modified Peri-insular Hemispherotomy

Shimizu and Maehara[28] described a modification of Villemure's peri-insular hemispherotomy technique in 2000. Information about the modified peri-insular hemispherotomy can be found in Chapter 29.

■ Special Considerations Regarding the Hemispheric Surgical Approaches

Anatomical hemispherectomy has regained its place among hemispherectomy techniques in recent years, thanks to significantly decreased complication rates in modern patient series.[16,17,22] However, many complications and concerns remain. Compared with other hemispherectomy techniques, anatomical hemispherectomy is associated with higher blood loss, the risk of coagulopathy, longer hospital stays, a higher rate of hydrocephalus, a lower seizure-free rate in

infarcti
with ex
reopera
Clinic F
underge
zures a
hemim
sphered
cal hen
some n
aly pati
cedures
horn w
mantle,
ACA tra
mally la

Com
nique o
significa
loss, an
higher r
ficult a
hemispl
able cor
for mul
cases. B
plicatio

Hem
requirir
time an
is also a
hydroce
tient.[4,24]
are sma
postope
tion, difl
and higl
are mos
tricles b
cases.[4,1]

■ Co

Althoug
tient sei
variatio
associat
death. A
operativ
experier
A postoj
tempora
before 3

28. Shimizu H, Maehara T. Modification of peri-insular hemispherotomy and surgical results. Neurosurgery 2000;47(2):367–372, discussion 372–373

29. Danielpour M, von Koch CS, Ojemann SG, Peacock WJ. Disconnective hemispherectomy. Pediatr Neurosurg 2001;35(4):169–172

30. Kestle J, Connolly M, Cochrane D. Pediatric peri-insular hemispherotomy. Pediatr Neurosurg 2000;32(1):44–47

31. Brian JE Jr, Deshpande JK, McPherson RW. Management of cerebral hemispherectomy in children. J Clin Anesth 1990;2(2):91–95

32. Carreño M, Wyllie E, Bingaman W, Kotagal P, Comair Y, Ruggieri P. Seizure outcome after functional hemispherectomy for malformations of cortical development. Neurology 2001;57(2):331–333

33. Kossoff EH, Vining EP, Pyzik PL, et al. The postoperative course and management of 106 hemidecortications. Pediatr Neurosurg 2002;37(6):298–303

34. Holthausen H, May TW, Adams TB, et al. Seizures post hemispherectomy. In: Tuxhorn I, Holthausen H, Boenigk H, eds. Pediatric Epilepsy Syndromes and Their Surgical Treatments. London, UK: John Libbey; 1997:749–773

35. Binder DK, Schramm J. Transsylvian functional hemispherectomy. Childs Nerv Syst 2006;22(8):960–966

36. De Almeida AN, Marino R Jr, Aguiar PH, Jacobsen Teixeira MJ. Hemispherectomy: a schematic review of the current techniques. Neurosurg Rev 2006;29(2):97–102, discussion 102

37. Devlin AM, Cross JH, Harkness W, et al. Clinical outcomes of hemispherectomy for epilepsy in childhood and adolescence. Brain 2003;126(pt 3):556–566

38. Villemure JG, Adams CBT, Hoffman HJ, Peacock WJ. Hemispherectomy. In: Engel J Jr, ed. Surgical Treatment of the Epilepsies. 2nd ed. New York, NY: Raven Press; 1993:511–518

25 Anatomical Hemispherectomy

Concezio Di Rocco, Kostas N. Fountas, and Luca Massimi

Anatomical hemispherectomy is the surgical procedure used to remove one cerebral hemisphere, with or without sparing the basal ganglia, in subjects with refractory hemispheric epilepsy. The procedure can be realized in a piecemeal fashion or en bloc.

Several variants of such a technique have been devised, mainly aimed at reducing the cranioencephalic disproportion resulting from the removal of the congenitally malformed or postnatally damaged cerebral hemisphere and at preventing the effects of the mechanical dislocation of the preserved normal hemisphere.

■ Historical Background

Anatomical hemispherectomy was introduced in 1928 by Dandy[1] for the treatment of a diffuse glial tumor of the nondominant hemisphere in a patient who survived the operation in good clinical conditions before dying from his disease. The technique consisted of the complete excision of the right hemisphere, including the basal ganglia, by means of a complete corpus callosotomy and opening of the lateral ventricle, after the exclusion of the anterior and middle cerebral arteries at the internal carotid bifurcation and coagulation of the veins. In the same year, Lhermitte[2] in France published a paper on the physiological features of this operation. A first modification of this procedure was proposed in 1933 by Gardner[3] to save the basal ganglia by occluding the middle and anterior cerebral arteries distally to the perforating lenticulostriate branches and to the Heubner's artery. Although originally conceived for the treatment of hemispheric gliomas, anatomical hemispherectomy was rapidly considered for the treatment of drug-resistant hemispheric epilepsy. In 1938, anatomical hemispherectomy was used by McKenzie[4] in a child with intractable epilepsy and infantile hemiplegia, obtaining the complete disappearance of the seizures. Later on, in 1950, Krynauw[5] reported on the favorable results he had obtained in a series of children in whom the procedure was specifically adopted to control seizures. The author, indeed, described 12 epileptic patients affected by infantile hemiplegia who showed not only an excellent epileptic outcome but also experienced a significant postoperative motor and cognitive improvement. On these grounds, during the following two decades, anatomical hemispherectomy gained an increasing popularity among the neurosurgical community because it allowed surgeons to obtain complete or nearly complete seizure control in 70 to 80% of patients with an acceptable surgical mortality rate (approximately 6 to 10%).[6] The procedure was performed according to two main techniques: the en bloc excision of the cerebral hemisphere and the piecemeal hemispherectomy, obtained through multiple lobectomies.[7–9]

During the late 1960s and the early 1970s, the interest in anatomical hemispherectomy rapidly declined because of the occurrence of late complications, as obstructive hydrocephalus and chronic subdural fluid collections accounted for a significantly high rate of late mortality (up to 25% of the cases).[7,10] These complications were interpreted on the grounds of chronic intracranial hemorrhages, secondary to the dislocation of the residual brain, resulting in repeated vascular tearings leading to neomembrane formation in the surgical cavity and chronic iron deposition on the cerebral structures. The acritical acceptance of late hemosiderosis as a frequent and unavoidable cause of late neurological deterioration led to the practical abandonment of the technique in favor of variants aimed at reducing the volume of the residual cavity after the excision of the epileptogenic cerebral hemisphere (subtotal hemispherectomy or functional hemispherectomy). In particular, in 1973, Rasmussen[11] introduced a promptly accepted technique consisting of the mere excision of portions of the central and temporal regions and disconnection of the remaining cerebral cortex, which was left in situ. Although functional hemispherectomy, compared with anatomical hemispherectomy, appeared to be weighted by a minor rate of complications while allowing comparable seizures control, some contemporary authors complained of the abandonment of anatomical hemispherectomy by considering its higher efficacy with regard to epilepsy control. In 1973, Northfield[12] writing about anatomical hemispherectomy, commented, in fact, "It is a pity that such a beneficial operation should be abandoned."

Anatomical hemispherectomy was revived in the 1980s when, after the introduction of the computed tomography (CT) scan, it was possible to identify the main cause of late neurologic deterioration, that is, the late occurrence of progressive hydrocephalus, a phenomenon that was difficult to recognize on the mere clinical ground before the wide availability of CT and magnetic resonance imaging (MRI). Silently, the demonstrations of hemosiderosis disappeared from the medical literature in the last decades. Nevertheless, it continued to be indicated in a nearly automatic fashion as one of the main factors in favor of the adoption of the functional hemispherectomy versus anatomical hemispherectomy.[13] Nowadays, hemosiderosis continues to be quoted in spite of reports that deny its occurrence in operated on patients observed for considerably long periods of time (definitively longer than the 8–10 years considered to be necessary in the past for the development of the complication).[14–17]

With the revival of the technique, new variants were introduced, all of them with the goal of counteracting the disproportion between the cranial and the brain volume brought about by the cerebral hemisphere excision and the occurrence of postoperative hydrocephalus. In 1983, Adams[18] introduced the *Oxford–Adams modification* consisting of the plugging of the homolateral foramen of Monro and a narrowing duraplasty. In the following years, other technical variants became available, such as hemidecortication and hemicorticectomy.[19,20] In the same time, the advances in neuroimaging diagnosis allowed surgeons to select better candidates for the procedure, namely those patients with hemimegalencephaly and diffuse cortical dysplasia in whom functional hemispherectomy may have some limitations because of the anatomical abnormalities of the midline structures and the huge volume of the malformed hemisphere.

■ Indications and Preoperative Evaluation

Candidates for anatomical hemispherectomy are those subjects suffering from intractable, catastrophic epilepsy caused by a diffuse lesion of one cerebral hemisphere. The anatomical substrates responsible for the seizure disorder are either congenital or acquired. Among the congenital disorders, the disturbances in neuronal migration and differentiation, namely hemimegalencephaly, plurilobar cortical dysplasia, Sturge-Weber syndrome, and perinatal occlusion of the middle cerebral artery, are the most frequent clinical entities. Posttraumatic and postinfective diffuse unilateral brain injuries and Rasmussen encephalitis account for nearly all the cases of acquired epileptogenic lesions, possibly requiring a resective or disconnective surgical treatment. All the types of unilateral hemispheric cerebral damage actually do respond quite satisfactorily to both anatomical hemispherectomy and functional hemispherectomy, the epileptic outcome being related to the effectiveness of the cortical disconnection and the psychomotor outcome to the "normality" of the contralateral hemisphere.[21–28] However, the results associated to the neuronal migration disorders are less rewarding than

those observed in subjects with other congenital anomalies or acquired lesions, whichever technique is adopted for the hemispherectomy.

The best candidates for disconnective procedures (functional hemispherectomy, hemispherotomy) are patients with atrophic brains and large ventricular cavities. Conversely, subjects with hypertrophic hemispheres, caused by diffuse migration disorders, and small, distorted cerebral ventricles may be the ideal candidates for anatomical hemispherectomy. Indeed, in these patients the anatomical resection of the malformed hemisphere ensures the complete excision of the epileptogenic substratum as well as the preservation of the integrity of the contralateral midline structures. These structures, in fact, are often dislocated from their normal position, because of the abnormally large malformed hemisphere and distorted so that they can be damaged by disconnective surgical maneuvers performed without an adequate exposure. Furthermore, by completely removing the hypertrophic hemisphere, anatomical hemispherectomy provides the space necessary to relieve the previously compressed residual healthy hemisphere and to allow its normal volumetric growth.

Several studies demonstrated that early hemispherectomy can give a significant advantage in favoring the psychomotor development.[17,29,30] Accordingly, patients undergoing hemispherectomy currently tend to be operated on in their infancy or young childhood. This trend involves in particular anatomical hemispherectomy because most of the children undergoing this procedure harbor a congenital cortical malformation producing early catastrophic seizures.[31] The young age of the candidates for anatomical hemispherectomy requires a careful and accurate preoperative evaluation for correct surgical planning (**Table 25.1**). To achieve this goal, the following preoperative steps are necessary:

- Perform a detailed epileptic history centered on the seizures' onset and semiology as well as their evolution and the development of drug resistance.
- Perform a careful neurological examination to verify the presence and the degree of the hemiparesis and of the possible visual field defect (hemianopsia).
- Perform neuropsychological assessment based on age-tailored scales. The target of this evaluation is to assess the developmental level in infants or children with severe mentally disabilities and to test the cognitive and behavioral skills in the older children (memory, language, visuospatial and perceptual–motor function, attention, executive function, behavioral features).
- Ensure adequate electroencephalographic (EEG) exploration to confirm the diagnosis of epilepsy and define a possible epileptic syndrome (e.g., Ohtahara syndrome, West syndrome, Lennox-Gastaut syndrome), to detect the epileptic foci, to analyze the interictal and the ictal patterns, and to confirm the ab-

Table 25.1 Selection Criteria for Epilepsy Surgery and Hemispherectomy

General Criteria for Epilepsy Surgery	Specific Criteria for Epilepsy Surgery	Specific Criteria for Hemispherectomy
1. Presence of symptomatic and drug resistant seizures 2. Compliance and motivation of the patient or the family 3. Possible social benefit from the surgical procedure	1. Presence of a localized and resectable lesion with clear correlation with the clinical picture 2. Absence of progressive neurological disease or chronic psychiatric disturbance	1. Presence of hemiparesis or hemiplegia 2. Seizures arising only from the affected hemisphere 3. Functional and anatomical integrity of the contralateral hemisphere 4. Lack of effectiveness of a more conservative brain resection 5. Prevention criterium*

*This criterion makes the others not absolute. For example, a patient with a mild but progressing unilateral motor deficit can be considered a candidate for hemispherectomy as well, if this procedure can prevent a further worsening of such a deficit.

sence of seizures arising from the contralateral hemisphere. Such a study is usually performed by using a long-term surface video-EEG recording. An invasive recording (stereo-EEG) may be required in case clinicoradiological discordance (e.g., MRI showing diffuse hemispheric alterations and clinical examination and surface EEG demonstrating only localized alterations).

• Detailed neuroimaging studies including structural and functional MRI with standard sequences, spectroscopy, diffusion and perfusion imaging, and angiographic sequences provide excellent anatomical details of the brain and the vascular structures, and they have paramount importance for the correct planning of anatomical hemispherectomy. Actually, in children with hemimegalencephaly, it is mandatory to preoperatively verify the presence of possible anatomical abnormalities, because distortion of the lateral ventricles, contralateral shift of the median vascular structures, hypertrophy of the veins draining into the sagittal sinus/hypoplasia of the deep venous system, abnormal extension of the sylvian veins up to the sagittal sinus, cortical hypervascularization, and so on. Functional studies (functional MRI, single photon emission computed tomography (SPECT), positron emission tomography (PET), and integration with magnetoencephalography) may be required to complete the preoperative neuroimaging assessment in selected cases.

■ Surgical Technique

Anesthesia and Perioperative Monitoring

Anatomical hemispherectomy requires a dedicated pediatric neuroanesthesiology team. The most frequently used anesthetic protocol consists of intravenously administered opioid (fentanyl or remifentanil) along with low-dose isoflurane or sevoflurane. Opioids have the advantage to induce sedation

and analgesia without major side effects and to reduce the oxygen cerebral metabolic rate and the intracranial pressure without significant changes on the cerebral perfusion pressure. Sevoflurane is suitable for pediatric anesthesia thanks to its short induction and recovery times.

The intraoperative intensive monitoring should include pulse oximetry, end-tidal-CO_2, invasive blood pressure, central venous pressure, core and peripheral body temperature, urine output, acid–base status, serum osmolality, and serial measurements of hematocrit and of serum proteins.

Operative Positioning and Opening

The patient lies on the operating table in supine position, with the shoulder homolateral to the affected hemisphere elevated and the torso mildly rotated to place the head in lateral decubitus (90-degree rotation toward the contralateral side). The head is fixed by the Mayfield head holder (Integra, Plainsboro, NJ) or, in very young children, by means of adhesive drapes.

The goal of the opening is to obtain an exposure of the abnormal hemisphere as wide as possible. For that reason a large skin incision and a large craniotomy are necessary. The skin incision is usually made in a question-mark fashion, starting from just above the zygomatic arch, extending posteriorly up to the occipital protuberance and then anteriorly up to cross the midline to reach the contralateral anterior frontal area just behind the hairline and approximately 1 to 2 cm from the midline. Alternatively, a T-shaped incision can be performed, the longer limb extending from the frontal region (behind the hairline) to the occipital protuberance, and the shorter one from the midline (2 cm posterior to the coronal suture) to the zygomatic arch. To reduce the bleeding from the skin, it can be infiltrated with a hemostatic mixture (e.g., 0.25–0.50% lidocaine hydrochloride with 1:200,000–400,000 epinephrine plus 0.25–0.50% bupivacaine with 1:400,000–800,000 epinephrine). However, this may not be necessary when a high-frequency coagulation needle is used for the skin incision. The skin flap is elevated and reflected anteriorly (anteriorly and posteriorly in case of T-incision). The temporal fascia is subsequently incised and reflected anteriorly without detaching it from the skin to preserve the frontal branch of the facial nerve. The temporal muscle is not dissected from the bone to realize an osteoplastic flap (**Fig. 25.1A**); it is incised anteriorly and posteriorly, leaving its base as large as possible to decrease the risk of denervation and devascularization.

The burr holes are made by using an air-driven skull perforator. They are placed as follows: one at the frontal key-hole point; one on the frontal bone, just over the beginning of the coronal suture; two or three along the midline but slightly contralateral to the sagittal suture; one or two along the lambdoid suture; one on the temporal squama. The midline burr holes are placed besides the midline to safely and completely expose the superior sagittal sinus (**Fig. 25.1A**). In case of hemimegalencephaly, the exact knowledge of the superior sagittal sinus is required to obtain a complete exposure of the enlarged abnormal hemisphere that may cross the midline. The burr holes over the sutures are used to carefully separate the dura mater from the overlying bone because these structures can be very adherent at this level. This can be performed with either a #3 Penfield dissector or a Yasargil dissector (Aesculap, Tuttlingen, Germany). The craniotomy is created by using a (high speed) air-driven craniotome to connect each burr hole. The bone flap is progres-

sively elevated through a delicate dissection from the dura mater, up to produce a fracture at the level of its temporal base, then it is reflected together with the temporal muscle and the periosteum. The craniotomy is completed by removing a certain amount of the anterior temporal bone with bone rongeurs to enhance the exposure of the temporal pole.

The dura mater is incised anteriorly, inferiorly, and posteriorly (that corresponds to the frontal, the temporo-occipital, and the parietooccipital ridges of the bone flap) and reflected with the base toward the midline. Alternatively, it can be opened in a starlike fashion.

Hemispherectomy

The anterior vascular deafferentation of the hemisphere is the first step of the procedure. Under magnification, the sylvian fissure is opened by a delicate microdissection, using arachnoid knife, microscissors, and #9 Rhoton dissector (Codman, Raynham, MA). After gentle retraction of the frontal and the temporal lobe (self-retained Greenberg retractor (Codman, Raynham, MA)), the internal carotid artery and its distal branches are visualized, dissected, and adequately exposed (**Fig. 25.1B**). The middle cerebral artery (MCA) is clipped and divided proximal to its bifurcation, thus sparing the perforating branches for the basal ganglia (**Fig. 25.2A**). The anterior cerebral artery (ACA) is clipped and divided proximal to the origin of the callosomarginal artery. To avoid

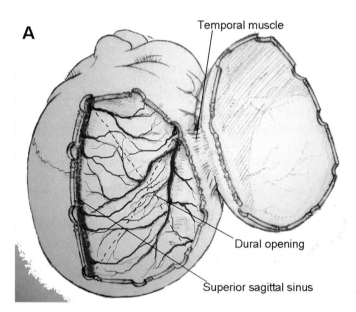

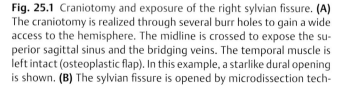

A

Temporal muscle

Dural opening

Superior sagittal sinus

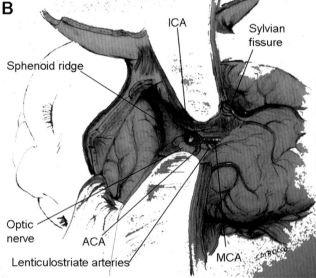

B

ICA

Sylvian fissure

Sphenoid ridge

Optic nerve

ACA

Lenticulostriate arteries

MCA

Fig. 25.1 Craniotomy and exposure of the right sylvian fissure. **(A)** The craniotomy is realized through several burr holes to gain a wide access to the hemisphere. The midline is crossed to expose the superior sagittal sinus and the bridging veins. The temporal muscle is left intact (osteoplastic flap). In this example, a starlike dural opening is shown. **(B)** The sylvian fissure is opened by microdissection tech-nique and gentle retraction of the frontal and temporal lobes. A wide opening of the sylvian fissure is required for correct identification of the main vascular, nervous, and bone landmarks, such as the internal carotid artery and its bifurcation into the anterior and middle cerebral arteries, with their perforating branches, the optic nerve, and the sphenoid ridge.

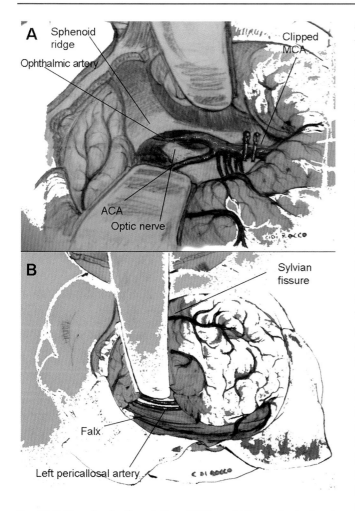

A Sphenoid ridge

Ophthalmic artery

Clipped MCA

ACA

Optic nerve

B

Sylvian fissure

Falx

Left pericallosal artery

Fig. 25.2 Vascular deafferentation. **(A)** The middle cerebral artery is closed proximally to its bifurcation. To save the basal ganglia vascularization, the artery is clipped distally to the lenticulostriate arteries. **(B)** The deep midline structures are reached by gentle retraction of the affected hemisphere and by progressive coagulation of the bridging veins to expose and to clip the homolateral pericallosal artery.

cortical veins are progressively dissected, coagulated, and divided to reach the underlying corpus callosum (**Fig. 25.2B**). In the case of hemimegalencephaly, the bridging veins may be abnormally enlarged and characterized by a more fragile wall than the normal veins and these features may make the vein coagulation quite tedious; in such cases, it is advisable to start the coagulation within the cortical surface rather than along the subarachnoid course of the vessels. Once the corpus callosum is exposed, the homolateral pericallosal artery should be coagulated (**Fig. 25.3A**). However, because the identification of contralateral pericallosal artery may be difficult, this coagulation can be more safely performed after opening the lateral ventricle, which allows the surgeon to visualize more anatomical landmarks. For the same reason, the corpus callosotomy is accomplished mainly by suction, avoiding, if possible, the use of the bipolar cautery (**Fig. 25.3A**). The corpus callosum is completely excised extending from the genu to the splenium. Once the lateral ventricle is entered, the foramen of Monro is plugged with a cottonoid to avoid the blood escaping into the contralateral ventricle and to protect the choroid plexus. The division of the frontobasal white matter is performed through a transventricular ependymal incision lateral and anterior to the basal ganglia and by suctioning the white matter to detach the frontal lobe to the basal nuclei (**Fig. 25.3B**). In case of piecemeal anatomical hemispherectomy, the frontal lobectomy is now completed by extending the ependymal incision up to the sylvian fissure and sectioning the cortical surface from the sylvian fissure to the midline. The piecemeal hemispherectomy is recommended for the excision of hemimegalencephalic hemispheres, which could be difficult to perform with an en bloc procedure. The advantage of performing multiple lobectomies is reducing the risk of distortion and traction of the brainstem during the dislocation of the affected hemisphere and enhancing the operating field exposure, thus making the procedure safer and more comfortable. The en bloc hemispherectomy, on the other side, has the advantage of reducing the bleeding caused by the multiple cortical incisions required by the piecemeal brain removal.

The procedure continues with the temporal and posterior lobe disconnection. Before this disconnection, however, the homolateral anterior choroidal artery, posterior communicating artery, and posterior cerebral artery (PCA) must be recognized. The PCA is divided at the level of its P3 segment to devascularize the temporo-occipital basal areas (**Fig. 25.4A**). The temporal stem is divided by extending the intraventricular ependymal incision posteriorly up to the trigonal area and the temporal horn and by aspirating the splenium remnants. After the coagulation of the posterior bridging veins, the parietooccipital lobe is freed and can be removed en bloc with the temporal lobe or in a piecemeal fashion through deep cortical incisions (**Fig. 25.4B**). If the small ventricular size prevents the possibility of entering the temporal horn from the tri-

the accidental clipping of the contralateral ACA, this vessel and the anterior communicating artery must be correctly identified before dividing the homolateral ACA. Finally, the arachnoid is incised along the basal surface of the frontal lobe up to reach the olfactory tract and along the temporal lobe up to visualize the tentorial notch. The opening of the sylvian fissure may be particularly hard in very young children or in case of brain hemimegalencephaly because of the tight interdigitation between the temporal and the frontal cortical gyri. In such circumstances, a standard frontal or temporal lobectomy can be performed as the first step of the hemispherectomy to gain enough space to reach the anterior part of the Willis circle.

After the vascular deafferentation and by gentle retraction of the mesial surface of the hemisphere, the bridging

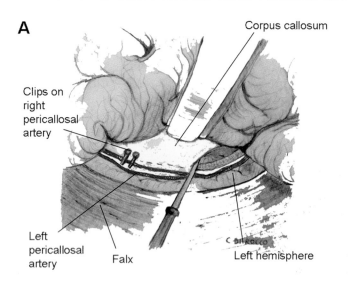

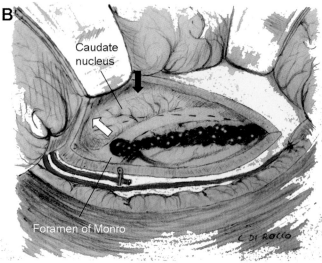

Fig. 25.3 Corpus callosotomy and access to the lateral ventricle. **(A)** The callosotomy is performed by microincision and suction. Care should be taken to avoid injuries to the contralateral hemisphere (which is visualized under the dural falx). **(B)** Once the lateral ventricle is entered, the foramen of Monro, the choroid plexus, and the caudate nucleus can be recognized. The frontobasal white matter is divided by an ependymal incision lateral and anterior to the basal ganglia. The lateral cut follows a 90-degree inclination (*black arrow*), whereas the anterior one is at a 45-degree inclination (*white arrow*).

gone, this cavity can be entered from the cortical surface, taking the sphenoidal wing as marker. The amygdalohippocampectomy can be made either by subpial dissection or by suctioning after the temporal horn is entered. Alternatively, it can be performed after the temporal lobectomy.

The basal ganglia and the thalamus may be excised or left in situ. The first option can be adopted in case of malformation of the cortical development where these deep structures are thought to influence the recurrence of seizures. Otherwise, the basal nuclei can be spared because they are

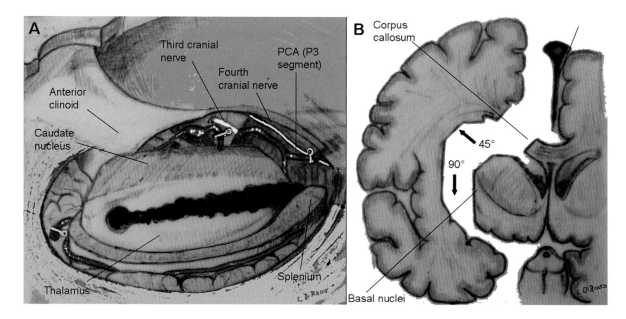

Fig. 25.4 Completion of the hemispherectomy. **(A)** The posterobasal white matter is divided after the closure of the P3 segment of the posterior cerebral artery. Care should be taken to not damage the third and fourth cranial nerves. **(B)** Coronal view of the surgical route used for the white matter disconnection.

believed to participate in the patient's motor residual activity. The coagulation of the choroid plexus is thought to reduce the risk of postoperative hydrocephalus.

Closure

The closure procedure begins after a meticulous hemostasis. Actually, because of the large residual dead space, even a small bleeding from the remaining basal nuclei or from the dural structures (falx, tentorium) may evolve into a voluminous subdural hematoma which may cause anemia or compression of the contralateral brain. A subdural external drainage can be left for the first few postoperative days to help the removal of surgical debris and to detect possible active bleedings.

In case of choroid plexus coagulation, the foramen of Monro is plugged with a small piece of muscle or Gelfoam (Pfizer, New York, NY), reinforced with fibrin glue. The basal ganglia are covered with Surgicel (Ethicon, Inc., Somerville, NJ). To reduce their possible dislocation related to the head movements, these structures can be anchored by suturing a constricting band of fascia or liophylized dura mater to the falx, the tentorium, and the basal dura mater.[32] A variety of techniques has been used since that described by Adams in 1983,[18] such as the use of different substitute dural patches, omentum vascularized free flap,[33] liophylized pig derma,[34] or even a Silastic prothesis to fill the subdural cavity.[35] The dural closure is obtained by reapproaching the dural flaps with running interlocking or interrupted 3–0 or 4–0 silk suture. After its closure, the dura mater is secured to the bone by multiple peripheral and central tack-up sutures to reduce the risk of epidural fluid collections. The osteosynthesis is made by multiple 0 silk stitches or by resorbable plates. Finally, the muscle, the muscular fascia, the galea, and the superficial layers are anatomically sutured with resorbable stitches. A subgaleal drain is usually left in place for the first 48 to 72 postoperative hours.

■ Complications

Anatomical hemispherectomy is a highly radical surgery technique more often required to treat very young patients with catastrophic epilepsy. Consequently, the related surgical risk is high. Nevertheless, thanks to the continuous improvement in the neurosurgical and neuroanesthesiologic techniques, the surgical risk is similar to that associated with other major neurosurgical operations. Actually, the operative mortality ranges from 1 to 7% and draws near the lower end of this range in the most recent and largest series.[13,14,17,36–38] Similarly, most of the nonspecific surgical complications [e.g., cerebrospinal fluid (CSF) leak from the surgical wound, superficial or deep infection of the surgical flap, postoperative hematomas] show approximately the same rate and severity as other neurosurgical procedures.[15]

Among more common complications, perioperative blood losses and secondary anemia are the most significant ones and represent the main cause of surgical mortality.[37,39] Significant blood losses are reported in approximately 10% of the operations[17,19,40]; the entire blood volume or more may needed to be replaced during the surgical procedure together with the clotting factors.[41] The blood losses are significant in patients affected by hemimegalencephaly or diffuse cortical dysplasia because of the abnormally rich and fragile vascular net. Occasionally, this subset of patients can require the replacement of their entire blood volumes even three to four times during a single operation.[40] Massive blood transfusion highly increases the risk of disseminated intravascular coagulation.[41] Disseminated intravascular coagulation is a potentially fatal complication in addition to being a possible cause of postoperative intraparenchymal hematoma.[34]

Some important intraoperative measures must be considered to reduce the perioperative bleeding. The first step is the occlusion of the major feeding arteries before starting the brain incision and removal. The second crucial step is the intraoperative control of the bleeding from the bridging veins. These veins may be fragile and very close to the superior sagittal sinus; thus, great care must be paid to avoid their accidental tearing during the surgical brain displacement. Moreover, they should be coagulated as close as possible to the cortical surface to ensure a more reliable closure and to avoid possible injuries to the sagittal sinus. The meticulous, step-by-step hemostasis is the third, mandatory intraoperative step. Actually, in children with small blood circulating volume, the intraoperative bleeding may become significant just during the opening procedure, because of the large skin and bone flaps, and it may insidiously persist after the closure. Finally, strict perioperative monitoring and timely blood replacement help prevent the previously mentioned hemorrhagic complications.

A further specific complication of anatomical hemispherectomy is represented by the ischemic lesions resulting from the accidental clipping of contralateral Willis circle arteries. For that reason, the MCA clipping is considered to be enough to decrease the risk of major blood losses. The occlusion of the ACA, indeed, is burdened by the risk of an improper closure of the contralateral artery, especially in hemimegalencephaly in which the two vessels may run one over the other in an abnormally verticalized interhemispheric commissure. In addition, the PCA closure may be difficult in hemimegalencephaly or posterior quadrantic dysplasia because of the resistance offered by the hypertrophic brain to reach the posterolateral surface of the midbrain.

A rare but possibly severe acute complication of anatomical hemispherectomy is represented by brainstem distortion or edema. This complication is usually related to the en bloc anatomical hemispherectomy because of the maneuvers of hemisphere dislocation required by this technique.[19] It presents as transient or persistent postoperative decline in consciousness with or without other signs of brainstem suffering.

Transient postoperative fever is very common after anatomical hemispherectomy, probably as result of the circulation of cellular and blood debris with the CSF.[17] It is characterized by an aseptic meningitis syndrome for 1 to 4 postoperative weeks, with negative systemic and CSF cultures. Making a prolonged irrigation of the residual cavity and leaving an external subdural drainage can help in limiting such a complication.

The circulation of surgical debris can also produce acute obstructive hydrocephalus, which occurs in approximately 7% of the cases.[42] A strict early clinical and radiological monitoring allows the surgeon to easily detect it. Persistent hydrocephalus is treated by a standard ventriculoperitoneal shunt.

Hydrocephalus may occur also as delayed complication in approximately 15 to 35% of the cases.[14,43] It is postulated that late hydrocephalus could share the same pathogenesis of the acute case or could arise from an impairment of the CSF dynamics resulting from the opening of the lateral ventricle and from the elimination of the pericephalic arachnoid spaces of one hemisphere. The analysis of several clinical series suggests a possible role of two factors: (1) the epileptogenic substratum more than the type of hemispherectomy technique used and (2) the age of the patient at the operation. Late hydrocephalus is, in fact, considerably more common in case of diffuse malformation of cortical development than in other congenital pathological conditions, namely Sturge-Weber syndrome or prenatal MCA ischemia.[13] Actually, this complication is reported after functional hemispherectomy/hemispherotomy,[25,26,28,37] with a higher incidence in hemimegalencephalic patients.[44,45] Because hemimegalencephaly usually causes catastrophic epilepsy early, it can be hypothesized to have a role of the immature CSF spaces, because late hydrocephalus is observed mainly in children less than 1 year old at the time of the operation.[13] It is possible that the long exposition to the environment of large portions of the dura mater in the very young patient can induce a functional damage of this structure, eventually limiting its absorptive capacity and leading to the hydrocephalus, because it often can be observed in infants and young children undergoing different type of neurosurgical operations. It is worth noting, however, that late hydrocephalus has been described even more than 30 years after the operation.[46]

Although it is an uncommon complication, the late occurrence of dystonic attacks or ballistic movements after anatomical hemispherectomy is reported in the literature.[47] Generally, this kind of complication is transient.

The herniation of the healthy hemisphere into the contralateral residual cavity is considered to be a potential cause of postoperative complications, mainly late hemorrhages resulting from the mechanical dislocation of the brain with the head movements.[35] We could not demonstrate such an association in any of our patients. On the contrary, the postoperative invasion of the surgical cavity by the progressively expanding healthy hemisphere was noted, in our experience, in the patients who showed the best postoperative psychomotor outcomes.[30]

■ Critical Analysis of Outcome

As to the complications, there are not significant differences among the different types of hemispherectomy in terms of surgical mortality[17,25,37] or postoperative aseptic meningitis.[13,48] Anatomical hemispherectomy is burdened by more abundant intraoperative blood losses (600–750 mL versus 250–350 mL), higher incidence of postoperative shunt (15–35% versus 0–15%), and longer operative times.[19,25,26,28,31,37] These figures are a result of the radical excision of one cerebral hemisphere, whereas a large portion of the hemisphere is spared by the disconnective procedures (especially hemispherotomies). It is worth noting, however, that the disconnected hemisphere undergoes a certain degree of late involution, in particular, if the branches of the MCA are ligated during the operation so that, according to Wen et al,[49] "in the long run, there will probably be little difference between the results of a hemispherotomy and those of an anatomical hemispherectomy regarding remaining brain tissue (p. 754)." The most important complication of functional hemispherectomy or hemispherotomy is the need of a second surgical procedure to complete the hemispheric disconnection, reported in up to 15 to 20% in some series,[17,37,50] and obviously unknown after anatomical hemispherectomy.

Anatomical hemispherectomy is very effective in the control of the epileptic seizures. The largest series in the literature shows a good epileptic outcome (Engel's Class I or II)[51] in approximately 80 to 90% of the cases,[13,17,19,20,36] even after more than 20 years follow-up.[14,52] In some cases, however, the control of seizures presents a deterioration with the time after surgery, so that the success rates generally ranges from 60 to 80% at late follow-up.[31,37] The more conservative functional hemispherectomies (standard or hemispherotomy) currently achieve outcomes with regard to the seizure control similar or only slightly lower than anatomical hemispherectomy.[25,28,53,54] The length of follow-up described in the literature, however, is usually longer in anatomical hemispherectomy than in the disconnective procedures.[14,25,38]

When comparing the surgical outcomes, however, the composition of the clinical series should be taken into account because, according to several studies, the epileptic outcome is influenced by the etiology more than by the surgical technique adopted. Patients affected by Sturge-Weber syndrome, porencephalic cysts, or Rasmussen encephalitis do much better than those affected by malformations of cortical development.[31,37,45,50,54] Further prognostic factors include the possible involvement of the healthy hemisphere, undetected by the currently available diagnostic tools, as well as possibly unfavorable anatomy that might prevent a correct surgical procedure.

Similar observations can be made with regard to motor and cognitive postoperative outcome. Cognitive performances generally present a significant postoperative improvement (up to 60–70% of the cases), especially in patients treated early.[30] Once again, patients affected by hemimegalencephaly or diffuse cortical dysplasia have a worse

psychomotor outcome,[29,31,50] probably as a result of an earlier catastrophic epilepsy, a less favorable epileptic outcome, and poorer psychomotor development. Only a small minority of hemispherectomized patients show a normal or quite normal psychomotor development at late follow-up, whatever the etiology or the surgical technique. Finally, the motor performances usually remain stable after surgery (50–60%) or improve mildly[14,55]; in case of postoperative worsening, motor function recovers within a few months whatever the type of hemispherectomy.[36,56]

References

1. Dandy WE. Removal of right cerebral hemisphere for certain tumors with hemiplegia. JAMA 1928;90:823–825
2. Lhermitte J. L'ablation complète de l'hemisphère droit dans les cas de tumeur cérébrale localisée conpliquée d'hémiplegie. La décérebration supra-thalamique unilaterale chez l'homme. Encephale 1928;23:314–323
3. Gardner WJ. Removal of the right cerebral hemisphere for infiltrating glioma. JAMA 1933;12:154–164
4. McKenzie KG. The present status of a patient who had the right cerebral hemisphere removed. JAMA 1938;111:168–183
5. Krynauw RA. Infantile hemiplegia treated by removing one cerebral hemisphere. J Neurol Neurosurg Psychiatry 1950;13(4):243–267
6. Wilson PJE. Cerebral hemispherectomy for infantile hemiplegia. A report of 50 cases. Brain 1970;93(1):147–180
7. Falconer MA, Wilson PJE. Complications related to delayed hemorrhage after hemispherectomy. J Neurosurg 1969;30(4):413–426
8. Griffith HB. Cerebral hemispherectomy for infantile hemiplegia in the light of the late results. Ann R Coll Surg Engl 1967;41(2):183–201
9. Obrador Alcalde S. About the surgical technique for hemispherectomy in cases of cerebral hemiatrophy. Acta Neurochir (Wien) 1952;3(1):57–63
10. Oppenheimer DR, Griffith HB. Persistent intracranial bleeding as a complication of hemispherectomy. J Neurol Neurosurg Psychiatry 1966;29(3):229–240
11. Rasmussen T. Postoperative superficial hemosiderosis of the brain, its diagnosis, treatment and prevention. Trans Am Neurol Assoc 1973;98:133–137
12. Northfield DWC. The Surgery of the Central Nervous System. Oxford, UK: Blackwell; 1973:570
13. Di Rocco C, Iannelli A. Hemimegalencephaly and intractable epilepsy: complications of hemispherectomy and their correlations with the surgical technique. A report on 15 cases. Pediatr Neurosurg 2000;33(4):198–207
14. Davies KG, Maxwell RE, French LA. Hemispherectomy for intractable seizures: long-term results in 17 patients followed for up to 38 years. J Neurosurg 1993;78(5):733–740
15. Fountas KN, Smith JR, Robinson JS, Tamburrini G, Pietrini D, Di Rocco C. Anatomical hemispherectomy. Childs Nerv Syst 2006;22(8):982–991
16. Kossoff EH, Vining EP, Pyzik PL, et al. The postoperative course and management of 106 hemidecortications. Pediatr Neurosurg 2002;37(6):298–303
17. Peacock WJ, Wehby-Grant MC, Shields WD, et al. Hemispherectomy for intractable seizures in children: a report of 58 cases. Childs Nerv Syst 1996;12(7):376–384
18. Adams CBT. Hemispherectomy—a modification. J Neurol Neurosurg Psychiatry 1983;46(7):617–619
19. Carson BS, Javedan SP, Freeman JM, et al. Hemispherectomy: a hemidecortication approach and review of 52 cases. J Neurosurg 1996;84(6):903–911
20. Winston KR, Welch K, Adler JR, Erba G. Cerebral hemicorticectomy for epilepsy. J Neurosurg 1992;77(6):889–895
21. Delalande O, Pinard JM, Basevant C, Gauthe M, Plouin P, Dulac O. Hemispherotomy: a new procedure for central disconnection. Epilepsia 1992;33:99–100
22. Kanev PM, Foley CM, Miles D. Ultrasound-tailored functional hemispherectomy for surgical control of seizures in children. J Neurosurg 1997;86(5):762–767
23. Morino M, Shimizu H, Ohata K, Tanaka K, Hara M. Anatomical analysis of different hemispherotomy procedures based on dissection of cadaveric brains. J Neurosurg 2002;97(2):423–431
24. Schramm J, Beherns F, Entzian W. Hemispherical deafferentation: a modified functional hemispherectomy technique. Epilepsia 1992;33:71
25. Schramm J, Kral T, Clusmann H. Transsylvian keyhole functional hemispherectomy. Neurosurgery 2001;49(4):891–900, discussion 900–901
26. Shimizu H, Maehara T. Modification of peri-insular hemispherotomy and surgical results. Neurosurgery 2000;47(2):367–372, discussion 372–373
27. Smith JR, Fountas KN, Lee MR. Hemispherotomy: description of surgical technique. Childs Nerv Syst 2005;21(6):466–472
28. Villemure JG, Mascott CR. Peri-insular hemispherotomy: surgical principles and anatomy. Neurosurgery 1995;37(5):975–981
29. Battaglia D, Di Rocco C, Iuvone L, et al. Neuro-cognitive development and epilepsy outcome in children with surgically treated hemimegalencephaly. Neuropediatrics 1999;30(6):307–313
30. Lettori D, Battaglia D, Sacco A, et al. Early hemispherectomy in catastrophic epilepsy: a neuro-cognitive and epileptic long-term follow-up. Seizure 2008;17(1):49–63

31. Di Rocco C, Battaglia D, Pietrini D, Piastra M, Massimi L. Hemimegalencephaly: clinical implications and surgical treatment. Childs Nerv Syst 2006;22(8):852–866

32. Di Rocco C. Surgical treatment of hemimegalencephaly. In: Guerrini R, ed. Dysplasias of the Cerebral Cortex and Epilepsy. Philadelphia, PA: Lippincott-Raven; 1996:295–304

33. Matheson JM, Truskett P, Davies MA, Vonau M. Hemispherectomy: a further modification using omentum vascularized free flaps. Aust N Z J Surg 1993;63(8):646–650

34. Dunn LT, Miles JB, May PL. Hemispherectomy for intractable seizures: a further modification and early experience. Br J Neurosurg 1995;9(6):775–783

35. Sorano V, Esposito S. Hemispherectomy complications in the light of craniocerebral disproportion: review of the literature and rationale for a filling-reduction cranioplasty. Childs Nerv Syst 1998;14(9):440–447

36. Adams CBT. Hemispherectomy. In: Kaye AH, Black PM, eds. Operative Neurosurgery. Edinburgh, UK: Churchill Livingstone; 2000:1285–1291

37. Cook SW, Nguyen ST, Hu B, et al. Cerebral hemispherectomy in pediatric patients with epilepsy: comparison of three techniques by pathological substrate in 115 patients. J Neurosurg 2004; 100(2, suppl Pediatrics)125–141

38. Schramm J. Hemispherectomy techniques. Neurosurg Clin North Am 2002, 13(1):113–134

39. Devlin AM, Cross JH, Harkness W, et al. Clinical outcomes of hemispherectomy for epilepsy in childhood and adolescence. Brain 2003;126(pt 3):556–566

40. Vining EP, Freeman JM, Pillas DJ, et al. Why would you remove half a brain? The outcome of 58 children after hemispherectomy-the Johns Hopkins experience: 1968 to 1996. Pediatrics 1997;100(2 pt 1):163–171

41. Piastra M, Pietrini D, Caresta E, et al. Hemispherectomy procedures in children: haematological issues. Childs Nerv Syst 2004;20(7):453–458

42. Montes JL, Farmer JP, Andermann F, Poulin C. Hemispherectomy: medications, technical approaches, and results. In: Wyllie E, Gupta A, Lachwani DK, eds. The Treatment of Epilepsy: Principles & Practice. Philadelphia, PA: Lippincott Williams & Wilkins; 2006: 1111–1124

43. Rasmussen T. Cerebral hemispherectomy: indications, methods and results. In: Schmidek HH, Sweet WH, eds. Operative Neurosurgical Techniques. New York, NY: Grune & Stratton; 1988:1235–1241

44. González-Martínez JA, Gupta A, Kotagal P, et al. Hemispherectomy for catastrophic epilepsy in infants. Epilepsia 2005;46(9):1518–1525

45. Kossoff EH, Vining EPG, Pillas DJ, et al. Hemispherectomy for intractable unihemispheric epilepsy etiology vs outcome. Neurology 2003;61(7):887–890

46. Kalkanis SN, Blumenfeld H, Sherman JC, et al. Delayed complications thirty-six years after hemispherectomy: a case report. Epilepsia 1996;37(8):758–762

47. Wroe S, Richens A, Compston A. Bilateral ballistic movements occurring as a late complication of hemispherectomy and responding to sulpiride. J Neurol 1986;233(5):315–316

48. Villemure JG. Cerebral hemispherectomy for epilepsy. In: Schmidek HH, Sweet WH, eds. Operative Neurosurgical Techniques. New York, NY: WB Saunders; 2000:1499–1510

49. Wen HT, Rhoton AL Jr, Marino R Jr. Anatomical landmarks for hemispherotomy and their clinical application. J Neurosurg 2004;101(5):747–755

50. Jonas R, Nguyen S, Hu B, et al. Cerebral hemispherectomy: hospital course, seizure, developmental, language, and motor outcomes. Neurology 2004;62(10):1712–1721

51. Engel J Jr. Outcome with respect to epileptic seizures. In: Engel J Jr, ed. Surgical Treatment of Epilepsies. New York, NY: Raven Press; 1987:553–571

52. Anderman F, Rasmussen TB, Villemure JG. Hemispherectomy: results for control of seizures in patients with hemiparesis. In: Lüders HO, ed. Epilepsy Surgery. Philadelphia, PA: Lippincott-Raven; 1991:625–632

53. Bittar RG, Rosenfeld JV, Klug GL, Hopkins IJ, Simon Harvey A. Resective surgery in infants and young children with intractable epilepsy. J Clin Neurosci 2002;9(2):142–146

54. Carreño M, Wyllie E, Bingaman W, Kotagal P, Comair Y, Ruggieri P. Seizure outcome after functional hemispherectomy for malformations of cortical development. Neurology 2001;57(2):331–333

55. Danielpour M, von Koch CS, Ojemann SG, Peacock WJ. Disconnective hemispherectomy. Pediatr Neurosurg 2001;35(4):169–172

56. Wyllie E. Surgical treatment of epilepsy in children. Pediatr Neurol 1998;19(3):179–188

26 Hemidecortication and Intractable Epilepsy

Adam L. Hartman, James Frazier, and George I. Jallo

Hemispherectomy in the treatment of intractable epilepsy was first reported by Krynauw in 1950 as an operative intervention for patients with infantile hemiplegia and intractable epilepsy.[1] Krynauw described this intervention as removal of the affected hemisphere, with the exception of the thalamus, caudate nucleus and its tail. Then hemidecortication (also known as hemicortectomy) was introduced by Ignelzi and Bucy in 1968 as an alternative surgical technique in the management of intractable epilepsy seen in infantile cerebral hemiatrophy.[2] This term now more commonly refers to resection of cortical gray matter and hippocampus, while leaving some white matter and nearly all subcortical gray structures intact.[3] Further case series confirmed the utility of this approach and reinforced the notion that certain aspects of cognitive and motor development even might improve postoperatively.[2]

■ Indications

Hemidecortication has been performed in a variety of clinical settings, ranging from congenital to acquired conditions. The overall goal in such a surgery is to remove cortex with pathology while allowing underlying white and deep gray matter to remain. This may be particularly useful when abnormal tissue is primarily located in the cortical gray matter. Given that seizures are generated by abnormal neuronal activity, hemidecortication may be useful for removing only the most affected tissue while preserving structures that still may be functioning normally.

In one large series of hemidecortications, the most common underlying pathology was Rasmussen syndrome.[4] Rasmussen syndrome is a progressive inflammatory condition of the brain characterized by intractable epilepsy and neurological impairments.[5] With a typical picture of early childhood onset, unilateral brain involvement, and a progressive nature, this syndrome appears to be quite amenable to hemispherectomy if medical management fails. The etiology of Rasmussen syndrome is not known; suggestions include a viral illness (including Epstein-Barr virus, cytomegalovirus, and herpes simplex-1 virus), antibodies (case reports and series include patients with antibodies against one subunit of the ionotropic glutamate receptor, GluR3, and the

presynaptic protein *munc-8*), or T-cell dysregulation.[5,6] No unifying hypothesis has emerged however, despite years of effort.[7] Clinically, the median age of presentation is 5 years, although adults present with Rasmussen syndrome, as well.[8] Three stages have been described: a *prodrome* characterized by seizures and a mild hemiparesis, followed by an *acute* stage characterized by more frequent seizures and progressive neurological deficits referent to one hemisphere, then a *residual* stage with fewer seizures but persistent functional deficits.[5] Any type of seizure may be seen, but focal motor seizures (including epilepsia partialis continua), sometimes appearing to represent a noncontiguous patchy distribution (e.g., face and leg), are most frequently noted.[7] Electroencephalography (EEG) can be confusing (i.e., abnormalities are sometimes seen bilaterally), but imaging typically shows unihemispheric atrophy over time.[7] The patchy nature of the seizures probably reflects the distribution of findings when pathological tissue is examined: perivascular cuffing, microglial nodules, and neuronal loss interspersed with areas of normal-appearing tissue.[9] This patchy involvement is one reason we avoid biopsies to diagnose Rasmussen syndrome in our practice. Diagnostic criteria based on a variety of clinical and paraclinical findings have been proposed.[5] Medical therapy includes anticonvulsants for controlling seizures (although this practice frequently is unsuccessful), immunotherapy (including intravenous immune globulin, corticosteroids, or plasmapheresis), and immune modulators (e.g., tacrolimus).[5] Some patients are helped to a limited extent by medical management, but the most effective therapy for control of the seizures (or relief from seizures in the context of unacceptable medication side effects), particularly if there is evidence of unilateral hemispheric dysfunction (e.g., hemiparesis, language involvement), is hemispherectomy.

Another common indication for hemidecortication is malformations of cortical development.[4] Cortical development can be affected adversely at any stage of development: cell proliferation, neuronal migration, or cortical organization.[10] Anomalies can range in size from heterotopias involving small areas of cortex to hemimegalencephaly, which involves the entire hemisphere. In addition to intractable epilepsy, these children may have developmental disabilities, contralateral motor deficits, associated neurocutaneous signs (e.g., epidermal nevi), and craniofacial anomalies (e.g., hemicrania). In those malformations not typically limited to one hemisphere, one of the greatest challenges in evaluation is ensuring that the contralateral hemisphere functions reasonably well. Some patients with Rasmussen syndrome have evidence of malformations of cortical development.[9] This might partly explain why EEG findings can be seen bilaterally; it also makes the preoperative assessment of risks and benefits critical in determining the likelihood of postoperative success.

Vascular injury (i.e., perinatal stroke) is another common pathology leading to hemidecortication.[4] Ischemic (arterial and venous) and hemorrhagic strokes may be seen in the neonatal period and can lead to seizures.[11] A variety of prenatal and perinatal events, coagulopathies, congenital cardiac lesions, infections, and metabolic abnormalities can lead to cerebrovascular cortical lesions that may eventually be amenable to surgical resection for control of seizures.

Much of the early literature on hemidecortication highlighted patients with Sturge-Weber syndrome.[12,13] Sturge-Weber syndrome is characterized by facial port-wine stains associated with leptomeningeal venous malformations and intracranial calcification in a gyriform pattern.[14] Many patients also suffer from intractable epilepsy, developmental delays, glaucoma, and cerebrovascular complications. Indications for and timing of hemispherectomy are somewhat controversial: patients with seizures starting younger than 1 year of age appear to have more intractable seizures, yet it is difficult to make early predictions of how intractable a given patient's seizures will become over time.[14] There is no solid evidence to indicate the best timing or the optimal choice of surgery (i.e., hemispherectomy versus focal resection), although seizure freedom is higher after hemispherectomy than after focal resections (although nonrandom choice of patients for each procedure may be a major confounder of this finding).[15,16]

Other pathologies in which hemidecortication may be useful include large tumors and tuberous sclerosis, both of which involve mass lesions associated with epileptogenic cortex, sometimes in the context of associated malformations of cortical development.

■ Presurgical Planning

The most important first step in the evaluation of a candidate for hemidecortication is diagnosing the correct epilepsy syndrome. When considering the removal of one hemisphere, several questions arise concerning the expected benefits of the surgery (i.e., seizure control and improved developmental outcomes after relief from seizures and medication side effects), potential risks (i.e., loss of full function in the contralateral hand and possibly partial visual field loss), freedom of the remaining hemisphere from seizure activity, the ability of the remaining hemisphere to assume new functions

postoperatively, and finally, the timing of the surgery (i.e., early in life versus later).[17] Several modalities exist to make some assessment of these parameters, although none have been completely predictive, based on clinical experience.[18] In the ideal situation, both structural and functional studies point to the remaining hemisphere as structurally normal, free from seizures, and fully capable of accommodating new function. Unfortunately, this is not always the case.

Imaging studies such as magnetic resonance imaging and computed tomography aid in the assessment of the structural characteristics such as the extent of pathology (i.e., involvement of gray or white matter, single versus multiple lobar involvement, and possibly involvement of the more normal side).[18] Magnetic resonance spectroscopy may contribute to the localization of involved cortex but rarely is the only abnormal study in a patient's evaluation. Functional magnetic resonance imaging may be useful for delineating the location of areas involved in critical language and motor function, particularly in patients with lesions thought to originate early in development, because their localization may be anomalous.[19] Positron emission tomography (PET) using radiolabeled fluorodeoxyglucose may identify areas of relative hypometabolism, indicating the extent of metabolic dysfunction in various regions.[20] We routinely obtain a concurrent EEG during PET studies to avoid false-negative tests (i.e., abnormal areas with epileptic foci that are active during the study—these areas may be more metabolically active than at baseline during an extended run of epileptiform activity, which would make them appear to be more normal than they actually are). EEG provides a functional picture of the source of epileptiform activity and can be useful for defining both the electrical source of seizures as well as one indication of the general electrical health of the presumably normal hemisphere before operation. Extended video-EEG monitoring in an epilepsy monitoring unit may be particularly useful if multiple different seizure types need to be characterized or if the nature of different types of events needs to be studied in the context of a question about whether a focal resection or hemispherectomy should be performed. Developmental screening or neuropsychological testing are invaluable tools in the assessment of a patient's current level of cognitive and language function. They may play a role in preparation of the patient for postoperative rehabilitation and serve as a baseline comparison for the postoperative evaluation.[20] We do not routinely use other studies such as the intracarotid amobarbital (Wada) test and magnetoencephalography in patients being considered for hemidecortication, given the high prevalence of developmental disabilities, lack of cooperation, and the fact that these studies rarely make a meaningful contribution to surgical decisions in this population. The importance of the assessment of the more normal side using various modalities cannot be overemphasized in their importance for presurgical counseling and prognostication (**Table 26.1**).

Table 26.1 Studies Useful before Hemidecorticectomy

Physiological Studies
Electroencephalography
　Scalp
　Intracranial

Anatomical and Metabolic Studies
Computed tomography
Magnetic resonance imaging
Positron emission tomography

Functional Studies
Functional magnetic resonance imaging
Developmental screening
Neuropsychological testing

Note: Choice of studies depends on the needs of the individual patient.

■ Surgery

As with any neurosurgical operation, positioning of the patient is of paramount importance when starting the surgery. The patient is placed in a semi-decubitus position, and the head is fixed in a Mayfield head holder (Integra, Plainsboro, NJ) followed by placement of the head parallel to the floor so that the hemisphere of interest is uppermost in the surgical field. A T-shaped incision is marked in which the midline incision begins behind the hairline and extends back to the occipital protuberance and the lateral incision begins anterior to the tragus of the ear at the zygomatic arch and extends to the midline incision approximately 2 cm behind the coronal suture.

After the patient is prepared and draped in a sterile fashion, the incision lines should be infiltrated with a mixture of lidocaine and epinephrine to assist in hemostasis. During incision of the skin, careful hemostasis must be a priority because small amounts of blood loss without replacement in infants and young children can have devastating consequences. Raney clips (Aesculap, Tuttlinger, Germany) and bipolar cautery are used to control bleeding. The temporalis muscle can be incised along with the skin for a myocutaneous flap, thus protecting the frontalis branch of the facial nerve from inadvertent injury. Once the underlying calvaria has been fully exposed, a perforator is used to drill multiple burr holes. Midline burr holes are placed slightly contralateral to the sagittal sinus. Once the burr holes are made, the dura is separated from the overlying bone with a #3 Penfield dissector (Codman, Raynham, MA). A craniotome with footplate is used to make the bone cuts between the burr holes. The surgeon should have immediate access to Gelfoam (Pfizer, New York, NY), Avitene (Darol, Warwick, RI), and vascular clips in the event of bleeding from the sagittal sinus and should be prepared to handle any violation of the sinus. The bone flap is gently elevated with simultaneous dissection of the dura with a periosteal elevator under direct visualization. After elevation of the bone flap, a temporal craniectomy can be performed to remove more bone and increase exposure. Dural tack-up 4–0 Nurolon sutures are then placed. The dura is opened with the flaps based toward the midline.

The operating microscope is brought into the surgical field for the hemidecortication. Attention is first aimed at the sylvian fissure, because a majority of hemispheric bleeding is from the middle cerebral artery (MCA). The sylvian fissure is dissected and opened carefully, and the MCA is identified back to the bifurcation of the internal cerebral artery. The MCA is clipped and divided lateral to the lateral lenticulostriate branches and proximal to its bifurcation. Next, attention is turned to the medial bridging cortical veins, which are coagulated or clipped and divided. Temporal decortication followed by frontal, parietal, and occipital decortication. Decortication is performed by using suction and bipolar coagulation to remove gray matter while leaving a mantle of white matter over the ependymal surface to preserve the ventricular system. The basal ganglia and thalamus are left intact. Because a temporal lobectomy is performed, the ventricular surface in the trigonal region is reconstructed with Gelfoam and Surgicel (Ethicon, Inc., Somerville, NJ) to prevent cerebrospinal fluid outflow.[21] During the frontal lobectomy, branches of the anterior cerebral artery (ACA) are coagulated and divided as they are encountered. If the surgeon wishes to clip and divide the ACA proximal to the callosomarginal artery, a preoperative imaging study is vital because accidental clipping of the contralateral ACA may occur in cases of abnormal patterns of the ACA complex.[22] The insular cortex is resected last, because manipulation of this area appears to be associated with cardiovascular instability in young children[21] (**Table 26.2**).

Meticulous hemostasis is performed, followed by copious irrigation of the resection cavity with normal saline. Gelfoam and Surgicel are placed over the residual surfaces to prevent any further bleeding. The dural flaps are reapproximated with 4–0 Nurolon sutures in a watertight fashion. A central dural tack-up suture is placed, followed by replacement and

Table 26.2 Major Steps in Hemidecortication

Positioning

Incision (myocutaneous flap)

Craniotomy and exposure

Dissection and decortication

- sylvian fissure and middle cerebral artery
- medial bridging cortical veins
- temporal lobectomy
- frontal, parietal, and occipital lobectomies
- reconstruction of ventricular surface in trigonal region
- insular decortication

Hemostasis

Closure

fixation of the bone flap. The temporalis muscle and fascial edges are reapproximated with 3–0 Vicryl sutures followed by the galea. A subgaleal drain may be left in place followed by closure of the skin with a 3–0 running nylon suture.

■ Complications

Hemidecortications may be associated with postoperative complications. Mortality has been reported to occur in 1 to 6.6% of hemispherectomy cases, although deaths likely occur at the lower end of this range because of improvements in surgical techniques.[23,24] In most cases, mortality is secondary to uncontrollable intraoperative bleeding, whereas significant postoperative brainstem shift and obstructive hydrocephalus have been found to be the cause of death in other cases.[23–26] Hydrocephalus can occur and has been extensively reported in the literature. The need for shunting has varied as documented in different series.[13,27–32] The persistence of elevated intracranial pressure indicates inadequate absorption of cerebrospinal fluid and requires prompt shunting to prevent any long-term effects.[21,30] In addition, cerebrospinal fluid leaks must be addressed promptly in an attempt to preempt infections, including meningitis.[21]

Although pediatric neuroanesthesia has made significant advancements, complications can arise from a large amount of intraoperative blood loss, hypothermia, and electrolyte changes in children.[33] These complications occur at a much lower rate as a result of these advances in anesthesia and surgical techniques. In the past, superficial cerebral hemosiderosis was a late postoperative complication, but recent series have not reported any cases.[24,34,35]

References

1. Krynauw RW. Infantile hemiplegia treated by removal of one cerebral hemisphere. S Afr Med J 1950;24(27):539–546
2. Ignelzi RJ, Bucy PC. Cerebral hemidecortication in the treatment of infantile cerebral hemiatrophy. J Nerv Ment Dis 1968;147(1):14–30
3. Binder DK, Schramm J. Multilobar resections and hemispherectomy. In Engel J, Pedley TA, eds. Epilepsy: A Comprehensive Textbook. 2nd ed. Philadelphia, PA: Lippincott, Williams & Wilkins; 2008:1879–1889.
4. Kossoff EH, Vining EP, Pyzik PL, et al. The postoperative course and management of 106 hemidecortications. Pediatr Neurosurg 2002;37(6):298–303
5. Bien CG, Granata T, Antozzi C, et al. Pathogenesis, diagnosis and treatment of Rasmussen encephalitis: a European consensus statement. Brain 2005;128(pt 3):454–471
6. Vining EPG. Rasmussen's syndrome. In: Singer HS, Kossoff EH, Hartman AL, et al., eds. Treatment of Pediatric Neurologic Disorders. Boca Raton, FL: Taylor & Francis; 2005:121–124
7. Vining EP. Struggling with Rasmussen's Syndrome. Epilepsy Curr 2006;6(1):20–21
8. Oguni H, Andermann F, Rasmussen TB. The syndrome of chronic encephalitis and epilepsy. A study based on the MNI series of 48 cases. Adv Neurol 1992;57:419–433
9. Pardo CA, Vining EP, Guo L, Skolasky RL, Carson BS, Freeman JM. The pathology of Rasmussen syndrome: stages of cortical involvement and neuropathological studies in 45 hemispherectomies. Epilepsia 2004;45(5):516–526
10. Barkovich AJ, Kuzniecky RI, Jackson GD, Guerrini R, Dobyns WB. A developmental and genetic classification for malformations of cortical development. Neurology 2005;65(12):1873–1887
11. Golomb MR, Garg BP, Carvalho KS, Johnson CS, Williams LS. Perinatal stroke and the risk of developing childhood epilepsy. J Pediatr 2007;151(4):409–413, 413, e1–e2
12. Hoffman HJ, Hendrick EB, Dennis M, Armstrong D. Hemispherectomy for Sturge-Weber syndrome. Childs Brain 1979;5(3):233–248
13. Ogunmekan AO, Hwang PA, Hoffman HJ. Sturge-Weber-Dimitri disease: role of hemispherectomy in prognosis. Can J Neurol Sci 1989;16(1):78–80
14. Comi AM. Update on Sturge-Weber syndrome: diagnosis, treatment, quantitative measures, and controversies. Lymphat Res Biol 2007;5(4):257–264
15. Kossoff EH, Buck C, Freeman JM. Outcomes of 32 hemispherectomies for Sturge-Weber syndrome worldwide. Neurology 2002;59(11):1735–1738
16. Bourgeois M, Crimmins DW, de Oliveira RS, et al. Surgical treatment of epilepsy in Sturge-Weber syndrome in children. J Neurosurg 2007;106(1, suppl)20–28
17. Lettori D, Battaglia D, Sacco A, et al. Early hemispherectomy in catastrophic epilepsy: a neuro-cognitive and epileptic long-term follow-up. Seizure 2008;17(1):49–63
18. Knowlton RC, Elgavish RA, Bartolucci A, et al. Functional imaging: II. Prediction of epilepsy surgery outcome. Ann Neurol 2008;64(1):35–41
19. Hartman AL, Lesser RP. Update on epilepsy and cerebral localization. Curr Neurol Neurosci Rep 2007;7(6):498–507
20. Cross JH. Epilepsy surgery in childhood. Epilepsia 2002;43(suppl 3):65–70
21. Carson BS, Javedan SP, Freeman JM, et al. Hemispherectomy: a hemidecortication approach and review of 52 cases. J Neurosurg 1996;84(6):903–911
22. Fountas KN, Smith JR, Robinson JS, Tamburrini G, Pietrini D, Di Rocco C. Anatomical hemispherectomy. Childs Nerv Syst 2006;22(8):982–991
23. Carmichael EA. The current status of hemispherectomy for infantile hemiplegia. Clin Proc Child Hosp Dist Columbia 1966;22(10):285–293
24. Di Rocco C, Iannelli A. Hemimegalencephaly and intractable epilepsy: complications of hemispherectomy and their correlations with the surgical technique. A report on 15 cases. Pediatr Neurosurg 2000;33(4):198–207
25. Cabieses F, Jeri R, Landa R. Fatal brain-stem shift following hemispherectomy. J Neurosurg 1957;14(1):74–91

26. White HH. Cerebral hemispherectomy in the treatment of infantile hemiplegia; review of the literature and report of two cases. Confin Neurol 1961;21:1–50

27. Chugani HT, Shewmon DA, Peacock WJ, Shields WD, Mazziotta JC, Phelps ME. Surgical treatment of intractable neonatal-onset seizures: the role of positron emission tomography. Neurology 1988; 38(8):1178–1188

28. Davies KG, Maxwell RE, French LA. Hemispherectomy for intractable seizures: long-term results in 17 patients followed for up to 38 years. J Neurosurg 1993;78(5):733–740

29. Mathew NT, Abraham J, Chandy J. Late complications of hemispherectomy: report of a case relieved by surgery. J Neurol Neurosurg Psychiatry 1970;33(3):372–375

30. Rasmussen T. Cerebral hemispherectomy: indications, methods, and results. In: Schmidek H, Sweet W, eds. Operative Neurosurgical Techniques: Indications, Methods, and Results. 2nd ed., Vol 2. New York, NY: WB Saunders; 1988:1235–1241

31. Strowitzki M, Kiefer M, Steudel WI. Acute hydrocephalus as a late complication of hemispherectomy. Acta Neurochir (Wien) 1994;131(3–4):253–259

32. Taha JM, Crone KR, Berger TS. The role of hemispherectomy in the treatment of holohemispheric hemimegaloencephaly. J Neurosurg 1994;81(1):37–42

33. J.L. M. Farmer JP, Andermann F, Poulin C. Hemispherectomy: medications, technical approaches, and results. In: Wyllie E, Gupta A, Lachhwani DK, eds. The Treatment of Epilepsy: Principles & Practice. 4th ed. Philadelphia, PA: Williams & Wilkins; 2006:1111–1124

34. Falconer MA. Delayed complications associated with ventricular dilatation following hemispherectomy. Dev Med Child Neurol Suppl 1969;20:96–97

35. Peacock WJ. Hemispherectomy for the treatment of intractable seizures in childhood. Neurosurg Clin N Am 1995;6(3):549–563

27 Functional Hemispherectomy at UCLA

Sandi Lam and Gary W. Mathern

Cerebral hemispherectomy remains one of the more common and conceptually dramatic types of pediatric epilepsy surgery. In the 2004 International League Against Epilepsy survey of 20 pediatric epilepsy surgery centers in Europe, the United States, and Australia, cerebral hemispherectomy accounted for 16% of all surgical procedures.[1] Even though cerebral hemispherectomy for epilepsy dates back to the early 1950s,[2] the idea that surgeons can remove half of the brain successfully still attracts the attention of the lay media as new and astounding. The public often assumes that children after this operation must be in a vegetative state without language or personalities and is amazed to find a smiling playful interactive child starting to walk and talk. Hence, even after 50 years there is still considerable interest in the techniques of cerebral hemispherectomy in the treatment of refractory epilepsy.

This chapter will focus on one type of cerebral hemispherectomy as developed and practiced at the University of California, Los Angeles (UCLA) since 1998.[3] Our procedure was designed for infants and small children with small malformed ventricular systems from severe cortical dysplasia and other malformations of cortical development. Initially, we outline the historical development and the rationale of the cerebral hemispherectomy performed at UCLA and describe the operative technique. This will be followed by presentation of the UCLA hemispherectomy cohort's clinical features and characteristics. The last section assesses UCLA's functional cerebral hemispherectomy along with ideas for future development.

■ History and Rationale for Cerebral Hemispherectomy at UCLA

The cerebral hemispherectomy technique performed at UCLA was developed based on the most common types of patients referred for the operation and our prior experience with anatomical[4,5] and Rasmussen functional procedures.[6] At UCLA, the typical patient referred for cerebral hemispherectomy is a child under the age of 3 years with severe cortical dysplasia and hemimegalencephaly (**Table 27.1**).[7] This patient population usually weighs less than 15 kg at surgery (some less than 6 kg) with a circulating blood volume of 500

mL to 1000 mL. Typically, the ventricular system is small or malformed, leading to challenges in operative dissection (**Fig. 27.1A–D**). Prior experience at our center with the anatomical cerebral hemispherectomy, in which the deep structures of the basal ganglia and thalamus were removed, was associated with the highest rate of seizure freedom. However, that procedure in small children with severe cortical dysplasia was also coupled with the most operative blood loss and complications.[3,8] With the Rasmussen functional cerebral hemispherectomy, fewer patients were seizure free postoperatively, many patients required second operations for removal of deep brain structures associated with generating seizures, and patients experienced operative blood loss comparable to those undergoing anatomical hemispherectomy. Based on our patient population and prior surgical experience, from 1997 to 1998 the senior author developed a modified version of the functional cerebral hemispherectomy that would address these issues.

The modified UCLA functional cerebral hemispherectomy was designed (1) to optimize the probability of postoperative seizure freedom by removing deep brain structures, (2) to restrict surgical blood loss, and (3) to reduce operative complications in young infants and children with large dysplastic brains. The key concept in the development of this modified procedure was the realization that from a technical perspective, the easiest cases were those cerebral hemispherectomy

Table 27.1 Histopathology of Hemispherectomy Cases at UCLA (1998 to 2008)

Histopathology	Percentage of Cases (*n* = 96)
Malformations of cortical development (58%)	
Hemispheric/multilobar cortical dysplasia	34%
Hemimegalencephaly	22%
Tuberous sclerosis complex	2%
Other substrates (42%)	
Rasmussen encephalitis	18%
Middle cerebral artery infarct/ hypoxia-ischemia	17%
Infections (herpes, bacterial)	3%
Tumor	2%
Trauma	1%
Sturge-Weber	1%

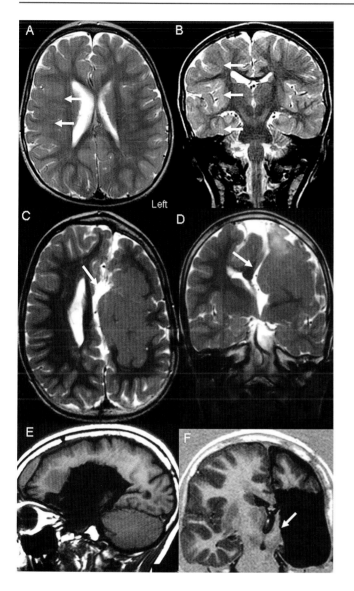

Fig. 27.1 Examples of magnetic resonance imaging (MRI) scans before and after hemispherectomy. **(A, B)** A relatively normal MRI. This 2.5-year-old began having seizures at 4 months of age and failed six antiepilepsy drugs. He neglected his left arm and leg even though he had fine finger dexterity of the left hand. Electroencephalography (EEG) lateralized to the right hemisphere. MRI shows decreased T2 signal of the white matter involving the frontal, temporal, and insular regions of the right hemisphere (*white arrows*). In addition, the cortex of the right insula is thicker than the opposite side. The right lateral ventricle is slightly larger than the left. Histopathology disclosed severe cortical dysplasia without balloon cells (Palmini Type IIA). This patient's operation is illustrated in **Figs. 27.2** and **27.3**. **(C, D)** Example of a malformed cerebral hemisphere. This 4-year-old began having seizures at 2 weeks of age and had failed more than 10 medications. MRI reveals a distorted left cerebral hemisphere from a large central heterotopia involving the basal ganglia and thalamus. The malformed left lateral ventricle opens directly into the 3rd ventricle (*white arrow*), there is heterotopic tissue in the anterior corpus callosum, and the left hemisphere crosses midline. Because of the distorted cerebral anatomy especially of the lateral ventricles, this child underwent an anatomical hemispherectomy in which the lobes were taken out separately so as not to damage the contralateral hemisphere. He is seizure free more than 5 years after surgery. **(E, F)** MRI 6 months after functional hemispherectomy. The sagittal view **(E)** shows the removal of the central operculum block with residual disconnected frontal, parietal, and occipital cortex. The coronal view **(F)** illustrates the corpus callosotomy, disconnection of the deep structures (*white arrow*), and removal of the mesial temporal structures.

patients with a prior history of perinatal middle cerebral artery (MCA) infarcts. In these cases, the ventricular system was enlarged, and the deeper structures were already atrophic.

The central idea for the UCLA operation was to create a similar operative field by dividing the MCA branches in the anterior sylvian fissure and removing the central operculum, including the lateral thalamus and basal ganglia.[9] Removal of the central operculum and deep structures disconnects almost all of the connections between the ipsilateral cerebral cortex to the ipsilateral thalamus and brainstem and provides ample exposure of the ventricular system for the intrahemispheric disconnections. The created space accommodates any postsurgical brain swelling. This technique reduces the size of the craniotomy compared with anatomical and Rasmussen cerebral hemispherectomy and, along with the early division of the MCA, minimized operative blood loss. This procedure was also designed to eliminate the need to retract firm dysplastic portions of the cerebral hemisphere with short friable veins to gain access to the anterior and posterior cerebral arteries, as necessary, for an anatomical hemispherectomy. Furthermore, the technique preserves the arachnoid granulations near the superior sagittal sinus aiming to reduce postsurgical hydrocephalus. Lastly, the functional hemispherectomy keeps enough tissue in the cerebral vault so that with growth the infant skull is less asymmetrical compared with children after anatomical hemispherectomy (**Figs. 27.1E** and **27.1F**).

The anatomical aims of the technique are the same as other cerebral hemispherectomy operations: remove or disconnect all the connections of the ipsilateral cortex to the ipsilateral thalamus and disconnect the connections between the two cerebral hemispheres. This is accomplished by removal of the central operculum and the mesial disconnection that follows the tentorium incisura. The therapeutic goal is to eliminate seizures as soon as possible to optimize cognitive and psychosocial development.[10]

■ Presurgery Evaluation

Chapter 24 provides a general overview of the presurgical evaluation of patients for cerebral hemispherectomy. At UCLA, the decision to offer cerebral hemispherectomy is a risk–benefit analysis addressing the risks of continued seizures including increased mortality and severe developmental delay from an epileptic encephalopathy versus the benefits of stopping the seizures early in life and risks of surgery.[11] There is no age or size that is too small for cerebral hemispherectomy if the seizures are severe enough. However, children generally weigh at least 5 kg or more before surgery.[3] Patients usually have tried three or more antiepilepsy drugs (AEDs) before presurgical evaluation. In infants and young children, the presurgical evaluation takes place within weeks to months prior to surgery. Children with refractory infantile spasms and status epilepticus are referred for presurgical evaluation promptly.[12,13] Standard presurgery evaluation includes scalp electroencephalography (EEG)/ video telemetry, magnetic resonance imaging (MRI), 2-deoxy-2-[^{18}F]fluoro-D-glucose (FDG)-positron emission tomography (PET), and, more recently, magnetoencephalography (MEG).[14–17] Even with high field strength MRI, we have found that FDG-PET is still very important in the presurgical evaluation, especially for infants and young children with cortical dysplasia, because the area of hypometabolism is often larger than the abnormality identified by structural MRI.[18] Hemiparesis is not a requirement before consideration of cerebral hemispherectomy at our institution.

■ Operative Technique

This section outlines the operative technique of functional hemispherectomy as performed at UCLA in 2008. As with any surgical technique, the operation has evolved over time, and additional subtle alterations can be expected as the team gains more experience.

Preincision

After induction of general anesthesia and endotracheal intubation, a transurethral catheter is inserted. The anesthesia team then inserts an arterial line, a central venous catheter (groin or neck placement), and two peripheral intravenous lines as large as the child's veins can tolerate. Laboratory parameters, including hematocrit, blood chemistry, acid–base

status, coagulation, and fibrinogen level, are performed throughout the surgery. For children weighing less than 10 kg, and especially for infants with hemimegalencephaly, blood must be available in the operating room before skin incision. Blood replacement begins with the skin incision in smaller children. Antibiotics, steroids (dexamethasone; 0.1 to 0.5 mg/ kg), and mannitol (1 g/kg) are given before skin incision.

Head position is lateral with the skull slightly higher than the chest, and the lateral frontal-temporal region is parallel to the floor (**Fig. 27.2A**). The patient is supine, and a small roll is placed to elevate the ipsilateral shoulder. The child is positioned on a sheepskin pad, and all pressure points of the heels and elbows are padded. In children older than 18 months, a Mayfield head holder (Integra, Plainsboro, NJ) is used; and in infants younger than 18 months of age, a pediatric horseshoe is preferred. When positioning on the horseshoe, particular attention is paid to the dependent pressure points over the contralateral eye, orbit, and ear. A T-shaped incision is marked on the skin (**Fig. 27.2A**). One arm of the incision is paramedian at the level of the ipsilateral midpupillary line, extending from the hairline to the parietal region, staying parallel to the sagittal suture. The other arm of the incision begins just in front of the tragus at the zygoma, extends vertically, and then curves slightly frontally to intersect with the first incision at a 90-degree angle at or near the coronal suture. Local anesthetic with epinephrine is infused into the skin incision and at the Mayfield pin sites.

Opening

The opening is a standard osteoplastic craniotomy with minor modifications to expose the anterior middle fossa and orbital frontal floor (**Fig. 27.2B–D**). We do not routinely use intraoperative neuronavigation. The skin flaps are elevated, preserving the temporalis muscle, fascia, and pericranium (**Fig. 27.2B**). In children, we use monopolar electrocautery sparingly. The skin flaps are wrapped in lap sponges and are held back with fishhooks and rubber bands are attached to the Greenberg retractor system (Codman, Raynham, MA). We elevate and incorporate into the skin flap the frontal-temporal fat pad and underlying fascia extending from the frontal portion of the zygomatic arch to the root of the zygoma (**Fig. 27.2B**; white asterisk). The temporalis muscle and fascia are incised along its fibers in the low temporal region to expose the zygomatic root and the frontal "keyhole" (**Fig. 27.2B**; black arrows).

Although the osteoplastic bone flap takes a bit more time, the exposure suits our purpose, and the cosmetic effect after surgery is superior. We also feel the risk of osteomyelitis is reduced with the osteoplastic bone flap, and, by retaining the blood supply, most children form a lifelong bony union. Burr holes are drilled just above and anterior to the zygomatic root, at the posterior margin where the ventricular catheter will eventually exit, behind the coronal suture, and

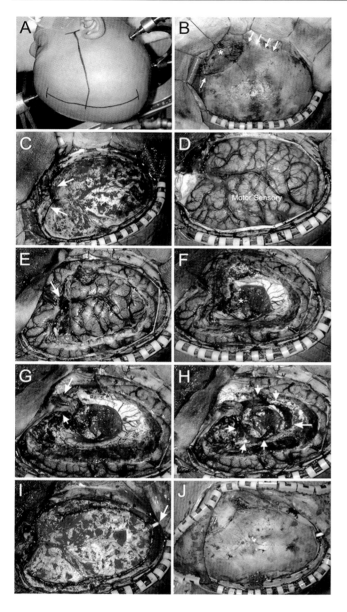

Fig. 27.2 Sequential steps in performing functional hemispherectomy at UCLA for a right-sided operation [see magnetic resonance imaging (MRI) in **Fig. 27.1A** and **1B**]. **(A)** Initial set-up before the drape is applied. A T-shaped incision is marked. Hair removal varies case to case depending on the preference of the patient and family. **(B)** After opening, the skin folds are held back with fish hooks and rubber bands. Notice the opening of the frontal-temporal fat pad and temporalis muscle fascia (*white asterisk*) in preparation for the osteoplastic bone flap. The muscle incisions are marked (*white arrows*). **(C)** View after craniotomy. The bone flap is wrapped in a moist lap sponge and secured with rubber bands. This allows for better exposure to the orbital floor and anterior temporal fossa (*white arrows*). Bone is removed to expose the floor of the middle fossa, anterior to the temporal tip, and from the lateral sphenoid to include the orbital floor. **(D)** View after opening the dura. The dura is tacked up to provide a fluid gutter along the anterior and middle temporal regions. The motor–sensory cortex is indicated. **(E)** Initial incisions over the lateral cerebral cortex. The first dissection goes through the anterior sylvian fissure to identify, coagulate, and ligate the branches of the middle cerebral artery and expose the arachnoid of the frontal and temporal circular sulcus. The cortical incision runs parallel to the ventricular system. **(F)** View after removal of the central operculum block. The ventricular system is exposed with the choroid lying over the top of the deep disconnection (*white asterisk*). **(G)** View before using the operative microscope. There are two additional cortical excisions on either side of the proximal sylvian fissure. This removes the anterior temporal pole and orbital frontal cortex to the level of the ventricle (*white arrows*). These resections provide exposure for the mesial disconnections. **(H)** View after the mesial disconnection performed under the operating microscope. The disconnection involves following the anterior cerebral artery from the genu of the corpus callosum to the anterior cerebral artery origin, the corpus callosotomy, and hippocampectomy (*white arrows*). **(I)** View after closure of the dura. Notice the exiting ventricular catheter at the posterior burr hole and out a separate skin incision (*white arrow*). **(J)** View after bony closure. Note the central tack-up sutures and use of plates to hold the bone securely in place.

in the frontal keyhole. The burr holes are connected with the drill paying attention to expose 2 to 3 cm of the orbital frontal floor, and the bone flap is "cracked" between the frontal and temporal burr holes. Additional bone is removed to expose the anterior middle fossa, middle fossa floor, and orbital frontal floor (**Fig. 27.2C**; white arrows). Bone wax is used sparingly and only in portions of bone edge that are bleeding to maximize postsurgical bony fusion. The dura is opened with the pedicle based between the frontal-temporal areas and tacked back (**Fig. 27.2D**). At this point, we inspect the lateral cortical surface of the brain for abnormal gyral patterns. We routinely perform intraoperative electrocorticography (ECoG) to identify sites to biopsy for research purposes. ECoG is performed under standard anesthetic conditions without inhalation anesthetics.[14]

Lateral Resection

Adequate exposure of the lateral surface of the brain to perform this operation includes the orbital frontal floor anteriorly, middle frontal gyrus superiorly, the midportion of the motor–sensory cortex, behind the Sylvian fissure above the trigone posteriorly, and temporally to the middle fossa floor and anterior temporal pole (**Fig. 27.2D**). For the cortical incisions, we use a 2-mm bipolar forceps set at 60 W, controllable suction tips, headlamps, and a surgical loupe magnification. We gently remove brain tissue using variable suction control to expose blood vessels and coagulate the veins and arteries before they rupture and bleed. We have abandoned the use of ultrasonic aspirators, which we find lead to too much bleeding, especially in infants and young children.

The lateral resection begins with a cortical incision perpendicular to the anterior sylvian fissure. We dissect the cerebral cortex on the temporal and frontal sides of the sylvian fissure and then identify and ligate the branches of the MCA at the bottom of the anterior third of the fissure (**Fig. 27.2E**; white arrow). Early control of the MCA greatly reduces blood loss in the subsequent portion of the dissection, especially for children with hemimegalencephaly in which the vessels on the cortical surface are often very friable. In addition, the dissection identifies the bottom of the sylvian fissure and exposes the frontal and temporal edges of the circular sulcus of the insula, which becomes a reference point for the anterior limb of the central operculum dissection. The incision over the lateral cortical surface follows the middle frontal gyrus around to the middle temporal gyrus, roughly parallel to and directly above the underlying ventricular system (**Fig. 27.2E**). The cortical incisions are sequentially deepened into the white matter of the corona radiata and, when necessary, the tissue block is held using self-retaining retractors. The ventricle is usually entered at its widest spot near the trigone, and the ventricular system is opened from posterior to anterior along the lateral and temporal ventricles.

Special care is taken to identify and coagulate veins along the ependymal walls of the ventricles because they can be very large, especially in infants with hemimegalencephaly or in children with periventricular nodular heterotopia. Once the ventricles are open, the anterior resection margin is deepened to the level of the ventricles on the frontal and temporal sides of the insula. During this portion of the resection, the surgeon begins to encounter small branches of the anterior cerebral artery (ACA) feeding the caudate nucleus and globus pallidus.

The central operculum block is gently lifted by the retractors to expose the choroid plexus. Staying just lateral to (above) the choroid fissure, the ependymal lining is incised, and the block of brain tissue is undercut, staying parallel to the choroid plexus in the frontal and temporal ventricles (**Fig. 27.2F**). This incision crosses the internal capsule, thalamus, globus pallidus, and caudate nucleus. In the anterior portions of the frontal and temporal regions, where the choroid plexus ends, we stay at the level of the ventricle and connect to the deep insular dissection. Perforating arteries into the deep caudate nucleus and basal ganglia structures need to be carefully identified, coagulated, and cut because they retract and bleed if ruptured. Once undercut, the central operculum is removed, exposing the ventricular system in a manner similar to what is seen in a patient after a MCA infarct (**Fig. 27.2F**). We remove most of the medial caudate nucleus to expose the anterior frontal ventricular system often revealing the foramen of Monro (**Fig. 27.3A**; white arrow). We also remove the amygdala to expose the anterior temporal horn.

Additional blocks of cortical tissue are removed on either side of the anterior sylvian fissure to assist with the mesial disconnections. This includes the orbital frontal cortex and the anterior temporal pole to the level of the ventricle (**Fig. 27.2G**; arrows). The cortex is removed in a subpial fashion on either side of the arachnoid covering the main trunk of the MCA. At this juncture, the patient's coagulation indexes such as prothrombin time, partial thromboplastin time, and fibrinogen level are assessed. After a large resection, it is not uncommon for the international normalized ratio to be greater than 1.2 or 1.3, especially in infants with hemimegalencephaly. If so, appropriate replacement with fresh frozen plasma, platelets, or cryoprecipitate is initiated.

Mesial Dissections under the Operating Microscopic

The disconnection of the two cerebral hemispheres and the ipsilateral mesial frontal connections into the ipsilateral thalamus are performed using the operating microscope. We begin by placing a retractor over the roof of the lateral ventricle, just opposite the caudate head, to expose the corpus callosum at the anterior body (**Fig. 27.3A**; black asterisks). Using suction and bipolar coagulation, the corpus callosum is resected, exposing, at a minimum, the arachnoid separating the callosum with the ipsilateral cingulate gyrus. We usually visualize the gray matter of the cingulate gyrus or the arachnoid plane overlying the pericallosal arteries. This plane is followed forward (anterior) around the genu of the corpus callosum, exposing the ACA, which is protected by a plane of arachnoid (**Fig. 27.3B**; white arrows). The ACA is followed from distal to proximal until the floor of the orbital frontal resection is reached. The mesial frontal disconnection of fibers into the ipsilateral anterior thalamus is the most difficult portion of the operation to understand conceptually and perform accurately. It is the most common place of an incomplete dissection leading to recurrent seizures after surgery. In infants with hemimegalencephaly, the ACA can be very deep and even dive toward the contralateral frontal lobe.

Once the anterior disconnection is complete, the body and tail of the corpus callosum are removed until the splenium is reached. Before surgery, the position of the vein of Galen is noted on the MRI, because it is sometimes very close to the undersurface of the splenium. We remove the pes, body, and tail of the hippocampus en bloc in a standard fashion along with the entorhinal and parahippocampal gyri for research purposes (**Figs. 27.3C** and **D**).[19,20] The final disconnection traces from the posterior hippocampus resection to the splenium by removing white matter and cortex to the arachnoid covering the falx cerebri (**Fig. 27.2H**; white arrows). This completes the mesial circle that disconnects the two hemispheres. The surgeon commonly encounters the posterior cerebral artery as it comes over the tentorium and penetrates the mesial temporal lobe. Care should be taken to avoid manipulation of the remaining cortical blocks at the midline, especially in children with stiff dysplastic brains, so

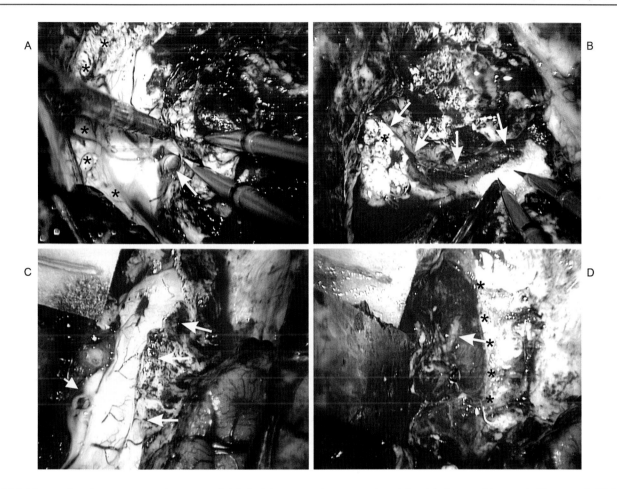

Fig. 27.3 Views using the operating microscope. **(A)** Subpial resection of the caudate nucleus in the frontal lateral ventricle exposes the foramen of Monro (*white arrow*). Note the choroid plexus entering the opening just behind the tip of the arrow. The un-resected corpus callosum is just under the retractor (*black asterisks*). **(B)** View after resection of the anterior corpus callosum and mesial frontal disconnection. The genu of the corpus callosum can be seen (*black asterisk*). The anterior cerebral artery is revealed covered by arachnoid from the genu to its origin with the carotid artery (*white arrows*). **(C)** Exposure of the hippocampus before resection. The body and pes of the hippocampus are seen (*long white arrows*) along with the fimbria just under the choroid plexus (*short white arrow*). **(D)** View after hippocampectomy shows the edge of the tentorium (*black asterisks*) with arachnoid protecting the brainstem and other structures. The 3rd nerve is visible through the arachnoid (*white arrow*).

as not to rupture the mesial parietal-occipital vein as it feeds into the vein of Galen.[21]

Closure

Closure follows standard neurosurgical practice. A ventricular catheter is placed into the resection cavity and tunneled through the posterior burr hole out a separate stab incision of the skin (**Fig. 27.2I**; white arrow). Anesthesia personnel are asked to give the patient a loading dose of AEDs as the dura is closed. Central tack-up sutures are placed, the bone is secured in place with plates and screws, and the temporalis muscle and fascia are reapproximated (**Fig. 27.2J**). The galea is closed with special attention directed toward reapproximating the skin edges at the intersection of the T, and the skin is closed with staples. We do not use epidural or subgaleal drains.

Immediate Postoperative and Intensive Care Unit Care

Patients are nearly always extubated in the operating room before transport to the postanesthesia recovery room. An exception would be a child taken to the operating room intubated in status epilepticus. For elective surgery, infants and children should be awake and interactive the night after surgery. Parents are informed that the level of interaction will decrease slightly by 48 hours after surgery during the period of peak brain swelling and then improve thereafter. Pain is treated by small doses of intravenous narcotics and from postoperative Day 5 to 7 onward with nonsteroidal antiinflammatory medications. The nonsteroidal medications also help in reducing the fever associated with the chemical meningitis that frequently occurs after surgery. Throughout the operation, in the recovery room, and for the first 3 days in the intensive care unit (ICU), the hematocrit is maintained from 28 to 32, the serum sodium from 136 to 140, and the international normalized ratio from 1.0 to 1.2. These values were selected based on the empirical observation that children appeared to have a better postoperative course with these measures. Infants with hemimegalencephaly can be expected to require additional blood and blood products in the ICU for the first 24 to 48 hours after surgery. Most commonly, children are drinking and starting foods within 48 hours after surgery. They are restarted on their standard AEDs once taking liquids by mouth.

The ventricular catheter is left open to drain at 5 to 6 cm of water. Despite confirming good hemostasis at surgical closure, the cerebrospinal fluid (CSF) often becomes cloudy and bloody for several days after surgery. At our institution, ventricular drains require patients to be in the ICU, and this mandates the length of time the child is in the ICU. CSF is drawn every other day for surveillance cultures. Once the CSF protein has fallen to less than 300 mg/dL we attempt to test-clamp the ventricular catheter overnight. If the intracranial pressure is less than 15 to 17 cm of water, the ventricular catheter is removed. If not, we resume ventricular drainage for another 12 hours and test-clamp overnight a second time. If the second test-clamp fails, the child is taken back to the operating room for a ventriculoperitoneal shunt. If a shunt is necessary, the ventricular catheter is placed within the resection cavity and not in the opposite hemisphere. We prefer to use nonprogrammable, antisiphon, low-pressure valves because they produce fewer artifacts on serial postoperative MRIs and are well suited to our patient population.

The first postoperative imaging is usually a head CT performed at the time the ventricles are best decompressed: when the ventricular catheter is removed or after the shunt is placed. It is very common to see a 1- to 2-cm epidural space filled with blood and air on this initial CT scan. The initial head CT is used as a reference should other scans be necessary in the postoperative period to determine whether hydrocephalus has developed. Determination of hydrocephalus on the head CT involves evaluation of the contralateral lateral and temporal ventricles along with the 3rd ventricle. Development of hydrocephalus can occur many years after cerebral hemispherectomy. Hence, should a child complain about headaches, not perform as well in school, show any signs of increased intracranial pressure , or develop new seizures after hemispherectomy, we immediately order neuroimaging to rule out late-acquired hydrocephalus.

Consultation with physical and occupational therapy determines whether the child will need inpatient or outpatient rehabilitation after cerebral hemispherectomy. Older children who were walking before surgery generally require inpatient rehabilitation. Fevers associated with chemical meningitis consisting of a stiff neck and malaise usually begin on postoperative Day 4 to 5 and can last several days to weeks. The fevers are easily controlled with antiinflammatory medications. Once the child is able to drink, eat, and has fevers less than 38.5°C, the patient is discharged from the hospital, which is usually within 7 to 14 days after surgery. Staples are removed 10 to 14 days after surgery.

Long-Term Follow-Up

Our typical schedule for follow-up visits is 6 and 12 months after surgery and then yearly thereafter. An MRI is performed as part of the 6-month visit to assess the surgical disconnection (**Fig. 27.1E,F**). The pediatric neurologist may begin tapering AEDs beginning 3 months after surgery. At each follow-up visit we assess the following: (1) seizure control, (2) number and amounts of AEDs, (3) motor development, (4) speech development, (5) psychosocial interactions and behavior, and (6) current physical and other therapies. Long-term follow-up over years is necessary, in our experience, to identify late recurrence of seizures or hydrocephalus and to understand whether the child is showing proper developmental milestones.

■ UCLA Cerebral Hemispherectomy Cohort Characteristics

General Description

Since the inception of this operation in 1998 to April 2008, 96 patients have undergone functional hemispherectomy at UCLA. This represents 38% of all resective operations for pediatric epilepsy surgery patients during this interval. A total of 166 patients have had cerebral hemispherectomy at UCLA since 1986. Four of the 96 patients had prior resections of the frontal and parietal lobes that were converted into a cerebral hemispherectomy with a second operation. Mean (± SD) age at seizure onset is 1.9 ± 3.3 years, with a median of 3 months, and a range from birth to 19 years. Mean age at surgery is 4.8 ± 5.6 years, with a median of 2.5 years and a range from 10 weeks to 36 years. Forty-seven percent of our cases had surgery before age 2 years with 28% before age 1 year. These features are generally younger than other cohorts of patients undergoing cerebral hemispherectomy at other institutions using other operative techniques.[22–24] Mean seizure duration is 2.9 ± 3.6 years, with a median of 1.25 years and a range from 1 month to 17 years. Ninety-one (95%) patients were having at least one seizure per day before surgery. The other 5% were having at least one seizure per week. There are 46 (48%) girls and 49 (51%) left-sided resections. A history of infantile spasms was noted in 44 (46%) patients, and 28

(29%) patients presented in acute status epilepticus requiring prompt surgery. The most common etiology was cortical dysplasia (34%), followed by hemimegalencephaly (22%) (**Table 27.1**).[25,26] Hence, in our hemispherectomy series, malformations of cortical development were the most frequent histopathological finding (58%), and this was mostly in children 2 years of age or less. In a prior retrospective study, we found that our procedure was associated with the least operative blood loss, shortest ICU stay, and lowest complication rate compared with anatomical and Rasmussen functional hemispherectomy techniques.[3]

Characteristics Based on Etiology

We and others have noted that operative risks and outcomes vary more by etiology and duration of seizures than by cerebral hemispherectomy technique, with children with hemimegalencephaly being the most challenging.[12,27,28] Patients with hemimegalencephaly and hemispheric cortical dysplasia are younger at age of seizure onset and surgery compared with patients with Rasmussen encephalitis and cerebral infarcts (**Table 27.2**). A history of infantile spasms and status epilepticus at the time of surgery is also more prevalent in children with malformations of cortical development (**Table 27.2**).[13] Likewise, children with hemimegalencephaly are reported to have the highest operative blood loss compared with other etiologies.[28]

Operation Time and Expected Blood Loss

In our experience, the length of the operation and blood loss varies, depending on the etiology.[29] Operative blood loss with the UCLA procedure ranges from 200 mL to 600 mL, with half of that loss on turning the bone flap. Blood loss

is highest for children with malformations of cortical development compared with Rasmussen encephalitis and infarcts.[30] For larger, older patients with atrophic etiologies, blood replacement is usually not necessary. However, children weighing less than 15 kg with cortical dysplasia, which makes up a large proportion of our cohort, can expect to receive blood replacement with cerebral hemispherectomy. Similarly, patients with large ventricles from perinatal infarcts will take less time to complete the operation (usually less than 5 hours) compared with infants less than 8 kg with hemimegalencephaly (10 to 12 hours).

Postoperative CSF Shunts

In our series, 31 (32%) patients have eventually had placement of a cerebral shunt for acquired hydrocephalus. Roughly half of the shunts were placed in the first 2 weeks after surgery, with the others placed months to years after the operation. In one case, hydrocephalus developed 4.5 years after cerebral hemispherectomy. The placement of shunts does not vary by etiology (**Table 27.2**), and no clinical factors have been identified to predict which patients will eventually require a CSF shunt ($p < .05$).

Operative Related Complications and Reoperations

Morbidity and mortality have been low with the UCLA functional hemispherectomy. There are no deaths in the 96 patients, and no patient has been left in a chronic vegetative condition. Serious complications lasting more than 3 months include two (2%) patients with partial 3rd nerve palsies. Minor complications (9%) include one patient reoperated for a partial osteomyelitis of the distal bone flap 3 months after

Table 27.2 Comparison of Clinical Features by Etiology in UCLA Hemispherectomy Series

Variable	Hemimeg. (n = 21)	Hemi CD (n = 24)	Rasmussen Syndrome (n = 17)	Infarct (n = 16)	p Value
Age at seizure onset (Yr)	0.2 ± 0.6	0.4 ± 0.8	5.7 ± 5.1	3.4 ± 2.8	< .0001
Age at surgery (Yr)	1.2 ± 2.1	3.1 ± 3.9	9.3 ± 8.2	7.8 ± 4.1	< .0001
Seizure duration (Yr)	1.1 ± 2.0	2.7 ± 3.4	3.6 ± 4.7	4.4 ± 3.0	.025
Seizure-free last follow-up	86%	81%	88%	100%	.16
Status epilepticus at surgery	52%	20%	41%	12%	.022
History of infantile spasms	71%	56%	6%	37%	.0004
Percentage with shunts	19%	38%	23%	31%	.45
Side (left/right)	16/5	15/19	6/11	10/6	.04
Gender (female/male)	9/12	13/21	10/7	9/7	.44

Abbreviations: Hemimeg., hemimegalencephaly; Hemi CD, hemispheric cortical dysplasia; Rasmussen, Rasmussen encephalitis; Infarct, MCA infarct, hypoxia-ischemia.

surgery (no fever or elevated serum white count), and eight patients treated for suspected postoperative CSF infections in the first 2 weeks after surgery (four culture positive). There have been three (3%) reoperations for persistent seizures, of which two became seizure free after further disconnection of the mesial frontal white matter tracts into the ipsilateral thalamus (**Fig. 27.3B**). There have been no cases of superficial hemosiderosis.

Outcome: Seizure Freedom, Use of AEDs, and Cognitive Development

At last follow-up, 86% of patients in the UCLA series reported that they were seizure free after cerebral hemispherectomy. This is comparable with other hemispherectomy techniques reported since 2004 in which more than 75% of patients are reported as seizure free.[22,24,31–33] In the UCLA cohort, the percentage of patients seizure free does not vary significantly with duration of follow-up (**Fig. 27.4A**) or etiology (**Table 27.2**). Use of AEDs, which averaged three agents before surgery, declined to an average of one AED at 2 and 5 years after cerebral hemispherectomy (**Fig. 27.4B**). In our hemispherectomy cohort, 17% of patients have stopped using AEDs at last follow-up. We and others have reported that longer seizure durations of more than 18 months and etiology (hemimegalencephaly) are associated with poorer Vineland developmental outcomes after cerebral hemispherectomy.[12,24,28]

Long-Term Studies: Motor Skills, Language, and Rehabilitation

Cohorts of patients after hemispherectomy offer the opportunity to study cerebral development with one half of the brain.[34] These studies have shown that motor recovery of the distal muscles of the arm and leg depends on the timing of surgery and etiology.[35] Younger children with perinatal strokes will develop more motor abilities than older children with Rasmussen syndrome.[36–38] However, even older children can show signs of functional plasticity many years after surgery. For example, we showed improvement in walking associated with functional MRI changes with intensive rehabilitation therapy in children many years after cerebral hemispherectomy.[39] For language, many children with hemimegalencephaly will not develop language compared with other etiologies of children undergoing cerebral hemispherectomy.[40,41] However, we have recently observed language in children with hemimegalencephaly if their cerebral hemispherectomy was performed before 6 months of age. Hence, children after cerebral hemispherectomy should continue to undergo physical and occupational therapies many years after surgery, and these patient groups offer a unique opportunity to study functional plasticity of the human cerebral cortex.

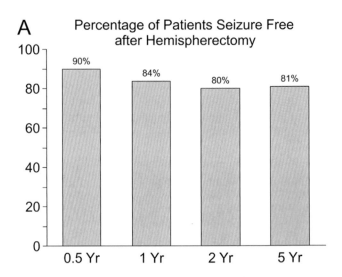

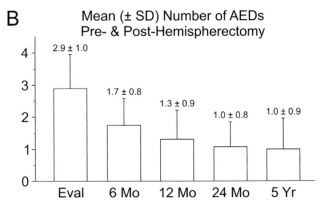

Fig. 27.4 Bar graphs illustrating the percentage of patients seizure free after cerebral hemispherectomy in the UCLA series, and number of antiepilepsy drugs (AED) **(A)** before and **(B)** after surgery. The percentage of patients seizure free after UCLA's functional cerebral hemispherectomy are shown based on duration of follow-up. Before surgery, 91% of patients were having daily or multiple seizures per day. Mean (± *SD*) number of AEDs used per patient before and after cerebral hemispherectomy.

■ Assessment and Conclusion

UCLA's cerebral hemispherectomy has fulfilled most of the objectives it was designed for. The technique is meant for infants and small children with large dysplastic brains and is associated with a high rate of seizure freedom, reduced operative blood loss, and minimal complication. Better postsurgery seizure control probably depends on removal of the thalamus and basal ganglia, especially in children with hemimegalencephaly and Rasmussen encephalitis. The amount of cerebral tissue removed is less than an anatomical hemispherectomy, but more than perisylvian hemispherotomy and some other techniques. There is still room for improvement with this operation. Blood loss could be reduced even more, and the rate of needing CSF shunts is disappointing given that the veins and arachnoid granulations at the midline are preserved. Further modifications of our and other cerebral hemispherectomy techniques can be expected as surgeons try new methods and ideas.

It is also worth pointing out that modified cerebral hemispherectomy techniques to reduce the amount of brain removal are not applicable for all patients. In the past 10 years, we have seen two patients in which the cortical dysplasia was so severe that the lateral ventricular system was obliterated (**Fig. 27.1C** and **D**). In such cases, we have performed anatomical cerebral hemispherectomy to define the mesial structures before removal. Hence, there is no perfect cerebral hemispherectomy technique applicable for all patients.

The technique applied should be one the surgeon is familiar and comfortable with and should be able to address the expected and unexpected anatomy that the patient presents with. Safety and efficacy are the most important factors to consider when selecting the cerebral hemispherectomy technique to apply to patients with refractory epilepsy, and this should take into consideration etiology, size, and position of the ventricular system and deep brain structures and age of the infant or child at surgery.

Acknowledgments This work was supported by the National Institutes of Health Grant R01 NS38992 to GWM.

References

1. Harvey AS, Cross JH, Shinnar S, Mathern BW; ILAE Pediatric Epilepsy Surgery Survey Taskforce. Defining the spectrum of international practice in pediatric epilepsy surgery patients. Epilepsia 2008;49(1):146–155

2. Krynauw RA. Infantile hemiplegia treated by removing one cerebral hemisphere. J Neurol Neurosurg Psychiatry 1950;13(4):243–267

3. Cook SW, Nguyen ST, Hu B, et al. Cerebral hemispherectomy in pediatric patients with epilepsy: comparison of three techniques by pathological substrate in 115 patients. J Neurosurg 2004; 100(2, suppl Pediatrics):125–141

4. Fountas KN, Smith JR, Robinson JS, Tamburrini G, Pietrini D, Di Rocco C. Anatomical hemispherectomy. Childs Nerv Syst 2006;22(8):982–991

5. Peacock WJ, Wehby-Grant MC, Shields WD, et al. Hemispherectomy for intractable seizures in children: a report of 58 cases. Childs Nerv Syst 1996;12(7):376–384

6. Rasmussen T. Hemispherectomy for seizures revisited. Can J Neurol Sci 1983;10(2):71–78

7. Salamon N, Andres M, Chute DJ, et al. Contralateral hemimicrencephaly and clinical-pathological correlations in children with hemimegalencephaly. Brain 2006;129(pt 2):352–365

8. Jahan R, Mischel PS, Curran JG, Peacock WJ, Shields DW, Vinters HV. Bilateral neuropathologic changes in a child with hemimegalencephaly. Pediatr Neurol 1997;17(4):344–349

9. Cats EA, Kho KH, Van Nieuwenhuizen O, Van Veelen CW, Gosselaar PH, Van Rijen PC. Seizure freedom after functional hemispherectomy and a possible role for the insular cortex: the Dutch experience. J Neurosurg 2007; 107(4, suppl)275–280

10. Battaglia D, Chieffo D, Lettori D, Perrino F, Di Rocco C, Guzzetta F. Cognitive assessment in epilepsy surgery of children. Childs Nerv Syst 2006;22(8):744–759

11. Cross JH, Jayakar P, Nordli D, et al; International League against Epilepsy, Subcommission for Paediatric Epilepsy Surgery; Commissions of Neurosurgery and Paediatrics. Proposed criteria for referral and evaluation of children for epilepsy surgery: recommendations of the Subcommission for Pediatric Epilepsy Surgery. Epilepsia 2006;47(6):952–959

12. Jonas R, Asarnow RF, LoPresti C, et al. Surgery for symptomatic infant-onset epileptic encephalopathy with and without infantile spasms. Neurology 2005;64(4):746–750

13. Koh S, Mathern GW, Glasser G, et al. Status epilepticus and frequent seizures: incidence and clinical characteristics in pediatric epilepsy surgery patients. Epilepsia 2005;46(12):1950–1954

14. Cepeda C, André VM, Flores-Hernández J, et al. Pediatric cortical dysplasia: correlations between neuroimaging, electrophysiology and location of cytomegalic neurons and balloon cells and glutamate/GABA synaptic circuits. Dev Neurosci 2005;27(1):59–76

15. Chandra PS, Salamon N, Huang J, et al. FDG-PET/MRI coregistration and diffusion-tensor imaging distinguish epileptogenic tubers and cortex in patients with tuberous sclerosis complex: a preliminary report. Epilepsia 2006;47(9):1543–1549

16. Mathern GW, Giza CC, Yudovin S, et al. Postoperative seizure control and antiepileptic drug use in pediatric epilepsy surgery patients: the UCLA experience, 1986-1997. Epilepsia 1999;40(12):1740–1749

17. Wu JY, Sutherling WW, Koh S, et al. Magnetic source imaging localizes epileptogenic zone in children with tuberous sclerosis complex. Neurology 2006;66(8):1270–1272

18. Chugani HT, Shields WD, Shewmon DA, Olson DM, Phelps ME, Peacock WJ. Infantile spasms: I. PET identifies focal cortical dysgenesis in cryptogenic cases for surgical treatment. Ann Neurol 1990;27(4):406–413

19. Mathern GW, Leite JP, Pretorius JK, Quinn B, Peacock WJ, Babb TL. Children with severe epilepsy: evidence of hippocampal neuron losses and aberrant mossy fiber sprouting during postnatal granule cell migration and differentiation. Brain Res Dev Brain Res 1994;78(1):70–80

20. Mathern GW, Leiphart JL, De Vera A, et al. Seizures decrease postnatal neurogenesis and granule cell development in the human fascia dentata. Epilepsia 2002;43(suppl 5):68–73

21. Di Rocco C, Battaglia D, Pietrini D, Piastra M, Massimi L. Hemimegalencephaly: clinical implications and surgical treatment. Childs Nerv Syst 2006;22(8):852–866

22. Villemure JG, Daniel RT. Peri-insular hemispherotomy in paediatric epilepsy. Childs Nerv Syst 2006;22(8):967–981

23. Schramm J, Kral T, Clusmann H. Transsylvian keyhole functional hemispherectomy. Neurosurgery 2001;49(4):891–900, discussion 900–901

24. Delalande O, Bulteau C, Dellatolas G, et al. Vertical parasagittal hemispherotomy: surgical procedures and clinical long-term outcomes

in a population of 83 children. Neurosurgery 2007; 60(2, suppl 1)ONS19–ONS32, discussion ONS32

25. Vinters HV, Fisher RS, Cornford ME, et al. Morphological substrates of infantile spasms: studies based on surgically resected cerebral tissue. Childs Nerv Syst 1992;8(1):8–17

26. Mischel PS, Nguyen LP, Vinters HV. Cerebral cortical dysplasia associated with pediatric epilepsy. Review of neuropathologic features and proposal for a grading system. J Neuropathol Exp Neurol 1995;54(2):137–153

27. Devlin AM, Cross JH, Harkness W, et al. Clinical outcomes of hemispherectomy for epilepsy in childhood and adolescence. Brain 2003;126(pt 3):556–566

28. Jonas R, Nguyen S, Hu B, et al. Cerebral hemispherectomy: hospital course, seizure, developmental, language, and motor outcomes. Neurology 2004;62(10):1712–1721

29. Piastra M, Pietrini D, Caresta E, et al. Hemispherectomy procedures in children: haematological issues. Childs Nerv Syst 2004;20(7):453–458

30. Pietrini D, Zanghi F, Pusateri A, Tosi F, Pulitanò S, Piastra M. Anesthesiological and intensive care considerations in children undergoing extensive cerebral excision procedure for congenital epileptogenic lesions. Childs Nerv Syst 2006;22(8):844–851

31. O'Brien DF, Basu S, Williams DH, May PL. Anatomical hemispherectomy for intractable seizures: excellent seizure control, low morbidity and no superficial cerebral haemosiderosis. Childs Nerv Syst 2006;22(5):489–498, discussion 499

32. Binder DK, Schramm J. Transsylvian functional hemispherectomy. Childs Nerv Syst 2006;22(8):960–966

33. Basheer SN, Connolly MB, Lautzenhiser A, Sherman EM, Hendson G, Steinbok P. Hemispheric surgery in children with refractory epilepsy: seizure outcome, complications, and adaptive function. Epilepsia 2007;48(1):133–140

34. de Bode S, Sininger Y, Healy EW, Mathern GW, Zaidel E. Dichotic listening after cerebral hemispherectomy: methodological and theoretical observations. Neuropsychologia 2007;45(11):2461–2466

35. van Empelen R, Jennekens-Schinkel A, Buskens E, Helders PJ, van Nieuwenhuizen O; Dutch Collaborative Epilepsy Surgery Programme. Functional consequences of hemispherectomy. Brain 2004;127(pt 9):2071–2079

36. de Bode S, Firestine A, Mathern GW, Dobkin B. Residual motor control and cortical representations of function following hemispherectomy: effects of etiology. J Child Neurol 2005;20(1):64–75

37. Wakamoto H, Eluvathingal TJ, Makki M, Juhász C, Chugani HT. Diffusion tensor imaging of the corticospinal tract following cerebral hemispherectomy. J Child Neurol 2006;21(7):566–571

38. Dijkerman HC, Vargha-Khadem F, Polkey CE, Weiskrantz L. Ipsilesional and contralesional sensorimotor function after hemispherectomy: differences between distal and proximal function. Neuropsychologia 2008;46(3):886–901

39. de Bode S, Mathern GW, Bookheimer S, Dobkin B. Locomotor training remodels fMRI sensorimotor cortical activations in children after cerebral hemispherectomy. Neurorehabil Neural Repair 2007;21(6):497–508

40. Curtiss S, de Bode S, Mathern GW. Spoken language outcomes after hemispherectomy: factoring in etiology. Brain Lang 2001;79(3):379–396

41. Liégeois F, Connelly A, Baldeweg T, Vargha-Khadem F. Speaking with a single cerebral hemisphere: fMRI language organization after hemispherectomy in childhood. Brain Lang; 2008:106(3):195–203

28 Transsylvian Hemispheric Deafferentation

Johannes Schramm

As outlined in Chapter 24, functional hemispherectomy, hemispherotomy, or hemispherical deafferentation are closely related surgical options for patients with medically intractable seizures resulting from one hemisphere, involving more than one lobe of that hemisphere. The co existence of these terms reflects the fact that in the past 25 years, a tendency toward less tissue removal and more extensive disconnection has taken place. After the introduction of Rasmussen's technique, which still consists of the removal of the whole temporal lobe and a large block of the central hemisphere, the next step in the development toward a very much less invasive technique was presented in 1992[1] followed by a first series of patients from Bonn in 1995.[2] Quite a different approach but using the same principle of transventricular deafferentation is described similarly early by Delalande et al with their parasagittal vertical hemispherotomy.[3] This was followed by a closely related technique.[4] The key element in these approaches is the deafferentation of the cortical mantle through a transventricular approach, whereby several variants related to that first description[1] followed.[5-7] Whereas the term *hemispheric deafferentation* does not suggest a large resection, hemidecortication or hemicorticectomy and some of the perisylvian hemispherectomy techniques[7] remove more brain and thus constitute a different class of intervention. This chapter focuses on the transsylvian/transventricular keyhole hemispherical deafferentation procedure, which may be called a transsylvian keyhole hemispherotomy.[6]

■ Indication and Presurgical Evaluation

The classic indication is for patients with severe hemispherical damage and drug-resistant epilepsy or drug-resistant epilepsy in early infancy known as catastrophic epilepsy. These patients usually are children or adolescents; in adults the procedure is performed les frequently.

This procedure is possible because these patients usually already have spastic hemiparesis, frequently partial hemianopia, and transferred of motor and language functions to the other (healthy) hemisphere either induced by the disease process or by the connatal condition. Diagnoses typi-

cally found in these patients may be classified into inborn, perinatal, or acquired conditions. In our series, these include intrauterine hemorrhages or perinatal injuries with brain defects ($n = 38$); multilobar cortical dysplasia, polymicrogyria, and other disorders of gyration (e.g., lissencephaly; $n = 8$); and hemimegalencephaly ($n = 9$). Other entities may present as progressive clinical pictures, like Rasmussen encephalitis ($n = 10$) or Sturge-Weber syndrome ($n = 4$)[8] (**Fig. 28.1**). Rarer acquired lesions include posttraumatic or postencephalitic hemispheric damage ($n = 8$), hemiatrophy ($n = 3$), and hemiconvulsion-hemiplegia-epilepsy syndrome ($n = 1$).

The indication is unproblematic if hemispheric damage is either congenital or occurred perinatally. An increase in the motor deficit usually is unlikely if the hemispheric damage happened in the first 3 years of life; here frequently only the fine pincer movements between index finger and thumb are lost postoperatively. Performing this surgery in children with a progressive disease that started to develop after the fourth year of life may be more difficult, although we have seen an initial postoperative deterioration of motor abilities in children between 4 and 8 years. A deterioration in motor function of the leg is usually transient. These children usually regain the ability to walk but frequently loose not only the pincer function between thumb and index finger but also grip function of their hand on the affected side. Deciding to perform hemispheric deafferentation in a progressive disease, such as Rasmussen's or Sturge-Weber, is made somewhat easier by the knowledge that these children will be progressively impaired by the epilepsy disorder itself eventually with the same type of deficit after a few years as to be expected from the surgery, with the additional damage to their functional and cognitive development by the affection of the healthy hemisphere.

Presurgical evaluation always tries to demonstrate that the disease process is limited to the abnormal hemisphere. Electroencephalography (EEG) studies consist of interictal and ictal video-EEG. In planned hemispherectomy cases, it is not important to localize ictal activity to certain areas of the affected hemisphere but, if possible, to lateralize it only to the affected side. In our experience, the use of invasive recordings in these patients is rarely necessary. The presence of epileptic EEG activity in the contralateral healthy hemisphere as observed in a minority of these cases is said to

241

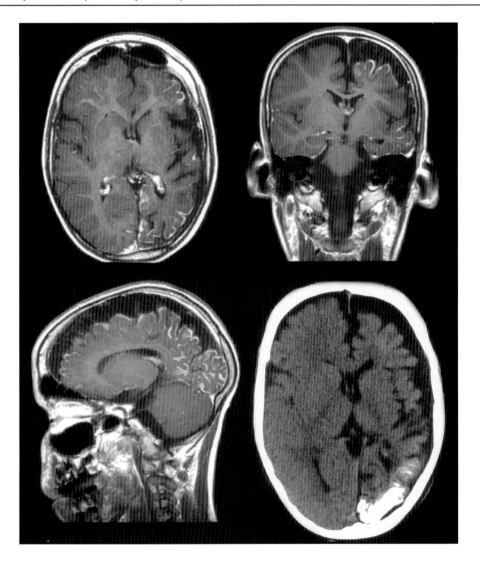

Fig. 28.1 Magnetic resonance images and computed tomography (CT) scan of a 10-year-old boy with Sturge-Weber syndrome associated with left-sided hippocampal sclerosis. Note the calcifications (bottom right) in the CT-scan. Although the manifestations of abnormal pial vessels is most marked in the occipitoparietal region, the whole hemisphere is atrophic. During the surgery, one pack of erythrocytes was given. The operation time from skin to skin was 225 minutes. Eight years after surgery, the patient is seizure free. (Copyright J. Schramm, reproduced with permission.)

indicate a lesser chance for seizure freedom[9]; however, this does not exclude the chance for seizure freedom after hemispherical deafferentation.[10] In one large series, 77% of those with suspected bilateral disease were either seizure free or had only "minor events."[11] Independently arising seizure activity from the healthy hemisphere clearly discernable from the EEG activity and the ictal picture originating from the affected hemisphere may be considered as a relative contraindication for surgery. When seizure activity is observed in the so-called healthy hemisphere only during seizure activity recorded from the affected hemisphere, the interpretation is more difficult; here one should keep in mind that

even a marked reduction in seizure activity after surgery is considered worthwhile by the families and the patients and may open the door for successful drug treatment, keeping in mind that there is a chance of perhaps 30 to 50% of seizure freedom despite the contralateral seizure activity in the EEG.

Of the various imaging modalities, the most important is magnetic resonance imaging (MRI), with computed tomography (CT) being mostly useful to demonstrate calcifications as in Sturge-Weber syndrome (**Fig. 28.1**). The value of MRI is particularly important for suspected malformations of cortical development. Disorders of gyration, irregularities or thickening of the cortical band, gross malformations of the brain, and ectopic gray matter are characteristic findings. Atrophy, ventricle size, hemispheric configuration, widespread posttraumatic or postencephalitic damage, as well as more subtle regional atrophy in the early stages of Rasmussen's may be demonstrable. In acute encephalitis and Sturge-Weber syndrome postcontrast MRI will show typical findings. In case of suspected Rasmussen encephalitis, it frequently is very helpful to carefully look at sequential MRIs over time, checking for developing atrophy and signs of regional inflammation.

In our hands positron emission tomography or single photon emission computed tomography is rarely indicated in these patients. The intracarotid amobarbital test (Wada test) is still used in unclear cases to lateralize language function or to demonstrate complete transfer of language function. To use functional MRI (fMRI) for speech localization is not as reliable, because it has been demonstrated in chronic epilepsy patients, that incorrect or unclear localization may occur in up to 28% of patients.[12,13] Neuropsychological assessment is performed as usual or as far as mental retardation allows.

The diagnosis of suspected Rasmussen encephalitis is not always that clear. If there is concern about the diagnosis, open brain biopsy, usually in the F1-gyrus though a fronto-dorsal-paramedian approach, is performed, delivering a tissue sample of 1 × 1 cm, without prior coagulation of the arachnoid, comprising pia mater, cortex, and white matter.

■ Advantages and Limitations of the Transsylvian Keyhole Deafferentation

Points that speak for this less invasive technique of transsylvian transventricular deafferentation are the proven reduction in blood loss, the reduced need for blood transfusion, and the reduction in operating room time.[14] Shimizu and Maehara,[5] Kestle et al,[15] and Cook et al[7] also demonstrated reduced need for blood replacement for their related techniques. The keyhole technique is well suited for hemispheres with large perinatal infarctions or large cysts in the territory of the middle cerebral artery (MCA), patients with enlarged ventricles, and patients with atrophic brains with a smaller-than-usual central bloc of insula-basal ganglia. The transsylvian transventricular approach is more difficult in hemimegalencephaly cases. The opercula may be much thicker, the configuration of the sylvian cistern is generally atypical, and thus orientation is much more difficult. One can still use the transsylvian transventricular deafferentation procedure in these cases; however, it is then advisable to combine it with a resection of the operculum, exposing the circular sulcus and facilitating the entry into the ven-

tricle considerably. This was done in seven of nine hemimegalencephaly cases of our series. One possible benefit of the keyhole technique, where the opercula are reflected and preserved compared with the perisylvian window techniques[4,5,7] in which they are resected, is that hardly any MCA branches and large sylvian veins have to be resected and there is a lesser chance for postoperative swelling because of circulation disturbances. Conversely, there may be some swelling from the manipulation of the operculum.

The limits of this approach include its limited applicability in hemimegalencephaly and the difficult anatomical orientation with an inherent risk of incomplete disconnection. So far, we have not observed a case of incomplete disconnection toward the midline or the fronto- and occipito-basal arachnoid, but we have seen a few cases in which the fronto-basal anterior disconnection line was not ideally placed as far posterior as the level of the anterior cerebral artery but slightly anterior to it.[16] Other authors have observed incomplete disconnection rates of 7, 19, 21, and 54%, even in Rasmussen-type surgeries.[17-20]

The high shunt rates known from anatomical resection do not seem to be reached by the transsylvian keyhole technique and related perisylvian or transventricular techniques. A certain percentage of shunt implantation appears unavoidable with all kinds of intraventricular procedures, as well as with these hemispherectomies. In more than 75 transsylvian procedures with 81 months mean follow-up on 56 transsylvian keyhole deafferentation procedures, we had 4 cases of hydrocephalus (5.4%), with only 2 of them needing a shunt (2.7%). The other 2 had cysto-ventriculostomy but no shunt. Shunt rates in related procedures[5,20,21] were 10/53 for Delalande's technique (19%), 5/63 for Villemure's perisylvian window technique (8%), 5/22 in the Cleveland series (23%), and 5/32 for Shimizu's and Maehara's series (16%). In the review of the Los Angeles series[7] in which three operation types were compared, the advantages of Mathern's modification of the peri-insular surgery variant are listed as: least operative blood loss, least overall complication rate, and even a greater seizure-free outcome rate. A brief review of the pros and cons of this procedure is given in recent book chapters.[22,23] A comparison of surgical techniques is given in Schramm 2002[16] and in adjoining chapters of this book.

■ Presurgical Management

The anticonvulsive medication is not withdrawn preoperatively. The laboratory evaluation includes the usual serum parameters including coagulation parameters and blood typing. Dexamethasone is given only preoperatively if a near normal or hemimegalencephalic brain volume is present, not in atrophic brains with large cysts or huge ventricles. Before skin incision, a prophylactic antibiotic is given. Two intravenous lines and one arterial line are placed; a central venous line is placed only in very small babies. After placement of a transurethral catheter, the patient is wrapped up carefully and kept warm using a Bair Hugger (Arizant Healthcare, Inc., Eden Prairie, MN).

■ Surgical Technique

The transsylvian transventricular hemispherical deafferentation through a small craniotomy may be called a keyhole approach because to achieve a disconnection around the corpus callosum, which is approximately 7 to 7.5 cm long in an adult, a craniotomy no larger than 4 to 5 cm in anterior–posterior-diameter is necessary (**Fig. 28.2**). Because the calvarial bone flap is approximately 5 to 6 cm away from the midline, it is easy to visualize the area from just anterior to the knee of the corpus callosum to just posterior of the splenium through this opening. This perspective leads to the analogy with the keyhole perspective or a keyhole approach. The small craniotomy flap is not a value per se, but bone flap

sizes ranging from 4 × 4 to 5 × 6 cm have been quite satisfactory. This approach includes four main features, which can be subdivided into five steps:

1. Transsylvian exposure via a small craniotomy following a curvilinear incision
2. Temporo-mesial disconnection via a transtemporal stem uncoamygdalohippocampectomy
3. Complete exposure of the whole ventricular system though the circular sulcus exposing the ventricle from the tip of the temporal horn to the tip of the frontal horn after a transcortical incision along the circular sulcus of the insular cistern
4. Basal and mesial disconnection
   a. Fronto-basal disconnection along the middle and anterior cerebral artery and postero-medial disconnection along the falcotentorial rim
   b. Paramesial callosal disconnection via an intraventricular approach by exposing the anterior cerebral and pericallosal arteries along the midline around the corpus callosum and posteriorly along the falcotentorial rim directly to the splenium

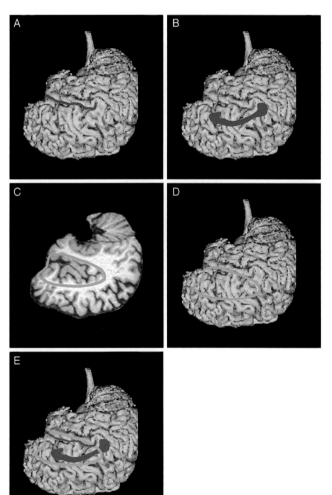

Fig. 28.2 Surgeon's view of surface projection of relevant structures for approach in keyhole transsylvian deafferentation as seen in a right-sided surgery. Magnetic resonance imaging taken from an unaffected brain. The position of the sylvian fissure is shown in red **(A)**, the surface projection of the corpus callosum is shown in blue **(B)**. The outline of the insular cistern is demonstrated as surface projection in **(D)** and from a parasagittal cut in **(C)**. In **(E)**, it becomes clear that to reach the anterior and posterior extent of the corpus callosum it is necessary to retract mainly the frontal operculum and to open the sylvian fissure to the very end. (Reproduced with permission by Lippincott Williams and Wilkins from Schramm J, Kral T, Clusmann H. Transsylvian keyhole functional hemispherectomy. Neurosurgery 2001; 49(4):891–900, discussion 900–901.)

Craniotomy and Transsylvian Exposure

The patient is placed in a lateral position or supine position with the shoulder elevated, so that the head is horizontal and slightly pointed downward. The skin incision is started right before the tragus and may be just a linear incision in case of a smaller craniotomy (4 × 4 cm) or slightly curvilinear for somewhat larger craniotomies (5 × 6 cm). The placement of the craniotomy is facilitated by the use of neuronavigation. The upper limit of the craniotomy should be at the level of the corpus callosum (not at the level of the roof of the lateral ventricle, because that may be higher than the level of the corpus callosum). The lower border of the craniotomy flap should be approximately 0.5 to 1 cm below the level of the ascending M1 branch. Thus, when the dura is opened, the craniotomy is usually placed 90% above the sylvian fissure and no more than 10% below the sylvian fissure (**Fig. 28.3**). Anteriorly, one should be able to see the basal aspect of the frontal lobe along the ascending M1. The size of the craniotomy can be enlarged if there is no adequate degree of atrophy or no porencephalic cyst, or if the basal ganglia-insular bloc is not atrophied.

After opening the dura, usually by two diagonal cuts, the sylvian fissure is opened through its entire length. The insular cortex is exposed by retracting the frontal operculum, which is overlying the insular cortex to a much larger extent than the temporal operculum (**Fig. 28.4**). The cortical surface of the insula corresponds to a triangle with its base located frontally and the narrow angle pointed posteriorly. The outline of the insular cortex corresponds to the circular sulcus. The normal anatomical lay-out of the insular topography may vary considerably in these patients. If atrophy is prominent, the bloc of basal ganglia and insular cortex may have shrunk surrounded by massively enlarged temporal horn, cella media, and frontal horn. The MCA and its branches may be considerably smaller than in healthy brains, the cortex of the insula may be much harder, or occasionally no longer recognizable as a distinct cortical layer separate from the

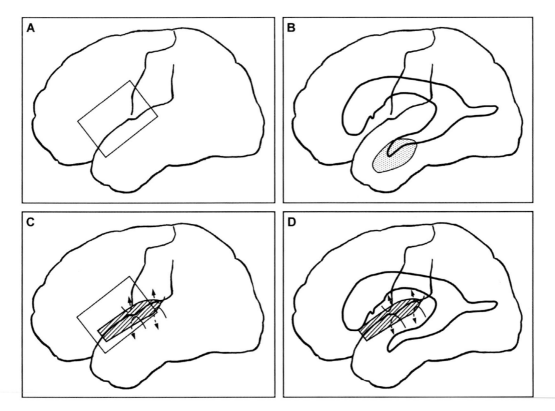

Fig. 28.3 Schematic outline of position of craniotomy over the sylvian fissure and its relationship to the ventricular system. **(A)** Outline of the brain surface with the projection of the craniotomy over the sylvian fissure. **(B)** Projection of the amygdalohippocampal complex onto the surface of the brain and a projection of the ventricular system on the brain surface. **(C)** Outline of the brain with slightly retracted frontal and temporal opercula. The *arrowheads* indicate the direction of the dissection toward the circular sulcus; the outline of the craniotomy is superimposed. **(D)** Brain contour with a projection of the ventricular system on the surface. The shaded area indicates the exposed sylvian cortex though the sylvian keyhole. The direction of the dissection through the circular sulcus into the ventricular system is indicated by the *arrowheads*. (Reproduced with permission by Lippincott Williams and Wilkins from Schramm J, Kral T, Clusmann H. Transsylvian keyhole functional hemispherectomy. Neurosurgery 2001; 49(4):891–900, discussion 900–901.)

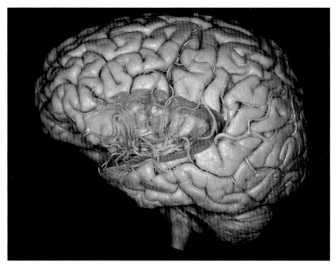 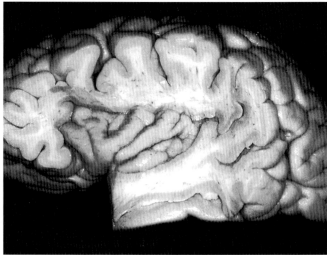

Fig. 28.4 Topography of the insular region. These two brain specimens illustrate the extent to which the opercula cover the insular cortex. At the same time, the abundance of those middle cerebral artery (MCA) branches that originate from the MCA over the insular cortex and then curve underneath the operculum to reach the surface through the sulci of the opercula can easily be seen. In the transsylvian keyhole exposure, most of these periopercular MCA branches can be preserved, whereas in those cases where the opercula are resected, it is more difficult to preserve all of these branches according to the experience in this series when the keyhole approach was supplemented by an opercular window. (Reproduced with permission from Yasargil: Microneurosurgery, Vol IV A, Thieme, Stuttgart-New York, 1994; 54–55)

basal ganglia bloc. In those patients in which intrauterine or perinatal infarction resulted in large cystic cavities, one should not expect to see one large cavity. Instead, there will be several cysts separated by membranes that usually have at least two layers, which still carry arteries and veins. Most likely, the multiplicity of cysts results from the preservation of arachnoidal layers that have sheathed the opercular gyri on the outside and on the inside as well as the insular cortex and the temporal operculum. It is frequently not easy to immediately find one's way through this maze of cysts, cyst walls, enlarged ventricles, and residual layers of brain tissue, which is usually gliotic and hardened. The choroid plexus, if preserved, is a good guide to recognize the ventricular cavity in these multicystic brains.

Temporomesial Disconnection and Uncoamygdalohippocampectomy

The hippocampal-parahippocampal area may be atrophic or may appear quite normal. The temporal horn is approached through the inferior limb of the circular sulcus, thus transecting the temporal stem (**Fig. 28.5**, lower). The uncus is emptied with the ultrasonic aspirator. The bulging amygdaloidal body with the entorhinal cortex is removed too. The fimbria are elevated along the choroidal fissure. The hippocampus-parahippocampus may be removed by ultrasonic aspiration or en bloc to have good histological diagnosis. Removal of the hippocampus may extend far posterior in the temporal horn,

much further than in the classic selective amygdalohippocampectomy. After completion of this step, the anterior and much of the posterior part of the temporal lobe are disconnected mesiobasally and at the level of the temporal stem. When removing the uncus, the amygdaloidal body, and the entorhinal cortex anterior to the choroidal fissure, the integrity of the mesial arachnoid over the large vessels running around the brainstem should be respected carefully.

Exposure of the Whole Ventricular System

Elevating the dorsal temporal and parietal opercula from the insular cortex with a self-retaining retractor, the circular sulcus is exposed in its posterior aspect, and a transcortical dissection to the lumen of the temporal horn and the trigone is performed. In these frequently atrophic brains, the layer of brain tissue may be very thin—sometimes only a few millimeters. Following the outline of the circular sulcus, the frontal operculum is now retracted and the transcortical opening of the ventricle is performed from the trigone anteriorly to the frontal horn. During this step, one will occasionally cross branches of the MCA, most of which are spared. The ependymal veins need to be coagulated and cut because the Cavitron Ultrasonic Surgical Aspirator does not necessarily transect them in the low setting used for this step. After the completion of this step, the U-shaped ventricle system is now completely opened via the similarly U-shaped incision through the circular sulcus (**Fig. 28.5**, upper).

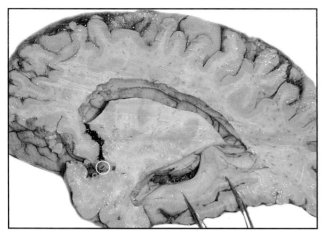

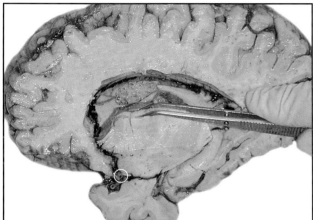

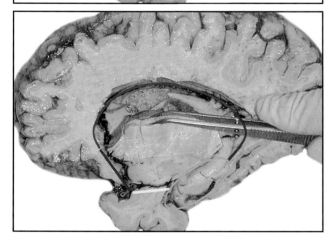

Fig. 28.5 Parasagittal cut through the ventricular system in a formalin-fixed brain exposing the ventricle from the frontal horn to the trigone and the tip of the temporal horn. The parasagittal cut is slightly oblique to simultaneously open the lateral ventricle from the frontal horn to the trigone but also the more laterally placed temporal horn. **Upper:** The dark line in the anterior aspect of the frontobasal lobe indicates the disconnection line from the tip of the frontal horn toward the ascending M1 branch (*white circle*). The forceps is rotating the hippocampus/parahippocampus away from the adhesion along the choroidal fissure. **Middle:** The forceps is elevating the basal ganglia/thalamus bloc. The *dark line* is indicating the transection in the ventricular system, through the fronto-basal matter and cortex, the temporal stem, and the trigone. The *white circle* marks the ascending M1 in front of the limen insulae. **Lower:** The temporo-mesial resection and different transection lines are delineated by different colors: the closed green oval around the hippocampus/parahippocampus bloc demonstrates the resection of these structures. The yellow transverse line across the temporal stem demonstrates the transection through the temporal stem between the temporo-mesial resection cavity and the limen insulae parallel to the ascending M1 branch. The fronto-basal–fronto-mesial disconnection is indicated by the anterior red line ascending from the middle cerebral artery to the tip of the frontal horn. The long blue line running parallel to the corpus callosum indicates the callosal disconnection. The posterior red line points to the occipito-mesial–temporo-mesial disconnection in the trigone. (Copyright J. Schramm, reproduced with permission.)

Basal and Mesial Disconnection

The mesial disconnection proper is mostly performed from within the ventricle except for the fronto-basal white matter. With one retractor reflecting the frontal opercula in the area of the frontal horn, the surgeon is able to simultaneously expose the lateral surface of the frontal lobe and the inner aspect of the frontal horn. The disconnection will run

at the level of the ascending M1-branch through the tissue of the basal frontal lobe ending at the interhemispheric fissure. The orientation is following the course of the MCA as it runs down vertically along the limen insulae. A coagulation of the pial surface of the frontal lobe is done along a line that is basally pointing to the M1 and upwardly pointing at the inferior end of the frontal horn inside the brain. Having opened the arachnoid on the lateral surface of the frontal lobe, the surgeon is working on the inner surface of the arachnoid, which is overlying the MCA immediately in front of the limen insulae. Working deeper and deeper, the surgeon follows the course of the MCA into the depth straight beyond the bifurcation where it turns into the A1 approximately half way down the base of the frontal lobe but still in the same direction. Always adjusting the line of disconnection between the deeper exposure along the A1 and the inner aiming point at the bottom of the frontal horn, the surgeon slowly works through the fronto-basal white matter and cortex. Usually it is possible to see the outline of the M1 or A1 leaving the arachnoid at the frontal base intact. Occasionally, the view is obscured, and then a tiny hole in the arachnoid allows the surgeon to verify that he or she is still following M1 or A1. In doing so, the surgeon automatically reaches the area where A1 turns around to become A2. This is the point where the surgeon has reached the midline. Now the disconnection line in the ventricle also changes a little bit because in following the A2 around the anterior knee of the corpus callosum, the surgeon will place the disconnection line in the frontal horn from its inferior point more upward and toward the area where the roof of the ventricle will finally be met. Following the A2, the surgeon will soon recognize that it is making an anterior bend around the callosal knee only to turn back again after approximately 2 cm, now making the exposure of the pericallosal artery at the roof of the corpus callosum possible. Because the roof of the ventricle in these atrophic brains is frequently positioned higher than the inferior margin of the corpus callosum, the callosotomy is not a callosotomy on the midline, but it is done paramesially where the fibers of the corpus callosum turn upward toward the roof of the enlarged lateral ventricle. Here, the tissue layer is frequently only a few millimeters, and this disconnection can be performed very quickly from the anterior horn backward to the trigonal area.

In the posterior part of the lateral ventricle where it slowly turns into the trigone, it is important not to turn basally into the trigonal area too early and thus end up in the splenium of the corpus callosum. An easy way not to loose orientation is to start looking for the inferior rim of the falx at approximately the middle or the posterior third of the callosal transection. This is the area where the pericallosal artery becomes thinner and may no longer be easily recognizable. In the end part of the callosal section, the surgeon is advised to follow the inferior falx margin, which far posterior slowly turns around basally and becomes the falcotentorial margin. This will lead the surgeon automatically posterior to the splenium through the posterior part of the trigone.

The only mesiobasal disconnection now left is through the mesial white matter of the trigonal area until the resection cavity of the hippocampus is reached. By just following the tentorial margin, the surgeon automatically ends up in the temporal resection cavity. Care has to be taken to not injure the posterior cerebral artery, which is found underneath the

area of the calcar avis, usually accompanied by one or two veins. If the arachnoid of the mesial surface of the occipital lobe is respected, the surgeon will not injure the posterior cerebral artery, and usually the veins can be preserved.

Hemostasis in the mesial disconnection line is usually uncomplicated with small strips of Surgicel (Ethicon, Somerville, NJ) placed there. The disconnection procedure in the last years has been followed by routine ablation of the insular cortex. Between the MCA branches overlying the insular cortex the pia mater is coagulated and incised and the cortex is removed by ultrasonic aspiration working between these branches. Keep in mind that the thickness of the cortex is usually no more than 4 to 5 mm, and the thin layer of white matter of the external capsule can easily be overlooked. In addition, in these sick brains, the architecture of the cortical layers may be quite abnormal because of atrophy, scarring, or fibrosis. By removing the insular cortex, the surgeon has excluded the theoretical chance that the insular cortex, which is still connected to the basal ganglia and thus to fiber tracts leading down to the spinal cord, may be responsible for persistent seizures. One should avoid getting too deep and entering the nuclei of the basal ganglia, because bleeding from these structures is more difficult to control.

When all retractors have been removed, Surgicel may be placed over injured surfaces of the opercula. Copious irrigation of the ventricular lumen is done removing some detritus and blood remnants until a relatively clear fluid is flowing back. The dura is closed in a water tight fashion. Bone flap replacement and closure of the wound follow the classic procedures.

◼ Postoperative Management

All patients go to the intensive care unit at least until the next morning. Usually, extubation takes place in the intensive care unit. Small infants and patients with hemimegalencephaly, in which the risk of brain swelling is bigger, may spend a second night on the intensive care unit.

The usual monitoring includes neurological parameters, such as verbal response, state of wakefulness, motor responses to commands and stimuli, and the classic parameters such as pulse frequency, temperature, and blood pressure. If not already done intraoperatively, fluid losses is replaced, urinary output monitored, and occasionally blood is given.

It is important to start early, that is, intraoperatively, particularly in babies and small infants with correction of abnormalities in serum electrolytes, coagulation parameters, and hemoglobin. This is completed in the postoperative period.

Anticonvulsive medication is kept at the same level as before surgery. Patients who experienced deterioration in their motor function usually are transferred to a rehabilitation unit. So far, we have not seen a single patient who lost the ability to walk independently from the surgical intervention. Careful monitoring for possible postoperative seizures, that may be different type than preoperatively present, is advisable, especially when preoperatively morphological or electroencephalographic involvement of the contralateral good hemisphere was suspected. All patients have early postoperative MRI in which the traces of fresh blood-tinged Surgicel act like a contrast medium indicating whether the transection reaches the fronto-basal, occipito-basal, and mesial arachnoid everywhere, thus proving the complete disconnection.

■ Complications

Intraoperative complications may include increased blood loss, not necessarily in Sturge-Weber syndrome, as frequently expected, but in hemimegalencephaly, because the field is deeper, the dissection is more complicated, and the orientation is more difficult. Thus, in these cases, more surgical time is needed and occasionally atypically large veins are encountered deep in the white matter. A potentially disastrous intraoperative complication would be transgression of the mesial arachnoid of the affected hemisphere into the healthy hemisphere or injury to the vessels in the interhemispheric fissure. This risk can be minimized if the surgeon follows the anterior cerebral and the pericallosal artery mostly along the closed arachnoid where it can usually be seen quite well. Typical operative complications include epi- or subdural hemorrhage, ventriculitis, bone flap infection, and cerebral edema in the operated or the contralateral hemisphere. So far, we have not had any hemispheric edema in the series. There was one bone flap infection appearing years later. A rare subgaleal cerebrospinal fluid collection resolved spontaneously. We observed one chronic subdural hematoma needing twist drill evacuation, two hygromas (one with twist drill), and one pneumonia that resolved uneventfully after treatment.

We frequently observe a raised temperature for a few days, sometimes for more than a week, associated with noninfectious elevated cell count in cerebrospinal fluid (CSF). This condition must be differentiated from infection of the intrathecal space, although normally cultures are negative, and the suspected diagnosis is based on a cell count considered to be higher than resulting just from intraventricular manipulation and detritus. We have seen meningitis, but we never observed a severe ventriculitis; cell counts normalized within 10 to 12 days in all cases. In more than 75 operations with this technique with good follow-up available for more than 1 year in 56 patients (mean > 84 months), we have so far seen four cases of hydrocephalus, one of which appeared late after surgery. Two were shunted, two had cystoventriculostomy. This is equivalent to a hydrocephalus rate of 5.4% and to a shunt rate of 2.7%. Severe intraoperative blood loss was only a problem with Rasmussen's technique, never with the transsylvian technique. We also did not see episodes of severe hypotension or even hemodynamic instability with the keyhole technique.

Unexpected neurological deteriorations were extremely rare. We had one patient with temporary memory disturbance lasting 3 days, most likely from touching the contralateral fornix when fenestrating the septum pellucidum, which was displaced from preexisting unilateral hydrocephalus. Otherwise, in a small proportion of the cases, some deterioration in lack of motor function is observed, mostly in patients in whom the disease started late and transfer to the other side was not complete. That should be considered an expected event and not necessarily a complication, just like complete homonymous hemianopsia, which is unavoidable. So far, there was one death among 78 keyhole cases or a mortality rate of 1.3%. After an uneventful early postoperative course, a severely handicapped 5-year-old boy was found dead in his bed in the morning after the fifth postoperative night with no apparent cause detectable on the immediate CT-scan.

■ Conclusion

The transsylvian hemispheric deafferentation procedure through the sylvian keyhole is one of the functional hemispherectomy procedures with very little resective surgery. So far, it can be confirmed by several authors that there is undoubtedly a shorter operation time, less blood loss, and, in our experience, no intraoperative dramatic episodes compared with other surgical techniques, both the anatomical resection and the Rasmussen technique. In our hands, the shunt rate was low, most likely lower than in related perisylvian techniques in which various parts of the opercula and the insular cortex are resected. The last word concerning complications that are well-known to appear late, such as hemosiderosis, cannot be spoken yet, because mean follow-up for the whole group of keyhole procedures is not yet long enough, that is, 20 years. The keyhole procedures should be supplemented with an opercular window for cases with hemimegalencephaly, and care should be taken to perform a really complete disconnection, because cases of incomplete disconnection have been described. It is the ideal procedure for cases with atrophic brains, very large ventricles, or porencephalic cysts in the MCA territory. In our own series, there is no evidence that the seizure freedom rate is lower than in Rasmussen's technique; the seizure freedom rates depend more on the etiology than on the procedure, as in many other series.

Acknowledgments

I thank C. E. Elger, Chief of the Department of Epileptology, and S. Kuczaty and R. Sassen, who have been neuropediatric and epileptological partners for these surgeries over the last years. S. Kuczaty reviewed the section on the presurgical procedures described in this chapter.

References

1. Schramm J, Behrens E, Entzian W. Hemispherical deafferentation: a modified functional hemispherectomy technique. Epilepsia 1992;33:71

2. Schramm J, Behrens E, Entzian W. Hemispherical deafferentation: an alternative to functional hemispherectomy. Neurosurgery 1995;36(3):509–515, discussion 515–516

3. Delalande O, Pinard J, Basevant C. Hemispherotomy: a new procedure for central disconnection. Epilepsia 1992;33(suppl 3): 99–100

4. Villemure JG, Mascott CR. Peri-insular hemispherotomy: surgical principles and anatomy. Neurosurgery 1995;37(5):975–981

5. Shimizu H, Maehara T. Modification of peri-insular hemispherotomy and surgical results. Neurosurgery 2000;47(2):367–372, discussion 372–373

6. Schramm J, Kral T, Clusmann H. Transsylvian keyhole functional hemispherectomy. Neurosurgery 2001;49(4):891–900, discussion 900–901

7. Cook SW, Nguyen ST, Hu B, et al. Cerebral hemispherectomy in pediatric patients with epilepsy: comparison of three techniques by pathological substrate in 115 patients. J Neurosurg 2004; 100(2, suppl Pediatrics):125–141

8. Arzimanoglou AA, Andermann F, Aicardi J, et al. Sturge-Weber syndrome: indications and results of surgery in 20 patients. Neurology 2000;55(10):1472–1479

9. Smith SJ, Andermann F, Villemure JG, Rasmussen TB, Quesney LF. Functional hemispherectomy: EEG findings, spiking from isolated brain postoperatively, and prediction of outcome. Neurology 1991;41(11):1790–1794

10. Döring S, Cross H, Boyd S, Harkness W, Neville B. The significance of bilateral EEG abnormalities before and after hemispherectomy in children with unilateral major hemisphere lesions. Epilepsy Res 1999;34(1):65–73

11. Kossoff EH, Vining EP, Pillas DJ, et al. Hemispherectomy for intractable unihemispheric epilepsy etiology vs outcome. Neurology 2003;61(7):887–890

12. Benke T, Köylü B, Visani P, et al. Language lateralization in temporal lobe epilepsy: a comparison between fMRI and the Wada Test. Epilepsia 2006;47(8):1308–1319

13. Woermann FG, Jokeit H, Luerding R, et al. Language lateralization by Wada test and fMRI in 100 patients with epilepsy. Neurology 2003;61(5):699–701

14. Schramm J. Hemispherectomy. In: Starr P, Barbaro N, Larson P, eds. Neurosurgical Operative Atlas 2E: Functional Neurosurgery. New York, NY: Thieme Medical Publishers; 2008;56–62

15. Kestle J, Connolly M, Cochrane D. Pediatric peri-insular hemispherotomy. Pediatr Neurosurg 2000;32(1):44–47

16. Schramm J. Hemispherectomy techniques. Neurosurg Clin N Am 2002;13(1):113–134, ix

17. Peacock WJ, Wehby-Grant MC, Shields WD, et al. Hemispherectomy for intractable seizures in children: a report of 58 cases. Childs Nerv Syst 1996;12(7):376–384

18. Kawai K, Shimizu H. Clinical outcome and comparison of surgical procedures in hemispherotomy for children with malformation of cortical. Epilepsia 2004;45(7):168

19. Shimizu H. Our experience with pediatric epilepsy surgery focusing on corpus callosotomy and hemispherotomy. Epilepsia 2005;46(suppl 1):30–31

20. González-Martínez JA, Gupta A, Kotagal P, et al. Hemispherectomy for catastrophic epilepsy in infants. Epilepsia 2005;46(9):1518–1525

21. Villemure JG, Vernet O, Delalande O. Hemispheric disconnection: callosotomy and hemispherotomy. Adv Tech Stand Neurosurg 2000;26:25–78

22. Browd SR, Kestle J. Periinsular hemispherotomy. In: Miller JW, Silbergeld DL, eds. Epilepsy Surgery: Principles and Controversies. New York, NY; London, UK: Taylor and Francis; 2006:585–588

23. Schramm J. Hemispherical deafferentation via the transsylvian keyhole. In: Miller JW, Silbergeld DL, eds. Epilepsy Surgery: Principles and Controversies. New York, NY; London, UK: Taylor and Francis; 2006:589–594

24. Yasargil MG. Microneurosurgery, Vol. IVA. Stuttgart-New York: Thieme, 1994;54–55.

29 Peri-insular Hemispherotomy

Nicholas M. Wetjen and John R. W. Kestle

Anatomical hemispherectomy has proven to be an effective surgical treatment for epilepsy when the epileptic pathology involves a large part of the cerebral hemisphere. Dandy[1] and L'hermitte[2] originally conceived of the use of hemispherectomy in the late 1920s as a treatment for malignant brain tumors and the procedure was first applied to the treatment of epilepsy by McKenzie[3] in Canada in 1938. In 1950, Krynauw et al[4] demonstrated control of epileptic seizures in a series of 12 patients with infantile hemiplegia treated by hemispherectomy. In anatomical hemispherectomy, the entire affected cerebral hemisphere is resected, and a large cerebrospinal fluid cavity is created postoperatively. Superficial cerebral hemosiderosis (SCH) secondary to repeated bleeding into the large subarachnoid space may occur in up to 33% of the patients.[5–7]

Rasmussen[8] introduced the functional hemispherectomy in the 1970s to achieve the goals of hemispheric disconnection while preventing SCH. In the functional hemispherectomy, the frontal and occipital poles are preserved but functionally disconnected from the rest of the brain. A temporal lobectomy with complete callosotomy and insular cortex resection is performed, along with the parasagittal frontal and parietal lobectomies to remove the central region. The benefits of the functional hemispherectomy are identical to those of the anatomical hemispherectomy, but by functionally disconnecting the hemisphere while leaving most of the brain intact, this technique avoids the complication of SCH. Other modifications of hemispherectomies have been developed to avoid late hemosiderosis, including reducing the subdural space by sewing the convexity dura to the falx, anterior and middle fossa dura, and tentorium,[9] plugging the foramen of Monro with muscle,[10] using postoperative subdural drainage and ventriculoperitoneal shunt placement,[11] or undertaking hemidecortication.[12,13]

More recently, other forms of the functional hemispherotomy have been conceived to minimize cortical resection further while still functionally disconnecting the affected hemisphere by transection of the neuronal fiber tracts.[14–16] These techniques have been described as hemispherotomy because the operative transection of fiber tracts predominantly occurs through a small peri-insular opening in the cerebral hemisphere. The advantages of these procedures include reduced operative time, reduced blood loss, better anatomical preservation of the surgically treated hemisphere, and decreased postoperative complications. Although other forms of functional hemispherectomy and the various hemispherotomy techniques are described in other chapters of this volume, our focus is the peri-insular hemispherotomy.

■ Preoperative Evaluation

The indications for peri-insular hemispherotomy are lesions that cause intractable epilepsy involving one cerebral hemisphere. The most common hemispheric syndromes include infantile hemiplegia, Sturge-Weber syndrome, Rasmussen encephalitis, atrophic cerebral hemisphere caused by vascular disorder or trauma, and cortical dysplasia involving a broad area of the cerebral hemisphere and hemimegalencephaly. These diseases, in most cases, lead to a hemispheric syndrome characterized by hemiplegia and hemianopsia. All patients undergo a detailed neurological evaluation, including multiple electroencephalographic evaluations, neuropsychological testing, and magnetic resonance imaging (MRI) studies, to confirm that the seizures originate from the diseased hemisphere.

■ Operative Procedure

The peri-insular hemispherotomy was first described by Villemure and Mascott[16] in 1995, and few modifications have been added since that time.[17,18] The procedure is performed under general endotracheal anesthesia, with the patient positioned supine and the head turned so the intended surgical hemisphere is facing upward. The head can be secured by Mayfield pin head holder (Integra, Plainsboro, NJ) or Sugita clamp (Mizuho, Tokyo, Japan) or positioned laterally on a horseshoe rest. A modified question mark- or U-shaped scalp incision provides the necessary exposure for the operation. The incision should be planned to reach the zygoma inferiorly, and the superior aspect of the incision need not extend above the mid-convexity level. The bone flap is designed so that the anterior extent reaches the coronal suture, the superior aspect is at the superior temporal line, and the posterior extent provides access to the posterior insular and extends inferiorly to the temporal floor. The preoperative MRI scan is useful to take into account the individual's anatomy, atrophy, and brain shift to plan the craniotomy. After the craniotomy, the dura mater is opened to expose the underlying frontal, parietal, and temporal lobe opercular cortex.

The peri-insular hemispherotomy involves disconnecting the operative hemisphere from the rest of the central nervous system, and the majority of the procedure is performed principally within the ventricular system. Access to the ventricle is gained primarily by two stages via (1) the superior insular window (suprainsular window) and (2) the inferior insular window (infrainsular window) **(Fig. 29.1)**.

The suprainsular window requires resection of the frontal and parietal opercular cortex to expose the upper insula and circular sulcus. The white matter is entered above the insula through the inferior frontal gyrus or superior circular sulcus until the lateral ventricle is entered. The approach to

the ventricle along this trajectory disrupts the corona radiata and the ascending and descending fibers of the internal capsule.

Development of the infrainsular window requires removal of the temporal opercular cortex to expose the inferior insula and inferior circular sulcus whereby the temporal horn of the lateral ventricle is entered. Once the temporal horn is entered and opened, the hippocampal formation and amygdala are visualized. The order of which window is to be opened first is at the discretion of the operating surgeon. Generally, it is easier to extend the opercular resection from the suprainsular window posterior and inferiorly around the insula to the temporal operculum with maintained visualization of the underlying lateral ventricle.

Suprainsular Window

After the dura mater is opened, the pia mater of the frontal and parietal opercular cortex is coagulated and incised approximately 5 mm above the sylvian fissure on the inferior frontal gyrus. The opercular cortex is removed by subpial aspiration using the operating microscope until the insular cortex and the superior circular sulcus that surrounds it are completely exposed **(Fig. 29.1A)**. The body of the lateral ventricle is entered through the white matter of the superior circular sulcus if the ventricles are large or entered with extension into the white matter of the corona radiata beneath the inferior frontal gyrus if the ventricles are small **(Fig. 29.1B)**. Once the ventricle is entered, the superior sylvian window is extended anteriorly to the frontal horn of the ventricle to open the superior circular sulcus completely and posteriorly to the ventricular trigone. It is important to limit the entry of blood into the remainder of the ventricular system by placing a Cottonoid patty over the foramen of Monro. After the lateral ventricle is opened along its anterior-to-posterior axis, the septum pellucidum and corpus callosum are visualized.

Corpus Callosotomy

Clear visualization of the septum pellucidum within the lateral ventricle is necessary to initiate the corpus callosotomy. Intraoperative ultrasonography or frameless stereotactic guidance may be used to identify the anterior cerebral arteries above the corpus callosum or the falx to clarify the trajectory for the corpus callosotomy. A small, 2-mm wide incision at the junction of the septum pellucidum with the roof of the ventricle in the coronal plane allows for identification of the corpus callosum. Occasionally, in patients with small ventricles, subpial resection of the most inferior aspect of the cingulate gyrus may be necessary to achieve exposure of the pericallosal arteries anteriorly along the corpus callosum. Once the corpus callosum has been identified and confirmed with subpial visualization of the pericallosal artery,

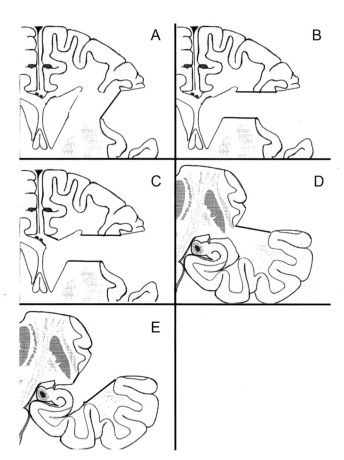

Fig. 29.1 **(A)** Suprasylvian–coronal–opercular resection. **(B)** Suprasylvian–coronal–section of corona radiata. **(C)** Suprasylvian–coronal–parasagittal callosotomy. **(D)** Infrasylvian–coronal–opercular resection. **(E)** Infrasylvian–coronal–section of corona radiata (temporal stem). *Source*: Reproduced with permission by Villemure JG, Daniel RT. Peri-insular hemispherotomy in paediatric epilepsy. Childs Nerv Syst 2006; 22(8):967–981.[17]

the ependyma of the ventricular roof is resected in an anterior-to-posterior direction while disconnecting the callosal fibers. The pericallosal arteries are used as a guide, and they are followed anteriorly by subpial aspiration of the corpus callosum from the rostrum to the splenium of the corpus callosum from within the lateral ventricle. This allows disruption of the fibers of the corpus callosum in a just slightly parasagittal plane (**Fig. 29.1C**). It is important not to actually enter the corpus callosum perpendicular to the midsagittal plane, because this could result in inadvertent entry into the contralateral hemisphere. Posteriorly, the pericallosal arteries course superiorly into the interhemispheric fissure so the dissection relies on visualization of the pia/arachnoid of the interhemispheric fissure and superior surface of the corpus callosum as landmarks.

Disruption of the frontal horizontal fibers is initiated after completion of the complete callosotomy. Attention is directed away from the inside of the lateral ventricle to the inferior and basal frontal lobe in the coronal plane at the anterior insula at the level of the sphenoid ridge. The pia over the frontal basal cortex is interrupted, and a corticectomy of the frontal lobe in the coronal plane is initiated at the level of the lesser wing of the sphenoid. The frontal basal corticectomy is extended into the white matter medially in the coronal plane and allows for visualization of the olfactory tract. The olfactory tract is preserved, and the subpial resection of the inferior frontal cortex continues until the pia begins to curve superiorly at the medial frontal lobe. Once this has been achieved, subpial aspiration of the white matter from the rostral callosotomy can be extended inferiorly just anterior to the rostrum of the corpus callosum and head of the caudate in the lateral wall of the ventricle in the coronal plane to connect the corticectomy across the frontobasal white matter of the frontal lobe. The corticectomy of the frontal basal cortex across the subcallosal, orbitofrontal, and gyrus rectus disrupts the commissural connections between the caudal orbitofrontal cortices, the ascending and descending projections of the frontobasal cortex via anterior sublenticular fibers, the connections between the orbitofrontal and insular cortex, and connections to the temporal lobe via the uncinate fasciculus.

Infrainsular Window

After the corpus callosotomy and disconnection of frontal horizontal fibers via the suprainsular window, attention is directed to the infrainsular window. The pia overlying the superior temporal gyrus is coagulated approximately 5 mm below the sylvian fissure. This is usually accomplished by starting in the superior temporal gyrus at the posterior margin of the insula. After creation of the suprainsular window, the lateral ventricle is opened posteriorly to the splenium of the corpus callosum. The opening into the lateral ventricle can be followed inferiorly by aspirating the cortex around

the posterior margin of the insular and posterior circular sulcus to the superior temporal gyrus (**Fig. 29.1D**). Extra care should be given to preserving middle cerebral artery (MCA) branches and large venous draining vessels when feasible to prevent postoperative infarcts and cerebral edema. This opening allows for continuous visualization of the ependyma and choroid plexus of the lateral ventricle from the frontal horn to the posterior temporal horn. The removal of the superior temporal gyrus proceeds from posterior to anterior from the level of the trigone of the lateral ventricle and by removing the cortex and underlying white matter along the inferior margin of the insula and inferior circular sulcus extending the opening into the lateral ventricle into the temporal horn. Once the temporal horn has been completely exposed, the hippocampus and amygdala can be easily visualized.

The choroid fissure extending from the temporal horn of the lateral ventricle is opened to the posterior extent of the complete callosotomy at the level of the splenium (**Fig. 29.2**). This incision disrupts parietooccipital connections via the short and long arcuate fibers of the superior longitudinal fasciculus, the cingulum, and fimbria fibers from the hippocampus. This resection of the medial white matter of the lateral ventricle inferiorly from the level of the splenium proceeds to the choroid fissure, and the basal vein and vein of Galen are often visualized through the arachnoid when this incision is completed.

After complete disconnection of parietooccipital fibers, the choroid fissure of the temporal horn is followed anteriorly to identify the anterior head of the hippocampus and amygdala (**Fig. 29.1E**). The amygdala is removed using a subpial aspiration. The superior extent of the amygdala

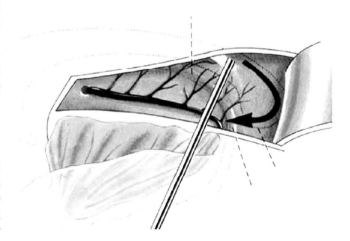

Fig. 29.2 Suprasylvian lateral site of posterior callosotomy, around the splenium, and posterior hippocampotomy. *Source:* Reproduced with permission from Villemure JG, Daniel RT. Peri-insular hemispherotomy in paediatric epilepsy. Childs Nerv Syst 2006; 22(8):967–981.[17]

resection proceeds to the level of the roof of the temporal horn. The resection may extend posteriorly into the hippocampus but is not necessary because the fimbria has been sectioned at the hippocampal tail. On completion of the inferior insular window and opening of the lateral ventricle from the atrium to the tip of the temporal horn, the retrolentiform and sublentiform internal capsule have been sectioned. Removal of the amygdala and anterior hippocampus disrupts the fibers of the posterior limb of the anterior commissure coursing between the superior amygdala and inferior lentiform body, the stria terminalis, and connections between the amygdala and basal ganglia. The hippocampal projections to the parahippocampal gyrus and then on to other cortical areas are disrupted by the opening of the infrainsular window and sectioning of the fimbria.

Fibers projecting from the insular cortex to the basal ganglia, thalamus, hypothalamus, and brainstem are disconnected by aspiration of the insular cortex (**Fig. 29.3**). At the conclusion of the procedure, the pia should be identified extending from along the floor of the anterior fossa and lesser sphenoid wing at the base of the frontal lobe over the

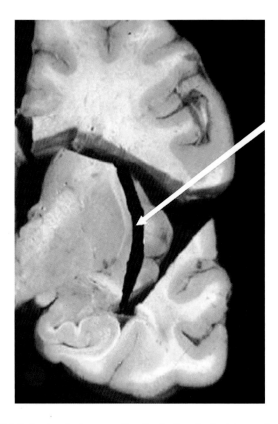

Fig. 29.3 Anatomical preparation illustrating the incision undermining the insula in the coronal plane (*white arrow*). (*Source:* Reproduced with permission by Villemure JG, Daniel RT. Peri-insular hemispherotomy in paediatric epilepsy. Childs Nerv Syst 2006; 22(8):967–981.[17])

olfactory tract, superiorly anterior to the insula and basal ganglia extending anterior to the genu and superior to the rostrum of the corpus callosum on the medial frontal lobe, posteriorly along the corpus callosum in a parasagittal plane to the splenium, and then inferiorly from the splenium to the choroid fissure of the temporal horn. It is important to identify this pial margin completely along its course as it is often difficult to visualize the disconnection on the postoperative MRI. At the conclusion of the procedure, a drain is left within the lateral ventricle and tunneled through the scalp to evacuate debris and bloody cerebrospinal fluid.

■ Modifications

There have been several modifications to the original procedure described by Villemure and Mascott[16] in 1995.[19–23] The fundamental concept of isolation of the cerebral hemisphere by disconnection of the medial temporal structures, internal capsule, corpus callosum, and horizontal frontal fibers is achieved by each of the techniques (**Fig. 29.4**). The steps in common to most hemispherotomy procedures include:

1. Interruption of the internal capsule and corona radiata
2. Resection of the medial temporal structures
3. Transventricular corpus callosotomy
4. Disruption of the horizontal fibers

Shimuzu and Maehara[22] introduced the first modification, termed the *transopercular hemispherotomy*, in 2000 (**Fig. 29.4C**). During this procedure, the upper half of the insula is exposed through a transsylvian approach. All of the ascending arteries over the insula are coagulated and divided. The frontoparietal operculum covering the insula, including the gray matter and underlying white matter, is resected en bloc along with the upper half of the insula. This creates a large cavity along the superior margin of the sylvian fissure. The upper limit of the resection cavity is parallel or slightly superior to the roof of the corpus callosum. The body of the lateral ventricle is entered through this opercular cavity, thereby sectioning the fibers of the internal capsule and corona radiata. The opening in the lateral ventricle is extended anteriorly to the lateral edge of the frontal horn and posteriorly to the trigone. An incision from the opercular cavity at the trigone is extended inferiorly toward the temporal horn of the lateral ventricle. This incision divides the fibers emerging from the inferior insula and temporal stem and allows for visualization of the hippocampus and amygdala. The head of the hippocampus is resected en bloc to examine it histologically along with the amygdala. The medial amygdala adjacent to the basal ganglia is left behind.[20] The transventricular corpus callosotomy is then completed from the genu to the splenium of the corpus callosum, and the horizontal frontal fibers are sectioned in the same manner as described by Villemure and Mascott.[16]

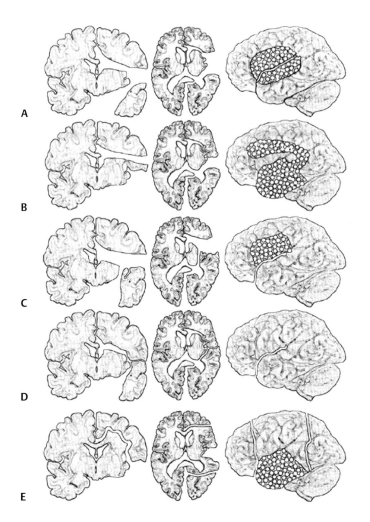

Fig. 29.4 Schematic view of hemispherectomies based on discon-nective techniques with the lateral approach. Dotted area delineates cortical resection. Group 2–subgroup C, lateral approach: **(A)** Ville-mure and Mascott[16]; **(B)** Schramm et al[15]; **(C)** Shimizu and Maehara[22]; **(D)** Schramm et al[21]; **(E)** Kanev et al[27] *Source:* Reproduced with per-mission by Springer from De Almeida AN, Marino R, Jr., Aguiar PH, Jacobsen Teixeira M. Hemispherectomy: a schematic review of the current techniques. Neurosurg Rev. 2006; 29(2):97–102; discussion 102.[19]

In 2003, Daniel and Villemure[24] published a description of surgical complications related to the hemispherotomy and described some additional modifications developed in an attempt to make the procedure safer. They no longer rec-ommended creating a continuous peri-insular window but instead advocated the use of multiple windows into the lat-eral ventricle around the insula to preserve as many MCA branches and sylvian venous structures as possible **(Fig. 29.5)**. They also recommended proceeding with the dis-section into the lateral ventricle through perisylvian cysts

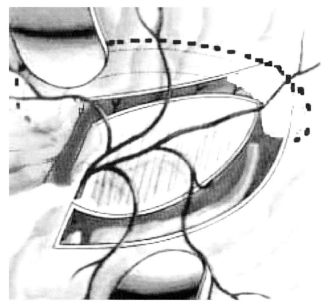

Fig. 29.5 Lateral view illustrating the peri-insular incision and pres-ervation of cortical vessels. (*Source:* Reproduced with permission by Villemure JG, Daniel RT. Peri-insular hemispherotomy in paediatric epilepsy. Childs Nerv Syst 2006; 22(8):967–981.[17])

if present. The insula is then disconnected anatomically through the claustrum or external capsule rather than pro-ceeding with resection of the insular cortex.

Comair[25] developed the transsylvian functional hemi-spherectomy as an extension of the transsylvian approach to the mesiotemporal lobe described by Yasargil.[26] Comair used this transsylvian approach to perform a peri-insular disconnection. In this approach, after the dura is opened, the sylvian fissure is opened under microscopic magnifica-tion. This procedure requires a wide exposure of the insula, and the authors describe opening the preinsular, insular, and retroinsular segments of the sylvian fissure. Once the sylvian fissure has been opened at the MCAs, insular gyri and the boundary of the circular sulcus around the insula are identi-fied. Once the sylvian fissure is opened and the MCA trunk has been mobilized lateral to medial, the inferior edge of the circular sulcus is coagulated and incised. The incision is then carried through the temporal stem in a plane parallel to the insula, down through the temporal lobe, into the temporal horn of the lateral ventricle. This results in entire transec-tion of the temporal stem from anterior to posterior and completely uncovers the underlying temporal horn posteri-orly into the trigone. Through this opening into the tempo-ral horn, an amygdalohippocampectomy is performed. The hippocampus is removed en bloc rather than transecting the fornix posteriorly in this procedure. Once the amygda-lohippocampectomy has been completed, the attention is directed to the central area and its inferior border. A 3- × 3-cm cortical incision is made at the inferior aspect of the central area to enter into the lateral ventricle superior to the insula. Through this opening, the callosotomy is performed, as has been described in the other peri-insular hemispherotomy techniques. After the corpus callosotomy is completed, disconnection of the frontal lobe is initiated from lateral to medial, toward the subcallosal area, using the A1 segment of the anterior cerebral artery as a landmark. The incision is performed from within the ventricle into the frontal lobe white matter, and the disconnection completes the anterior corpus callosal incision at the level of the rostrum through to the basal frontal area. Once this portion is completed, the insula is removed or disconnected by subpial aspiration.

In 1997, Kanev et al[27] introduced a variation of the hemispherotomy that does not require a transventricular corpus callosotomy and relies heavily on intraoperative ultrasound to identify anatomical landmarks **(Fig. 29.4E)**. The skin incision and craniotomy are similar to those in the other procedures. After the dura is open, the ultrasound is brought into the operative field and used to identify the ventricular landmarks. First, the ultrasound probe is placed over the posterior superior temporal lobe to identify the atrium of the lateral ventricle. A coronal incision is made in the temporal lobe posterior to the atrium, and this serves as the posterior limit of the temporal lobectomy. The temporal lobectomy proceeds with an en bloc removal of the lateral temporal gyri followed by ultrasound-guided entrance into the temporal horn and exposure of the hippocampus. The medial temporal structures, including the hippocampus, amygdala, and uncus, are resected by subpial dissection. The occipital horn is then identified by ultrasound, and the coronal incision that marked the posterior limit of the temporal lobectomy is extended in the coronal plane superiorly across the lateral parietooccipital cortex to the interhemispheric fissure behind the occipital horn across the forceps major and behind

the splenium to avoid entry into the occipital horn. The ultrasound probe is again used to identify the frontal horn of the lateral ventricle, and another coronal incision is made in the lateral neocortex of the frontal lobe in a plane anterior to the rostrum of the corpus callosum avoiding the frontal horn toward the interhemispheric fissure across the forceps minor. Next, the distal MCA branches coursing superiorly out of the sylvian fissure are divided, a subpial resection of the lateral cerebral cortex proceeds toward the midline, and the pia of the corpus callosum is identified. This incision across the lateral neocortex extends from the frontal coronal incision anteriorly to the occipital coronal incision posteriorly to complete the hemispheric disconnection.

In 2001, Schramm and colleagues[21] described the transsylvian keyhole functional hemispherectomy **(Fig. 29.4D)**. It is very similar to the procedure described by Comair[25] because the approach to disconnect the hemisphere is via opening of the sylvian fissure. Once the sylvian fissure is opened and the entire anterior posterior and superior inferior extent of the superior sulcus is identified, the dissection proceeds by outlining the entire circular sulcus into the lateral ventricle. Special care is taken to preserve most of the peripheral MCA branches in this procedure. Through the inferior limb of the inferior sulcus, the temporal horn is opened transcortically. A biopsy of the temporal lobe is usually taken, and an amygdalohippocampectomy with removal of lateral nuclei and uncus of the amygdala is then performed. The transcortical incision into the temporal horn is extended posteriorly, outlining the lower limb of the insular sulcus, and enlarged posteriorly to the posterior end of the sylvian cistern; it then enters the ventricle posterior to the pulvinar exposing the trigone. The transcortical dissection into the ventricular system is then extended superiorly around and anterior into the tip of the frontal horn and proceeds to the most anterior aspect of the superior limb of the circular sulcus. It is usually necessary to tilt the microscope to expose the most posterior

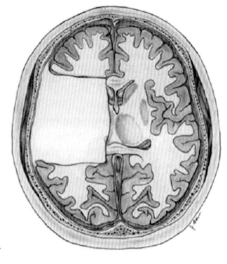

A

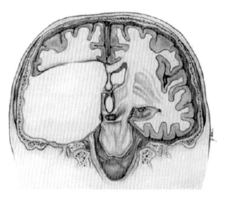

B

Fig. 29.6 Line drawings in the axial **(A)** and coronal **(B)** planes illustrating the anatomical structures removed and disconnected in the modified lateral hemispherotomy. Reproduced with permission by *Journal of Neurosurgery* from Cook SW, Nguyen ST, Hu B, et al. Cerebral hemispherectomy in pediatric patients with epilepsy: comparison of three techniques by pathological substrate in 115 patients. J Neurosurg 2004;100(2 suppl Pediatrics):125–141.[28]

and anterior aspects of the ventricular system, and gentle retraction on the opercula, as well as the basal ganglia and insula, may be required to complete the dissection into the ventricular system. After this step of the procedure, the insula cortex is aspirated subpially.

Cook and colleagues[28] developed the "modified lateral hemispherotomy" to reduce the intraoperative blood loss of the anatomical hemispherectomy and reduce the reoperation rate of the functional hemispherectomy. The operation develops a working space around the ventricles by removing the thalamus, basal ganglia, caudate nucleus, and other deep hemisphere structures as a standard part of the procedure (**Fig. 29.6**). The authors describe ligating the MCA proximally in the sylvian fissure as an early step to prevent excessive blood loss. They believe removal of the deep hemisphere structures may reduce recurrent seizures leading to reoperation in functional hemispherectomy.

■ Surgical Outcome

Intractable epilepsy from diffuse hemispheric disorders responds well to hemispherotomy. There have been no randomized clinical trials to compare the various procedures; most reports are retrospective reviews of an institution's or surgeon's experience and are subject to differential selection bias and compensatory equalization. The success rate for seizure control is usually good, and the results among different series are similar.[13,16–18,22,27–39] Most authors report their outcomes in series with mixed pathological conditions, which likely influence the success of surgery.[12,29,40–42] In the review of seizure outcome after hemispherectomy by Holthausen et al,[12] the success rate for seizure control was highest in the group of patients with Sturge-Weber syndrome (82.1%), followed by those with infantile hemiplegia (77.3%), Rasmussen encephalitis (77.1%), vascular causes (76.1%), other causes (67.9%), and cortical dysplasia (56.6%).

In a 2006 series of 34 patients who underwent peri-insular hemispherotomy with up to 9 years follow-up,[17] 90% of patients achieved Engel Class I seizure outcome. The best results were obtained in children with infantile hemiplegia secondary to prenatal vascular occlusion of the carotid or MCA (93%) and Rasmussen encephalitis (90%). Patients who underwent surgery for cortical migration disorders (75%) or hemimegalencephaly (67%) did not fare as well.

In another combined series from Primary Children's Medical Center and British Columbia Children's Hospital, the results of 16 operations for diffuse hemispheric disorders were described.[18] The first 5 patients in the series underwent hemidecortication and the remainder underwent peri-insular hemispherotomy; 8 of 11 patients who underwent peri-insular hemispherotomy had Class I outcome, and 4 of the 5 who underwent hemidecortication had Class I outcome. Seizure outcomes were not divided with respect to

presenting diagnosis because of the small number of patients in the series overall.

In a follow-up article by Basheer and colleagues in 2007,[31] with median 6-year follow-up compared with 3 years in the first study, 79% of the patients continued to have complete seizure control, and more than 90% of these patients were no longer on antiepileptic medications. Of the other five patients, four were on antiepileptic monotherapy and one patient with Rasmussen encephalitis was on two antiepileptic medications. Four of the five patients with poor seizure control had bilateral MRI abnormalities. Twelve of 14 patients with preoperative slowing of epileptiform activity in the contralateral hemisphere were seizure free.

The authors of most published series reporting results for peri-insular hemispherotomy discuss seizure outcomes and postoperative complications. More recently, results of the level of adaptive function postoperatively are being examined with aspects of cognitive behavioral motor outcomes being reported. For instance, Basheer and colleagues[31] measured the level of adaptive functioning using the Scales of Independent Behavior–Revised (SIB-R). This test assesses motor skills, social interaction, communication skills, personal living skills, and community living skills based on parent ratings. In addition, tests of cognitive function as assessed by the Peabody Picture Vocabulary Test-Third Edition and the Beery Developmental Test of Visual Motor Integration were also reported. The mean age of adaptive and cognitive assessment was 10.5 years old, and the median time to the most recent follow-up examination was 5.5 years. The mean SIB-R broad independent score was very low in the overall group at 45.5. This measure is recorded in the standard score format like IQ with a mean of 100 and a standard deviation of 15, with higher scores indicating better functional independence. The patients undergoing surgery for hemispheric seizure disorders had severe impairment in carrying out all age-appropriate activities of daily living. Only 14% had a score greater than 80, which is probably within normal limits. Mean scores on the Peabody test and social communication skill were consistent with borderline to mild impairment in language skills. As expected, the SIB-R motor scale was the lowest score overall, with 82% of the children scoring below the first percentile, reflecting their severe pain and poor functional motor skills. The duration of epilepsy was significantly related to the overall SIB-R broad independence score in all four SIB-R skill scores with shorter duration of epilepsy associated with higher scores in each case. Age at surgery was also significantly related to these scores, with younger children having better functioning.

Health-related quality of life (HR-QOL) is another important outcome measure as an index of objective and subjective well-being, particularly in children with chronic health conditions. The elevated incidence of behavioral and adjustment problems in epilepsy as reflected in the recent study by Basheer et al[31] emphasized the importance of considering these impairments on life quality. Griffiths and colleagues,[43] also from the University of British Columbia and British Columbia Children's Hospital, undertook a cross-sectional study of patients who had undergone hemispherectomy to describe the postsurgical HR-QOL and then compared the HR-QOL of patients after hemispherectomy with the HR-QOL of patients who underwent temporal or frontal resections as well as that of nonsurgical pediatric epilepsy patients. An examination of the baseline characteristics revealed that the children who underwent hemispheric surgery were typically younger than those who had temporal or frontal resections. Those that were in the nonsurgical group were younger at assessment than those who underwent temporal or frontal resections and had a shorter duration of illness. Those in the frontal resection group were taking the most antiepileptic medications. The hemispherectomy group had lower full-scale IQs and lower SIB-R than all of the other groups. In addition, 11 members of the hemispherectomy group were untestable because of low functional levels. The HR-QOL ratings were obtained from the parents by completion of the Impact of Childhood Illness scale (ICI) and the Hague Restrictions in Childhood Epilepsy Scale (HARCES). The ICI is not epilepsy specific and was originally designed for pediatric patients with various illnesses and disabilities. The ICI assesses the impact of the disorder and its treatment, the impact of the child's development and adjustment, the impact on the parents, and the overall impact on the family. In addition, for each of these items, the parent rates how often the specified problem or situation occurs and the amount of concern each problem causes. The HARCES assesses the child's disability related to the restrictions imposed by seizure disorders. There are two general scale items that reflect global restrictions and activities and eight items pertaining to specific daily activities. Both the ICI and the HARCES are structured with higher scores denoting more health-related difficulties, usually adversely affecting life quality, as indicated by lower HR-QOL scores. Interestingly, parents of hemispherectomy, temporal resection, frontal resection, and nonsurgical patients reported generally similar HR-QOL on both scales. There is only one group difference in HR-QOL, with a trend for parents of patients who underwent temporal resection to report fewer epilepsy-related physical limitations for the children than parents of nonsurgical patients. A linear regression analysis was used to evaluate whether hemispherectomy was an independent risk factor for poorer HR-QOL. Female gender, higher antiepileptic medications, and lower functional independence on the SIB-R predicted a lower HR-QOL.

■ Complications

The surgical complications that may be encountered after peri-insular hemispherotomy include intraoperative blood loss requiring transfusion, postoperative fever, incomplete disconnection, hydrocephalus, remote hemorrhage, infarction, cerebral edema, and death.

The overall operative time and intraoperative blood loss are considerably lower than in other hemispherectomy techniques. In one study, the mean estimated blood loss was 1300 mL in hemidecortication cases, with all 5 patients requiring blood transfusion, compared with 462 mL blood loss and 8 of 11 patients requiring transfusion in the peri-insular hemispherotomy cases.[18] In 14 of 16 patients, immediate postoperative hemiparesis was worse than before the operation. In the 2 that did not worsen, there was already a long-standing, stable hemiparesis: 1 attributable to a large perinatal infarct and the other to a hemispheric cortical dysplasia. The functional ability in the affected arm and leg recovered to the preoperative status in all but 2 patients, and no patients had a decrease in ambulatory status as a result of surgery. Three patients who had incomplete hemianopsia had a complete anopsia after surgery, and no patients had a change in their speech function after surgery. When comparing the postoperative course of the hemidecortication with that of the peri-insular hemispherotomy, the incidence of postoperative fever, meningismus, and irritability is significantly less after peri-insular hemispherotomy. This sometimes lasts as long as 3 weeks despite no evidence of progressive ventriculomegaly or infection to account for their symptoms. This syndrome has also been described by other groups and found to be less prevalent in patients who undergo peri-insular hemispherotomy compared with other techniques of hemispherectomy.

The incidence of hydrocephalus requiring ventriculoperitoneal shunting after peri-insular hemispherotomy ranges from 0 to 4%.[17,18,21,24] Most patients only require ventricular drainage for a few days to remove blood and tissue debris. Shimizu and Maehara[22] reported that 15% of patients required a ventriculoperitoneal shunt in their transopercular hemispherotomy series; this result was very similar to the rates reported by Delalande et al[44] for vertical parasagittal hemispherotomy (15.7%), Cook et al[28] for modified lateral hemispherotomy (22%), and Schramm et al[15] for hemispherical deafferentation (8%). The incidence of hydrocephalus is significantly improved over anatomical hemispherectomy (10–78%),[8,28,36,37,45–47] functional hemispherectomy (5–12%),[8,33] and hemidecortication (9–40%).[13,18,32]

Significant neurological morbidity and death are rare after peri-insular hemispherotomy (3–4%).[17,18,24] Deaths, when they have occurred, were secondary to cerebral edema from infarction and remote hemorrhage. One death was related to an infarct in the disconnected hemisphere. The edema secondary to infarct in this case was attributed to sacrifice of arteries and veins while developing a continuous suprainsular and infrainsular window. For this reason, Villemure and Daniel[17] recommend preservation of MCA branches and venous structures from the sylvian fissure. In another patient, a remote hemorrhage occurred contralateral to an atrophic operated hemisphere resulting in death. A clear explanation for the second complication was not found but was hypothesized to be attributed to excessive loss of cerebrospinal fluid from the operated side resulting in brain shift.[24] For this reason, attention should be paid to prevent excessive cerebrospinal fluid loss both during the procedure and postoperatively when patients have an external ventricular drain.

References

1. Dandy W. Removal of right cerebral hemisphere for certain tumors with hemiplegia: Preliminary report. JAMA 1928;90:823–828
2. L'hermitte J. L'ablation complete de l'hemisphere droit dans les cas de temeur cerebrale localisee compliquee d'hemiplegia. La decerebration supra-thalamique unilaterale chez l'homme. Encephale 1928;23:314–323
3. McKenzie K. The present status of a patient who had the right cerebral hemisphere removed. Am Med Assoc Chicago. 1938;111:168-183
4. Krynauw RA. Infantile hemiplegia treated by removing one cerebral hemisphere. J Neurol Neurosurg Psychiatry 1950;13(4):243–267
5. Laine E, Pruvot P, Osson D. [Ultimate Results of Hemispherectomy in Cases of Infantile Cerebral Hemiatrophy Productive of Epilepsy.]. Neurochirurgie 1964;10:507–522
6. Feichtinger M, Schröttner O, Eder H, et al. Efficacy and safety of radiosurgical callosotomy: a retrospective analysis. Epilepsia 2006;47(7):1184–1191
7. Oppenheimer DR, Griffith HB. Persistent intracranial bleeding as a complication of hemispherectomy. J Neurol Neurosurg Psychiatry 1966;29(3):229–240
8. Rasmussen T. Hemispherectomy for seizures revisited. Can J Neurol Sci 1983;10(2):71–78
9. Adams CB. Hemispherectomy—a modification. J Neurol Neurosurg Psychiatry 1983;46(7):617–619
10. Wilson PJ. Cerebral hemispherectomy for infantile hemiplegia. A report of 50 cases. Brain 1970;93(1):147–180
11. Andermann F, Rasmussen T, Villemure JG. Hemispherectomy: results for control of seizures in patients with hemispherectomy. In: Luders H, ed. Epilepsy Surgery. New York, NY: Raven Press; 1991:625–632
12. Holthausen H, May TW, Adams CTB, et al. Seizures post hemispherectomy. In: Tuxhorn I, Holthausen H, Boenigk H, eds. Pediatric Epilepsy Syndromes and Their Surgical Treatment. London, UK: John Libbey & Co.; 1997:749–773
13. Winston KR, Welch K, Adler JR, Erba G. Cerebral hemicorticectomy for epilepsy. J Neurosurg 1992;77(6):889–895
14. Delalande O, Pinard J, Basevant C. Hemispherotomy: a new procedure for central disconnection. Epilepsia 1992;33(suppl 3):99–100
15. Schramm J, Behrens E, Entzian W. Hemispherical deafferentation: an alternative to functional hemispherectomy. Neurosurgery 1995;36(3):509–515, discussion 515–516
16. Villemure JG, Mascott CR. Peri-insular hemispherotomy: surgical principles and anatomy. Neurosurgery 1995;37(5):975–981
17. Villemure JG, Daniel RT. Peri-insular hemispherotomy in paediatric epilepsy. Childs Nerv Syst 2006;22(8):967–981
18. Kestle J, Connolly M, Cochrane D. Pediatric peri-insular hemispherotomy. Pediatr Neurosurg 2000;32(1):44–47
19. De Almeida AN, Marino R Jr, Aguiar PH, Jacobsen Teixeira M. Hemispherectomy: a schematic review of the current techniques. Neurosurg Rev 2006;29(2):97–102, discussion 102
20. Morino M, Shimizu H, Ohata K, Tanaka K, Hara M. Anatomical analysis of different hemispherotomy procedures based on dissection of cadaveric brains. J Neurosurg 2002;97(2):423–431
21. Schramm J, Kral T, Clusmann H. Transsylvian keyhole functional hemispherectomy. Neurosurgery 2001;49(4):891–900, discussion 900–901
22. Shimizu H, Maehara T. Modification of peri-insular hemispherotomy and surgical results. Neurosurgery 2000;47(2):367–372, discussion 372–373
23. Wen HT, Rhoton AL Jr, Marino R Jr. Anatomical landmarks for hemispherotomy and their clinical application. J Neurosurg 2004;101(5):747–755
24. Daniel RT, Villemure JG. Peri-insular hemispherotomy: potential pitfalls and avoidance of complications. Stereotact Funct Neurosurg 2003;80(1–4):22–27
25. Comair YG. The transsylvian functional hemispherectomy: patient selection and results. In: Luders HO, Comair YG, eds. Epilepsy Surgery. 2nd ed. Philadelphia, PA: Lippincott Williams & Wilkins; 2001:699–704
26. Yaşargil MG, Teddy PJ, Roth P. Selective amygdalo-hippocampectomy. Operative anatomy and surgical technique. Adv Tech Stand Neurosurg 1985;12:93–123
27. Kanev PM, Foley CM, Miles D. Ultrasound-tailored functional hemispherectomy for surgical control of seizures in children. J Neurosurg 1997;86(5):762–767
28. Cook SW, Nguyen ST, Hu B, et al. Cerebral hemispherectomy in pediatric patients with epilepsy: comparison of three techniques by pathological substrate in 115 patients. J Neurosurg 2004; 100(2, suppl Pediatrics)125–141
29. Jonas R, Nguyen S, Hu B, et al. Cerebral hemispherectomy: hospital course, seizure, developmental, language, and motor outcomes. Neurology 2004;62(10):1712–1721
30. Terra-Bustamante VC, Inuzuka LM, Fernandes RM, et al. Outcome of hemispheric surgeries for refractory epilepsy in pediatric patients. Childs Nerv Syst 2007;23(3):321–326
31. Basheer SN, Connolly MB, Lautzenhiser A, Sherman EM, Hendson G, Steinbok P. Hemispheric surgery in children with refractory epilepsy: seizure outcome, complications, and adaptive function. Epilepsia 2007;48(1):133–140
32. Carson BS, Javedan SP, Freeman JM, et al. Hemispherectomy: a hemidecortication approach and review of 52 cases. J Neurosurg 1996;84(6):903–911
33. Davies KG, Maxwell RE, French LA. Hemispherectomy for intractable seizures: long-term results in 17 patients followed for up to 38 years. J Neurosurg 1993;78(5):733–740
34. Lindsay J, Ounsted C, Richards P. Hemispherectomy for childhood epilepsy: a 36-year study. Dev Med Child Neurol 1987;29(5):592–600
35. Morino M, Shimizu H, Uda T, et al. Transventricular hemispherotomy for surgical treatment of intractable epilepsy. J Clin Neurosci 2007;14(2):171–175
36. Ogunmekan AO, Hwang PA, Hoffman HJ. Sturge-Weber-Dimitri disease: role of hemispherectomy in prognosis. Can J Neurol Sci 1989;16(1):78–80

37. Peacock WJ, Wehby-Grant MC, Shields WD, et al. Hemispherectomy for intractable seizures in children: a report of 58 cases. Childs Nerv Syst 1996;12(7):376–384

38. Vigevano F, Di Rocco C. Effectiveness of hemispherectomy in hemimegalencephaly with intractable seizures. Neuropediatrics 1990;21(4):222–223

39. Villemure JG, Rasmussen T. Functional hemispherectomy in children. Neuropediatrics 1993;24(1):53–55

40. Bourgeois M. Crimmins DW, de Oliveira RS, et al. Surgical treatment of epilepsy in Sturge-Weber syndrome in children. J Neurosurg 2007; 106(1, suppl)20–28

41. Di Rocco C, Battaglia D, Pietrini D, Piastra M, Massimi L. Hemimegalencephaly: clinical implications and surgical treatment. Childs Nerv Syst 2006;22(8):852–866

42. Tubbs RS, Nimjee SM, Oakes WJ. Long-term follow-up in children with functional hemispherectomy for Rasmussen's encephalitis. Childs Nerv Syst 2005;21(6):461–465

43. Griffiths SY, Sherman EM, Slick DJ, Eyrl K, Connolly MB, Steinbok P. Postsurgical health-related quality of life (HRQOL) in children following hemispherectomy for intractable epilepsy. Epilepsia 2007;48(3):564–570

44. Delalande O, Bulteau C, Dellatolas G, et al. Vertical parasagittal hemispherotomy: surgical procedures and clinical long-term outcomes in a population of 83 children. Neurosurgery 2007; 60(2, suppl 1): ONS19–ONS32, discussion ONS32

45. Taha JM, Crone KR, Berger TS. The role of hemispherectomy in the treatment of holohemispheric hemimegaloencephaly. J Neurosurg 1994;81(1):37–42

46. Villemure JG. Anatomical to functional hemispherectomy from Krynauw to Rasmussen. Epilepsy Res Suppl 1992;5:209–215

47. Nieuwenhuys R, Voogd J, van Huijzen C. The Human Central Nervous System. 3rd ed. Berlin, Germany: Springer-Verlag; 1988

30 Corpus Callosotomy

Tai-Tong Wong, Shang-Yeong Kwan, and Kai-Ping Chang

Approximately 10% of children with newly diagnosed epilepsy develop intractable seizures.[1,2] Surgical management of children with medically intractable seizures includes resective and palliative surgical interventions. For patients who are not good candidates for resective surgery, palliative procedures such as disconnection surgeries (corpus callosotomy) and neuromodulation procedures (vagus nerve stimulation) are considered. Corpus callosotomy consists of partial or total disconnection of the corpus callosum and aims to block interhemispheric spread of secondary generalized seizures. It is an effective palliative, although not curative, surgical intervention that is particularly useful for atonic, tonic–clonic, and tonic seizures from different types of medically refractory epilepsies and epilepsy syndromes.

■ Histological Refinement of Corpus Callosotomy

Corpus callosotomy in the surgical management for epilepsy patients was first reported by van Wagenen and Herron in the 1940s.[3] They ligated the anterior one third of the superior sagittal sinus, divided the corpus callosum in various extents, sectioned the anterior commissure, and, in some cases, also divided the fornix unilaterally or bilaterally.[3,4] This approach was complicated with significant morbidity and did not gain any popularity. Approximately 20 years later in 1960s, Bogen and his colleagues revived the operation again.[5] They performed two different approaches: complete and partial disconnection. Complete disconnection was performed by dividing the entire corpus callosum, anterior commissure, unilateral fornix, hippocampal commissure, and even massa intermedia in some patients. The partial disconnection was performed by dividing the anterior one third of the corpus callosum, unilateral fornix, and anterior commissure in patients with bilateral independent seizure discharges with seizure foci restricted to frontal or temporal lobes.[5,6] In 1970, Luessenhop et al reported their experience with corpus callosotomy in the treatment of intractable seizures in children.[7] Then, again in 1970s, Wilson applied an operating microscope during this procedure, and he limited the operation to divide only the corpus callosum and hippocampal commissure. He did not enter the ventricles to avoid postoperative hydrocephalus.[6,8,9] Thereafter, in the 1980s, the staged callosotomy concept was introduced in the field by Maxwell, and corpus callosotomy started to be used more frequently in epilepsy patients.[6] The anterior two thirds to three quarters callosotomy was performed in the first stage, and the remaining posterior corpus callosum was divided in the second stage if the patient did not have much benefit from anterior two thirds callosotomy.[6] In 1993, Wyler described his technique for anterior callosotomy.[10] He split the corpus callosum from midline in between two pericallosal arteries to enter the cavum septum pellucidum. He advocated sectioning most of the corpus callosum and left only the splenium intact.[10] Later, although not commonly used, callosotomy with gamma knife radiosurgery was also described as a novel technique.[11,12] After introduction of the vagal nerve stimulator, corpus callosotomy lost its popularity somewhat, but it is still an effective procedure in a well selected patient population.[13–15]

■ Anatomical and Physiological Basis and Rational

Several midline commissural structures connect two cerebral hemispheres. The corpus callosum is the largest commissure and principal anatomical and neurophysiological connection pathway between the two hemispheres. The others include the anterior commissure, posterior commissure, hippocampal commissure, and massa intermedia. The corpus callosum can be divided into four parts: rostrum, genu, body (anterior and posterior), and splenium. The anterior half of the corpus callosum starts from the rostrum and includes the genu and the anterior half of the body and carries fibers projecting from premotor, supplementary motor, motor, anterior insular, and anterior cingulated cortical areas. Thus, it is essential for the generalization of tonic and tonic–clonic convulsions and atonic drops. The posterior half of the corpus callosum includes the posterior half of the callosal body, isthmus, and splenium and connects cortical areas from the parietal, temporal, and occipital lobes. The posterior midbody and isthmus carries fibers from parietal, superior temporal, posterior insula, and posterior cingulate. The splenium interconnects occipital lobe, caudal portion of

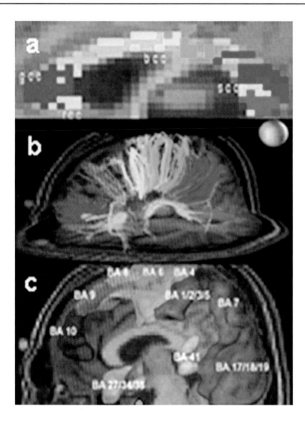

Fig. 30.1 Using diffuse tensor tractography–magnetic resonance imaging for topography study of the corpus callosum, **(A)** the parcellation of the corpus callosum, **(B)** the cortical associated tracts, and **(C)** the related cerebral cortex can be defined. (Courtesy of Ching-Po Lin, Institute of Neuroscience, National Yang-Ming University, Taiwan)

inferotemporal region, and lateral to caudal portions of the parahippocampal gyrus. The corpus callosum contains topographically organized fibers covering very large parts of the cerebral hemispheres, and these fiber tracts can be seen with current magnetic resonance imaging (MRI) techniques, such as diffuse tensor tractography (DT-MRI).[16–18] (**Fig. 30.1**). This topographical distribution is also significant from the surgical approach standpoint. A clinically sufficient number of fibers for interhemispheric transfer of some perceptual information can be preserved by sparing splenium during callosotomy and related complications occurring after complete callosotomy can be diminished.[19,20] This is one of the major advantages of the anterior two thirds corpus callosotomy approach.

Patient Selection Criteria, Surgical Indications, and Preoperative Assessment

Patient selection criteria for corpus callosotomy in children include several factors: clinically having documented resistance to major antiepileptic medications (AEDs), not being a candidate for curative surgical procedures, having certain

types of seizures (described later) and epilepsy syndromes, having disabling seizures with high risk of injury, experiencing a decreased quality of life secondary to seizures, and, finally, parents' preference among the available management options.

At Taipei Veterans General Hospital (Taipei VGH), the main indication for callosotomy is having medically refractory seizures without an identifiable or resectable epileptogenic focus. Sometimes, children with unilateral hemispheric lesions or bihemispheric malformation of cortical development are also considered as candidates for corpus callosotomy. Our criteria for clinically documented medical intractability of seizures are as follows: (1) presence of medically intractable seizures in a patient who has been treated by a pediatric epileptologist for at least 1 year, (2) poor response to currently available major AEDs with sufficient treatment dosages and serum levels, and (3) having more than two disabling seizures within a month. We do not accept mental retardation as a contraindication.[21] Currently, we perform corpus callosotomy in the amelioration of medically refractory seizures of some generalized epileptic syndromes such as Lennox-Gastaut syndrome (LGS), infantile spasms, severe epilepsy with multiple independent spike foci, and hemiconvulsion-hemiplegia-epilepsy syndrome. LGS patients constitute the largest group in our series, and they usually present with multiple seizure types including drop attacks, generalized tonic–clonic seizures (GTCS), partial seizures, and atypical absence. Drop attacks are the most responsive seizure type to callosotomy.[22–24]

At Taipei VGH, the preoperative evaluation of the patients for callosotomy includes the following:

- Detailed history and documentation of seizure semiology,
- Physical and neurological examinations,
- electroencephalography (EEG) and long-term video/EEG monitoring,
- MRI of brain, and
- Neuropsychological tests for intelligence scale and psychosocial behavior evaluation.

MR-venography for presurgical planning may also be obtained; however, it is not an absolute necessity.[23]

Surgical Technique

The operation is performed under general anesthesia. The patient's head is placed on a headrest with the sagittal plane perpendicular to the floor. A curvilinear, right-sided scalp incision is made along the coronal sutures by crossing midline approximately 2 cm. A right frontal craniotomy is performed with a midline cut on the left side of the sagittal sinus and the posterior edge of the skull flap stays just behind the coronal suture on the right and extends 6 to 7 cm anteriorly. Then a free skull flap is removed by exposing the right fron-

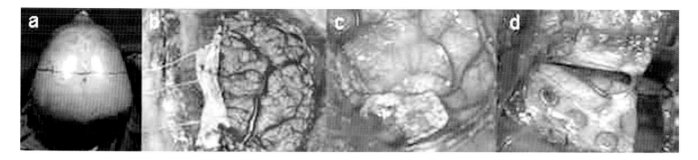

Fig. 30.2 **(A)** Curvilinear scalp incision along coronal suture for a 2-cm crossing midline frontal craniotomy. **(B–D)** Different patterns of cortical drainage veins to the sagittal sinus at the frontal region encountered during callosotomy. **(C)** Early attachment and entrance to dural sinus of a major cortical vein. The dura is cut laterally and along it to reach the edge of the sagittal sinus. **(D)** An alternative approach through the left side through a crossing midline right frontal craniotomy. Reprinted from: Wong TT, Kwan SY, Chang KP, et al. Corpus callosotomy in children. Childs Nerv Syst 2006;22(8): 999–1011.

tal region, and the dura is opened by coming as close to the sagittal sinus as much as possible. The dural flap is reflected over the sagittal sinus. Although the location of cortical bridging veins varies patient to patient, it rarely constitutes an obstruction to the surgeon in front of the coronal suture. If any dural venous lake or large drainage vein is encountered, the dural incision is extended accordingly along these bridging veins to avoid any injury and to reach the edge of the sagittal sinus. If it is unexpectedly difficulty to make a right interhemispheric approach because of large bridging veins or venous lakes, in our experience, it is always possible to do the procedure through the other side (**Fig. 30.2**). We cover the exposed cortical veins with Gelfoam strips (Pfizer,

New York, NY), and Cottonoids to avoid any accidental injury during the procedure. Before starting interhemispheric dissection, we obtain precallosotomy electrocorticography (ECoG). Then, the interhemispheric microdissection assisted by microscope or binocular loupes is performed. First, the arachnoid attachments are divided and the interhemispheric fissure is gradually exposed by draining cerebrospinal fluid (CSF). While dissection continues, the brain can be further relaxed by suctioning CSF from interhemispheric space. Gradually, the brain becomes relaxed enough to retract it sufficiently to be able to perform the procedure without any need for lumbar drainage or application of osmotic agents. The next step is dividing the interhemispheric adhesions

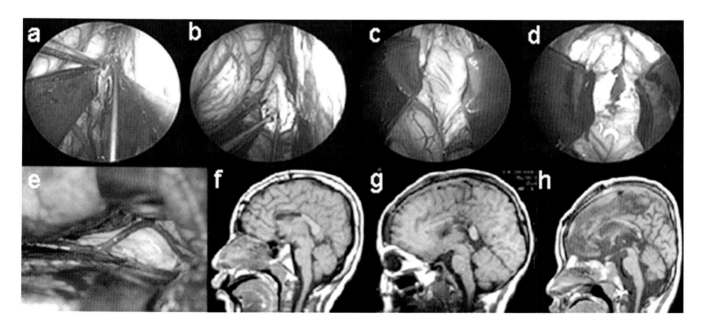

Fig. 30.3 **(A)** Interhemispheric microdissection and splitting of the body of the corpus callosum in between the pericallosal arteries. **(B–D)** Splitting of genu and body of the splenium and counting the length of callosal section by using 1-cm blade of the retractor. **(E)** The rare single pericallosal artery and its branches. **(F–H)** Postoperative magnetic resonance images showing different extents of the callosotomy. Reprinted from: Wong TT, Kwan SY, Chang KP, et al. Corpus callosotomy in children. Childs Nerv Syst 2006;22(8):999–1011.

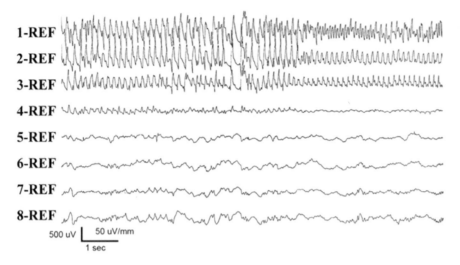

1-REF

2-REF

3-REF

4-REF

5-REF

6-REF

7-REF

8-REF

500 uV | 50 uV/mm

1 sec

Fig. 30.4 The postcallosotomy electrocorticography in an 18-year-old boy with chronic generalized tonic–clonic seizures. The upper four channels (1-REF, 2-REF, 3-REF and 4-REF) showed isolation of electroencephalography (EEG) seizure at the left frontal cortex recorded via a 4 × 1 electrode strip. The lower four channels (5-REF, 6-REF, 7-REF and 8-REF) represented EEG recording by another 4 × 1 electrode strip over the right frontal cortex. Reprinted from: Wong TT, Kwan SY, Chang KP, et al. Corpus callosotomy in children. Childs Nerv Syst 2006;22(8):999–1011.

adequately to avoid injury to the mesial frontal cortex before stepwise hemispheric retraction. This also provides a good exposure to pericallosal arteries and their branches. As the dissection is advanced toward the callosum, the retractor blade is further replaced to expose the cingulum. The cingular gyri can be quite adherent and difficult to separate in some cases because of arachnoid adhesions; in these cases, the trajectory is redirected to a portion where dissection can easily be performed and then extended further using fine-tipped bipolar forceps and appropriate dissectors. The supracallosal cistern is opened, and the underlying glistening white corpus callosum and the pericallosal arteries are exposed. Although rare, it can be seen in some cases that a single pericallosal artery supplies both hemispheres. Pericallosal arteries are gently separated with bipolar tips and dissectors and Cottonoid micropatties were placed on both ends to keep them separated. The corpus callosum is then divided between the pericallosal arteries at the midline of the rostral midbody of corpus callosum by a microspatula. The grayish-blue color of the ependymal lining of the ventricle can be easily appreciated while deepening the callosal dissection, and it is preferable not to enter the ventricle by opening the ependyma to avoid risk of chemical meningitis. If the goal is anterior two-thirds callosotomy, then the challenge at this stage is translating the planned length of the callosotomy on the surgical field. As the midline cleft between the roofs of the lateral ventricles is exposed, we follow this cleft to split the genu anteriorly down to the anterior commissure and then to divide the caudal part of body of the corpus callosum posteriorly to reach the splenium as much as possible (**Fig. 30.3**). In selected patients with severe mental retardation, single-stage total callosotomy may be performed. Sometimes, we tilt the table up or down to elevate or lower the head a bit to gain space to see the genu or posterior part of the corpus callosum better. After the callosotomy, a postdivision ECoG is performed (**Fig. 30.4**). Then the surgical area is irrigated with saline, and meticulous hemostasis is obtained. Then the entry points of cortical drainage veins are rechecked, and Gelfoam pieces are packed around them, if needed. Then the dura is closed primarily and the skull flap is replaced. Postoperatively, the extent of corpus callosum division is assessed by MRI. We recently started to use a special software package for this purpose.

■ Complications and Disconnection Syndromes

Common complications of corpus callosotomy are cerebral edema, infarction, bleeding, meningitis (septic/aseptic), and hydrocephalus. These complications generally develop secondary to brain retraction, injury of bridging veins, and entering the ventricles. Postoperative epidural and subdural hematoma were also reported, although they are rare.[23] Postoperative deficits may occur with both partial and total corpus callosotomy procedures.[25] The most often reported adverse events of callosal sectioning are related to the separation of the hemispheres and include speech-related problems, such as a brief period of mutism.[26] Sussman et al indicated that this syndrome might be the result of disruption of interhemispheric connections when both hemispheres are required for speech production.[27] Sass et al also suggested that speech and language deficits are prone to present after callosotomy in patients with crossed dominance or patients with bilateral speech representation.[28] Manual dexterity contralateral to a dysfunctional hemisphere may decline, or there may be gradual deterioration in manipulospatial skills.[29] In Andersen's series, four patients suffered from symptoms of cerebral disconnection syndrome that interfered with activities of daily living.[26] Several older patients in Lassonde's series also showed prolonged apraxia of the nondominant hand, which resulted in reduced bimanual coordination and a mild decline in performance IQ.[30] However, previous reports indicated that children, especially those younger than age 13 years, adapt more easily to callosal section than do adults. It has been suggested that there is greater cerebral plasticity of the immature brain, which allows for significant adjustment after brain surgery.[27]

Disconnection syndromes can be categorized as acute disconnecting syndrome (ADS), posterior disconnection syndrome, split-brain syndrome, and deficit reinstatement. Difficulty of initiating speech, mutism, various degrees of left leg paresis, left forced grasp, and urgency incontinence may be caused by traction of the nondominant parasagittal cortex or ADS. ADS is usually temporary and may last for days to weeks. Transient increase of local motor seizures is occasionally observed. Posterior (sensory) disconnection syndrome may occur after splenium section or posterior section for staged posterior callosotomy. Patients may exhibit deficits of tactile and visual transfer. Split-brain syndrome may be seen after total or near total callosotomy. Patients may show language impairment, hemisphere competition, and disordered attention–memory sequencing. Patients with split-brain syndrome usually improve with time. Deficit reinstatement occurs in certain patients who have early hemispheric injury with transcallosal compensation or mixed cerebral dominance. In staged anterior callosotomy, these complications have been seen less, especially in children.[31–33]

Postoperative Assessment

Postoperative MRI is performed to assess and document the extent of corpus callosum division. The patients are followed postoperatively in the pediatric epilepsy clinic for AED adjustment and seizure outcome evaluation. Postoperative EEG follow-up studies are performed at the 3rd, 6th, and 12th month after surgery. Neuropsychological assessment is also repeated at the 6th and 12th month after callosotomy. The seizure outcome is classified into six grades: grade 1, seizure free without AED; grade 2, seizure free with AED; grade 3, seizures reduced by more than 50%; grade 4, seizures reduced by less than 50%; grade 5, no change in either frequency or severity of seizures; grade 6, worsening of seizures. Favorable improvement is defined as more than 50% reduction in seizure frequency after the operation, which includes grade 1, grade 2, and grade 3.

Outcome

Satisfactory seizure control (> 50% reduction of seizures) rates after corpus callosotomy was reported to be between 66.2 and 79.5% in several studies.[31,34,35] Contrary to resective epilepsy surgery procedures, seizure-free outcome is quite rare after corpus callosotomy. It was found to be 13% in Fuiks

series and 18.9% in our series.[34,36] However, this was closely related to duration of postoperative follow-up period and decreased from 18.9% to 9.3% with longer durations of follow-up.[23] In our series, approximately 80% of corpus callosotomy procedures were performed in children with LGS.[23] Children with LGS usually present with multiple seizure types, including absence, drop attacks (axial tonic, massive myoclonic, and atonic seizures), and other seizure types (GTCS and partial seizures). Corpus callosotomy is most effective in drop attacks. Maehara and Shimizu reviewed the seizure outcome in 52 patients with drop attacks and reported more than 90% seizure reduction in 85% of patients.[24] In our series of 48 cases of LGS, 31 patients (64.6%) achieved significant improvement (> 50% reduction of seizure frequency) after anterior two-thirds to four-fifths callosotomy with a mean follow-up of 5.8 years (range from 4 to 7.5 years).[22]

In addition to improved seizure control, corpus callosotomy positively affects the neuropsychological function level of the patients. In most studies, improved attention, behavior, and performance in daily activities were reported.[29] Andersen et al indicated that 10 of 20 patients had a favorable seizure outcome; and of these, 50% noticed an improved quality of life and were satisfied with the treatment.[26] In Gilliam's series, most parents reported satisfaction with the outcome of callosotomy, and the satisfaction is reported by improvement in other aspects of daily function and behavior in addition to seizure reduction. Improved alertness and responsiveness are most closely associated with satisfaction.[37] From the postoperative questionnaire survey of Shimizu, of the 22 responders, 77% reported improvement in overall behavior, 60% indicated expansion of vocabulary, and none detected worsening of mental functions.[38] Nordgren et al indicated that there was no postoperative deterioration in behavior, memory, or language function and many patients have had marked improvement in their behavior and alertness after callosotomy, presumably on the basis of decreased seizures and lower levels of anticonvulsant medications.[27] Our previous study suggested that the greatest improvement of life domains after callosotomy included level of self-care, family life, and school performance. Hyperactivity, attention span, and social skills also improved significantly in 11 of 25 patients after callosotomy. In this study, we found that callosotomy did not improve mental performance.[39] Lassonde et al suggested that higher IQ was associated with better outcome in the group of patients younger than 13, mainly because this group was more severely retarded and had more to gain from the surgery than the older group.[30]

■ Taipei VGH Study

In 2000, we studied 127 cases of anterior corpus callosotomy to assess the effect of the procedure and the clinical factors influencing seizure outcome. In this series, 122 patients were younger than 18 years old; 80% of these patients had LGS and the mean follow-up period was 3.9 years. The mean age at corpus callosotomy was 8.2 years. Two-thirds anterior callosotomy was performed in 17.3% of the patients, and four-fifths callosotomy was performed in 77.2% of the patients. With AED, 16.5% of the patients were seizure free, 38.6% had significant seizure reduction (> 50%), 16.5% had seizure reduction (< 50%), and 18.9% of the patients had no seizure reduction after callosotomy. In this study, we found that there was no statistical significance for the following clinical factors to affect seizure outcome after anterior callosotomy: age of onset of epilepsy, duration of epilepsy, age at callosotomy, degree of mental retardation, extent of callosotomy (< ⅔ vs. > ⅔ callosal section), etiology of epilepsy, and types of epilepsy (LGS versus other types of epilepsy). Because only five patients had a complete callosotomy in this series, we could not assess the clinical significance of complete callosotomy on seizure outcome.

■ Conclusion

The concept and technique of corpus callosotomy has been well established since the 1980s. It is a palliative procedure that is applied predominantly in children with LGS and drop attacks. Compared with partial division, complete callosotomy is more effective for seizure control in drop attacks. Improved seizure control after callosotomy is always associated with improved quality of life, satisfaction of parents, and improvement in the family's quality of life. Significant neuropsychological changes are evident only on formal testing, are usually ignored by patient and family members, and rarely affect daily life. The surgical procedure is quite safe in experienced hands with minimal surgical complications and acceptable adverse events. Early identification of medically resistant epilepsy and appropriate selection of the surgical candidates for corpus callosotomy are important for satisfactory outcome.

References

1. Berg AT, Shinnar S, Levy SR, Testa FM, Smith-Rapaport S, Beckerman B. Early development of intractable epilepsy in children: a prospective study. Neurology 2001;56(11):1445–1452

2. Czochańska J, Losiowski Z, Langner-Tyszka B, et al. Intractable epilepsy in children who develop epilepsy in the first decade of life—a prospective study. Mater Med Pol 1996;28(4):133–137

3. van Wagenen WP, Herren RY. Surgical division of commissural pathways in the corpus callosum. Arch Neurol Psychiatry 1940;44:740–759

4. Mathews MS, Linskey ME, Binder DK. William P. van Wagenen and the first corpus callosotomies for epilepsy. J Neurosurg 2008;108(3):608–613

5. Bogen JE, Fisher ED, Vogel PJ. Cerebral commissurotomy. A second case report. JAMA 1965;194(12):1328–1329

6. Maxwell RE, Gates JR, Gumnit RJ. Corpus callosotomy at the University of Minnesota. In: Engel J Jr, ed. Surgical Treatment of the Epilepsies. New York, NY: Raven Press; 1986:659–666

7. Luessenhop AJ, Dela Cruz TC, Fenichel GM. Surgical disconnection of the cerebral hemispheres for intractable seizures. Results in infancy and childhood. JAMA 1970;213(10):1630–1636

8. Wilson DH, Reeves A, Gazzaniga M. Division of the corpus callosum for uncontrollable epilepsy. Neurology 1978;28(7):649–653

9. Wilson DH, Reeves AG, Gazzaniga MS. "Central" commissurotomy for intractable generalized epilepsy: series two. Neurology 1982;32(7):687–697

10. Wyler AR. Corpus callosotomy. In: Wyllie E, ed. The Treatment of Epilepsy—Principles and Practice. Philadelphia, PA; London, UK: Lea & Febiger; 1993:1120–1125

11. Nádvornik P, Krupa P, Chrastina J, Smrcka V, Novák Z, Zborilová E. Circular stereotactic callosotomy: a preliminary report. Technical note. Acta Neurochir (Wien) 1997;139(4):359–360

12. Pendl G, Eder HG, Schroettner O, Leber KA. Corpus callosotomy with radiosurgery. Neurosurgery 1999;45(2):303–307, discussion 307–308

13. Wheless JW, Maggio V. Vagus nerve stimulation therapy in patients younger than 18 years. Neurology 2002;59(6, suppl 4):S21–S25

14. Frost M, Gates J, Helmers SL, et al. Vagus nerve stimulation in children with refractory seizures associated with Lennox-Gastaut syndrome. Epilepsia 2001;42(9):1148–1152

15. Fandiño-Franky J, Torres M, Nariño D, Fandiño J. Corpus callosotomy in Colombia and some reflections on care and research among the poor in developing countries. Epilepsia 2000;41(suppl 4):S22–S27

16. Witelson SF. Hand and sex differences in the isthmus and genu of the human corpus callosum. A postmortem morphological study. Brain 1989;112(pt 3):799–835

17. Pandya DN, Yeterian EH. Hodology of limbic and related structures: Cortical and commissural connections. In: Wiesser HG, Elger CE, eds. Presurgical Evaluation of Epileptics. Berlin, Germany; Heidelberg, Germany; New York, NY: Springer; 1987:3–14

18. Park HJ, Kim JJ, Lee SK, et al. Corpus callosal connection mapping using cortical gray matter parcellation and DT-MRI. Hum Brain Mapp 2008;29(5):503–516

19. Risse GL, Gates J, Lund G, Maxwell R, Rubens A. Interhemispheric transfer in patients with incomplete section of the corpus callosum. Anatomic verification with magnetic resonance imaging. Arch Neurol 1989;46(4):437–443

20. Funnell MG, Corballis PM, Gazzaniga MS. Cortical and subcortical interhemispheric interactions following partial and complete callosotomy. Arch Neurol 2000;57(2):185–189

21. Sussman NM, Gur RC, Gur RE, O'Connor MJ. Mutism as a consequence of callosotomy. J Neurosurg 1983;59(3):514–519

22. Kwan SY, Lin JH, Wong TT, Chang KP, Yiu CH. Prognostic value of electrocorticography findings during callosotomy in children with Lennox-Gastaut syndrome. Seizure 2005;14(7):470–475

23. Wong TT, Kwan SY, Chang KP, et al. Corpus callosotomy in children. Childs Nerv Syst 2006;22(8):999–1011

24. Maehara T, Shimizu H. Surgical outcome of corpus callosotomy in patients with drop attacks. Epilepsia 2001;42(1):67–71

25. Sass KJ, Spencer DD, Spencer SS, Novelly RA, Williamson PD, Mattson RH. Corpus callosotomy for epilepsy. II. Neurologic and neuropsychological outcome. Neurology 1988;38(1):24–28

26. Andersen B, Rogvi-Hansen B, Kruse-Larsen C, Dam M. Corpus callosotomy: seizure and psychosocial outcome. A 39-month follow-up of 20 patients. Epilepsy Res 1996;23(1):77–85

27. Nordgren RE, Reeves AG, Viguera AC, Roberts DW. Corpus callosotomy for intractable seizures in the pediatric age group. Arch Neurol 1991;48(4):364–372

28. Sass KJ, Novelly RA, Spencer DD, Spencer SS. Postcallosotomy language impairments in patients with crossed cerebral dominance. J Neurosurg 1990;72(1):85–90

29. Duchowny MS. Surgery for intractable epilepsy: issues and outcome. Pediatrics 1989;84(5):886–894

30. Lassonde M, Sauerwein C. Neuropsychological outcome of corpus callosotomy in children and adolescents. J Neurosurg Sci 1997;41(1):67–73

31. Cendes F, Ragazzo PC, da Costa V, Martins LF. Corpus callosotomy in treatment of medically resistant epilepsy: preliminary results in a pediatric population. Epilepsia 1993;34(5):910–917

32. Spencer SS, Williamson P, Spencer DD, Maxwell R, Roberts D. Corpus callosotomy section. In: Engel J, ed. Surgical Treatment of the Epilepsies. New York, NY: Raven Press; 1987:425–444

33. Pilcher WH, Roberts DW, Flanigin HF, et al. Complications of epilepsy surgery. 2nd ed. In: Engel J Jr, ed. Surgical Treatment of the Epilepsies. New York, NY: Raven Press; 1993;565–581

34. Kwan SY, Wong TT, Chang KP, et al. Seizure outcome after corpus callosotomy: the Taiwan experience. Childs Nerv Syst 2000;16(2):87–92

35. Nei M, O'Connor M, Liporace J, Sperling MR. Refractory generalized seizures: response to corpus callosotomy and vagal nerve stimulation. Epilepsia 2006;47(1):115–122

36. Fuiks KS, Wyler AR, Hermann BP, Somes G. Seizure outcome from anterior and complete corpus callosotomy. J Neurosurg 1991;74(4):573–578

37. Gilliam F, Wyllie E, Kotagal P, Geckler C, Rusyniak G. Parental assessment of functional outcome after corpus callosotomy. Epilepsia 1996;37(8):753–757

38. Shimizu H, Maehara T. Neuronal disconnection for the surgical treatment of pediatric epilepsy. Epilepsia 2000;41(suppl 9):28–30

39. Yang TF, Wong TT, Kwan SY, Chang KP, Lee YC, Hsu TC. Quality of life and life satisfaction in families after a child has undergone corpus callostomy. Epilepsia 1996;37(1):76–80

31 Multiple Subpial Transections in Children with Refractory Epilepsy

Zulma Tovar-Spinoza and James T. Rutka

The multiple subpial transection (MST) technique was described by Frank Morrell as a new surgical procedure to treat patients with epileptogenic zones in functionally critical cortical areas where resective surgery can cause unacceptable neurological deficits.[1-3] In theory, the MST procedure is based on selective destruction of the short horizontal fiber connections and aims to prevent synchronization and spread of epileptogenic discharges while allowing preservation of the normal cortical functions.[1-4]

■ Fundamentals

The rationale for MST is based on the following facts and assumptions:

- Columnar organization of the cortex: MST was based on experimental evidences describing functional cortical units composed of vertically oriented neuronal elements and vertical afferent and efferent fibers.[5-9]
- Synchronized neuronal discharges: An epileptogenic focus requires paroxysmal synchronous discharges from a critical volume of neurons and tangential-horizontal interneuronal projections to spread seizure activity.[10-13]
- The critical mass of cortical cells: A critical volume of contiguous neurons (1 cm^2) is necessary to sustain synchronous spikes. It is believed that cortical areas greater than 5 mm width or tangential connections greater than 5 mm are indispensable for the generation of paroxysmal neuronal discharges.[14-16] This observation explains the transection interval of 5 mm classically suggested for MST.
- Spread of epileptogenic discharges: The lateral radiating cortical-cortical interneuronal connections in all cortical layers—but mainly in layers IV through V of the cerebral cortex—are the main projections of spreading the seizure activity.[17,18] Morrell reasoned that interrupting this pattern of propagation of seizure activity might eliminate the spread of the epileptic discharges.[11-13]
- Preservation of cortical blood supply. Anatomically, the gyral blood supply enters perpendicularly to the cortical surface, and the arterial flow and venous drainage have a parallel trajectory with the axonal fibers. Thus, MST technique would not disrupt the vascular supply to the cortex and preserve the integrity of the subpial bank.[2]

■ Indications

Although MST is a well-known technique, its application is still not widespread. MST was the least frequently performed epilepsy surgery procedure (on the order of 0.6%) among all cases reported by Harvey et al in their recently published survey from the Pediatric Epilepsy Surgery Subcomission of the International League Against Epilepsy.[19]

Focal Seizures Located in the Eloquent Cortex

Currently, this is the main indication for MST. In children, as in adults, the MST can be performed as a stand-alone procedure or can be combined with cortical resection or lesionectomy.[20-22] In one of the largest series, Shimizu and Machara[23] presented their experience with 31 children who underwent MST. The procedure was performed along with resective surgeries (lobectomy, corticectomy, or lesionectomy) in 25 patients and as a stand-alone procedure in the remaining 6 patients. Of 25 patients who were followed for more than 1 year, 10 of them had Engel Class I or II outcome, but no details were provided as to whether these patients had MST alone or combined with cortical resection. No mortality or morbidity was encountered during surgery or postoperatively. Later, Blount et al[20] described their series of 30 consecutive children who underwent MST. The procedure was performed as a stand-alone therapy (4 patients) or in conjunction with cortical excisions (26 patients). Twenty-three children underwent invasive monitoring with subdural grid electrodes, and intraoperative electrocorticography was performed in the remaining 7 children. The mean follow-up period for the group was 3.5 years (minimum 30 months in all cases). All 20 patients in whom MST was performed in the primary motor cortex experienced transient hemiparesis lasting up to 6 weeks. No patient suffered a permanent motor deficit in the long-term follow-up period. In the 26 patients who underwent cortical resections followed by MST, 12 children (46%) were seizure free (Engel Class I) after surgery. Eleven patients (42%; Engel Classes II and III) continued to suffer seizures but the improvement in seizures was still acceptable. In the 23 patients in whom subdural grids were placed to capture the ictal onset zone by invasive video-electro-encephalography (VEEG), MST area consisted of a mean of 37% of the surgically treated area under the grid. It is difficult to assess the effectiveness of MST as a distinct surgical procedure because the majority of published series include patients in whom MST is combined with lesionectomy or cortical resection. The use of MST as a stand-alone therapy has been described by Schramm et al,[24] Smith,[25] Lui et al,[26] and Whisler et al.[27] These series addressed both adult and pediatric populations. Schramm obtained 45% and 50% good results according to Engel's and Spencer's classifications, respectively. Seizure-free outcome was 5% in Schramm's series, 37.5% in Smith's series, and 63% in Whisler's series. Téllez-Zenteno et al[28] published a meta-analysis of several series of patients with MST, both pure and combined with resective surgery. The mean follow-up period was 5 years in this study. They concluded that MST has the lowest rate of long-term, seizure-free outcome (16%) among all epilepsy surgical procedures. Previously, Spencer et al[29] reported their meta-analysis from six series and reviewed the data covering 211 patients collected from six different centers. Fifty-five patients in this study underwent pure MST, and 156 patients had MST and resection combined procedures. The overall seizure outcome was similar in the patients with partial seizures whether the patient had pure MST or MST with cortical resection. However, the patients with generalized seizures had better outcome if the MST was combined with cortical resections. Unfortunately, this study did not specify the postsurgical follow-up period for outcome analysis. This report and others concluded that MST could be considered an effective surgical treatment alternative for uncontrolled seizures arising in eloquent brain areas.[22,25,30–34]

Landau-Kleffner Syndrome

Landau-Kleffner Syndrome (LKS) has been considered as another main indication for MST in children.[3] This rare syndrome consists of an acquired epileptic aphasia or verbal auditory agnosia that may start abruptly or gradually and occurs in children with previously normal developmental history. A well-defined electrophysiological profile underlying this condition consists of frequent epileptiform discharges when awake, and generalized slow spike-wave discharges over the perisylvian region during slow wave sleep.[35] Antiepileptic drugs can improve clinical seizures but EEG findings can be frequently resistant to treatment.[36]

The MST technique was initially applied to the LKS patients by Morrell et al,[3] and they reported their experience with 14 patients. Seven recovered age-appropriate speech ability and

no longer needed speech therapy or special education classes. Another four had marked improvement in their speech but still required speech therapy. Three children had no changes in their preoperative conditions. Sawhney et al[34] reported improvement in all three of their patients with LKS who underwent MST. Neville et al[37] reported one case that had marked postoperative improvement in reading, vocabulary, sign language, and nonverbal subtests. Nass et al[38] described their experience in seven patients with atypical forms of LKS and reported mild improvement in receptive language functions. Irving et al.[39] reported five children with this condition who underwent MST and reported improvement in their language skills. Although none of them improved to an age-appropriate level, seizures and behavior disturbances were immediately improved in all cases. Castillo et al[35] reported one case with significant linguistic improvement after a 2-year follow-up.

In summary, MST application in LKS can result in improvements in communication skills and behavior after surgery. However, improvement in speech takes a considerably longer period of time.[40,41] Use of MST for severe autistic regression in childhood epilepsy is not always associated with improvement in cognitive and behavioral function. At best, gains observed are temporary, and further studies are needed to prove its worth in this condition.[38]

Syndrome of Malignant Rolandic-Sylvian Epilepsy

This nonlesional syndrome described by Otsubo et al[42] relates to children who have intractable rolandic partial seizures that progress to secondary generalization, fronto-centro-temporal spikes on EEG, localized spike sources in the rolandic-sylvian regions on magnetoencephalography (MEG), and neurocognitive problems. Resective surgery is required in nonfunctional cortex and as an additional management strategy. MSTs are also recommended throughout the eloquent cortex. The series included seven patients and reported that the combination of techniques could reduce or eliminate seizure activity, avoiding postoperative permanent motor deficits or further language deficits.

Other Indications

MST has been reported in the treatment of patients with cortical dysplasia, epilepsia partialis continua (EPC), and Rasmussen encephalitis. Molyneux et al described the successful treatment of one patient with EPC using MST on epileptogenic focus over the left central cortex.[43] This patient had a normal magnetic resonance imaging (MRI) scan, but a diagnosis of cortical dysplasia was made by biopsy. MSTs have also been attempted with variable results for EPC caused by Rasmussen encephalitis.[34,44]

Presurgical Evaluation

Defining the seizure focus is the main goal of the presurgical evaluation for all patients who are candidates for epilepsy surgery procedures, including MST. Although different protocols exist depending on the institution, most epilepsy centers use many common techniques to assess the surgical candidates. Harvey et al[19] recently published a survey collecting data from 20 programs in the United States, Europe, and Australia on 543 patients and all 20 centers reported using scalp EEG, VEEG, and MRI in the presurgical evaluation of all patients. Eight percent of the centers used ictal single-proton emission computed tomography (SPECT), 85% used 2-deoxy-2[^{18}F]fluoro-D-glucose (FDG)-positron emission tomography (PET), 70% used functional MRI (fMRI), usually for language localization, 35% used MEG/magnetic source imaging (MSI), and 50% performed an intracarotid amobarbital procedure (IAP; Wada test). Only three centers used all presurgical tests (ictal-SPECT, FDG-PET, fMRI, MEG, and IAP).

The epilepsy surgery protocol at the Hospital for Sick Children in Toronto includes ictal and interictal scalp EEG, ictal and interictal VEEG, and MRI with special sequences to evaluate myelination, cortical pathways, and to rule out neoplasms.[21] In addition to these, formal neurological and neuropsychological evaluations are performed to determine preoperative levels of verbal and memory functions and their lateralization. Language dominance is determined by Wada testing, fMRI, or functional MEG. MEG spikes source localization can be overlaid onto MRIs to generate an MSI.[45] MSI can also be incorporated into neuronavigation systems to localize the focus of spike-wave disturbances at the time of surgery. The merging of the data from all of these evaluations will help to define the epileptogenic focus amenable to surgical treatment.

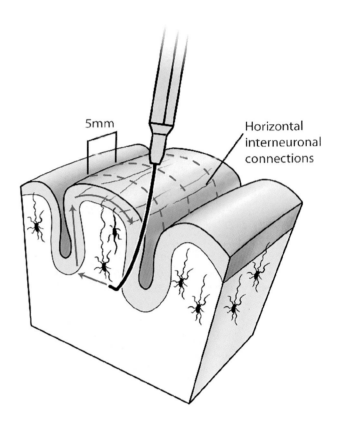

Fig. 31.1 The multiple subpial transection (MST) knife is introduced through the incised pial hole and is subpially directed toward the sulcal margin, making a right-angle cut to the long axis of the gyrus to a depth of approximately 5 to 7 mm. The blade of the MST knife is maintained in a strictly vertical orientation and the tip of the MST knife is visualized through the pia mater as it is drawn back along the subpial space completing the transection. (Reproduced with permission by McGraw-Hill Companies from Tovar-Spinoza ZS, Rutka JT. Multiple subpial transections. In: Textbook of Stereotactic and Functional Neurosurgery. Lozano A, Gildengerg P, Tasker R, eds. (2nd ed) Berlin Heidelberg: Springer: 2009)

Surgical Technique

The original technique of MST was described and developed by Morrell and Whisler.[27,46,47] The bipolar electrocautery is used to cauterize a small pial point on the defined epileptogenic focus either at the side of the gyrus or at the crest.[48] Then, the cortex is penetrated at this site with the tip of an 11 blade scalpel. A right angle blunt dissector is introduced through the incised pial hole and it is subpially directed toward the sulcal margin, making a right-angle cut to the long axis of the gyrus to a depth of approximately 5 to 7 mm (**Fig. 31.1**). The blade of the MST knife (**Fig. 31.2**) should be maintained in a strictly vertical orientation to avoid undercutting the cortex. The tip of the MST knife is visualized through the pia mater as it is drawn back along the subpial space completing the transection. The surgeon should avoid disrupting the pia matter or injuring sulcal vessels during

the procedure. If the insertion point is made in the center of the gyrus, after the first half cut, the instrument is removed and reinserted, aiming in the opposite direction, and the remainder of the transection is completed. Another variation on the technique is to point the MST knife downward using sharpened rather than blunt knives to diminish the damage of using blunt instruments.[48]

Parallel cuts (spaced 5 mm apart) are then made from this cut until the entire proposed epileptogenic zone has been transected. Pial bleeding at the blade insertion point can be controlled with a bipolar or a small piece of thrombin-soaked Gelfoam. Intraoperative ultrasound has been useful when MST is performed in extensive areas of the brain to rule out the presence of an acute intracerebral hematoma.[21]

The efficacy and extent of the procedure are judged intraoperatively by using electrocorticography before and after MST. However, the role of electrocorticography in predicting

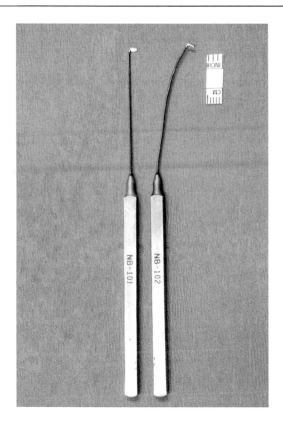

Fig. 31.2 Multiple subpial transection knives.

seizure outcome has been the subject of some controversy.[20,21,49]

■ Complications

In general, MST is associated with low morbidity. Although transient postoperative neurological deficits are common, permanent deficits lasting longer than 3 months are rare even when extensive regions of cortex are transected.[20,24,27,30,33] Some of these complications include hemiparesis,[25,27,29,34,50,51] hemisensory deficits, memory deficits, visual field deficits,[29] alteration in proprioception,[31] aphasia/dysphasia,[24,27,29] and dysdiadochokinesis.[50] Children usually show clinical improvement within 1 week of the procedure. In addition to small subarachnoid and intracerebral hemorrhages,[27,52] some unusually large and symptomatic hematomas have been reported.[24,27] Mild brain swelling is expected, but excessive brain swelling not related to hematoma formation has only been reported once.[24]

■ Surgical Technique

There are many reasons for the wide range of variations in the application and results of MST. Differences in the presur-

gical evaluation, definition of the epileptogenic focus, indications, and surgical technique can considerably affect the seizure outcome.[53]

The surgical technique in MST is not standard. Different surgeons perform the procedure with some variations that can also potentially influence the outcome. Transection intervals and depth, transecting just the crown, or transecting the entire gyrus may easily affect the result of the procedure. Again failure to keep the transection perfectly vertical with respect to the gyral surface may result in sparing of the cortical tissue at the sulcus and the U fibers.[31] Nontransected tissue bridges in layers IV and V or V and VI could allow for seizure propagation.[18] Differences in the length of the curved MST dissectors might also play a factor in the completion of the transection appropriately.[54]

Another reason for variable results is patient selection. Although there is not a full consensus on the benefit of MST, the most common two indications for MST in children are epileptogenic focus in an eloquent area of the brain and LKS. The other indications are significantly more controversial, and the surgical criteria variable depending on the individual centers.

One other reason for variable results is using MST technique as a stand-alone procedure or combined with resective surgeries. As discussed earlier, the role of the MST as standalone therapy is still controversial, and further studies are needed to clarify this controversy.

In published studies, several authors have presented their outcome data based on different follow-up periods. It is a well-known fact that seizures may change over time.[24,47,55] Whether or not the initial seizure improvement seen in the first 1 to 2 years after surgery will persist over subsequent years is unclear. In addition, the lack of an accepted and standardized seizure outcome scale, and the use of different scales such as the Engel,[56] modified Engel,[55] or Spencer classification[24] in series makes comparisons difficult.

■ Conclusion

Current advances in the preoperative evaluation techniques in children with refractory epilepsy clearly show that pediatric patients benefit from definitive surgeries if the procedure is performed as early as possible. Certain groups advocate more aggressive approaches in children even if the epileptogenic focus is located in functionally critical cortical areas. However, frequently, the risk of a resective surgery in eloquent cortex is high and functionally unacceptable. MST constitutes a relatively safe surgical alternative in this patient group. Current data also suggest that MST is probably more effective when combined with cortical resection compared with its application as a stand-alone procedure. However, prospective studies are needed to assess the full potential of MST as stand-alone therapy in children.

References

1. Morrell F, Hanbery W. A new surgical technique for the treatment of focal cortical epilepsy. Electroencephalogr Clin Neurophysiol 1969;26:120

2. Morrell F, Whisler WW, Bleck TP. Multiple subpial transection: a new approach to the surgical treatment of focal epilepsy. J Neurosurg 1989;70(2):231–239

3. Morrell F, Whisler WW, Smith MC, et al. Landau-Kleffner syndrome. Treatment with subpial intracortical transection. Brain 1995;118(pt 6):1529–1546

4. Kaufmann WE, Krauss GL, Uematsu S, Lesser RP. Treatment of epilepsy with multiple subpial transections: an acute histologic analysis in human subjects. Epilepsia 1996;37(4):342–352

5. Asanuma H, Sakata H. Functional organization of a cortical efferent system examined with focal depth stimulation in cats. J Neurophysiol 1967;30:35–54

6. Asanuma H, Stoney SD Jr, Abzug C. Relationship between afferent input and motor outflow in cat motorsensory cortex. J Neurophysiol 1968;31(5):670–681

7. Hubel DH, Wiesel TN. Receptive fields, binocular interaction and functional architecture in the cat's visual cortex. J Physiol 1962;160:106–154

8. Mountcastle VB. Modality and topographic properties of single neurons of cat's somatic sensory cortex. J Neurophysiol 1957;20(4):408–434

9. Powell TP, Mountcastle VB. Some aspects of the functional organization of the cortex of the postcentral gyrus of the monkey: a correlation of findings obtained in a single unit analysis with cytoarchitecture. Bull Johns Hopkins Hosp 1959;105:133–162

10. Tharp BR. The penicillin focus: a study of field characteristics using cross-correlation analysis. Electroencephalogr Clin Neurophysiol 1971;31(1):45–55

11. Reichenthal E, Hocherman S. The critical cortical area for development of penicillin-induced epilepsy. Electroencephalogr Clin Neurophysiol 1977;42(2):248–251

12. Lueders H, Bustamante L, Zablow L, Krinsky A, Goldensohn ES. Quantitative studies of spike foci induced by minimal concentrations of penicillin. Electroencephalogr Clin Neurophysiol 1980;48(1):80–89

13. Lueders H, Bustamante LA, Zablow L, Goldensohn ES. The independence of closely spaced discrete experimental spike foci. Neurology 1981;31(7):846–851

14. Dichter M, Spencer WA. Penicillin-induced interictal discharges from the cat hippocampus. II. Mechanisms underlying origin and restriction. J Neurophysiol 1969;32(5):663–687

15. Dichter M, Spencer WA. Penicillin-induced interictal discharges from the cat hippocampus. I. Characteristics and topographical features. J Neurophysiol 1969;32(5):649–662

16. Goldensohn ES, Zablow L, Salazar A. The penicillin focus. I. Distribution of potential at the cortical surface. Electroencephalogr Clin Neurophysiol 1977;42(4):480–492

17. Ebersole J, Chatt A. The laminar susceptibility of cat visual cortex to penicillin induced epileptogenesis. Neurology 1980;30:355

18. Telfeian AE, Connors BW. Layer-specific pathways for the horizontal propagation of epileptiform discharges in neocortex. Epilepsia 1998;39(7):700–708

19. Harvey AS, Cross JH, Shinnar S, Mathern BW; ILAE Pediatric Epilepsy Surgery Survey Taskforce. Defining the spectrum of international practice in pediatric epilepsy surgery patients. Epilepsia 2008;49(1):146–155

20. Blount JP, Langburt W, Otsubo H, et al. Multiple subpial transections in the treatment of pediatric epilepsy. J Neurosurg 2004;100(2, suppl Pediatrics):118–124

21. Benifla M, Otsubo H, Ochi A, Snead OC III, Rutka JT. Multiple subpial transections in pediatric epilepsy: indications and outcomes. Childs Nerv Syst 2006;22(8):992–998

22. Guenot M. [Surgical treatment of epilepsy: outcome of various surgical procedures in adults and children]. Rev Neurol (Paris) 2004;160(spec no 1):5S241–50

23. Shimizu H, Maehara T. Neuronal disconnection for the surgical treatment of pediatric epilepsy. Epilepsia 2000;41(suppl 9):28–30

24. Schramm J, Aliashkevich AF, Grunwald T. Multiple subpial transections: outcome and complications in 20 patients who did not undergo resection. J Neurosurg 2002;97(1):39–47

25. Smith MC. Multiple subpial transection in patients with extratemporal epilepsy. Epilepsia 1998;39(suppl 4):S81–S89

26. Liu Z, Zhao Q, Li S, Tian Z, Cui Y, Feng H. Multiple subpial transection for treatment of intractable epilepsy. Chin Med J (Engl) 1995;108(7):539–541

27. Whisler WW. Multiple subpial transection. Tech Neurosurg 1995;1:40–44

28. Téllez-Zenteno JF, Dhar R, Wiebe S. Long-term seizure outcomes following epilepsy surgery: a systematic review and meta-analysis. Brain 2005;128(pt 5):1188–1198

29. Spencer SS, Schramm J, Wyler A, et al. Multiple subpial transection for intractable partial epilepsy: an international meta-analysis. Epilepsia 2002;43(2):141–145

30. Mulligan LP, Spencer DD, Spencer SS. Multiple subpial transections: the Yale experience. Epilepsia 2001;42(2):226–229

31. Pacia SV, et al. Multiple subpial transections for intractable partial seizure: seizures outcome. J Epilepsy 1997;10:86–91

32. Liu Z, Zhao Q, Li S, Tian Z, Cui Y, Feng H. Multiple subpial transection for treatment of intractable epilepsy. Chin Med J (Engl) 1995;108(7):539–541

33. Rougier A, Sundstrom L, Claverie B, et al. Multiple subpial transection: report of 7 cases. Epilepsy Res 1996;24(1):57–63

34. Sawhney IMS, Robertson IJ, Polkey CE, Binnie CD, Elwes RD. Multiple subpial transection: a review of 21 cases. J Neurol Neurosurg Psychiatry 1995;58(3):344–349

35. Castillo EM, Butler IJ, Baumgartner JE, Passaro A, Papanicolaou AC. When epilepsy interferes with word comprehension: findings in Landau-Kleffner syndrome. J Child Neurol 2008;23(1):97–101

36. Buelow JM, Aydelott P, Pierz DM, Heck B. Multiple subpial transection for Landau-Kleffner syndrome. AORN J 1996;63(4):727–729, 732–735, 737–739, quiz 741–744

37. Neville BG, Harkness WF, Cross JH, et al. Surgical treatment of severe autistic regression in childhood epilepsy. Pediatr Neurol 1997;16(2):137–140

38. Nass R, Gross A, Wisoff J, Devinsky O. Outcome of multiple subpial transections for autistic epileptiform regression. Pediatr Neurol 1999;21(1):464–470

39. Irwin K, Birch V, Lees J, et al. Multiple subpial transection in Landau-Kleffner syndrome. Dev Med Child Neurol 2001;43(4):248–252

40. Harkness W. How to select the best surgical procedure for children with epilepsy. In: Epilepsy Surgery. Luders H, ed. Philadelphia, PA: Lippincott Williams & Wilkins; 2001:767–780

41. Grote CL, Van Slyke P, Hoeppner JA. Language outcome following multiple subpial transection for Landau-Kleffner syndrome. Brain 1999;122(pt 3):561–566

42. Otsubo H, Chitoku S, Ochi A, et al. Malignant rolandic-sylvian epilepsy in children: diagnosis, treatment, and outcomes. Neurology 2001;57(4):590–596

43. Molyneux PD, Barker RA, Thom M, van Paesschen W, Harkness WF, Duncan JS. Successful treatment of intractable epilepsia partialis continua with multiple subpial transections. J Neurol Neurosurg Psychiatry 1998;65(1):137–138

44. Nakken KO, Eriksson AS, Kostov H, et al. [Epilepsia partialis continua (Kojevnikov's syndrome)]. Tidsskr Nor Laegeforen 2005;125(6): 746–749

45. Otsubo H, Oishi M, Snead OCI. Magnetoencephalography. In: Epilepsy Surgery: Principles and Controversies Neurological Disease and Therapy. Miller J, Silbergeld D, eds. New York, NY: Mercel Decker Inc; 2007:752–767

46. Morrell F, Hanbery JW. A new surgical technique for the treatment of focal cortical epilepsy. Electroencephalogr Clin Neurophysiol 1969;26(1):120

47. Morrell F, Whisler WW, Bleck TP. Multiple subpial transection: a new approach to the surgical treatment of focal epilepsy. J Neurosurg 1989;70(2):231–239

48. Wyler AR. Multiple subpial transections in neocortical epilepsy: Part II. Adv Neurol 2000;84:635–642

49. Wennberg R, Quesney LF, Lozano A, Olivier A, Rasmussen T. Role of electrocorticography at surgery for lesion-related frontal lobe epilepsy. Can J Neurol Sci 1999;26(1):33–39

50. Hufnagel A, Zentner J, Fernandez G, Wolf HK, Schramm J, Elger CE. Multiple subpial transection for control of epileptic seizures: effectiveness and safety. Epilepsia 1997;38(6):678–688

51. Patil AA, Andrews R, Torkelson R. Isolation of dominant seizure foci by multiple subpial transections. Stereotact Funct Neurosurg 1997;69(1–4 pt 2):210–215

52. Shimizu H, Suzuki I, Ishijima B, Karasawa S, Sakuma T. Multiple subpial transection (MST) for the control of seizures that originated in unresectable cortical foci. Jpn J Psychiatry Neurol 1991;45(2): 354–356

53. Wyler A. Multiple subpial transections: a review and arguments for use. In: Epilepsy Surgery. Miller J, Silbergeld D, eds. New York, NY: Taylor & Francis Group, LLC; 2006:524–529

54. Patil AA, Andrews RV, Torkelson R. Surgical treatment of intractable seizures with multilobar or bihemispheric seizure foci (MLBHSF). Surg Neurol 1997;47(1):72–77, discussion 77–78

55. Orbach D, Romanelli P, Devinsky O, Doyle W. Late seizure recurrence after multiple subpial transections. Epilepsia 2001;42(10): 1316–1319

56. Engel J, et al. Outcome with respect to epileptic seizures. In: Surgical Treatment of the Epilepsies. Engel J Jr, ed. New York, NY: Raven Press; 1993:609–621

57. Tovar-Spinoza ZS, Rutka JT. Multiple subpial transections. In: Textbook of Stereotactic Neurosurgery. Lozano A, Gildenberg P, Tasker R, eds. (2nd ed). Berlin Heidelberg: Springer; 2009:2715–2727

32 Hippocampal Transection
Hiroyuki Shimizu

Hippocampal transection was first reported in 2006 as a new surgical treatment for temporal lobe epilepsy.[1] Using this method, postoperative verbal memory can be preserved even in patients with left mesial temporal lobe epilepsy without hippocampal atrophy. Verbal memory disturbances after left temporal lobectomy can be observed in pediatric patients as well as in adults.[2–4] We applied this new surgical technique to pediatric patients and obtained good seizure outcome and preservation of verbal function. The overall surgical technique and surgical outcomes, including adult and pediatric patients, are presented, and a representative pediatric case is illustrated.

■ Surgical Rationale and Method

Exposure of the Hippocampus

The hippocampal pathway, closely related with verbal memory, originates in the inferior temporal association cortex and projects directly onto CA1 pyramidal neurons, after running through the perirhinal cortex.[5] Therefore, access to the inferior horn via the basal temporal lobe area can compromise this neuronal connection. Zola-Morgan et al demonstrated that bilateral temporal stem can be transected without causing memory disturbance in monkeys, using a task known to be sensitive to human amnesia.[6]

Based on the previously mentioned neurofunctional data, we place a small corticotomy within 4.5 cm from the temporal tip. After aspirating the gray matter of the superior temporal gyrus along the sylvian fissure, the temporal stem is exposed. If the temporal stem is aspirated just beneath the gray matter of the insula, the temporal horn can be easily opened (**Fig. 32.1A**). The anterolateral part of the ventricle is suctioned as widely as possible and the hippocampal head and amygdala are fully exposed.

Electrocorticography over the Hippocampus and Amygdala

Before starting surgical procedures, specially designed electrodes are placed over the hippocampus and amygdala. Elec-

trocorticography (ECoG) is recorded in many points over the hippocampus. For this purpose, two small strip electrodes with four contacts for exploring the hippocampal body and tail and two square electrodes with four contacts for recording in the hippocampal head and amygdala are applied. Therefore, ECoG is recorded at 12 contacts all over the hippocampus and the amygdala (**Figs. 32.1B,C**).

Hippocampal Transection

The rationale of hippocampal transection is based on the theory of multiple subpial transection (MST) developed by Morrell et al.[7] Because the pyramidal cell layer of the hippocampus is within 2 mm from the surface,[5] we devised a ring transector 2 mm in diameter (**Fig. 32.2A**). Because the alveus covering the pyramidal layer is a very firm, fibrous tissue, the alveus is sharply cut with microscissors. A 2-mm ring transector is inserted through this slit and the pyramidal layer is transected 4 mm apart using the same distance used for MST. At the bilateral corners of the CA4 portion and near the subiculum, the pyramidal layer becomes deeper and a 4-mm ring transector is used for transection. Toward the posterior portion of the hippocampus, the width of the hippocampus becomes narrower and an oval-formed transector with a 4-mm long diameter is applied for transection of the bilateral corners (**Figs. 32.2B**).

The transection areas of the pyramidal cell layer are determined based on the results of intraoperative ECoG. After areas with epileptic discharges are transected, ECoG is repeated to detect residual epileptic activity. If residual spikes are found, transection is also performed until prominent spike areas completely disappear (**Fig. 32.2C**).

■ Seizure Outcome

Between January 2001 and February 2008, we performed hippocampal transection in 45 patients, left side in 23 and right side in 22. The patients consisted of 22 men and 23 women. Patient ages ranged from 2 to 42 years, with a mean of 25 years old. In all patients, preoperative MRI did not demonstrate any sign of atrophy or asymmetry of the hippocampus (**Fig. 32.3**). In six patients, organic lesions were

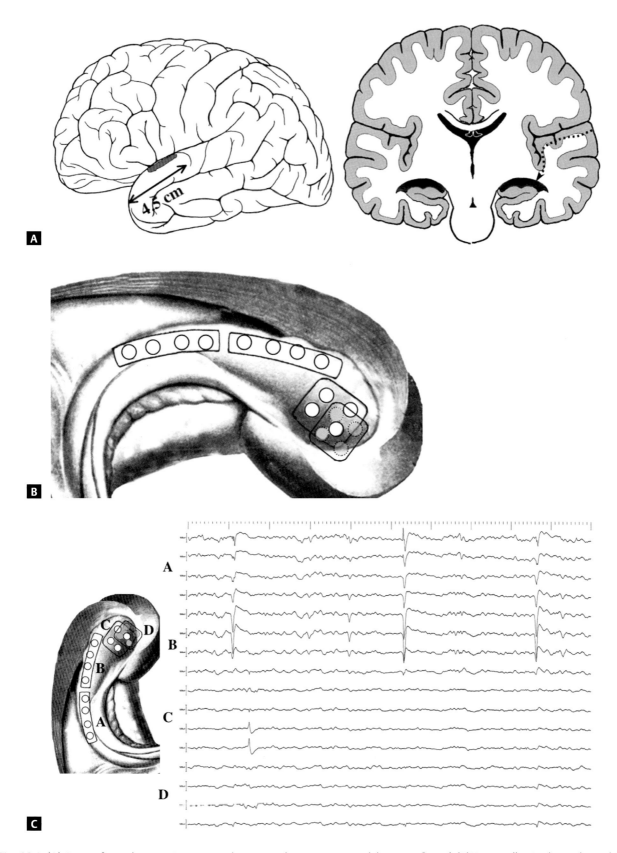

Fig. 32.1 **(A)** Access from the superior temporal gyrus to the temporal horn is shown. First a small corticotomy is made on the surface of the superior temporal gyrus within 4.5 cm from the tip. Along the sylvian fissure (*dotted line*), the gray matter of the superior temporal gyrus is aspirated to reach the temporal stem. By sectioning the temporal stem, the temporal horn is opened, and the hippocampus and amygdala are confirmed. **(B)** Two small strip electrodes with four contacts and two square plate electrodes with four contacts are arrayed over the hippocampus and the amygdala to record electrocorticography (ECoG). **(C)** Intraoperative ECoG demonstrated distribution of epileptic discharges.

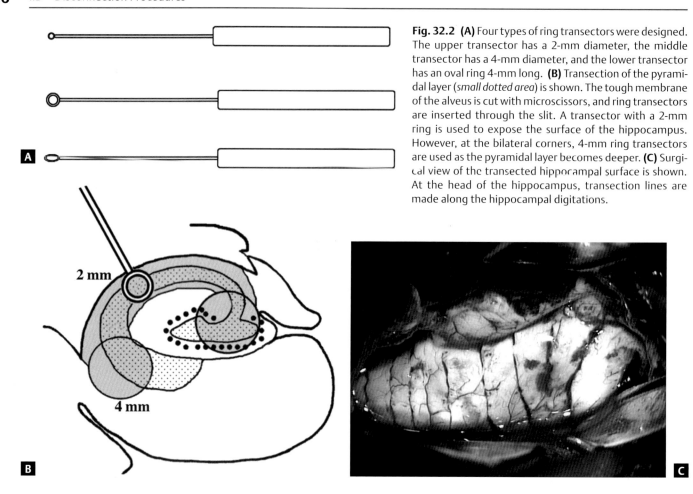

Fig. 32.2 (A) Four types of ring transectors were designed. The upper transector has a 2-mm diameter, the middle transector has a 4-mm diameter, and the lower transector has an oval ring 4-mm long. **(B)** Transection of the pyramidal layer (*small dotted area*) is shown. The tough membrane of the alveus is cut with microscissors, and ring transectors are inserted through the slit. A transector with a 2-mm ring is used to expose the surface of the hippocampus. However, at the bilateral corners, 4-mm ring transectors are used as the pyramidal layer becomes deeper. **(C)** Surgical view of the transected hippocampal surface is shown. At the head of the hippocampus, transection lines are made along the hippocampal digitations.

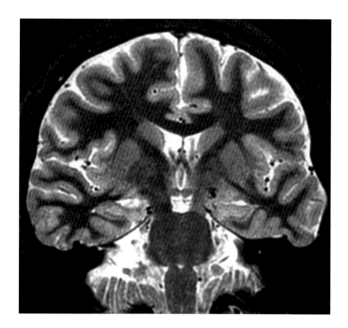

Fig. 32.3 In our series of hippocampal transection, preoperative magnetic resonance imaging did not show any hippocampal atrophy or asymmetry in any of the patients.

confirmed in front of the hippocampus. In 12 cases, intracranial subdural electrodes were inserted, and laterality of the mesial temporal focus was determined. In the remaining patients, laterality was diagnosed based on scalp electroencephalography (EEG) with sphenoidal lead, single photon emission computed tomography (SPECT), and neuropsychometry data.

Within 2 weeks after surgery, postoperative magnetic resonance imaging (MRI) was examined. Compared with preoperative MRIs, a tract along the sylvian fissure aspirating the gray matter of the superior temporal gyrus was confirmed. However, there was no deformity of the hippocampus after hippocampal transection (**Fig. 32.4**). In 36 patients who were followed for more than 1 year, 28 (78%) patients were categorized in Engel Class I, 4 (11%) patients were categorized in Class II, 3 patients (8%) were categorized in Class III, and 1 patient (3%) was categorized in Class 4.

■ Postoperative Verbal Memory

The auditory verbal learning test (AVLT) is known as a very sensitive test for evaluating short-term verbal memory.[8]

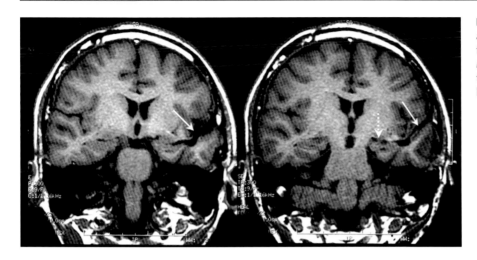

Fig. 32.4 On magnetic resonance imaging after hippocampal transection, the tract from the surface to the inferior horn (*arrows*) could be demonstrated. However, there was no deformity of the transected hippocampus (*dotted arrow*).

AVLT was used as an objective index for evaluation of pre- and postoperative hippocampal function. In cases of left hippocampal transection, AVLT scores showed a transient decrease immediately after surgery. However, within 6 months, decreased scores generally recovered to preoperative levels. Approximately 6 months after surgery, transected hippocampus usually showed slight atrophy. However, memory function recovered despite this atrophy and there was no decline of memory thereafter. In some cases, there was no worsening of AVLT even immediately after surgery. This may be because of the extent of surgical procedures added to hippocampal transection. If surgical procedures were confined to hippocampal transection only, postoperative AVLT scores were generally kept at preoperative levels. However, when other procedures, such as MST of the lateral temporal cortex or resection of the temporal basal area, were performed in addition to hippocampal transection, there was a greater tendency toward immediate decline of AVLT scores and later recovery.

■ Pediatric Data and Case Report

We performed hippocampal transection in eight pediatric patients (18 years or less). Subjects consisted of six boys and two girls, with ages ranging from 2 to 17 years (mean age = 10 years). Postoperative follow-up ranged from 1.7 to 5.8 years. All patients became seizure free except for one patient who demonstrated rare residual seizures. Because AVLT examination was difficult to perform in most of the children, their

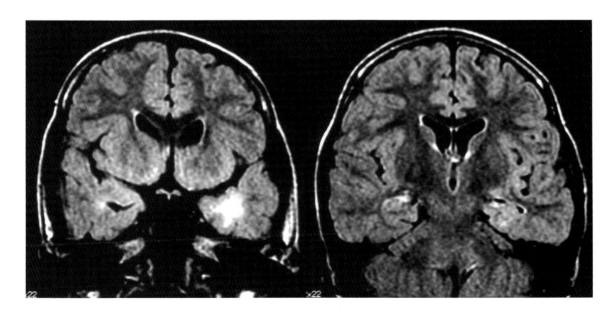

Fig. 32.5 Preoperative magnetic resonance imaging showing a dysplastic lesion in the left temporal pole (*left*). However, there was no atrophy of the hippocampus on the same side (*right*).

verbal memory function was evaluated by developmental quotient. Most patients showed various degrees of improvement in the speech–social category.

■ Case Study

The representative case study is of a 5-year-old boy with no history contributory to the present illness. His development had been normal until he had his first seizure at the age of 2 years and 11 months. Thereafter, habitual seizures started with blank staring, followed by meaningless manual movements. Seizures usually continued for approximately 1 minute. When the patient was standing, he often collapsed gradually after the start of seizures. Seizures mainly occurred in the morning 5 to 10 times every day. He had speech delay, and he often showed aggressive behaviors.

He was referred to our clinic to evaluate the possibility of surgical treatment. Neurological examination did not detect any abnormality. Scalp EEG showed high-amplitude multiple spikes in the left temporal area. MRI showed abnormal intensity in the left temporal pole, suggestive of cortical tu-

ber or other type of dysgenesis. There was no asymmetry of the hippocampus (**Fig. 32.5**). SPECT demonstrated low perfusion in the left temporal area. According to neuropsychological examination, he showed developmental delay with a developmental quotient of 49 for both speech–social and cognition–adaptation ability.

Based on the previously mentioned data, left temporal lobe epilepsy was diagnosed. On September 2, 2005, he underwent left temporal lobe surgery. According to intraoperative ECoG, epileptic areas were treated with preservation of brain functions. The left hippocampus was transected, and the temporal tip with an temporal horn area on MRI was resected in front of the inferior ventricle. MST was applied extensively over the lateral temporal cortex. The postoperative course was uneventful. The histopathology of the resected temporal pole showed cortical dysplasia.

Since surgery, he has been completely seizure free for more than 2 years. He is now able to concentrate more in class, and his mental state has become calmer and more stable. His neuropsychological evaluation 2 years after surgery showed development in speech ability with a developmental quotient of 58 compared with a preoperative score of 49.

References

1. Shimizu H, Kawai K, Sunaga S, Sugano H, Yamada T. Hippocampal transection for treatment of left temporal lobe epilepsy with preservation of verbal memory. J Clin Neurosci 2006;13(3):322–328
2. Szabó CA, Wyllie E, Stanford LD, et al. Neuropsychological effect of temporal lobe resection in preadolescent children with epilepsy. Epilepsia 1998;39(8):814–819
3. Dlugos DJ, Moss EM, Duhaime AC, Brooks-Kayal AR. Language-related cognitive declines after left temporal lobectomy in children. Pediatr Neurol 1999;21(1):444–449
4. Gleissner U, Sassen R, Lendt M, Clusmann H, Elger CE, Helmstaedter C. Pre- and postoperative verbal memory in pediatric patients with temporal lobe epilepsy. Epilepsy Res 2002;51(3):287–296
5. Duvernoy H. The Human Hippocampus. Berlin, Germany: Springer; 1998;26–37
6. Zola-Morgan S, Squire LR, Mishkin M. The neuroanatomy of amnesia: amygdala-hippocampus versus temporal stem. Science 1982;218(4579):1337–1339
7. Morrell F, Whisler WW, Bleck TP. Multiple subpial transection: a new approach to the surgical treatment of focal epilepsy. J Neurosurg 1989;70(2):231–239
8. Rosenberg SJ, Ryan JJ, Prifitera A. Rey Auditory-Verbal Learning Test performance of patients with and without memory impairment. J Clin Psychol 1984;40(3):785–787

33 Vagus Nerve Stimulation

David D. Limbrick Jr. and Matthew D. Smyth

Implantable devices for chronic vagal nervous stimulation (VNS) have been used since 1988 as an adjunct in the treatment of medically refractory epilepsy.[1] Over the intervening 20 years, a substantial body of literature, including several randomized, controlled trials[2,3] has confirmed the usefulness of VNS in refractory epilepsy. In this chapter, we review the historical and scientific basis of VNS and its application in pediatric epilepsy and other neurological disorders.

■ History of VNS

The first description of VNS for seizure control was by James Corning in 1884.[4] Based on the hypothesis that cerebral hyperemia produced seizures, Corning devised an "electrocompressor" combined with a transcutaneous vagal nerve stimulator with mechanical carotid compression. Despite simultaneously decreasing cardiac output and occluding carotid flow, Corning's results were inconsistent, and his techniques were abandoned.

In the 1930s, Bailey and Bremer first demonstrated that stimulation of the vagal nerve affected electroencephalography (EEG) patterns in cats.[5] Several subsequent reports confirmed that manipulation of the vagus by ligation[6] or stimulation[7–11] decreased EEG spikes in various animal models of seizures. Based largely on these studies, safety and efficacy studies were conducted in primates[12] before proceeding with implanting the first VNS devices in human subjects.[1,13]

■ Anatomy and Physiology of Vagal Nerve Stimulation

Approximately 80% of the vagus is composed of afferent fibers,[14] including myelinated A and B fibers and unmyelinated C fibers. General sensory afferents from the pharynx and larynx, external auditory apparatus, and posterior fossa meninges travel through the vagus en route to the spinal trigeminal tract and nucleus. Perhaps more relevant to VNS physiology, visceral sensory fibers ascending through the vagus project diffusely throughout the central nervous system.[15] Although

many of these fibers synapse in the nucleus of the tractus solitarius, others travel directly to their target in a monosynaptic pathway. Several of the targets of these projections, which include the dorsal raphe, locus ceruleus, nucleus ambiguus, cerebellum, parabrachial nucleus, hypothalamus, amygdala, thalamus, hippocampus, and insular cortex, are involved in pathways for rhythmic excitability or have the potential for epileptogenicity themselves.[16,17] Indeed, recent work using positron emission tomography, single photon emission computed tomography, and functional magnetic resonance imaging to evaluate VNS-related changes in the brain showed variable alterations in frontal, parietal, and temporal activity but consistent, widespread limbic involvement (reviewed in Barnes et al[18]), including ipsilateral brainstem, cingulate, amygdala, and hippocampus, as well as the contralateral thalamus and cingulate.[18] Further, in a single patient, high-frequency VNS produced a measurable decrease in hippocampal sharp waves.[19] Preliminary animal studies have confirmed the inhibitory effect of VNS on hippocampal activity but have not yet been published.[20]

Although the precise mechanism of seizure suppression by VNS remains to be elucidated, progress has been made in identifying central effects of peripheral VNS. VNS has been shown to increase neuronal discharges from the locus ceruleus[21] and dorsal raphe nucleus,[22] and chemically induced lesions of the locus ceruleus attenuate VNS-induced seizure suppression.[23] Cross-modulatory pathways exist between the nucleus of the tractus solitarius, the locus ceruleus, and the dorsal raphe nucleus,[24] implicating ascending transmitter pathways in the action of VNS. Recent microdialysis experiments have demonstrated that VNS increases norepinephrine levels in the amygdala,[25] hippocampus, and cerebral cortex.[26] Indeed, the data showing that locus ceruleus neurons are the primary source of norepinephrine to the hippocampus[27] and the cortex,[28] strongly implicates the role of this nucleus in the mechanism of action of the VNS.

The effect of VNS on cerebrospinal fluid concentrations of amino acid neurotransmitters is less clear. γ-aminobutyric acid (GABA) has been shown to increase in all patients with VNS implanted for seizure control, including patients who did not have a clinical response to the VNS.[29] The excitatory amino acid aspartate was noted to decrease in these patients, consistent with an overall inhibitory condition. The serotonin metabolite 5-HIAA also was elevated. In patients who underwent VNS placement for depression, the results were quite different, with no observed change in GABA, 5-HIAA, or norepinephrine.[30] Whether the differences in these studies are due to indication for VNS (epilepsy or depression), anticonvulsant or antidepressant medications, or experimental technique or aberration is unknown. Further investigation will be required to parse out these differences.

Acute and long-term alterations in genetic expression have been identified in animal models of VNS. Cunningham et al (2008) reported increased c-Fos expression acutely after initiation of VNS in the nucleus of the tractus solitarius, hypothalamus, stria terminalis, and locus ceruleus. Both expression of c-Fos and the long-term neuronal activation biomarker delta-FosB were observed in the cingulate cortex and dorsal raphe nucleus with chronic VNS only.[31] Moreover, long-term changes in GABA(A) receptor density have been found in patients with chronically implanted VNS compared with matched control subjects.[32]

■ Evidence for VNS in Epilepsy

After the initial case series describing the use of VNS in humans with intractable partial seizures[1] and several other studies reporting favorable outcomes,[13,33-35] the Vagus Nerve Stimulation Study Group formed to investigate the safety and efficacy of VNS. In conjunction with Cyberonics, Inc., three open-label and two double-blind randomized controlled trials were conducted. The first trial (EO3) included 114 patients older than 12 years of age with at least six seizures per month while on antiepileptic drugs.[36] Subjects were randomized to receive low-stimulation (30-second VNS every 90 minutes; 1 Hz; 130 µs; ≤ 3.5 mA) or high-stimulation (30 second VNS every 5 minutes; 30 Hz; 500 µs; up to 3.5 mA) VNS. After 14 weeks of VNS, the high-stimulation group exhibited a 30.9% reduction in seizure frequency compared with an 11.3% reduction in the low-stimulation group, a statistically significant difference.

The second major trial (EO5) enrolled 199 patients older than 12 years with intractable partial-onset seizures.[3] Patients were again randomized to low- or high-stimulation for 3 months and evaluated for seizure reduction and device safety. The high-stimulation group exhibited a 28% reduction in seizure frequency versus a 15% decrease in the low-stimulation group. In addition, the high-stimulation group demonstrated improved global evaluation scores, but dysphonia and dyspnea also were more common in this group.

In 1999, long-term efficacy and safety results from the five Vagus Nerve Stimulation Study Group clinical trials (EO1-EO5)[2,3,36-39] were reported in a meta-analysis.[40] A total of 454 patients were followed for up to 3 years using one of three methods for data analysis (last visit carried forward method, constant cohort method, or declining N method). Although only 1 to 2% of patients become seizure free, many derived long-term benefit from VNS. Median reduction of seizure frequency was 35% at 1 year after VNS initiation, 44.3% at 2 years, and 44.1% at 3 years. More than 50% seizure reduction was seen in 23% at 3 months, 37% of patients at 1 year, 43% at 2 years, and 43% at 3 years after VNS initiation. Adverse effects, including hoarseness, decreased over the follow-up period. Additional studies have reported similar results in terms of safety and efficacy of VNS over even longer durations, further confirming the long-term benefits of VNS in select patients.[41,42]

The U.S. Food and Drug Administration (FDA) approved VNS (Cyberonics, Inc., Houston, TX, USA) in 1997 as an adjunctive therapy for use in medically refractory epilepsy patients older than 12 years with partial-onset seizures. FDA approval for VNS therapy for the indication of depression came in 2001.

■ VNS in Pediatric Patients

As noted previously, the studies conducted by the Vagus Nerve Stimulation Study Group enrolled only patients at least 12 years of age. Based on preliminary results from a small series of children in which VNS was placed for medically and surgically refractory seizures,[43] the Pediatric VNS Group performed a compassionate use prospective open safety study (EO4).[44] A total of 60 pediatric patients (younger than 18 years) with various seizure types were included in EO4, with 16 patients younger than 12 years old. The median reduction in seizure frequency was 23, 42, 34, and 42% at 3, 6, 12, and 18 months, respectively. Two years later, a multi-institutional, retrospective study of 95 pediatric VNS patients reported favorable results for safety and efficacy, with a mean seizure reduction of 36% at 3 months and 45% at 6 months.[45]

Several reports have now been published that consistently demonstrate the utility of VNS in the pediatric epilepsy population in terms of seizure control[46-48] and overall quality of life.[49-54] The majority of these studies reported results for all seizure types (absence, atonic, simple partial, complex partial, generalized tonic–clonic, Lennox-Gastaut syndrome) and were not restricted to partial-onset seizures as had been the Vagus Nerve Stimulation Study Group studies. One group reported seizure reduction rates for atonic (80%), absence (65%), complex partial (48%), and generalized tonic–clonic (45%) seizures.[49]

Although the previously mentioned data are compelling, there have been no prospective, randomized, controlled trials to rigorously evaluate VNS in children. Currently, FDA approval for VNS in the pediatric epilepsy population is limited to adolescents older than 12 years of age with medically refractory partial-onset seizures. Nonetheless, because many children are refractory to anticonvulsants and are not candidates for resective neurosurgical procedures, VNS remains an important adjunctive therapeutic option and is frequently used in an "off-label" capacity.

Relatively little data exist regarding the safety and efficacy of VNS in the very young. Although several studies have enrolled patients younger than 2 years of age as part of a larger series, only one report has evaluated children of this age exclusively. Blount et al described their experience with VNS in six children with a mean age of 20.5 months.[55] Of the six patients, five (83%) had a significant decrease in seizure frequency, and there was no treatment-related morbidity. Although preliminary, these data suggest that VNS may be a viable treatment option in very young children with refractory, catastrophic epilepsy.

■ Pediatric VNS and Specific Seizure Types

Several case series have been published providing early insight into the efficacy of VNS in specific epilepsy types. A multicenter retrospective study of 10 patients with tuberous sclerosis and refractory epilepsy fared particularly well, with 9 of 10 patients experiencing at least 50% reduction in seizure frequency, and half of the patients had at least 90% reduction.[56] In a series of six patients with hypothalamic hamartomas, three patients had significant reduction in seizure frequency (25% to more than 90% reduction).[57] Interestingly, four of four patients in this series with autism demonstrated improvements in autistic behaviors.[57]

The efficacy of VNS in Lennox-Gastaut syndrome has been evaluated by several studies. One multicenter retrospective investigation included 50 patients, 36% of whom had tried the ketogenic diet and 10% of whom had previously had a corpus callosotomy.[58] Median seizure reduction was 58% at both 3 and 6 months after VNS. Other series have shown similar encouraging results in this difficult patient population, with 25 to 90% seizure reduction.[52,59,60] In these patients, response to VNS was found to be best in those with the highest frequency of background EEG activity.[46] It should be noted that one group did report disappointing results for Lennox-Gastaut syndrome.[61]

Two case reports have been published regarding the use of VNS in the setting of status epilepticus. One reported the implementation of VNS in a young adult with status epilepticus elicited by anticonvulsant withdrawal.[62] The second case was a 13-year-old boy with status epilepticus in the setting of a long-standing history of epilepsy. In both cases, the status epilepticus was terminated by VNS, and in the second case, available follow-up demonstrated that the patient experienced significant seizure reduction in long-term.[63]

■ Operative Technique for VNS Placement

Surgical implantation of VNS is performed under general anesthesia and generally requires 1 to 2 hours of surgical time. At our institution, the operation is performed as an outpatient procedure, although other facilities admit patients overnight for observation. Unless there are special considerations, the VNS is placed on the left side. The reason for choosing the left side is based on the asymmetrical vagal innervation of the heart. Whereas the right vagus is responsible for innervation of the sinoatrial node, the left vagus innervates the cardiac atrioventricular node.[64] Stimulation of the left vagus is thus less likely to actively modulate heart rate.

The patient is positioned supine with his or her neck in a neutral position. A gel roll is placed transversely under the shoulders to gently extend the neck. The operating room table is turned 90 degrees clockwise, allowing the surgeon access to the left side of the neck and chest. Before skin incision, 25 mg/kg intravenous cefazolin is administered, and the skin is prepared with antiseptic solution. The surgery begins with a transverse 2 to 3 cm incision placed, when possible, in a natural skin fold located along the mid portion of the sternocleidomastoid muscle (SCM; **Fig. 33.1A**). The incision itself is located one third lateral and two thirds medial to the medial border of the SCM and is similar to that used in an anterior cervical discectomy. The platysma is then divided transversely and undermined superiorly and inferiorly to assist with exposure and retraction. The dissection is carried down through the cervical fascia and along the medial border of the SCM. The SCM is then retracted laterally, and the carotid pulse is used to locate the carotid sheath. The sheath is then opened sharply and the vagus nerve is located with the neurovascular bundle. The position of the vagus varies considerably with respect to the carotid artery and internal jugular vein, but generally the nerve is located posteriorly within the sheath and medial to the jugular. A vessel loop is then passed underneath to assist with mobilization of the nerve and subsequent placement of the VNS electrodes (**Fig. 33.1B**). Careful dissection and isolation at least 3 to 4 cm of nerve provides sufficient room for wrapping the two electrodes and anchoring coil.

Once the cervical dissection is complete, a subcutaneous pocket is made in the chest to accommodate the VNS pulse generator. Although the location for this pocket varies with surgeon preference, we use an incision along the lateral border of the pectoralis major muscle to create a subcutaneous pocket directly over the pectoralis fascia in the infraclavicular fossa (**Fig. 33.1A**). The electrodes are then tunneled from the superior limit of the pocket over the clavicle to the cervical incision (**Fig. 33.1C** and **33.2A**).

With care to minimize manipulation of the vagus, the helical electrodes are applied to the nerve by grasping the

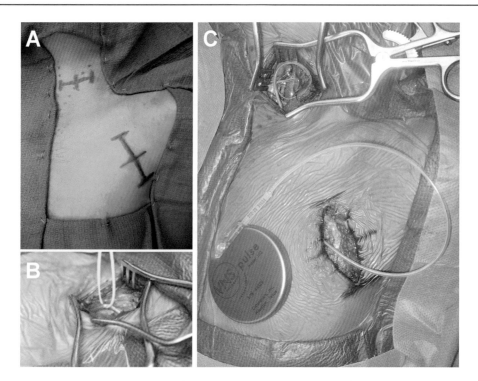

Fig. 33.1 Typical locations for the cervical **(A)** and chest **(B)** incisions used for implantation of a left-sided vagus nerve stimulator. The cervical incision is oriented transversely and, when possible, is made within a natural skin fold located along the midportion of the sternocleidomastoid muscle. To create a subcutaneous pocket for the vagus nerve stimulation pulse generator, an incision is made along the lateral border of the pectoralis major muscle. The electrodes are then tunneled from the superior limit of the pocket over the clavicle to the cervical incision **(C)**.

suture ends of each coil to open the configuration (**Figs. 33.1C, 33.2B,** and **33.2C**). Once the coil has been unfurled, the electrode is wrapped around the nerve. This application process is performed first for the anchoring coil, then the positive electrode, and lastly the negative electrode (**Fig. 33.2C**). The vagus, with electrodes applied, is then replaced as close as possible to its original anatomical position within the carotid sheath with care to minimize tension on the leads. A strain-relief loop is then fashioned (**Fig. 33.1C** and **33.2A**) and sutured with nonabsorbable material to the SCM muscle.

The connector pins located at the distal end of the VNS lead are then inserted into the pulse generator and secured with the manufacturer's hexagonal torque wrench (**Fig. 33.2D**). The pulse generator is then inserted into the subcutaneous pocket. Any excess length of the lead is coiled directly on the pectoralis fascia deep to the pulse generator to prevent hardware injury if revision surgery is required. Finally, a silk suture is used to secure the pulse generator within its pocket. Both incisions are then irrigated with copious antibiotic-containing saline and closed in layers with absorbable suture and liquid skin adhesive.

■ Special Considerations in VNS Surgery

As noted previously, because of asymmetric cardiac innervation by the vagus,[64] the left side is preferred for placement of the VNS. In fact, the VNS manufacturer Cyberonics cautions that "the safety and efficacy . . . have not been established for stimulation of the right vagus nerve."[65] However, clinical scenarios exist in which placement of the VNS on the right side may be considered. VNS hardware infections occur in approximately 3 to 6% of cases and generally require removal of the hardware.[66,67] In those patients who experience a significant reduction in seizure frequency but require VNS hardware explantation because of infection, placement of a right-sided VNS may be considered.[68] A small series of right-sided VNS implantations performed under these conditions showed efficacy in reducing seizure frequency with no cardiac complications.[68] Two of the three patients did experience respiratory side effects with reactive airway disease.[68]

Variations in the surgical technique for VNS implantation have been described to streamline the procedure or to avert predictable surgical complications. Cognitively impaired

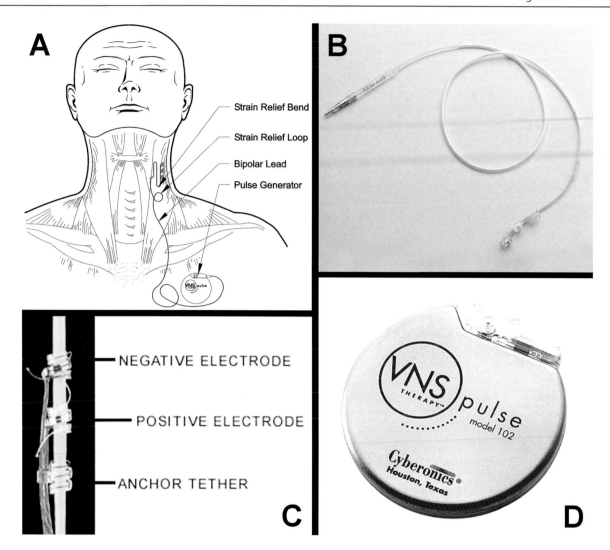

Fig. 33.2 Implanted device hardware required for vagus nerve stimulation (VNS). **(A)** Cartoon depicting the configuration of the implanted VNS hardware. In the device construct shown, the lead extends from the electrode attachment on the left vagus, through a strain-relief loop, to the pulse generator in an infraclavicular subcutaneous pocket. **(B)** The VNS lead (VNS Therapy Model 302; Cyberonics, Inc., Houston, TX, USA), with proximal helical electrodes and anchoring coil and a distal lead connector pin. **(C)** Close-up view of anchoring coil and positive and negative helical electrodes with their respective positions along the vagus nerve. **(D)** VNS pulse generator (VNS Therapy Model 102; Cyberonics, Inc., Houston, TX, USA). (Images courtesy of Cyberonics, Inc., Houston, TX, USA. Used with permission.)

children undergoing VNS placement frequently tamper with their surgical wounds, increasing the risk of wound infection. To address this concern, alternative locations for the position of the pulse generator, including subpectoral[69] or interscapular[70] placement, have been reported. In addition, an alternative technique using a single, low-cervical, transverse incision for implantation of both the vagal nerve electrodes and the pulse generator obviates the need for a second incision or the tunneling of electrodes.[71]

In some cases of revision VNS surgery, particularly in caring for patients transferred from other facilities, the components of the VNS system may not be known. In such cases, routine x-rays of the chest and neck may be helpful not only in detecting clear fractures or disconnections but also in determining the existing VNS hardware and thus which components will be needed for the revision. For example, a chest x-ray will show the number of lead connector pins necessary for interfacing with the pulse generator. VNS Therapy Models 101 and 102R both accommodate two lead connector pins, whereas Model 102 accepts a single lead connector pin input only.

■ Surgical Complications of VNS

Complications of VNS include those related to the surgery and hardware implantation and those resulting from the stimulation itself. Stimulation-related complications will be covered in a subsequent section. In children, and especially in very young children, one might expect that complication rates would be higher than that in the general adult VNS patient population. The tendency of mentally delayed children to obsessively tamper with their wounds and the relatively large size of the pulse generator in relation the child's body are two obvious possible causes for wound infection, erosion of hardware through the skin, or hardware failure.[70]

Smyth et al reported on a series of 74 patients younger than 18 years who were followed for a minimum of 1 year (mean 2.2 years).[66] Seven patients (9.4%) ultimately required explantation of the hardware, three (3.5%) for deep wound infections and four (5.4%) for device intolerance or lack of benefit. Three patients had superficial wound infections that did not require removal of the hardware. Two patients required hardware revision for lead fracture, one of which was believed to be caused by the child repeatedly rotating the pulse generator within the infraclavicular pocket.

Similar to the previously mentioned reported results, Kirse et al described deep VNS infections requiring hardware removal in 3 of 102 pediatric patients (2.9%).[72] By contrast, Rychlicki et al reported no cases of wound infection in a series of 36 pediatric patients.[73] Hardware revision was required in three patients (8.3%; two lead fractures, one case of poor electrical contact), and one device was removed because of lack of effect. Rychlicki et al also reported a single case of transient unilateral vocal paresis, a finding that has been described infrequently in the adult literature as well.[3]

The previously mentioned data demonstrate that VNS implantation is well tolerated in pediatric patients. In all of the previously discussed reports, the surgical complication rate requiring hardware revision or explantation was less than 10%. Even in children younger than 5 years old, minimal surgical morbidity was observed.[55] Thus, from a surgical standpoint, VNS is safe and well tolerated in children.

■ VNS Hardware and Simulation Parameters

The current VNS implantable unit used at our institution is the VNS Therapy Model 102. In addition to the implanted hardware, Cyberonics provides a personal digital assistant/computer with proprietary software and a radiofrequency telemetry wand for noninvasive, remote interrogation and programming of the device. The implanted pulse generator is powered by a lithium carbon battery with an approximate battery life of 6 years, depending on stimulation parameters.[65]

Before beginning surgery, it is wise to verify that the appropriate VNS leads and pulse generator are in the operating room and that the personal digital assistant telemetry unit is functional. The pulse generator should be interrogated and

Table 33.1 Typical Settings for Vagus Nerve Stimulation[a]

Parameter	Initial Setting Standard	Initial Setting Rapid Cycling
Normal mode		
Output current	0.25 mA	0.25 mA
Signal frequency	20 Hz	20 Hz
Pulse width	250 ms	250 ms
Signal on time	30 s	7 s
Signal off time	5 min	1.8 min
Magnet mode		
Output current	0.5 mA	0.5 mA
Pulse width	250 ms	250 ms
Signal on time	60 s	60 s

[a]VNS Therapy Model 102; Cyberonics, Inc., Houston, TX, USA.

pass a system check before opening the package. Cyberonics, Inc., recommends activating the VNS 2 weeks after surgery to minimize the risk of cardiac or other adverse events.[65] However, it has been our practice to activate the VNS at low settings while the patient is still in the operating room with cardiac monitoring, and we have not encountered any adverse events. Starting stimulation parameters are verified with the patient's treating neurologist before surgery. Typical parameters programmed at the time of implantation for both standard and rapid-cycling VNS modes are listed in **Table 33.1**. The output current is increased from 0.25 mA to 0.5 mA at the postoperative wound check 2 weeks after surgery. Subsequent changes in the parameters are generally performed by the treating neurologist on an outpatient basis.

Each patient is supplied with a handheld magnet, which allows the patient control over the device if needed in particular clinical situations.[74] With this magnet, the patient or parent can deliver on-demand stimulation to prevent or abort seizure activity. This is performed by passing the magnet over the pulse generator for at least 1 second and then removing the magnet from the field. This action converts the device to a "magnet mode" that delivers a single preprogrammed, patient-specific stimulation. The magnet may also be used to terminate all stimulation by holding the magnet over the pulse generator for at least 65 seconds. Finally, the VNS may be reset entirely by using the magnet in conjunction with the programming wand.

■ Adverse Effects from Vagus Nerve Stimulation

Stimulation-related adverse effects were investigated in adolescents and adults in the studies EO1 through EO5[40] and have been reviewed in detail.[17] With the notable rare exception of cardiac asystole or dysrhythmias during intra-operative device testing (five reported cases in total),[75,76] no dysautonomia has been noted with VNS. In addition, sudden unexplained death rates with VNS are equivalent to or lower than similar groups of patients without VNS.[77] Other stimulation-related adverse effects observed at 3 months after implantation include voice alteration (62%), throat paresthesias (25%), cough (21%), headache (20%), throat pain (17%), dyspnea (16%), pharyngitis (9%), and depression (3%).[40] All of these effects improved over time, and 5 year follow-up showed that the most common long-term side effect was voice alteration (18.7%).[40] The rates of all other adverse effects fell to less than 5% by 5 years after operation. The observed adverse effects were typically mild to moderate and only rarely required stimulation parameter changes or device explantation.[17]

In children, VNS-related adverse effects have been less well studied; however, it is has been shown that stimulation also may cause voice alterations, throat pain, or paresthesias, and cough in children.[17] Lower facial paresis, drooling, dysphagia, aspiration, sleep apnea, torticollis, headache, involuntary movements, inappropriate laughter, urinary retention, and fever have also been reported.[66,78–80] Rychlicki et al found hoarseness to be the most common complaint in pediatric VNS, occurring in 39% of patients.[73] Several studies have investigated aspiration as an adverse effect in children treated with VNS.[78,81] These studies concluded that patients with previous swallowing difficulties and those with decreased level of alertness (from sedative medications or disability) may be at a slightly increased risk of aspiration.

The long-term effect of VNS on nerve physiology remains unclear. One case report described the histological changes observed at autopsy in a vagus nerve stimulated for more than 1 year.[82] The patient was a 5-year-old boy who underwent placement of a VNS for intractable seizures and recurrent episodes of status epilepticus. He was found dead from asphyxia more than 1 year after VNS implantation. The autopsy specimen demonstrated fibrosis grossly, and the histopathology showed perineural edema and focal inflammation in the stimulated segment. Myelin loss was estimated at 90% with preservation of the axons. Although two other reports indicate that VNS does not cause neuropathological changes in the nerve,[83,84] clinical experience argues otherwise. In VNS revision cases, we have universally found fibrosis and scarring around the stimulated segment, complicating and often precluding revision of the helical electrodes. Although no definitive statements regarding nerve anatomy or physiology can be made on the basis of this limited information, it is likely that some pathological changes do occur with long-term VNS. In fact, it has been suggested that these changes may account for the improvement in hoarseness and other stimulation-related adverse effects that are observed over time.[82]

■ Nonpharmacological Treatments for Intractable Seizures

In those children with medically refractory seizures and who are not candidates for resective epilepsy surgery (diffuse, multifocal, or bihemispheric seizure onset), relatively few treatment options exist. Nonpharmacological interventions include the ketogenic diet, corpus callosotomy, and VNS.[85] The ketogenic and Atkins diets, which involve fasting followed by a diet high in fat and low in carbohydrates, generate a ketotic state, which has been shown to be useful in the management of some patients with intractable epilepsy.[86–88] Selected patients may experience reductions in seizure frequency of at least 90% with these dietary changes alone.[89] Using ketogenic diets in appropriate patients obviates surgical risks but can produce significant metabolic derangements, including acidosis, hypoglycemia, dehydration, hyperlipidemia, and renal stones.[90] Recent observations suggest that combining a ketogenic diet with other treatments, specifically VNS, may have a synergistic effect, with a rapid decrease in seizure frequency.[91]

Surgical options in this difficult group of patients include VNS and corpus callosotomy. Corpus callosotomy is a disconnective operation designed to interrupt interhemispheric spread of seizure activity. Callosotomy has proven particularly useful in the surgical treatment of drop attacks and atonic seizures, tonic seizures, and tonic–clonic seizures.[92,93] The operation involves a craniotomy and intradural, interhemispheric dissection, and potential complications include severe neurological deficit or death. Although VNS and callosotomy are approximately equivalent in seizure reduction and palliation, the surgical risks are relatively lower in VNS. This fact, coupled with the evidence demonstrating improved quality of life with VNS, has prompted many surgeons to favor VNS as a first-line surgical option in the nonpharmacological management of refractory epilepsy.[94]

■ Alternative Indications for VNS

As noted previously, VNS was approved initially by the FDA in 1997 as an adjunctive therapy for use in medically refractory epilepsy patients older than 12 years. After use of the device began, patients began reporting long-term improvements in mood with VNS.[95,96] This observation, in conjunction with the increased recognition that anticonvulsant medications were effective in treating mood disorders and the finding that VNS altered central nervous system monoamine concentrations and modulated prefrontal and limbic activity, prompted several investigations into the use of VNS in refractory depression.[97–101] This evaluation culminated in approval for the use of VNS in the treatment of chronic, refractory, or recurrent depression in Europe in 2001 and in the United States in 2005.

Research is now under way investigating the use of VNS in the treatment of refractory headaches and in chronic pain syndromes. Several case series have reported observations of decreased pain perception in patients undergoing VNS for seizures[102] or depression,[103,104] and studies are ongoing to investigate the mechanism of the antinociceptive role of VNS.[105] Similarly, VNS is being evaluated as a treatment for medically refractory migraine and cluster headaches. Preliminary studies have demonstrated promising results.[106,107]

Various other conditions have been proposed as potential indications for VNS. VNS may improve cognition and could potentially benefit people with Alzheimer's disease or other dementias.[108,109] Postural cerebellar tremors observed in multiple sclerosis have responded to VNS,[110] but despite promising results in animal studies,[111] VNS thus far has produced disappointing results in essential tremor.[112] Finally, animal studies[113] and observations in humans treated with VNS for depression[114,115] indicate that VNS may modulate satiety signals and modify eating behaviors, suggesting a possible role for VNS in the treatment of obesity.

■ Conclusion

VNS is a useful adjunct in the treatment of children with medically refractory epilepsy who are otherwise not candidates for focal cortical resection. Although still considered off label in children younger than 12, VNS has been shown to be of benefit in a variety of types of partial and generalized seizures, including the catastrophic pediatric epilepsies such as Lennox-Gastaut syndrome. The benefit of VNS also appears to increase over time, with progressive reductions in seizure frequency over successive years of follow-up. VNS is safe and well tolerated, and many children actually enjoy improvements in quality of life with VNS. Further investigation is needed to develop and validate criteria identifying those patients who will have a significant response to VNS; this subset may benefit from earlier consideration of VNS in the treatment of their epilepsy. Currently, VNS is an important tool in the management of children with refractory epilepsy, but the list of potential pediatric neurological and neuropsychological applications for VNS is likely to expand as research of the device continues.

References

1. Penry JK, Dean JC. Prevention of intractable partial seizures by intermittent vagal stimulation in humans: preliminary results. Epilepsia 1990;31(suppl 2):S40–S43
2. The Vagus Nerve Stimulation Study Group. A randomized controlled trial of chronic vagus nerve stimulation for treatment of medically intractable seizures. Neurology 1995;45(2):224–230
3. Handforth A, DeGiorgio CM, Schachter SC, et al. Vagus nerve stimulation therapy for partial-onset seizures: a randomized active-control trial. Neurology 1998;51(1):48–55
4. Lanska DJ. J.L. Corning and vagal nerve stimulation for seizures in the 1880s. Neurology 2002;58(3):452–459
5. Bailey P, Bremer F. A sensory cortical representation of the vagus nerve. With a note on the effects low blood pressure on the cortical electrogram. J Neurophysiol 1938;1:405–412
6. Zanchetti A, Wang SC, Moruzzi G. The effect of vagal afferent stimulation on the EEG pattern of the cat. Electroencephalogr Clin Neurophysiol 1952;4(3):357–361
7. Chase MH, Sterman MB, Clemente CD. Cortical and subcortical patterns of response to afferent vagal stimulation. Exp Neurol 1966;16(1):36–49
8. Chase MH, Nakamura Y, Clemente CD, Sterman MB. Afferent vagal stimulation: neurographic correlates of induced EEG synchronization and desynchronization. Brain Res 1967;5(2):236–249
9. Stoica I, Tudor I. Vagal trunk stimulation influences on epileptic spiking focus. Rev Roum Neurol 1968;5:203–210
10. Koo B. EEG changes with vagus nerve stimulation. J Clin Neurophysiol 2001;18(5):434–441
11. Woodbury DM, Woodbury JW. Effects of vagal stimulation on experimentally induced seizures in rats. Epilepsia 1990;31(suppl 2):S7–S19
12. Lockard JS, Congdon WC, DuCharme LL. Feasibility and safety of vagal stimulation in monkey model. Epilepsia 1990;31(suppl 2):S20–S26
13. Uthman BM, Wilder BJ, Hammond EJ, Reid SA. Efficacy and safety of vagus nerve stimulation in patients with complex partial seizures. Epilepsia 1990;31(suppl 2):S44–S50
14. Foley JO, DuBois F. Quantitative studies of the vagus nerve in the cat: I, the ratio of sensory to motor fibers. J Comp Neurol 1937;67:49–97
15. Rhoton AL Jr, O'Leary JL, Ferguson JP. The trigeminal, facial, vagal, and glossopharyngeal nerves in the monkey. Afferent connections. Arch Neurol 1966;14(5):530–540
16. Amar AP, Levy ML, Apuzzo MLJ. Vagus nerve stimulation for Intractable Epilepsy. In: Winn HR, ed. Youmans Neurological Surgery. Vol 2. 5th ed. Philadelphia, PA: Saunders; 2004:2643–2650
17. Ben-Menachem E. Vagus-nerve stimulation for the treatment of epilepsy. Lancet Neurol 2002;1(8):477–482
18. Barnes A, Duncan R, Chisholm JA, Lindsay K, Patterson J, Wyper D. Investigation into the mechanisms of vagus nerve stimulation for the treatment of intractable epilepsy, using 99mTc-HMPAO SPET brain images. Eur J Nucl Med Mol Imaging 2003;30(2):301–305
19. Olejniczak PW, Fisch BJ, Carey M, Butterbaugh G, Happel L, Tardo C. The effect of vagus nerve stimulation on epileptiform activity recorded from hippocampal depth electrodes. Epilepsia 2001;42(3):423–429
20. Groves DA, Brown VJ. Vagal nerve stimulation: a review of its applications and potential mechanisms that mediate its clinical effects. Neurosci Biobehav Rev 2005;29(3):493–500
21. Groves DA, Bowman EM, Brown VJ. Recordings from the rat locus coeruleus during acute vagal nerve stimulation in the anaesthetised rat. Neurosci Lett 2005;379(3):174–179

22. Dorr AE, Debonnel G. Effect of vagus nerve stimulation on serotonergic and noradrenergic transmission. J Pharmacol Exp Ther 2006;318(2):890–898

23. Krahl SE, Clark KB, Smith DC, Browning RA. Locus coeruleus lesions suppress the seizure-attenuating effects of vagus nerve stimulation. Epilepsia 1998;39(7):709–714

24. Van Bockstaele EJ, Peoples J, Telegan P. Efferent projections of the nucleus of the solitary tract to peri-locus coeruleus dendrites in rat brain: evidence for a monosynaptic pathway. J Comp Neurol 1999;412(3):410–428

25. Hassert DL, Miyashita T, Williams CL. The effects of peripheral vagal nerve stimulation at a memory-modulating intensity on norepinephrine output in the basolateral amygdala. Behav Neurosci 2004;118(1):79–88

26. Roosevelt RW, Smith DC, Clough RW, Jensen RA, Browning RA. Increased extracellular concentrations of norepinephrine in cortex and hippocampus following vagus nerve stimulation in the rat. Brain Res 2006;1119(1):124–132

27. Loy R, Koziell DA, Lindsey JD, Moore RY. Noradrenergic innervation of the adult rat hippocampal formation. J Comp Neurol 1980;189(4):699–710

28. Loughlin SE, Foote SL, Fallon JH. Locus coeruleus projections to cortex: topography, morphology and collateralization. Brain Res Bull 1982;9(1–6):287–294

29. Ben-Menachem E, Hamberger A, Hedner T, et al. Effects of vagus nerve stimulation on amino acids and other metabolites in the CSF of patients with partial seizures. Epilepsy Res 1995;20(3):221–227

30. Carpenter LL, Moreno FA, Kling MA, et al. Effect of vagus nerve stimulation on cerebrospinal fluid monoamine metabolites, norepinephrine, and gamma-aminobutyric acid concentrations in depressed patients. Biol Psychiatry 2004;56(6):418–426

31. Cunningham JT, Mifflin SW, Gould GG, Frazer A. Induction of c-Fos and DeltaFosB immunoreactivity in rat brain by vagal nerve stimulation. Neuropsychopharmacology 2008;33(8):1884–1895

32. Marrosu F, Serra A, Maleci A, Puligheddu M, Biggio G, Piga M. Correlation between GABA(A) receptor density and vagus nerve stimulation in individuals with drug-resistant partial epilepsy. Epilepsy Res 2003;55(1–2):59–70

33. Uthman BM, Wilder BJ, Penry JK, et al. Treatment of epilepsy by stimulation of the vagus nerve. Neurology 1993;43(7):1338–1345

34. Landy HJ, Ramsay RE, Slater J, Casiano RR, Morgan R. Vagus nerve stimulation for complex partial seizures: surgical technique, safety, and efficacy. J Neurosurg 1993;78(1):26–31

35. Holder LK, Wernicke JF, Tarver WB. Treatment of refractory partial seizures: preliminary results of a controlled study. Pacing Clin Electrophysiol 1992;15(10 pt 2):1557–1571

36. Ben-Menachem E, Mañon-Espaillat R, Ristanovic R, et al; First International Vagus Nerve Stimulation Study Group. Vagus nerve stimulation for treatment of partial seizures: 1. A controlled study of effect on seizures. Epilepsia 1994;35(3):616–626

37. Ramsay RE, Uthman BM, Augustinsson LE, et al; First International Vagus Nerve Stimulation Study Group. Vagus nerve stimulation for treatment of partial seizures: 2. Safety, side effects, and tolerability. Epilepsia 1994;35(3):627–636

38. George R, Salinsky M, Kuzniecky R, et al; First International Vagus Nerve Stimulation Study Group. Vagus nerve stimulation for treatment of partial seizures: 3. Long-term follow-up on first 67 patients exiting a controlled study. Epilepsia 1994;35(3):637–643

39. Salinsky MC, Uthman BM, Ristanovic RK, Wernicke JF, Tarver WB; Vagus Nerve Stimulation Study Group. Vagus nerve stimulation for the treatment of medically intractable seizures. Results of a 1-year open-extension trial. Arch Neurol 1996;53(11):1176–1180

40. Morris GL III, Mueller WM. Long-term treatment with vagus nerve stimulation in patients with refractory epilepsy. The Vagus Nerve Stimulation Study Group E01-E05. Neurology 1999;53(8):1731–1735

41. De Herdt V, Boon P, Ceulemans B, et al. Vagus nerve stimulation for refractory epilepsy: a Belgian multicenter study. Eur J Paediatr Neurol 2007;11(5):261–269

42. Ardesch JJ, Buschman HP, Wagener-Schimmel LJ, van der Aa HE, Hageman G. Vagus nerve stimulation for medically refractory epilepsy: a long-term follow-up study. Seizure 2007;16(7):579–585

43. Murphy JV, Hornig G, Schallert G. Left vagal nerve stimulation in children with refractory epilepsy. Preliminary observations. Arch Neurol 1995;52(9):886–889

44. Murphy JV; The Pediatric VNS Study Group. Left vagal nerve stimulation in children with medically refractory epilepsy. J Pediatr 1999;134(5):563–566

45. Helmers SL, Wheless JW, Frost M, et al. Vagus nerve stimulation therapy in pediatric patients with refractory epilepsy: retrospective study. J Child Neurol 2001;16(11):843–848

46. Majoie HJ, Berfelo MW, Aldenkamp AP, Renier WO, Kessels AG. Vagus nerve stimulation in patients with catastrophic childhood epilepsy, a 2-year follow-up study. Seizure 2005;14(1):10–18

47. Farooqui S, Boswell W, Hemphill JM, Pearlman E. Vagus nerve stimulation in pediatric patients with intractable epilepsy: case series and operative technique. Am Surg 2001;67(2):119–121

48. Saneto RP, Sotero de Menezes MA, Ojemann JG, et al. Vagus nerve stimulation for intractable seizures in children. Pediatr Neurol 2006;35(5):323–326

49. Patwardhan RV, Stong B, Bebin EM, Mathisen J, Grabb PA. Efficacy of vagal nerve stimulation in children with medically refractory epilepsy. Neurosurgery 2000;47(6):1353–1357, discussion 1357–1358

50. Wheless JW, Maggio V. Vagus nerve stimulation therapy in patients younger than 18 years. Neurology 2002; 59(6, suppl 4)S21–S25

51. Lundgren J, Amark P, Blennow G, Strömblad LG, Wallstedt L. Vagus nerve stimulation in 16 children with refractory epilepsy. Epilepsia 1998;39(8):809–813

52. Hornig GW, Murphy JV, Schallert G, Tilton C. Left vagus nerve stimulation in children with refractory epilepsy: an update. South Med J 1997;90(5):484–488

53. Hallböök T, Lundgren J, Stjernqvist K, Blennow G, Strömblad LG, Rosén I. Vagus nerve stimulation in 15 children with therapy resistant epilepsy; its impact on cognition, quality of life, behaviour and mood. Seizure 2005;14(7):504–513

54. Kang HC, Hwang YS, Kim DS, Kim HD. Vagus nerve stimulation in pediatric intractable epilepsy: a Korean bicentric study. Acta Neurochir Suppl (Wien) 2006;99:93–96

55. Blount JP, Tubbs RS, Kankirawatana P, et al. Vagus nerve stimulation in children less than 5 years old. Childs Nerv Syst 2006;22(9):1167–1169

56. Parain D, Penniello MJ, Berquen P, Delangre T, Billard C, Murphy JV. Vagal nerve stimulation in tuberous sclerosis complex patients. Pediatr Neurol 2001;25(3):213–216

57. Murphy JV, Wheless JW, Schmoll CM. Left vagal nerve stimulation in six patients with hypothalamic hamartomas. Pediatr Neurol 2000;23(2):167–168

58. Frost M, Gates J, Helmers SL, et al. Vagus nerve stimulation in children with refractory seizures associated with Lennox-Gastaut syndrome. Epilepsia 2001;42(9):1148–1152

59. Wakai S, Kotagal P. Vagus nerve stimulation for children and adolescents with intractable epilepsies. Pediatr Int 2001;43(1):61–65

60. Majoie HJ, Berfelo MW, Aldenkamp AP, Evers SM, Kessels AG, Renier WO. Vagus nerve stimulation in children with therapy-resistant epilepsy diagnosed as Lennox-Gastaut syndrome: clinical results, neuropsychological effects, and cost-effectiveness. J Clin Neurophysiol 2001;18(5):419–428

61. Rychlicki F, Zamponi N, Trignani R, Ricciuti RA, Iacoangeli M, Scerrati M. Vagus nerve stimulation: clinical experience in drug-resistant pediatric epileptic patients. Seizure 2006;15(7):483–490

62. Patwardhan RV, Dellabadia J Jr, Rashidi M, Grier L, Nanda A. Control of refractory status epilepticus precipitated by anticonvulsant withdrawal using left vagal nerve stimulation: a case report. Surg Neurol 2005;64(2):170–173

63. Winston KR, Levisohn P, Miller BR, Freeman J. Vagal nerve stimulation for status epilepticus. Pediatr Neurosurg 2001;34(4):190–192

64. Randall WC, Ardell JL. Differential innervation of the heart. In: Sipes D, Jalife J, eds. Cardiac Electrophysiology and Arrhythmias. New York, NY: Grune and Stratton; 1985:137–144

65. Cyberonics Inc. Physician's Manual for the VNS Therapy Pulse Model 102 Generator. Houston, TX: Cyberonics; 2003.

66. Smyth MD, Tubbs RS, Bebin EM, Grabb PA, Blount JP. Complications of chronic vagus nerve stimulation for epilepsy in children. J Neurosurg 2003;99(3):500–503

67. Ramani R. Vagus nerve stimulation therapy for seizures. J Neurosurg Anesthesiol 2008;20(1):29–35

68. McGregor A, Wheless J, Baumgartner J, Bettis D. Right-sided vagus nerve stimulation as a treatment for refractory epilepsy in humans. Epilepsia 2005;46(1):91–96

69. Bauman JA, Ridgway EB, Devinsky O, Doyle WK. Subpectoral implantation of the vagus nerve stimulator. Neurosurgery 2006; 58(4 suppl 2):ONS-322–ONS-325

70. Le H, Chico M, Hecox K, Frim D. Interscapular placement of a vagal nerve stimulator pulse generator for prevention of wound tampering. Technical note. Pediatr Neurosurg 2002;36(3):164–166

71. Patil A, Chand A, Andrews R. Single incision for implanting a vagal nerve stimulator system (VNSS): technical note. Surg Neurol 2001;55(2):103–105

72. Kirse DJ, Werle AH, Murphy JV, et al. Vagus nerve stimulator implantation in children. Arch Otolaryngol Head Neck Surg 2002;128(11):1263–1268

73. Rychlicki F, Zamponi N, Cesaroni E, et al. Complications of vagal nerve stimulation for epilepsy in children. Neurosurg Rev 2006;29(2):103–107

74. Technical Information. In: Physician Manual VNS Therapy System Pulse Model 102 Generator and Pulse Duo model 102R Generator. Houston, TX: Cyberonics, Inc; 2008.

75. Tatum WO IV, Moore DB, Stecker MM, et al. Ventricular asystole during vagus nerve stimulation for epilepsy in humans. Neurology 1999;52(6):1267–1269

76. Asconapé JJ, Moore DD, Zipes DP, Hartman LM, Duffell WH Jr. Bradycardia and asystole with the use of vagus nerve stimulation for the treatment of epilepsy: a rare complication of intraoperative device testing. Epilepsia 1999;40(10):1452–1454

77. Annegers JF, Coan SP, Hauser WA, Leestma J. Epilepsy, vagal nerve stimulation by the NCP system, all-cause mortality, and sudden, unexpected, unexplained death. Epilepsia 2000;41(5):549–553

78. Lundgren J, Ekberg O, Olsson R. Aspiration: a potential complication to vagus nerve stimulation. Epilepsia 1998;39(9):998–1000

79. Murphy JV, Hornig GW, Schallert GS, Tilton CL. Adverse events in children receiving intermittent left vagal nerve stimulation. Pediatr Neurol 1998;19(1):42–44

80. Valencia I, Holder DL, Helmers SL, Madsen JR, Riviello JJ Jr. Vagus nerve stimulation in pediatric epilepsy: a review. Pediatr Neurol 2001;25(5):368–376

81. Schallert G, Foster J, Lindquist N, Murphy JV. Chronic stimulation of the left vagal nerve in children: effect on swallowing. Epilepsia 1998;39(10):1113–1114

82. Tubbs RS, Patwardhan R, Palmer CA, et al. Histological appearance of a chronically stimulated vagus nerve in a pediatric patient. Pediatr Neurosurg 2001;35(2):99–102

83. Tougas G, Fitzpatrick D, Hudoba P, et al. Effects of chronic left vagal stimulation on visceral vagal function in man. Pacing Clin Electrophysiol 1992;15(10 pt 2):1588–1596

84. Tarver WB, George RE, Maschino SE, Holder LK, Wernicke JF. Clinical experience with a helical bipolar stimulating lead. Pacing Clin Electrophysiol 1992;15(10 pt 2):1545–1556

85. Wheless JW. Nonpharmacologic treatment of the catastrophic epilepsies of childhood. Epilepsia 2004;45(suppl 5):17–22

86. Freeman JM, Kossoff EH, Hartman AL. The ketogenic diet: one decade later. Pediatrics 2007;119(3):535–543

87. Kossoff EH. More fat and fewer seizures: dietary therapies for epilepsy. Lancet Neurol 2004;3(7):415–420

88. Kossoff EH, McGrogan JR, Bluml RM, Pillas DJ, Rubenstein JE, Vining EP. A modified Atkins diet is effective for the treatment of intractable pediatric epilepsy. Epilepsia 2006;47(2):421–424

89. Groesbeck DK, Bluml RM, Kossoff EH. Long-term use of the ketogenic diet in the treatment of epilepsy. Dev Med Child Neurol 2006;48(12):978–981

90. Wilong AA. Complications and consequences of epilepsy surgery, ketogenic diet, and vagus nerve stimulation. Semin Pediatr Neurol 2007;14(4):201–203

91. Kossoff EH, Pyzik PL, Rubenstein JE, et al. Combined ketogenic diet and vagus nerve stimulation: rational polytherapy? Epilepsia 2007;48(1):77–81

92. Gates JR, Wada JA, Reeves AG, et al. Reevaluation of corpus callosotomy. In: Engel JJ, ed. Surgical Treatment of the Epilepsies. New York, NY: Raven Press; 1993:637–648

93. Cendes F, Ragazzo PC, da Costa V, Martins LF. Corpus callosotomy in treatment of medically resistant epilepsy: preliminary results in a pediatric population. Epilepsia 1993;34(5):910–917

94. Wong TT, Kwan SY, Chang KP, et al. Corpus callosotomy in children. Childs Nerv Syst 2006;22(8):999–1011

95. Hoppe C, Helmstaedter C, Scherrmann J, Elger CE. Self-reported mood changes following 6 months of vagus nerve stimulation in epilepsy patients. Epilepsy Behav 2001;2(4):335–342

96. Elger G, Hoppe C, Falkai P, Rush AJ, Elger CE. Vagus nerve stimulation is associated with mood improvements in epilepsy patients. Epilepsy Res 2000;42(2–3):203–210

97. Ansari S, Chaudhri K, Al Moutaery KA. Vagus nerve stimulation: indications and limitations. Acta Neurochir Suppl (Wien) 2007;97(pt 2):281–286

98. Rush AJ, George MS, Sackeim HA, et al. Vagus nerve stimulation (VNS) for treatment-resistant depressions: a multicenter study. Biol Psychiatry 2000;47(4):276–286

99. Marangell LB, Rush AJ, George MS, et al. Vagus nerve stimulation (VNS) for major depressive episodes: one year outcomes. Biol Psychiatry 2002;51(4):280–287

100. George MS, Sackeim HA, Marangell LB, et al. Vagus nerve stimulation. A potential therapy for resistant depression? Psychiatr Clin North Am 2000;23(4):757–783

101. Sackeim HA, Rush AJ, George MS, et al. Vagus nerve stimulation (VNS) for treatment-resistant depression: efficacy, side effects, and predictors of outcome. Neuropsychopharmacology 2001;25(5):713–728

102. Kirchner A, Birklein F, Stefan H, Handwerker HO. Left vagus nerve stimulation suppresses experimentally induced pain. Neurology 2000;55(8):1167–1171

103. Borckardt JJ, Kozel FA, Anderson B, Walker A, George MS. Vagus nerve stimulation affects pain perception in depressed adults. Pain Res Manag 2005;10(1):9–14

104. Borckardt JJ, Anderson B, Andrew Kozel F, et al. Acute and long-term VNS effects on pain perception in a case of treatment-resistant depression. Neurocase 2006;12(4):216–220

105. Kirchner A, Stefan H, Bastian K, Birklein F. Vagus nerve stimulation suppresses pain but has limited effects on neurogenic inflammation in humans. Eur J Pain 2006;10(5):449–455

106. Hord ED, Evans MS, Mueed S, Adamolekun B, Naritoku DK. The effect of vagus nerve stimulation on migraines. J Pain 2003;4(9):530–534

107. Mauskop A. Vagus nerve stimulation relieves chronic refractory migraine and cluster headaches. Cephalalgia 2005;25(2):82–86

108. Merrill CA, Jonsson MA, Minthon L, et al. Vagus nerve stimulation in patients with Alzheimer's disease: additional follow-up results of a pilot study through 1 year. J Clin Psychiatry 2006;67(8):1171–1178

109. Sjögren MJ, Hellström PT, Jonsson MA, Runnerstam M, Silander HC, Ben-Menachem E. Cognition-enhancing effect of vagus nerve stimulation in patients with Alzheimer's disease: a pilot study. J Clin Psychiatry 2002;63(11):972–980

110. Marrosu F, Maleci A, Cocco E, Puligheddu M, Barberini L, Marrosu MG. Vagal nerve stimulation improves cerebellar tremor and dysphagia in multiple sclerosis. Mult Scler 2007;13(9):1200–1202

111. Krahl SE, Martin FC, Handforth A. Vagus nerve stimulation inhibits harmaline-induced tremor. Brain Res 2004;1011(1):135–138

112. Handforth A, Ondo WG, Tatter S, et al. Vagus nerve stimulation for essential tremor: a pilot efficacy and safety trial. Neurology 2003;61(10):1401–1405

113. Bugajski AJ, Gil K, Ziomber A, Zurowski D, Zaraska W, Thor PJ. Effect of long-term vagal stimulation on food intake and body weight during diet induced obesity in rats. J Physiol Pharmacol 2007;58(suppl 1):5–12

114. Bodenlos JS, Kose S, Borckardt JJ, et al. Vagus nerve stimulation acutely alters food craving in adults with depression. Appetite 2007;48(2):145–153

115. Pardo JV, Sheikh SA, Kuskowski MA, et al. Weight loss during chronic, cervical vagus nerve stimulation in depressed patients with obesity: an observation. Int J Obes (Lond) 2007;31(11):1756–1759

34 Cortical and Deep Brain Stimulation

Eric H. Kossoff and George I. Jallo

Throughout Part II of this textbook, the risks and benefits of surgical procedures to either remove an epileptic focus or palliate intractable multifocal epilepsy have been discussed. As the reader is well aware, there are situations in which a child has epilepsy that is generalized in onset, focal but localized to a region of the brain that would cause significant functional morbidity, or the child is at too high of a surgical risk because of medical co morbidities. In addition to this, as is discussed in Chapter 36, surgical failures do occur, and further nonsurgical (but nonpharmacological) therapies are requested by parents.

What other options do parents and their children have? At this time, the two major nonpharmacological therapies that are reliably proven to reduce seizure frequency are the ketogenic diet and vagus nerve stimulation. Both of these therapies have had an incredible growth in both clinical and research interest over the past decade, even considering the near doubling in the number of anticonvulsant drugs available.

One of the most exciting areas of research in epilepsy is the use of electricity to abort seizures, not just by continuous stimulation of the vagus nerve but also through direct brain stimulation to the cortex as well as deeper brain structures. Although innovative and likely more advantageous than vagus nerve stimulation, primarily because of closer proximity to the epileptic foci or circuits, the time involvement and preparation of both the epileptologist and neurosurgeon are exponentially greater to use these new technologies. This chapter discusses the current methods under investigation to provide electrical stimulation to the brain. Most of the research to date involves adults, but limited data do exist for children, and future directions of these therapies in the pediatric age range will be presented at the conclusion of this chapter.

■ Brain Stimulation Regions

Subcortical Structures

Perhaps the most frequently studied regions of the brain for direct neurostimulation have been the subcortical structures, most notably the thalamus, caudate, and cerebellum. Advances in safety and accuracy of the stereotactic place-

ment of deep brain electrodes, especially for movement disorders such as Parkinson disease, has led to a strong interest in this technique to reach brain structures that animal research has identified as involved in the spread of seizures. These structures, although not typically the exact epileptic focus, have widespread excitatory and inhibitory connection and are safe to stimulate without causing a loss of function.

Cerebellum and Caudate

Both controlled and uncontrolled trials of stimulation to the cerebellum and caudate nucleus have shown mixed results.[1-4] The caudate nucleus is a theoretically attractive target for stimulation because of its connectivity with the thalamus and neocortex. Only one study from 1997 showed benefits, but it has not been confirmed to date with a controlled trial.[4] The cerebellum also has excitatory connections to the thalamus, which can be theoretically inhibited by neurostimulation. One relatively large study of 32 adults from 1992 reported 23 patients (85%) with seizure reduction as a result of cerebellar stimulation.[1] A double-blind study from 2005 of five patients demonstrated a mean 67% seizure reduction in patients with active therapy versus 7% reduction in those with therapy not turned on ($p = .02$).[3] Interestingly, seizure improvement continued to occur in patients over the 2-year study period.

Thalamus

Studies of the caudate and cerebellum have been less frequent in the past decade, as alternative subcortical structures have been identified as perhaps more promising. The thalamus specifically appears to be the most likely subcortical structure to result in seizure reduction when stimulated because of its widespread inhibitory connections with the cortex and evidence for possible indirect stimulation by vagus nerve stimulation over the past two decades of use. One of the first thalamic nuclei studied was the centromedian nucleus, because of its projections to the entire cerebral cortex from ascending brainstem regions. The efficacy of this approach is unclear, however, with both positive (for Lennox-Gastaut syndrome)[5] and negative (for complex partial seizures) results.[6] The subthalamic nucleus has also been stimulated in small studies, with only modest results.[7,8] One case report included a child with a focal centroparietal dysplasia who received benefit from stimulation of this nucleus.[9]

In recent years, there has been significant interest in stimulation of the anterior nucleus of the thalamus. This small structure is distant from basal vascular structures yet has connections to the limbic system via the circuit of Papez, which connects the hippocampus, fornix, and mammillary bodies to the cingulum and parahippocampal cortex in a functional loop.[10] The first pilot study of five patients who underwent bilateral anterior thalamic stimulation demonstrated a mean seizure reduction of 54%; however, patients who were implanted but not stimulated had similar responses interestingly.[11] Other small studies have mostly replicated these results; one of the more recent studies of four adults demonstrated a slightly higher mean reduction of 76% in monthly seizure frequency.[12]

On the basis of these early results, this thalamic nucleus has been recently investigated in a multicenter study for intractable partial epilepsy sponsored and just completed by Medtronics, Inc., titled SANTE (Stimulation of the Anterior Nucleus of the Thalamus for Epilepsy). The surgical procedure to implant these electrodes is described well in a recent review by Halpern, et al[13] and the device in an adult subject is depicted in **Fig. 34.1**. For inclusion, patients were required to be between the ages of 18 and 65 years, have failed 12 to 18 months trial of at least two anticonvulsant drugs, and have at least six partial and disabling seizures per month. Study results should be forthcoming soon.

Hippocampus

The hippocampus is another target for neurostimulation because of its association with temporal lobe epilepsy and connections to the circuit of Papez. Several small, uncontrolled studies showed modest levels of improvement, including one demonstrating four of seven patients with more than 50% seizure reduction and one who became seizure free.[14] However, a recent double-blind, controlled study of hippocampal stimulation for four patients with mesial temporal lobe epilepsy showed a minimal seizure reduction of 15% with stimulation, and improvement also occurred during periods without active stimulation.[15]

Cortex

The deep brain structures mentioned previously are all potential targets for neurostimulation that can be accessed with stereotactical placement of electrodes and their stimulation may suppress seizures by increasing inhibitory neuronal activity through epileptic circuits. However, the majority of epilepsy does not start in subcortical structures but rather in the cortex itself. Providing stimulation directly to the cortical regions of epileptogenicity is theoretically attractive. Ideal subjects have had their epilepsy localized to one cortical region, yet surgery is either not recommended because of presumed functional morbidity or the patient has either failed or only had partial seizure reduction after a previous resection to that area. In these situations, stimulating one discrete region of the cortex would not cause further morbidity. Current methods of stimulating the cortex are magnetic, nonresponsive, and open-loop stimulation (transcranial magnetic stimulation) as well as electrical, responsive, and closed-loop stimulation (NeuroPace Inc., Mountain View, CA).

■ Transcranial Magnetic Stimulation

Transcranial magnetic stimulation (TMS) is a method of stimulation using magnetic fields rather than electricity to reduce seizure frequency. Using either a handheld magnet or an aligned frame, TMS has been used at frequencies of 0.5 to 1.0 Hz over the cortical region of epileptogenicity for typically 15 to 30 minutes twice daily for several days.[16] In one study of 24 patients randomly assigned to placebo (TMS angled away from the patient) or therapy, there was a mean of 16% seizure reduction only in the first 2 weeks with the

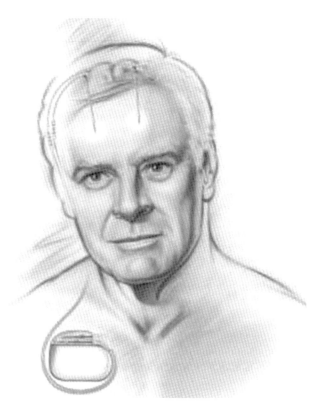

Fig. 34.1 Depiction of the stimulator device and electrodes to the anterior nucleus of the thalamus as used in the Stimulation of the Anterior Nucleus of the Thalamus for Epilepsy (SANTE) trial. (Courtesy of Dr. Robert Fisher.)

active group, with no change in the placebo.[17] A study from Japan of seven patients with extratemporal epilepsy showed similar results, with a 19% seizure reduction after 2 weeks, although this finding did not reach statistical significance.[18] One randomized study from Brazil of 21 patients, comparing sham to active stimulation, showed improvement both immediately and after 4 weeks.[19]

■ Responsive Neurostimulation

Whereas all of the previously described methods of neurostimulation, both subcortical and cortical, are nonrespon-

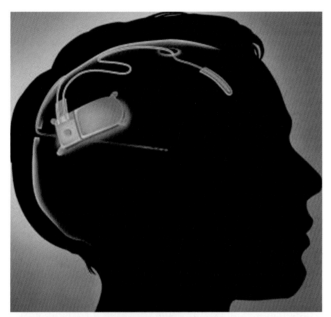

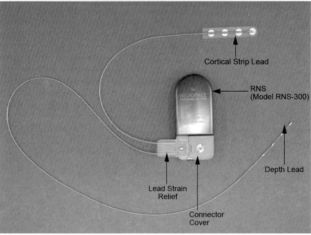

Fig. 34.2 Responsive neurostimulator (NeuroPace) as depicted in a patient with both surface cortical and depth electrodes (*top*). Photograph of actual device (*bottom*). (Courtesy Dr. Martha Morrell and NeuroPace, Inc.)

sive, ongoing studies using direct cortical stimulation to epileptic foci using a responsive stimulator.[20,21] In this regard, stimulation is delivered by a computerized device only in response to the patient's individual seizure activity. Advances in seizure detection algorithms and microcomputers have led to the development of a responsive neurostimulator (NeuroPace) that is implanted into the skull with a metal clamp securing it in place (**Fig. 34.2**). Two electrode leads, which can be surface or depth contacts, are then placed over the region(s) of suspected epileptogenicity and connected to the stimulator at the time of surgery. When the battery needs to be replaced, without breaching the dura by a scalp incision, the device can be removed by temporary disconnection of the electrodes, and then reinsertion and connection of a new device. The responsive neurostimulator detects seizure activity and subsequently disrupts it via electrical stimulation to the cortex, saving several second intervals of electroencephalography (EEG) in the memory for later review. This memory of both EEG and stimulation frequency is then downloaded for analysis using a wand in a similar manner to vagus nerve stimulation as well as via a home laptop computer and phone modem lines. Early studies of this technology for adults and adolescents using the seizure detection and stimulation algorithms via implanted subdural electrode grids showed promising results.[22]

The NeuroPace device is currently in a blinded and controlled multicenter clinical trial for adults with intractable partial epilepsy who are having at least eight seizures in a 3-month period (www.seizurestudy.com). Early results are encouraging, as are safety findings.

■ Surgical Technique

The surgical technique for the NeuroPace device requires planning for the craniotomy, placement of the cortical or depth electrodes, and placement of the ferrule and the neurostimulator. Thus the placement of the neurostimulator must be coordinated with the implantation of possibly bilateral depth electrodes or subdural strip electrodes or a combination, which are applied to the seizure focus site. Before the surgical incisions, the location of the ferrule and the arrangement of the leads so that they do not traverse any surgical incisions must be planned before positioning. As an example, a patient with bilateral medial temporal lobe focus would need to be positioned prone with fixation pins. A preoperative stereotactic image guidance magnetic resonance image would be performed to assist in the bilateral depth electrode placement. After adequate prone positioning, three incisions would need to be planned to encompass the burr holes and the location of the ferrule. Two straight incisions for the occipital trajectory and stereotactic placement of the depth electrodes must be planned such that the leads do not cross the incision because they are connected to the neuroresponsive stimulator. An S-shaped or horseshoe incision then needs to be planned so that the craniectomy or craniotomy for the ferrule is created. The neuroresponsive stimulator is secured into the ferrule after connection of the two leads. The detection algorithms are then programmed to enable detection of the seizure activity.

■ Use in Pediatric Subjects

At this time, both of the ongoing multicenter studies (SANTE and NeuroPace) are open to enrollment only for adults older than 18 years of age. However, most pediatric epileptologists involved in cortical and deep brain stimulation trials are anxious to potentially use these therapies in children should they receive U.S. Food and Drug Administration (FDA) approval. Many children have intractable epilepsy that is either multifocal or only resectable if a significant motor deficit would be tolerated, such as because of a large hemispheric dysplasia. It is not uncommon for many parents to defer permanent surgical treatment because of limited impact of seizures on quality of life in young children, the possibly unclear localization in magnetic resonance imaging or positron emission tomography–negative subjects, and the inherent hope of natural remission that many parents have for children. Vagus nerve stimulation and the ketogenic diet are frequently used to buy time and defer an irreversible surgery until a child is older.[23] Deep brain stimulation may therefore become widely used in these intractable pediatric epilepsy cases because of its relatively low risk, inherent reversibility, and ability to theoretically disrupt the widespread epileptic circuits (especially in the subcortical stimulation techniques) believed to be problematic in many young children with epilepsy. As these therapies become FDA approved for adults in the coming years, it is highly likely they will be used initially on an investigative basis in children in academic centers with trained pediatric epilepsy neurosurgeons.

■ Conclusion

The use of both cortical and deep brain stimulation is an exciting and growing field in the treatment of intractable epilepsy. Using electricity to disrupt electricity has been practiced for many decades and continues to be actively investigated. As new computer technology, stereotactic techniques, seizure detection algorithms, and battery life evolve, these methods of seizure control will continue to evolve and become more widely used. Although nearly universally studied in adults at this time, look for expanded uses in children with multifocal or surgically inaccessible epilepsy in years to come.

References

1. Davis R, Emmonds SE. Cerebellar stimulation for seizure control: 17-year study. Stereotact Funct Neurosurg 1992;58(1-4):200–208

2. Wright GD, McLellan DL, Brice JG. A double-blind trial of chronic cerebellar stimulation in twelve patients with severe epilepsy. J Neurol Neurosurg Psychiatry 1984;47(8):769–774

3. Velasco F, Carrillo-Ruiz JD, Brito F, et al. Double-blind, randomized controlled pilot study of bilateral cerebellar stimulation for treatment of intractable motor seizures. Epilepsia 2005;46(7):1071–1081

4. Chkhenkeli SA, Chkhenkeli IS. Effects of therapeutic stimulation of nucleus caudatus on epileptic electrical activity of brain in patients with intractable epilepsy. Stereotact Funct Neurosurg 1997;69(1-4 pt 2):221–224

5. Velasco AL, Velasco F, Jiménez F, et al. Neuromodulation of the centromedian thalamic nuclei in the treatment of generalized seizures and the improvement of the quality of life in patients with Lennox-Gastaut syndrome. Epilepsia 2006;47(7):1203–1212

6. Fisher RS, Uematsu S, Krauss GL, et al. Placebo-controlled pilot study of centromedian thalamic stimulation in treatment of intractable seizures. Epilepsia 1992;33(5):841–851

7. Loddenkemper T, Pan A, Neme S, et al. Deep brain stimulation in epilepsy. J Clin Neurophysiol 2001;18(6):514–532

8. Däuper J, Peschel T, Schrader C, et al. Effects of subthalamic nucleus (STN) stimulation on motor cortex excitability. Neurology 2002;59(5):700–706

9. Benabid AL, Koudsie A, Benazzouz A, et al. Deep brain stimulation of the corpus luysi (subthalamic nucleus) and other targets in Parkinson's disease: extension to new indications such as dystonia and epilepsy. J Neurol 2001;248(suppl 3):III37–III47

10. Papez JW. A proposed mechanism of emotion. Arch Neurol Psychiatry 1937;38:725–743

11. Hodaie M, Wennberg RA, Dostrovsky JO, Lozano AM. Chronic anterior thalamus stimulation for intractable epilepsy. Epilepsia 2002;43(6):603–608

12. Osorio I, Overman J, Giftakis J, Wilkinson SB. High frequency thalamic stimulation for inoperable mesial temporal epilepsy. Epilepsia 2007;48(8):1561–1571

13. Halpern CH, Samadani U, Litt B, Jaggi JL, Baltuch GH. Deep brain stimulation for epilepsy. Neurotherapeutics 2008;5(1):59–67

14. Vonck K, Boon P, Claeys P, Dedeurwaerdere S, Achten R, Van Roost D. Long-term deep brain stimulation for refractory temporal lobe epilepsy. Epilepsia 2005;46(suppl 5):98–99

15. Tellez-Zenteno JF, McLachlan RS, Parrent A, Kubu CS, Wiebe S. Hippocampal electrical stimulation in mesial temporal lobe epilepsy. Neurology 2006;66(10):1490–1494

16. Theodore WH, Fisher RS. Brain stimulation for epilepsy. Lancet Neurol 2004;3(2):111–118

17. Theodore WH, Hunter K, Chen R, et al. Transcranial magnetic stimulation for the treatment of seizures: a controlled study. Neurology 2002;59(4):560–562

18. Kinoshita M, Ikeda A, Begum T, Yamamoto J, Hitomi T, Shibasaki H. Low-frequency repetitive transcranial magnetic stimulation for seizure suppression in patients with extratemporal lobe epilepsy–a pilot study. Seizure 2005;14(6):387–392

19. Fregni F, Otachi PT, Do Valle A, et al. A randomized clinical trial of repetitive transcranial magnetic stimulation in patients with refractory epilepsy. Ann Neurol 2006;60(4):447–455

20. Morrell M. Brain stimulation for epilepsy: can scheduled or responsive neurostimulation stop seizures? Curr Opin Neurol 2006;19(2):164–168

21. Sun FT, Morrell MJ, Wharen RE Jr. Responsive cortical stimulation for the treatment of epilepsy. Neurotherapeutics 2008;5(1):68–74

22. Kossoff EH, Ritzl EK, Politsky JM, et al. Effect of an external responsive neurostimulator on seizures and electrographic discharges during subdural electrode monitoring. Epilepsia 2004;45:1560–1567

23. Stainman RS, Turner Z, Rubenstein JF, Kossoff EH. Decreased relative efficacy of the ketogenic diet for children with surgically approachable epilepsy. Seizure 2007;16(7):615–619

35 Radiosurgical Treatment for Epilepsy

Jean Régis, Marc Lévêque, Fabrice Bartolomei, Didier Scavarda, and Patrick Chauvel

Radiosurgery is, by definition, a neurosurgical procedure that uses stereotactically focused, converging, narrow ionizing beams to induce a desired biological effect in a predetermined target, with minimal radiation to the surrounding tissues and without opening the skull. The increased worldwide use of gamma knife surgery (GKS) to treat various pathologies has rendered the side-effect profile of radiosurgery rare, generally transient, and quite easily predictable.[1] Once it is established that resection of a small deeply seated lesion has a significant risk for surgical complications or functional worsening, GKS must be discussed as an alternative.

The first radiosurgical treatments for epilepsy surgery were performed by Talairach in the 1950s.[2] As early as 1974, Talairach reported on the use of radioactive yttrium implants in patients with mesial temporal lobe epilepsy (MTLE) without space-occupying lesions and showed a high rate of seizure control in patients with epilepsies confined to the mesial structures of the temporal lobe.[2] In 1980, Elomaa[3] promoted the idea of the use of focal irradiation for the treatment of temporal lobe epilepsy based on the preliminary reports of Tracy, Von Wieser, and Baudouin.[4,5] Furthermore, clinical experience of the use of GKS and linac-based radiosurgery in arteriovenous malformations and cortico-subcortical tumors revealed an anticonvulsive effect of radiosurgery in the absence of tissue necrosis.[6-8] A series of experimental studies in small animals confirmed this effect[9,10] and emphasized a relationship to the dose delivered.[11,12]

The Department of Functional Surgery in Marseille is a major referral center for epilepsy surgery and radiosurgery and has reported the first comprehensively evaluated series of MTLE successfully operated by GKS. The first case of GKS for MTLE was treated in 1993 and reported in 1994 by this group.[13] Several prospective trials from this group have demonstrated

1. The safety efficacy of this approach,[14,15]
2. A very specific timetable of the clinical and radiological events,[14,16]
3. The importance of the anterior parahippocampal cortex for seizure cessation,[17,18]
4. The importance of the marginal dose (24 Gy) for efficacy,[18]

5. The feasibility of sparing verbal memory with GKS in dominant-side epilepsy,[15] and
6. The nonlesional mechanism of action of radiosurgery.[19]

Recently, all these findings have been confirmed by a prospective trial in the United States.[20] The Marseille group has treated 155 patients with epilepsy surgery using GKS radiosurgery among a total of 8,590 GKS procedures since 1993. The majority of these patients presented with MTLE (56 patients) and hypothalamic hamartoma (HH, 77 patients). The rest of the patients had severe epilepsy associated with small benign lesions such as cavernous malformations (42 patients) for which an epileptic zone was considered to be confined to the surrounding cortex.[21]

Seizure cessation may be generated by a specific neuromodulatory effect of radiosurgery, without induction of a significant amount of histological necrosis.[13,16,19,22,23] The selection of the appropriate technical parameters (e.g., dose, volume target) allowing us to accurately obtain the desired functional effect without histological damage remains an important challenge. A detailed review of these cases, as well as other clinical and experimental data, suggests that the use of radiosurgery is beneficial only to those patients in whom a strict preoperative definition of the extent of the epileptogenic network has been achieved,[24] and where strict rules of dose planning have been followed.[25] The strategy must be to define the patients in whom the safety/efficacy ratio makes radiosurgery advantageous or at least comparable to craniotomy and cortical resection.

■ Mesial Temporal Lobe Epilepsy

The first GKS operations for MTLE were performed in Marseille in March 1993. Because there was no similar experience available in the literature at that time, we were obliged to define our treatment criteria and technical choices based on present experience of radiosurgery for other pathological conditions at that time. We treated four patients with different technical choices in terms of dose, volume, and target definition. Then we observed some significant radiological changes in these patients several months after radiosurgery.[16] This finding led us to stop such treatment, and we decided to follow the long-term results of these first four patients. Long-term results in these patients were re-assuring with documented clinical safety of the procedure and gradual disappearance of the acute magnetic resonance imaging (MRI) changes several months later. Therefore, we again decided to treat a new series of patients under strict prospective controlled trial conditions. This classic planning (**Fig. 35.1**) was based on the use of two 18-mm shots, covering a volume of around 7 mL at the 50% isodose (24 Gy). The results were impressive with a high rate of seizure cessation.[14,26] Then, we redefined our treatment target by focus-

ing it on the parahippocampal cortex and sparing significant parts of the amygdaloidal complex and hippocampus to decrease morbidity. We further reduced the dose from 24 Gy to 20 and 18 Gy at the margin to find a dose that would create smaller amount of transient acute MRI changes to further refine our GKS technique. However, we observed that this reduction in the dose also caused a significant decrease in the rate of seizure cessation. We currently use 24 Gy for MTLE and recently reviewed our long-term follow-up data of our first 15 patients who were operated by GKS for MTLE

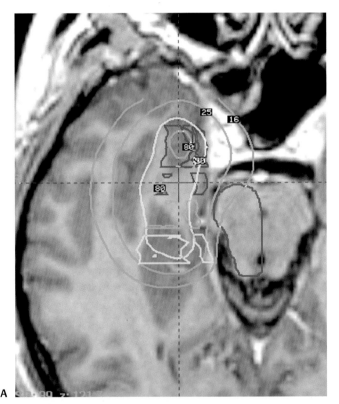

A

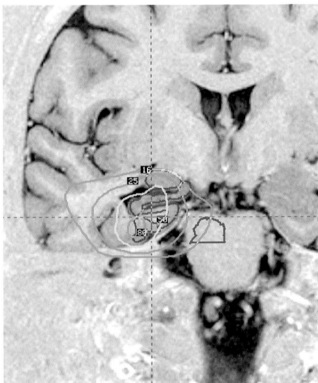

B

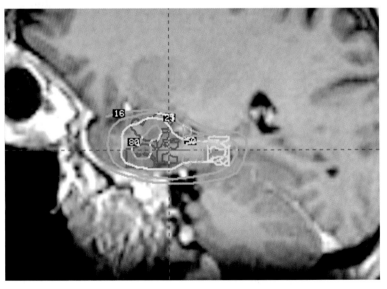

C

Fig. 35.1 Gamma Knife radiosurgery planning for a right mesial temporal lobe epilepsy with axial **(A)**, coronal **(B)**, and sagittal **(C)** images. The dose is 24 Gy at the 50% isodose line (yellow). Doses to the brainstem are less than 12 Gy (25%), and the dose to the optic chiasm less than 8 Gy (16%). Complete seizure cessation occurred 12 months after radiosurgery with no complication and no (even transient) side effects.

at the state of the art (24 Gy). The mean follow-up in this group was 8 years and the seizure-free outcome rate was 73%, which is comparable with open surgery. We found no permanent neurological deficit except some visual field deficits in nine patients.[27]

We inform our patients before the procedure regarding the delayed efficacy of radiosurgery as its main drawback and define the typical course of the seizures after GKS treatment in three stages: no significant change in seizure frequency for the first few months, then a rapid and dramatic increase in auras for several days or weeks, and finally disappearance of the seizures. We observed that seizure cessation mostly occurred around the 8th to 18th month, although it may occur as late as 26 months after GKS, as we saw in one patient. We usually consider minimum duration after radiosurgery to assess the effect of GKS as 2 years. We observed the same pattern of MRI changes in all our patients unrelated to the amount of marginal dose (18–24 Gy) and volume of treatment (5–8.5 mL). However, the degree of these changes and the delay in their onset may vary according to the dose delivered to the margin, the volume treated, and the individual patient. If there is no or minimal initial radiological changes or clinical benefit, then the recommendation is to wait for the onset of the MRI changes and their subsequent disappearance. To allow an optimal evaluation, we recommend that subsequent microsurgery should not be considered before the third year after radiosurgery. If this is the case, then the reason for the treatment failure should be investigated carefully. We identified likely causes for GKS failure based on our file review as follows:

1. Poor patient selection (e.g., patients with epilepsy involving more than the MTL structures),
2. Too early surgical intervention with a diagnosis of "treatment failure" (< 3 years after radiosurgery),[28]
3. Targeting the amygdala and hippocampus instead of parahippocampal cortex,[29] and
4. Insufficient dosage.[28–30]

Dose

Initially the targets in functional GKS radiosurgery (capsulotomy, thalamotomy of ventral intermediate (VIM) or the centromedian nuclei, pallidotomy) were treated using a high dose (300–150 Gy nuclei) delivered in very small volumes (3–5 mm in diameter).[31] Then Barcia-Salorio et al documented a small and heterogeneous group of patients treated with different types of radiosurgical techniques and variable dosimetry according to the patient.[32] Some of these patients were treated with very large volumes and very low dosage (approximately 10 Gy). These results led several other teams to consider using very low doses, as low as 10 Gy to 20 Gy at the margin, but to expect the same efficacy as the 24 Gy protocol (at the margin). This was the dose that we used for our

first series of patients with MTLE.[14] However the real rate of seizure cessation was only 36% (4/11) among the 11 patients reported by Barcia-Salorio et al, and this was much lower than what we would expect with resection in MTLE.[32,33] In another study, Yang et al confirmed that only a very low rate of seizure control is achieved when low doses (from 9 to 13 Gy at the margin) are used based on the result of a heterogeneous group of 176 patients.[30] Again, a recent de-escalation study has demonstrated poorer results in patients receiving doses of 18 or 20 Gy at the margin compared with 24 Gy.[17,34] This finding is significant because any radiosurgical strategy associated with a much lower rate of seizure cessation in MTLE is unacceptable because of the high rate of seizure freedom achievable by surgical resection. Fractionated stereotactically guided radiotherapy was used by Grabenbauer et al in 12 patients; none of the patients become seizure free and only seizure reduction has been obtained in this series.[35,36]

Target

If the radiosurgical target is a lesion, then it can be precisely defined radiologically and the question of the selection of the marginal dose can be quite easily addressed by correlating safety and efficacy with individual outcome to the marginal dose and can be refined based on stratification according to volume, location, age, etc. However, this is not the case in patients presenting with MTLE for two reasons: there is no consensus regarding the required extent of mesial temporal lobe resection for good seizure control, and the concept of MTLE syndrome with a stable extent of the epileptogenic zone that can be defined as surgical target is controversial.[37,38] The volume, in association with marginal dose, is well known to be a major determinant of the tissue effect in radiosurgery, as shown in integrated risk/dose volume formulas.[39] Therefore, target determination is critical in the effectiveness of GKS in MTLE patients. In the first series of patients we treated, our marginal isodose volume was ~7mL (range 5–8.5 mL). In a recent published study, authors tried to correlate dose/volume, degree of MRI changes, and seizure control rates.[34] In this study, it was shown that the higher the dose and the volume were, the higher the risk was of having more severe MRI changes, as well as the higher the chance was of achieving seizure cessation. It is clear that efficacious dose-planning strategies with smaller prescription isodose volumes need more precise definition of the essential targets in mesial temporal lobe. However this is a difficult task. There is growing evidence in the current literature that defines the organization of the epileptogenic zone as a network. According to this hypothesis, epileptogenic zone includes several different and possibly distant structures that discharge simultaneously at the onset of the electroclinical seizures. This perspective helps to explain the high failure risk in a simple lesionectomy without preoperative investigations in the management of severe drug-resistant epilepsies associated with a benign lesion.[40] This has been also reported in MTLE cases.[37,38] Therefore precise definition of target in radiosurgery is very critical. Wieser et al analyzed the postoperative MRIs of patients who were operated by Yasargil and had amygdalohippocampectomy.[41] In this study, they were able to correlate the degree of the resection of each substructure of the mesial temporal lobe and correlate the result with the seizure outcome.[41] They reported that only the resection amount of the anterior parahippocampal cortex was correlated strongly with a higher chance of seizure cessation.[41] We also tried to perform a similar study in patients treated with GKS radiosurgery.[34]

Patient Selection

In a previously published study, Whang and Kwon reported seizure cessation in only 38% (12/31) of the patients who were treated for epilepsy associated with slowly growing lesions.[42] This observation as well as the arguments we summarized previously emphasizes the importance of preoperative definition of the extent of the epileptic zone and its relationship with the lesion.[40,43] Therefore, the philosophy in our institution is to choose appropriate investigation techniques and management strategies in each case individually. In some patients, the electroclinical data, structural and functional imaging, and neuropsychological examination may be sufficiently concordant, and surgery of the temporal lobe is proposed without depth electrode recording. In other cases, preoperative assessment results may be discordant to define MTLE reliably, and a stereoelectroencephalographic (stereo-EEG) study is performed. Stereo-EEG implantation is used to assess the reliability of the primary hypothesis (mesial epileptogenic zone) or alternative hypothesis (early involvement of the temporal pole, lateral cortex, basal cortex, insular cortex, or other cortical areas). The purpose is to record the patient's habitual seizures to define the temporo-spatial pattern of cortical involvement during these seizures. In these patients, depth electrode recording allows us precise tailoring of the extent of surgical resection according to the temporo-spatial course of the seizures. Furthermore, if depth electrode investigation enables us to define a particular subtype of MTLE, then further tailoring of the treatment volume, even reducing it, becomes feasible. Because the main limitation of radiosurgery is the size of the target (prescription isodose volume), the requirement for precision and accuracy to define the epileptogenic zone is higher in this technique. Although this requirement makes the GKS planning for MTLE very challenging, it also makes it the most selective surgical therapy modality for this patient group.

Complications

It is well known that the radiotherapy in young patients has been associated with a significant rate of cognitive de-

cline[44,45] and tumorogenesis,[46] including some carcinogenesis.[47] However, such reported cases[48-50] are extremely rare and frequently do not meet the classic criteria to define the tumors as radiation induced.[51] Even if this risk exists, it is most likely approximately 1/10 000, which is far lower than the mortality risk associated with temporal lobectomy.[52-56] Epilepsy may cause sudden unexplained death in epileptic patients, and the death rate among epilepsy patients is higher than in the general population.[57,58] This risk is especially higher in patients treated with more than two antiepileptic drugs and with a lower IQ (<70). The surgical treatment of epilepsy provides a possibility of immediate seizure cessation and reduces the mortality risk to that of the general population.[58] Conversely, this risk persists for a longer period of time in the patients who received GKS treatment because of the delayed benefits of radiosurgical treatment in the epilepsy patient. Therefore, we systematically inform our patients about this disadvantage of radiosurgery.

Current Indications

Radiosurgery for MTLE is still an investigational treatment. The advantages of radiosurgery are the comfort and noninvasiveness of the procedure; avoiding general anesthesia and surgical complications, including mortality; the very short hospital stay; and, finally, the immediate return to the previous function level and employment. Whether or not radiosurgery provides a better result in sparing memory function is still a matter of debate and needs to be confirmed with further comparative studies. Long-term efficacy and safety of radiosurgery also needs to be documented. Microsurgical management of MTLE provides very satisfactory results because of the rarity of surgical complications and the high rate of seizure freedom. Therefore, the most appropriate treatment modality should be chosen carefully, and the patient should clearly understand the advantages, disadvantages, and limitations of both modalities. The patient should be able to understand the limits and constraints of radiosurgery very well. In our opinion, the most important selection parameter for GKS is the demonstration of the purely mesial location of the epileptogenic zone. Another good candidate for GKS is the patient with proven MTLE who has had a surgical failure because of insufficient extent of resection. Overall, the best candidates are young patients with moderately severe epilepsy, socially well-adapted people with a high functioning level and quite a high risk of memory deficit with open surgery (such as MTLE on the dominant side with a subtle hippocampal atrophy and slight preoperative deficit in verbal memory). Postoperative memory deficit exposes these patients to potentially huge social and professional consequences; therefore, GKS constitutes a very good alternative treatment modality for this patient group.

◼ Hypothalamic Hamartomas

HHs are rare, congenital heterotopic lesions that are intrinsically epileptogenic when closely connected to the mammillary bodies.[59,60] Patients classically present with gelastic seizures during the first years of life.[61] In the more severe forms of the disease, affected patients develop an epileptic encephalopathy during the following years that is characterized by drug resistance, various types of seizures including generalized seizures and drop attacks,[61] cognitive decline,[62–64] and severe psychiatric co-morbidity.[65] Usually the seizures begin early in life and are often particularly drug resistant from the onset. Commonly, seizure semiology suggests the involvement of temporal or frontal lobe region and even secondary epileptogenesis. HHs may also be asymptomatic or associated with precocious puberty, associated with neurological disorders (including epilepsy, behavior disturbances, and cognitive impairment), or both.

The natural history is unfavorable in the majority of the patients because of behavioral symptoms (particularly aggressive behavior) and mental decline, which occur as a direct effect of the seizures.[66] Interestingly, in our experience, the reversal of these behavioral symptoms after radiosurgery appears to begin even before complete cessation of the seizures and appears to be correlated to the improvement in background EEG activity. It is the authors' speculation that these continuous discharges lead to the disorganization of several systems, including the limbic system, and that their disappearance accounts for the improvement seen in attention, memory, cognitive performance, and impulsive behavior. In these cases, the role of radiosurgery in the reversal of the behavioral symptoms may be as or more important than its effect on decreasing seizure occurrence. Consequently, we consider that it is essential to operate on these young patients as early as possible, whatever the surgical approach considered (resection or radiosurgery).

Even though the first successful and safe removal of an HH was reported by Paillas et al in 1969,[59] the interest for the surgical cure of this specific group of patients developed only in the 1990s. According to Valdueza et al, epilepsy in HH is observed only in medium/large sessile HH broadly attached to tuber cinereum or mammillary body.[67] The microsurgical resection in this critical area is related to a significant risk of oculomotor palsy, hemiparesis, and visual field deficit.[68,69] The first clinical series evaluating microsurgical resection using pterional and midline frontal approaches did not emphasize complications.[67,70–73] However, in 2002, Palmini and coworkers analyzed the patients with HH who were treated in several of the best centers for epilepsy surgery around the world, and they reported severe complications after microsurgical resection in 7 of 13 patients.[74] These complications included four thalamocapsular infarcts with contralateral hemiplegia, transient third nerve paresis in four subjects, a central diabetes insipidus, and a nonreversible hyperpha-

gia.[74] Conversely, they also confirmed the efficacy of surgery in this pathological condition. More specifically, 3 patients showed complete seizure cessation and the remaining 10 subjects had more than 90% reduction in the frequency of their seizures.

The rationale for the application of disconnective surgeries in the treatment of HH is that the lesion is not a neoplasm, and its removal is therefore not mandatory. Another factor favoring disconnection technique is the possibility of avoiding the complications that may occur during the dissection in the cisterns, a maneuver necessary for the microsurgical resection. Delalande et al[68] actually stressed this point as favoring the simple disconnection of an HH instead of its complete excision because of the occurrence of severe complications in their first patient. When the clinical result is not satisfactory and the upper part of the lesion is mainly in the third ventricle, Delalande proposed a second step via an endoscopic approach to the third ventricle. In 2003, the same author published a series of 17 patients with a follow-up between 1 month and 5.4 years.[68] A second intervention (usually endoscopic) was necessary in 8 patients. In this excellent series, 47% of the patients (8 of 17) were seizure free, including three patients who were operated on twice. The author reported some permanent severe complications, namely, one case of hemiplegia, one case of hemiparesis, two cases of hyperphagia, one case of panhypopituitarism, one case of hypothyroidism, and another case with growth hormone deficiency. Transient morbidity included one case of meningitis and two cases of diabetes insipidus. In addition, the author reported a postoperative frontal lobe ischemic complication, which was apparently asymptomatic. In conclusion, only six patients (35%) were seizure free with no permanent deficit. Contrary to the other reports describing the results with transcallosal approach, Delalande did not observe any memory deficit. Finally, the author observed a correlation between completeness of disconnection and control of the seizures.

We retrospectively analyzed the results of radiosurgical management in a series of 10 HH patients collected from centers around the world.[75] The excellent safety–efficacy ratio (all improved, 50% cured, and no adverse effects except one case of poikilothermia) in this series led us to organize a prospective multicenter trial. In this trial, we prospectively evaluated 55 patients and published the results in a preliminary report.[60] In this study, preoperative cognitive deficits and behavioral disturbances were investigated, and the relationship of seizure severity and anatomical type as well as cognitive abilities were characterized.[62] The goal of the preoperative workup was to adequately select the candidates for inclusion and to evaluate the baseline neurological and endocrinological functions. All radiosurgical procedures were performed using the Leksell 201-source Cobalt 60 Gamma Knife (Elekta Instrument, Stockholm, Sweden). We consistently used multi-isocentric complex dose planning of high conformity and selectivity. We also used low peripheral doses to take into account the close relationship with optic pathways and hypothalamus (median 17 Gy; range 13 to 26 Gy). We paid special attention to the dose delivered to the mamillary body and to the fornix, and we tried to tailor the dose plan for each patient on the basis of the use of a single run of shots with the 4-mm collimator. The lesions were generally small (median 9.5 mm; range 5–26). Patients were evaluated with respect to seizures, cognition, behavior, and endocrine status at 6, 12, 18, 24, and 36 months after radiosurgery and then every year. There was satisfactory follow-up for 27 patients. Among these patients, 10 were seizure free (37%) and 6 were very much improved (22.2%) with a significant seizure reduction (usually only rare residual gelastic seizures) associated with a dramatic behavioral and cognitive improvement. Overall, an excellent result was obtained in 60% of the patients. According to our policy, the patient and the family are offered a second radiosurgery in case of partial benefit when the lesion is anatomically small and well defined. Five patients (18.5%) with small hamartomas were only modestly improved and are being considered for a second session of radiosurgery. Two of them reported no significant improvement until now. A microsurgical approach has been performed in 4 patients (14.8%) with quite large HH and poor efficacy of radiosurgery. Of these patients,

2 are cured and 2 failed to respond. The radiosurgical treatment has been performed twice in 9 patients.

HH Classification and Treatment Strategy

Topological classification of the lesion is a key feature in the decision-making process[60] (**Fig. 35.2**). This should be done based on a good, high-resolution MRI study. Previous classifications have been based on anatomical[76-78] or surgical[76] considerations. These classifications failed to describe the large diversity of these lesions and their therapeutic consequences. As underlined by Palmini and coworkers, the exact location of the lesion and its relation with interpeduncular fossa and third ventricle walls is critical. These topographical characteristics correlate with the extent of excision, seizure control, and complication rate.[12] Because of this, we classify the HH according to its topology based on our original classification.[45] In our experience, this classification correlates very well with the clinical semiology and its severity. It is especially critical for determining the appropriate surgical strategy. According to this classification, six types of HH have been described.

Type I lesions correspond to small HHs located inside the hypothalamus that also extend more or less in the third ventricle. This group includes the best candidates for GKS,

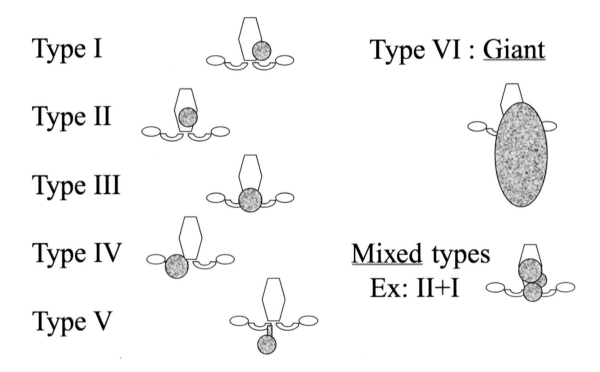

Fig. 35.2 Classification of hypothalamic hamartomas into these five categories based on magnetic resonance imaging findings resulted in a clear correlation between symptoms and the subsequent clinical course and is pertinent for clinical management.[60]

because the morbidity of microsurgical removal in this group of patient is potentially high.

In type II, the lesions are small and mainly located in the third ventricle. Radiosurgery is again certainly a safer alternative in this group of patients (**Fig. 35.3**). Even though the endoscopic and transcallosal interforniceal approaches have been well described, the risks of short-term memory worsening, endocrinological disturbance (hyperphagia with obesity, low thyroxin, sodium metabolism disturbance), and thalamic or thalamocapsular infarcts have been reported even in the hands of highly skilled and experience neurosurgeons. However, in exceptional cases with a very severe recurrent status epilepticus, we still recommend open surgery through either a transcallosal interforniceal approach or an endoscopic approach for these patients. If the lesion is small and the third ventricle is large, then an endoscopic approach is a reasonable option.

In type III, the lesions are located essentially in the floor, and we prefer GKS for these patients because of the extremely close relationship between the mammillary body the fornix and the lesion. We believe that sessile HHs always more or less have an extension into the hypothalamus close to the mammillary body. Thus, when a lesion is classified as a type II or III, that means that the lesion appears on the MRI as being located in the third ventricle and is likely to have a root in the hypothalamus.

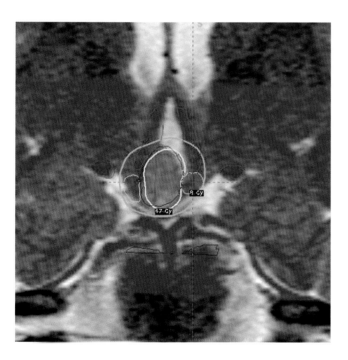

Fig. 35.3 Radiosurgery planning for a hypothalamic hamartoma, type II, according to our original classification. The marginal isodose (17 Gy) is displayed in yellow. The green line corresponds to the 25% isodose line and is illustrating the very good fall-off of the dose gradient. Five months after radiosurgery, seizures have disappeared completely and there are no magnetic resonance imaging changes.

In type IV, the lesion is generally sessile in the cistern, and surgical disconnection can be preferred using pterional approach with or without orbitozygomatic osteotomy. However, if the lesion is small, GKS can be recommended because of its safety and its ability to simultaneously treat the small associated part of the lesion in the hypothalamus itself that is frequently visible on the high-resolution MRI. In Delalande's series, only two patients among 14 are seizure free after a single disconnection through a pterional approach.[76] Consequently, we only recommend this approach in the cases with too large lesions for GKS and as a first step of a staged approach. In most circumstances, the patient is improved but stays still not seizure free after the first surgical step and GKS is planned at 3 months as a second step in the treatment of these cases.

Type V constitutes a group of lesions with pedicle. These lesions are rarely epileptic and can be easily cured by radiosurgery or disconnection through a pterional approach. In cases of severe epilepsy, surgical disconnection will certainly allow a faster seizure cessation than GKS. However, a distant extension of the lesion in the hypothalamus must be cautiously searched on high-resolution MRI, because the presence of an extension close to the mammillary bodies will eventually lead to recommending GKS that would provide treatment for both parts of the lesion. This is especially true in cases in which the cisternal component is small.

Type VI includes giant HHs. These patients are not good candidates for up-front radiosurgery, and a combination of several therapeutic modalities should be used in nearly all cases. Even if GKS does not appear to be suitable when the lesion is large, radiosurgical disconnection can be considered. The result of radiosurgical targeting of only the superior part of the lesion located in the hypothalamus or the third ventricle and leaving the lower part of the lesion below the floor untreated has been uniformly disappointing. In our opinion, this strategy may result in a loss of a precious developmental stage of a child, and we do not recommending this approach. Again a staged approach can be considered if microsurgical resection leaves a small remnant in the third ventricle, and the patient is still not seizure free. We do recommend GKS in these patients as well.

Effect of GKS on Behavior and Cognitive Functions

We observed dramatic improvement in nine of our patients. All patients with paroxysmal aggressivity improved substantially, and some patients who previously exhibited excessive behavioral inhibition experienced increased alertness, elevated mood, and greater speech production. A positive effect on sleep was frequently reported by the parents. Finally, dramatic developmental acceleration was observed in three young patients. Because of the very critical location of these lesions, we always try to tailor the dose plan for each patient individually, based on the use of a single run of shots with the 4-mm collimator, and we pay special attention to the dose delivered to the mamillary body and to the fornix. The early effect on subclinical EEG discharges appears to play a major role in the dramatic benefit to sleep quality, behavior, and cognitive developmental improvement. GKS can safely lead to the reversal of the epileptic encephalopathy.

Limits and Strengths of Radiosurgery in HH

Although significant progress has been made in the management of HH, two major questions remain: First, we know that complete treatment or resection of the lesion is not always necessary for seizure control,[79–81] but we still do not know how to predict the amount of the HH that must be treated to obtain a complete seizure control in each patient. The second question is related to the extent of the involvement of epileptogenic zone, because these patients frequently present with electrical and clinical–semiological findings suggestive for involvement of the temporal or frontal lobe.[82,83] In our experience, although some of these patients can be completely cured by the isolated treatment of the HH, incomplete results are obtained with persisting residual seizures in some others, despite significant psychiatric and cognitive improvement.

Our initial results indicate that GKS is as effective as microsurgical resection in the management of HH patients, with reduced morbidity. GKS also avoids the risks seen with radiofrequency lesioning or stimulation. The disadvantage of radiosurgery is again its delayed action; therefore, longer follow-up is mandatory for proper evaluation of the effectiveness of GKS in this patient group. Results are faster and more complete in a subset of patients with smaller lesions located inside the III ventricle (type II). Because of the poor clinical prognosis of a majority of patients with HH and the invasiveness of microsurgical resection, GKS can now be considered as a first-line intervention for small- to medium-sized HH associated with epilepsy. However, the role of secondary epileptogenesis or of widespread cortical dysgenesis in these patients needs to be further evaluated and understood to optimize patient selection and define the best treatment strategy.

■ Cavernous Malformations

Cavernous malformations (CMs) are congenital vascular malformations of the brain. They may cause hemorrhage and neurological deficits, but the most frequent presenting symptom is epilepsy.[84] The epileptogenicity of these lesions results from the ongoing deposition of iron and blood products at the margin of the lesion.[85] The incidence of medically refractory epilepsy associated with these lesions is not well

known. However, in one large recent series, 40% of patients with a supratentorial CM presented with medically refractory epilepsy.[86] GKS treatment of CMs is a controversial topic, and only a few studies are available, with conflicting results concerning GKS's effect on protection from hemorrhage.[87–90] Because of the relatively high rate of radiation-induced side effects[87] of radiation therapy and the safety and efficacy of microsurgical excision,[85] the latter technique is usually recommended for this indication. Nevertheless, the risk of bleeding secondary to CM is different based on the lesion location, and a low risk of clinical bleeding[91] is associated with CMs located in cortical/subcortical sites as opposed to deep-seated lesions. Therefore, the main indication for surgery in these lesions is frequently seizure control, and microsurgery is considered the best treatment in patients with intractable epilepsy. However, in some series, a beneficial effect of GKS was also reported for seizures secondary to supratentorial CMs.[88] Because GKS is usually associated with a minimal risk of injury to the surrounding nontarget neural tissue, this technique could be a good alternative for these patients, particularly when the CM is located in a brain region associated with a high surgical risk.

The effectiveness of GKS in the management of medically refractory seizures associated with CMs has been evaluated in a retrospective multicenter study (Marseille, France; Graz, Austria; Komaki, Japan; Sheffield, England; and Prague, Czech Republic).[40] Forty-nine patients with cortical/subcortical CMs with severe long-term drug-resistant epilepsy were included and had been followed for more than 1 year after GKS. The mean duration of epilepsy before GKS procedures was 7.5 (±9.3) years. The mean frequency of seizures was 6.9/month (±14). The mean marginal radiation dose was 19.17 Gy ± 4.4. Among the 49 patients, 35% had a CM located in or adjacent to a highly functional area. Follow-up examinations revealed 53% seizure-free outcome (Engel's Class I), including 49% in Class IA and 4% of the patients with occasional auras. A highly significant decrease in the number of seizures was also achieved in an additional 20% of the patients (Class II). The remaining 26% patients showed little or no improvement. The mediotemporal site was associated with a higher risk of failure in these patients. One patient had hemorrhage during the observation period, and another experienced radiation-induced edema with transient aphasia. Postradiosurgery excision was performed in five patients, and a second radiosurgical treatment was performed in one patient.

Prognostic Factors

Type of seizure and location of the CM were found to be important prognostic factors. The outcome was better for patients with simple partial seizures than for those with complex partial seizures. Location of the CM, which is probably related to the type of seizure, appeared to be the most valuable prognostic factor. Location in the mesial temporal region was associated with a poor outcome (12 of 14 patients), whereas location in the lateral temporal region was associated with a good outcome (6 of 7 patients). Location in the central region was also associated with an excellent outcome; all four patients in this group were seizure free. Results were unpredictable for other locations. The morbidity was found to be low. Radiologically, seven patients presented major reactional edema during the first year after GKS. In two of these patients, there were clinical manifestations with severe hemiparesis and speech impairment, but both patients fully recovered during the follow-up period.

Management Strategy

Management strategy for CM is complex, but the general consensus is that microsurgical resection of the lesion is the best treatment for patients with intractable epilepsy. Two surgical strategies can be applied, depending on the date of onset and features of the seizures.[92] For patients with recent onset seizures and with good correlation between symptoms and location of the CM, lesionectomy is the best method. Epilepsy surgery strategies should be preferred for patients with a long history of chronic epilepsy in whom correlation of clinical and EEG findings are unclear. In these cases, a multimodal approach including invasive techniques should be considered. In this context, surgery should aim to control epilepsy rather than to remove the lesion. The appropriate use or nonuse of these criteria probably explains why the success rate for surgical excision of CM varies from 20 to 80% in the literature.[85,86,91–99] The effect of GK surgery on epilepsy in patients with CM is probably quite different than its effect on the prevention of bleeding. Of the 11 patients presenting with intractable epilepsy before GKS in the series of Kida et al, 7 patients (65%) achieved good seizure control after GKS even though there was no apparent change in the size of the CM.[88] The apparent size of a CM appears to fluctuate and depend on the production and absorption of blood pigments.

Although a reliable prospective study with long-term follow-up is still needed, this retrospective series indicates that GKS can be effective for seizure control in CM patients with a low morbidity. It should be emphasized that the GKS procedure targets the lesion and immediate surrounding tissue. With this approach, the results observed in this study were comparable with those reported in the recent literature for lesionectomy.[85,86,91 99] The most valuable prognostic factor for seizure outcome after GKS was lesion location. A probable explanation for this finding is that the relationship between the lesion and the epileptogenic zone is particularly more intimate in certain regions. This is especially true for simple partial motor seizures associated with CMs in the rolandic region. By contrast, when a CM is located in the

mesial temporal region, a more complex organization probably accounts for the extended epileptogenic zone, and epilepsy surgery strategies should be preferred in these cases. This probably explains why patients with complex partial seizures have a less favorable outcome than patients with simple partial seizures in our study.

We lack convincing data concerning the efficacy of GKS in the prevention of bleeding risk associated with CMs. Early authors reported no effect.[87,88,90] Recently, some authors have reported a decrease in bleeding 2 years after GKS,[89,100] but the majority reported no effect. Thus, the role of radiosurgery in the management of these lesions remains controversial.[89] Moreover, in some studies, the incidence of radiation-induced complications was particularly high after radiosurgery of the CM.[87,101] This is perhaps explained by poor radiological localization and available dose-planning software at that time. This problem was countered by the use of a lower radiation dose than is usually applied for other vascular targets.

■ Technical Questions

Target Definition

Some articles reporting microsurgical resection of occult malformations suggest that resection of the hemosiderin-stained tissue surrounding the lesion is critical for eliminating seizures.[102] Obviously, the reason for seizure cessation is not the dose received by the margin of the target (even if defined generously) but the ionizing radiation received by the epileptogenic zone located close to the CM. The aim of management of patients with cavernomas who present with a major hemorrhage is to control and prevent future hemorrhages, and the best method is usually microsurgery. However, for patients presenting with seizures arising from eloquent cortex surrounding the lesion, GK treatment appears to be a suitable alternative. It is essential that close electroclinical correlation be established for this strategy to work. Microsurgical excision remains the preferred approach for cortical/subcortical epileptogenic CMs that are not located in functional cortex. Considering that image-guided microsurgical excision can be performed safely for the majority of patients, a comparative prospective trial is necessary to establish the possible role of GKS for this indication.

Dose Selection

Various doses have been tested in experimental studies on animals[23,103,104] and clinical experience with GKS on epileptic lesions.[75,105,106] There is clearly a relationship between dose and effectiveness on seizures. Depending on the dose, animals undergo seizure cessation, seizure reduction, no change, or worsening of epilepsy.[104] Dose selection is obviously crucial for clinical control of seizures. We consider that, at present, satisfactory evidence is lacking for recommendation of the systematic use of GKS for cortical/subcortical CM associated with drug-resistant epilepsy. Although the result of this series is very encouraging, the aim of this chapter is not to promote widespread use of GKS. Our main interest is to gain insight into the relationships between dose selection, target volume, and effectiveness on epilepsy in this unique population.

■ Conclusion

The field of epilepsy surgery is a new and promising one for radiosurgery. However, determination of the extent of the epileptogenic zone, which is crucial to achieve a reasonable rate of seizure cessation, requires specific expertise. In addition, the huge impact of fine technical detail on the efficacy and eventual toxicity of the procedure means that, at present, its use for these indications remains under investigation, and further prospective work remains necessary.

References

1. Flickinger JC, Kondziolka D, Lunsford LD. Clinical applications of stereotactic radiosurgery. Cancer Treat Res 1998;93:283–297
2. Talairach J, Bancaud J, Szikla G, et al. Approche nouvelle de la neurochirurgie de l'epilepsie. Méthodologie stéréotaxique et résultats thérapeutiques. Neurochirurgie 1974;20 (suppl 1):1–240
3. Elomaa E. Focal irradiation of the brain: an alternative to temporal lobe resection in intractable focal epilepsy? Med Hypotheses 1980;6(5):501–503
4. Baudouin M, Stuhl L, Perrard A. Un cas d'épilepsie focale traité par la radiothérapie. Rev Neurol 1951;84:60–63
5. Von Wieser W. Die Roentgentherapie der traumatischen Epilepsie. Mschr Psychiat Neurol 1939;101:422–424
6. Heikkinen ER, Konnov B, Melnikov L, et al. Relief of epilepsy by radiosurgery of cerebral arteriovenous malformations. Stereotact Funct Neurosurg 1989;53(3):157–166
7. Rogers LR, Morris HH, Lupica K. Effect of cranial irradiation on seizure frequency in adults with low-grade astrocytoma and medically intractable epilepsy. Neurology 1993;43(8):1599–1601
8. Rossi GF, Scerrati M, Roselli R. Epileptogenic cerebral low-grade tumors: effect of interstitial stereotactic irradiation on seizures. Appl Neurophysiol 1985;48(1–6):127–132
9. Barcia Salorio JL, Roldan P, Hernandez G, Lopez Gomez L. Radiosurgical treatment of epilepsy. Appl Neurophysiol 1985;48(1–6):400–403
10. Gaffey CT, Montoya VJ, Lyman JT, Howard J. Restriction of the spread of epileptic discharges in cats by means of Bragg peak, intracranial irradiation. Int J Appl Radiat Isot 1981;32(11):779–784
11. Chen ZF, Kamiryo T, Henson SL, et al. Anticonvulsant effects of gamma surgery in a model of chronic spontaneous limbic epilepsy in rats. J Neurosurg 2001;94(2):270–280
12. Maesawa S, Kondziolka D, Dixon CE, Balzer J, Fellows W, Lunsford LD. Subnecrotic stereotactic radiosurgery controlling epilepsy produced by kainic acid injection in rats. J Neurosurg 2000;93(6):1033–1040
13. Régis J, Peragui JC, Rey M, et al. First selective amygdalohippocampal radiosurgery for 'mesial temporal lobe epilepsy.' Stereotact Funct Neurosurg 1995;64(suppl 1):193–201
14. Régis J, Bartolomei F, Rey M, et al. Gamma knife surgery for mesial temporal lobe epilepsy. Epilepsia 1999;40(11):1551–1556
15. Régis J, Rey M, Bartolomei F, et al. Gamma knife surgery in mesial temporal lobe epilepsy: a prospective multicenter study. Epilepsia 2004;45(5):504–515
16. Regis J, Semah F, Bryan RN, et al. Early and delayed MR and PET changes after selective temporomesial radiosurgery in mesial temporal lobe epilepsy. AJNR Am J Neuroradiol 1999;20(2):213–216
17. Hayashi M, Régis J, Hori T. [Current treatment strategy with gamma knife surgery for mesial temporal lobe epilepsy]. No Shinkei Geka 2003;31(2):141–155
18. Regis J, Levivier M, Hayashi M. Radiosurgery for intractable Epilepsy. Tech Neurosurg 2003;9(3):191–203
19. Régis J, Bartolomei F, Hayashi M, Chauvel P. Gamma Knife surgery, a neuromodulation therapy in epilepsy surgery! Acta Neurochir Suppl 2002;84:37–47
20. Yang I, Barbaro NM. Advances in the radiosurgical treatment of epilepsy. Epilepsy Curr 2007;7(2):31–35
21. Régis J, Bartolomei F, Hayashi M, Roberts D, Chauvel P, Peragut JC. The role of gamma knife surgery in the treatment of severe epilepsies. Epileptic Disord 2000;2(2):113–122
22. Régis Y, Roberts DW. Gamma Knife radiosurgery relative to microsurgery: epilepsy. Stereotact Funct Neurosurg 1999;72(suppl 1):11–21
23. Régis J, Kerkerian-Legoff L, Rey M, et al. First biochemical evidence of differential functional effects following Gamma Knife surgery. Stereotact Funct Neurosurg 1996;66(suppl 1):29–38
24. Rheims S, Fischer C, Ryvlin P, et al. Long-term outcome of gamma-knife surgery in temporal lobe epilepsy. Epilepsy Res 2008;80(1):23–29
25. Régis J, Hayashi M. The dose selection issue in epilepsy surgery. In: International Stereotactic Radiosurgery Symposium. Kyoto, Japan: Karper; 2003:190–196
26. Régis J, Bartolomei F, Rey M, Hayashi M, Chauvel P, Peragut JC. Gamma knife surgery for mesial temporal lobe epilepsy. J Neurosurg 2000;93(suppl 3):141–146
27. Bartolomei F, Hayashi M, Tamura M, et al. Long-term efficacy of gamma knife radiosurgery in mesial temporal lobe epilepsy. Neurology 2008;70(19):1658–1663
28. Cmelak AJ, Abou-Khalil B, Konrad PE, Duggan D, Maciunas RJ. Low-dose stereotactic radiosurgery is inadequate for medically intractable mesial temporal lobe epilepsy: a case report. Seizure 2001;10(6):442–446
29. Kawai K, Suzuki I, Kurita H, Shin M, Arai N, Kirino T. Failure of low-dose radiosurgery to control temporal lobe epilepsy. J Neurosurg 2001;95(5):883–887
30. Yang KJ, Wang KW, Wu HP, Qi ST. Radiosurgical treatment of intractable epilepsy with low radiation dose. Di Yi Jun Yi Da Xue Xue Bao 2002;22(7):645–647
31. Lindquist C, Kihlström L, Hellstrand E. Functional neurosurgery—a future for the gamma knife? Stereotact Funct Neurosurg 1991;57(1–2):72–81

32. Barcia-Salorio JL, Barcia JA, Hernández G, López-Gómez L. Radiosurgery of epilepsy. Long-term results. Acta Neurochir Suppl 1994;62:111–113

33. Barcia Salorio JL, et al. Radiosurgery in epilepsy and neuronal plasticity. Adv Neurol 1999; 81:299–305

34. Hayashi M, et al. MR changes after gamma knife radiosurgery for mesial temporal lobe epilepsy: an evidence for the efficacy of subnecrotic doses. In: Kondziolka D, ed. Radiosurgery. Basel, Switzerland: Karger; 2002:192–202

35. Grabenbauer GG, Reinhold Ch, Kerling F, et al. Fractionated stereotactically guided radiotherapy of pharmacoresistant temporal lobe epilepsy. Acta Neurochir Suppl (Wien) 2002;84:65–70

36. Stefan H, Hummel C, Grabenbauer GG, et al. Successful treatment of focal epilepsy by fractionated stereotactic radiotherapy. Eur Neurol 1998;39(4):248–250

37. Bartolomei F, Wendling F, Bellanger JJ, Régis J, Chauvel P. Neural networks involving the medial temporal structures in temporal lobe epilepsy. Clin Neurophysiol 2001;112(9):1746–1760

38. Spencer SS, Spencer DD. Entorhinal-hippocampal interactions in medial temporal lobe epilepsy. Epilepsia 1994;35(4):721–727

39. Flickinger JC. An integrated logistic formula for prediction of complications from radiosurgery. Int J Radiat Oncol Biol Phys 1989;17(4):879–885

40. Régis J, Bartolomei F, Kida Y, et al. Radiosurgery for epilepsy associated with cavernous malformation: retrospective study in 49 patients. Neurosurgery 2000;47(5):1091–1097

41. Wieser HG, Siegel AM, Yaşargil GM. The Zürich amygdalo-hippocampectomy series: a short up-date. Acta Neurochir Suppl (Wien) 1990;50:122–127

42. Whang CJ, Kwon Y. Long-term follow-up of stereotactic Gamma Knife radiosurgery in epilepsy. Stereotact Funct Neurosurg 1996;66(suppl 1):349–356

43. Kitchen N. Experimental and clinical studies on the putative therapeutic efficacy of cerebral irradiation (radiotherapy) in epilepsy. Epilepsy Res 1995;20(1):1–10

44. Glosser G, McManus P, Munzenrider J, et al. Neuropsychological function in adults after high dose fractionated radiation therapy of skull base tumors. Int J Radiat Oncol Biol Phys 1997;38(2):231–239

45. McCord MW, Buatti JM, Fennell EM, et al. Radiotherapy for pituitary adenoma: long-term outcome and sequelae. Int J Radiat Oncol Biol Phys 1997;39(2):437–444

46. Strasnick B, Glasscock ME III, Haynes D, McMenomey SO, Minor LB. The natural history of untreated acoustic neuromas. Laryngoscope 1994;104(9):1115–1119

47. Simmons NE, Laws ER Jr. Glioma occurrence after sellar irradiation: case report and review. Neurosurgery 1998;42(1):172–178

48. Kaido T, Hoshida T, Uranishi R, et al. Radiosurgery-induced brain tumor. Case report. J Neurosurg 2001;95(4):710–713

49. Shamisa A, Bance M, Nag S, et al. Glioblastoma multiforme occurring in a patient treated with gamma knife surgery. Case report and review of the literature. J Neurosurg 2001;94(5):816–821

50. Yu JS, Yong WH, Wilson D, Black KL. Glioblastoma induction after radiosurgery for meningioma. Lancet 2000;356(9241):1576–1577

51. Cahan WG, Woodard HQ, et al. Sarcoma arising in irradiated bone; report of 11 cases. Cancer 1948;1(1):3–29

52. Ganz JC. Gamma knife radiosurgery and its possible relationship to malignancy: a review. J Neurosurg 2002; 97(5, suppl):644–652

53. Rowe J, Grainger A, Walton L, Silcocks P, Radatz M, Kemeny A. Risk of malignancy after gamma knife stereotactic radiosurgery. Neurosurgery 2007;60(1):60–65, discussion 65–66

54. Muracciole X, Cowen D, Régis J. [Radiosurgery and brain radio-induced carcinogenesis: update]. Neurochirurgie 2004;50(2–3 pt 2):414–420

55. Loeffler JS, Niemierko A, Chapman PH. Second tumors after radiosurgery: tip of the iceberg or a bump in the road? Neurosurgery 2003;52(6):1436–1440, discussion 1440–1442

56. Lunsford LD, Niranjan A, Flickinger JC, Maitz A, Kondziolka D. Radiosurgery of vestibular schwannomas: summary of experience in 829 cases. J Neurosurg 2005;102(suppl):195–199

57. Ficker DM, So EL, Shen WK, et al. Population-based study of the incidence of sudden unexplained death in epilepsy. Neurology 1998;51(5):1270–1274

58. Sperling MR, Feldman H, Kinman J, Liporace JD, O'Connor MJ. Seizure control and mortality in epilepsy. Ann Neurol 1999;46(1):45–50

59. Paillas JE, Roger J, Toga M, et al. Hamarthome de l'hypothalamus. Rev Neurol 1969;120:177–194

60. Régis J, Hayashi M, Eupierre LP, et al. Gamma knife surgery for epilepsy related to hypothalamic hamartomas. Acta Neurochir Suppl (Wien) 2004;91:33–50

61. Tassinari CA, et al. Gelastic seizures. In Tuxhorn I, Holthausen H, Boenigk H, eds. Current Problems in Epilepsy. London, UK: John Libbey; 1997:429–446

62. Frattali CM, Liow K, Craig GH, et al. Cognitive deficits in children with gelastic seizures and hypothalamic hamartoma. Neurology 2001;57(1):43–46

63. Nguyen D, Singh S, Zaatreh M, et al. Hypothalamic hamartomas: seven cases and review of the literature. Epilepsy Behav 2003;4(3):246–258

64. Quiske A, Frings L, Wagner K, Unterrainer J, Schulze-Bonhage A. Cognitive functions in juvenile and adult patients with gelastic epilepsy because of hypothalamic hamartoma. Epilepsia 2006;47(1):153–158

65. Weissenberger AA, Dell ML, Liow K, et al. Aggression and psychiatric comorbidity in children with hypothalamic hamartomas and their unaffected siblings. J Am Acad Child Adolesc Psychiatry 2001;40(6):696–703

66. Deonna T, Ziegler AL. Hypothalamic hamartoma, precocious puberty and gelastic seizures: a special model of "epileptic" developmental disorder. Epileptic Disord 2000;2(1):33–37

67. Valdueza JM, Cristante L, Dammann O, et al. Hypothalamic hamartomas: with special reference to gelastic epilepsy and surgery. Neurosurgery 1994;34(6):949–958, discussion 958

68. Delalande O, Fohlen MJ, Jalin C, et al. Surgical treatment of epilepsy due to hypothalamic hamartoma: technique and preliminary results in five cases. Epilepsia 1998;39(suppl 6):90–91

69. Stewart L, Steinbok P, Daaboul J. Role of surgical resection in the treatment of hypothalamic hamartomas causing precocious puberty. Report of six cases. J Neurosurg 1998;88(2):340–345

70. Machado HR, Hoffman HJ, Hwang PA. Gelastic seizures treated by resection of a hypothalamic hamartoma. Childs Nerv Syst 1991;7(8):462–465

71. Nishio S, Fujiwara S, Aiko Y, Takeshita I, Fukui M. Hypothalamic hamartoma. Report of two cases. J Neurosurg 1989;70(4):640–645

72. Nishio S, Morioka T, Fukui M, Goto Y. Surgical treatment of intractable seizures due to hypothalamic hamartoma. Epilepsia 1994;35(3):514–519

73. Nishio S, Shigeto H, Fukui M. Hypothalamic hamartoma: the role of surgery. Neurosurg Rev 1993;16(2):157–160

74. Palmini A, Chandler C, Anderman F, et al. Resection of the lesion in patients with hypothalamic hamartomas and catastrophic epilepsy. Neurology 2002;58(9):1338–1347

75. Régis J, Bartolomei F, de Toffol B, et al. Gamma knife surgery for epilepsy related to hypothalamic hamartomas. Neurosurgery 2000;47(6):1343–1351, discussion 1351–1352

76. Delalande O, Fohlen M. Disconnecting surgical treatment of hypothalamic hamartoma in children and adults with refractory epilepsy and proposal of a new classification. Neurol Med Chir (Tokyo) 2003;43(2):61–68

77. Feiz-Erfan I, Horn EM, Rekate HL, et al. Surgical strategies for approaching hypothalamic hamartomas causing gelastic seizures in the pediatric population: transventricular compared with skull base approaches. J Neurosurg 2005; 103(4, suppl):325–332

78. Maixner W. Hypothalamic hamartomas—clinical, neuropathological and surgical aspects. Childs Nerv Syst 2006;22(8):867–873

79. Pascual-Castroviejo I, Moneo JH, Viaño J, García-Segura JM, Herguido MJ, Pascual Pascual SI. [Hypothalamic hamartomas: control of seizures after partial removal in one case]. Rev Neurol 2000;31(2):119–122

80. Rosenfeld JV, Harvey AS, Wrennall J, Zacharin M, Berkovic SF. Transcallosal resection of hypothalamic hamartomas, with control of seizures, in children with gelastic epilepsy. Neurosurgery 2001;48(1):108–118

81. Watanabe T, Enomoto T, Uemura K, Tomono Y, Nose T. [Gelastic seizures treated by partial resection of a hypothalamic hamartoma]. No Shinkei Geka 1998;26(10):923–928

82. Cascino GD, Andermann F, Berkovic SF, et al. Gelastic seizures and hypothalamic hamartomas: evaluation of patients undergoing chronic intracranial EEG monitoring and outcome of surgical treatment. Neurology 1993;43(4):747–750

83. Munari C, Kahane P, Francione S, et al. Role of the hypothalamic hamartoma in the genesis of gelastic fits (a video-stereo-EEG study). Electroencephalogr Clin Neurophysiol 1995;95(3):154–160

84. Maraire JN, Abdulrauf SI, Berger S, Knisely J, Awad IA. De novo development of a cavernous malformation of the spinal cord following spinal axis radiation. Case report. J Neurosurg 1999; 90(2, suppl):234–238

85. Maraire JN, Awad IA. Intracranial cavernous malformations: lesion behavior and management strategies. Neurosurgery 1995; 37(4):591–605

86. Casazza M, Broggi G, Franzini A, et al. Supratentorial cavernous angiomas and epileptic seizures: preoperative course and postoperative outcome. Neurosurgery 1996;39(1):26–32, discussion 32–34

87. Karlsson B, Kihlström L, Lindquist C, Ericson K, Steiner L. Radiosurgery for cavernous malformations. J Neurosurg 1998;88(2):293–297

88. Kida Y, Kobayashi T, Tanaka T. Radiosurgery of symptomatic angiographically occult vascular malformations with Gamma Knife. In: Radiosurgery. Kondziolka D, ed. Basel, Switzerland: Karger; 1995:207–217

89. Kondziolka D, Lunsford LD, Flickinger JC, Kestle JR. Reduction of hemorrhage risk after stereotactic radiosurgery for cavernous malformations. J Neurosurg 1995;83(5):825–831

90. Seo Y, Fukuoka S, Takanashi M, et al. Gamma Knife surgery for angiographically occult vascular malformations. Stereotact Funct Neurosurg 1995;64(suppl 1):98–109

91. Porter PJ, Willinsky RA, Harper W, Wallace MC. Cerebral cavernous malformations: natural history and prognosis after clinical deterioration with or without hemorrhage. J Neurosurg 1997;87(2):190–197

92. Kahane P, et al. Approche chirurgicale multimodale des angiomes caverneux épileptogènes. Epilepsies 1994;6:113–130

93. Engel J, et al. Outcome with respect to epileptic seizures. In: Engel J, ed. Surgical treatment of the Epilepsies. New York, NY: Raven Press; 1993:609–622

94. Dodick DW, Cascino GD, Meyer FB. Vascular malformations and intractable epilepsy: outcome after surgical treatment. Mayo Clin Proc 1994;69(8):741–745

95. Acciarri N, Giulioni M, Padovani R, Galassi E, Gaist G. Surgical management of cerebral cavernous angiomas causing epilepsy. J Neurosurg Sci 1995;39(1):13–20

96. Cohen DS, Zubay GP, Goodman RR. Seizure outcome after lesionectomy for cavernous malformations. J Neurosurg 1995;83(2):237–242

97. Giulioni M, Acciarri N, Padovani R, Galassi E. Results of surgery in children with cerebral cavernous angiomas causing epilepsy. Br J Neurosurg 1995;9(2):135–141

98. Schroeder H, Gaab M, Runge U. Supratentorial cavernous angiomas and epileptic seizures: preoperative course and post-operative outcome. Neurosurgery 1997;40:885

99. Zevgaridis D, van Velthoven V, Ebeling U, Reulen HJ. Seizure control following surgery in supratentorial cavernous malformations: a retrospective study in 77 patients. Acta Neurochir (Wien) 1996;138(6):672–677

100. Kondziolka D, Lunsford D, Flickinger J. Stereotactic radiosurgery for cavernous malformations. In: Lunsford D, ed. Gamma Knife Brain Surgery. Basel, Switzerland: Karger; 1998:78–88

101. Amin-Hanjani S, Ogilvy CS, Candia GJ, Lyons S, Chapman PH. Stereotactic radiosurgery for cavernous malformations: Kjellberg's experience with proton beam therapy in 98 cases at the Harvard Cyclotron. Neurosurgery 1998;42(6):1229–1236, discussion 1236–1238

102. Kraemer DL, Griebel ML, Lee N, Friedman AH, Radtke RA. Surgical outcome in patients with epilepsy with occult vascular malformations treated with lesionectomy. Epilepsia 1998;39(6):600–607

103. Barcia Salorio JL, Vanaclocha V, Cerda M, et al. Response of experimental epileptic focus to focal ionizing radiation. Appl Neurophysiol 1987;50:359–364

104. Kondziolka D, et al. Stereotactic radiosurgery for the treatment of epilepsy evaluated in the rat kainic acid model. Paper presented at: 8th international Leksell Gamma Knife Society. June 22–25, 1997. Marseille, France.

105. Régis J, Bartolomei F, Metellus P, et al. Radiosurgery for trigeminal neuralgia and epilepsy. Neurosurg Clin N Am 1999;10(2):359–377

106. Régis J, et al. Role of Gamma knife surgery in the treatment of severe epilepsies. In: Wyllie E, ed. The Treatment of Epilepsy: Principle and Practice. Baltimore, MD: William & Wilkins; 2000:1185–1192

III Outcome

36 Surgical Failure and Reoperation

Jeffrey P. Blount, Hyunmi Kim, Curtis J. Rozzelle, and Pongkiat Kankirawatana

In children, localization-related medically refractile epilepsy (LRMRE) is inherently neocortical in origin. By far the most common structural anomaly encountered in pediatric surgical epilepsy specimens is malformations of cortical development (MCDs) which are also known as cortical dysplasias (CDs).[1] Although complex, they can be suitably and summarily considered structural aberrations of normal neocortex.[2,3] The human cerebral neocortex is remarkable in the breadth and extent of its projections and axonal arborizations. Such an inherently robust projection pattern of the neocortex makes initial localization difficult and increases the likelihood of failure of long-term seizure control with focal neocortical resections. As a result, epilepsy surgery in children has traditionally been a time and resource consumptive undertaking that has only enjoyed a fraction of the success of adult epilepsy surgery (in which temporal resection is the most common intervention). Surgical series in children have traditionally demonstrated rates of failure of 40 to 50%. Technologic and conceptual advances over the past two decades have resulted in better outcomes but surgical failure, and reoperation, has long been an inherent issue within pediatric epilepsy surgery.[4–6] Reoperation can be highly effective but has inherent risks that are often higher than the initial operation.[7,8]

■ Surgical Failure

Defining Surgical Failure

Although different neurosurgical operations for epilepsy have different objectives, the overarching principle is the elimination of seizures and the attainment of a seizure-free outcome. Clearly the objective of palliative procedures such as corpus callosotomy is more modest and usually includes an elimination of drop events and decrease in overall generalized seizures. Surgical failure is the lack of attainment of the specific objective for a given procedure and usually implies the return of seizures after an operation designed to eliminate or reduce them. The rate of surgical failure varies between procedures and the timeframe of the operative intervention. For example, grid-based focal cortical resections for CD now show an approximately 70 to 75% incidence of seizure-free outcome and a 90%

likelihood of marked seizure reduction, whereas large series from the 1970s showed seizure-free outcomes in the 50 to 60% range.[1,4,9–12] Hemispherectomy has always been a highly effective procedure with seizure-free outcomes of 80 to 85%.[1,13,14] Temporal resection has similarly been highly effective, with 80 to 85% seizure-free rates for adults with mesial temporal sclerosis who undergo anterior temporal lobectomy. Temporal lobe surgery in children is somewhat different in that neocortical and lesional epilepsy predominates, but outcomes in general are similarly good.[1,15,16]

The traditional definition of surgical failure as a lack of seizure-free outcome must be carefully considered in pediatric epilepsy surgery. Although it is unequivocal that the best outcomes arise from seizure freedom, many of the pediatric epilepsy syndromes are so severe that outcomes other than absolute seizure freedom can be associated with markedly improved quality of life for patients and families. As such, these procedures may fail by conventional analyses that emphasize degree of seizure freedom, yet they are highly successful in substantially reducing the burden of clusters and flurries of daily seizures. It is inaccurate and inappropriate to consider a procedure a surgical failure that reduces a child's seizure burden from hundreds of events per day to small numbers of events per month for the singular reason that the child is not rendered seizure free. Seizure freedom will always represent the gold standard for epilepsy surgery (and must remain the standard toward which operative intervention strives to achieve). However, for some severe pediatric epilepsy syndromes, it is an artificial gold standard that underestimates the profound impact that reduction of seizure burden may play.

Recognition of Surgical Failure

Acute postoperative seizures (APOSs) are seizures that occur within the immediate 7 to 14 days after surgery.[17–19] Traditionally, these events have been attributed to transient local phenomena that have occurred as a result of surgery, such as brain edema, local hemorrhage, or metabolic disturbances. APOSs often have a particularly devastating impact on the patient and the family. As a result, several reports have attempted to determine the predictive capability of APOSs to predict long-term seizure control. Unfortunately, the majority of these studies incorporate adult patients, and a limited number of purely pediatric series exist.[18–21] Mani et al showed that APOSs were an independent predictor of poor surgical outcome in a group of 132 pediatric patients undergoing extratemporal resections for intractable epilepsy.[18] Extratemporal resection was more frequently associated with the occurrence of APOSs, and long-term seizure control was 27%, 22%, and 13% at 6, 12, and 24 months postoperatively in the group that had demonstrated APOSs. The incidence of APOSs was found to be significantly higher after extratemporal resection than after hemispherectomy.[18]

Park and colleagues demonstrated that APOSs predicted a lower postoperative seizure-free rate in a group of 148 children and adolescents.[21] Twenty-five percent of the patients had APOSs, and this group demonstrated only a 51% rate of long-term seizure control, which contrasted sharply with the 81% rate of seizure freedom seen in non-APOS group. Risk factors included extratemporal lobe surgery, postoperative fever, postoperative interictal activity, and seizures other than partial seizures.[21] By contrast, no difference in long-term seizure control was noted between a group of 17 patients (26%) who had APOSs after frontal resection and a larger group (48 patients or 74%) who did not have APOSs in a group of 65 adults reported by Tigaran et al.[19] In another study, it was found that more than five seizures within 7 to 10 days of hemispherectomy has been correlated with long-term failure of control and a more complicated hospital course.[17]

Little other evidence currently exists regarding the timing of surgical failure, although it is increasingly clear that rates of postoperative seizure freedom decline gradually for the first several years after surgery. Thus, it would appear a reasonable response to address the occurrence of postoperative seizures as a significant, but not catastrophic, event. A straightforward, compassionate approach that shares the best available evidence with the family by explaining that postoperative seizures are associated with poorer long-term control yet emphasizes that not all patients having postoperative events demonstrate poor long-term control is the most appropriate response. It is essential that the patient and family understand that the epilepsy team will continue to follow, assess, and treat the patient over time until the epilepsy is controlled or the family and treating team agree that further treatment incorporates unacceptable risk to the patient. When the seizures occur acutely after cortical resection surgery (APOS), it is better to allow the patient time to recover from surgery, re-evaluate seizure frequency and semiology, relocalize if necessary, and then reconsider further medical or surgical therapeutic options. Assurance of commitment to this process on the part of the treating epilepsy team goes a long way toward easing patient and family disappointment, fear, and anxiety and is instrumental in building confidence

in the team for the long-term relationship that is often necessary for success in pediatric neocortical epilepsy. Disconnection surgeries constitute an exception to this approach. If the seizures occur initially right after surgery in which disconnection is the primary surgical technique, such as functional hemispherectomy or corpus callosotomy, then prompt consideration for imaging to identify regions of insufficient or failed disconnection would be more appropriate. If a clear, failed area of disconnection can be identified, prompt return to the operating room may prove the easiest and safest route to seizure control or seizure freedom in these patients. Conversely, identifying a singular area of failed resection or disconnection is rarely the case for neocortical grid-based resections.

Prediction of Surgical Failure

No consistent and reliable clinical, electrophysiological, or radiological preoperative indicator of surgical failure has been reported. Cohen-Gadol et al found that normal pathological findings, male gender, prior surgery, and an extratemporal origin for seizures were factors associated with poor outcomes.[22] When substratified for CD-induced epilepsy, the same authors found that only a clear and complete resection of all the regions of CD was predictive of good outcome.[22] Kim and colleagues defined the extent of resection of CD as an important correlate of surgical outcome.[4] The extent of resection of the CD was also found to be the only feature correlating with surgical outcome in pediatric CD in a study published by Krsek and colleagues.[23] These investigators reviewed a large cohort of 149 patients with histologically confirmed MCD and specifically surveyed whether age, duration of epilepsy, seizure characteristics (infantile spasms, status epilepticus, secondarily generalized tonic-clonic seizures (SGTCS), neurological or neuropsychological findings, EEG, or MRI characteristics predicted surgical outcome. The only factor found in this series (which is the largest such series to date) was the extent of resection of the region of CD.[23] The extent of resection of a CD is conceptually and intellectually important, yet its practical implication is substantially limited because the extent of many CDs is not discernable either by magnetic resonance imaging (MRI) or under the operating microscope. Clearly, for those situations in which the limits of the CD may be defined, it is optimal for seizure control that the entire region of dysplasia be resected. Of course, individual circumstances, such as the relationship of the dysplasia to eloquent cortex, will determine whether all of the dysplastic cortex can be safely removed.

The concept of completeness of resection or disconnection is also a central theme and predictor of failure in other operations as well. The principle cause of surgical failure for corpus callosotomy and functional hemispherectomy is incomplete disconnection.

Patterns of Surgical Failure

Patterns of surgical failure can be characterized according to localization and extent of surgical resection. Preoperative localization is either correct and sufficient or incorrect. Similarly resection may be sufficient or insufficient to achieve seizure freedom.

Localization Correct—Resection Insufficient

Situations in which localization is correct yet seizure-free (or markedly improved) outcomes are not attained often involve cases in which epileptogenic tissue overlaps eloquent cortex. In such a scenario, the resection must be limited to avoid irreversible, severe neurological injury. Such decisions are not always straightforward and must be made carefully; the surgically induced deficit should be less severe than predicted or the fixed deficit induced should have less adverse impact on the child's overall quality of life than that imparted by the seizure disorder. This is particularly the case for motor deficits and markedly less so for crucial and delicate functions such as memory, speech and language, and frontal disinhibition. Neurological deficits related to these functions can be profoundly serious and are less amenable to postoperative intensive therapy to obtain meaningful improvement in the child's capability. Often a fixed motor deficit can be readily accommodated (particularly if mild to moderate), whereas insults to memory, speech, and frontal executive function are far more disabling. As such, when the issue of proximity to eloquent tissue arises as a cause for surgical failure, the surgeon and epileptologist must consider whether additional technological adjuncts such as awake techniques with real-time evaluation of function, improved functional imaging on frameless navigation platforms, or surgical techniques such as multiple subpial transections or intragyral resections may play a role to extend the resection safely and meaningfully.[24]

Another scenario in which surgical failure can follow correct localization is that of technical failure in surgical resection. If the surgical resection is improperly or incompletely performed, it is possible to leave tissue in place that has been localized and implicated as epileptogenic in character. Such an example would be the incomplete resection of an MRI-evident lesion by leaving a portion of the lesion in place. At times, the lesional tissue can blend imperceptibly with surrounding brain, and determination of exact extent of the lesion may be very difficult intraoperatively. Frameless navigation may be useful in preventing such problems, yet it is not an absolute protection because tissue shifts can occur when large lesions are removed that can render initial registration relatively inaccurate. Displacement or mislabeling of subdural grids or misinterpretation or mislabeling of grid maps are uncommon other sources of technical error that can result in surgical failure after correct localization.

Initial Localization and Resection Are Correct and Sufficient, but Evolution of the Epilepsy Induces Surgical Failure

Neocortical epilepsy is notorious in its capability to establish new regions of epileptogenesis and propagation. Although the process of surgical localization is aimed inherently at defining a focal or local region implicated in epileptogenesis, CDs likely involve vast regions of neocortex. After resection, new pathological circuitry can become established that frequently has its epicenter at the margin of the previous resection cavity (**Fig. 36.1**). The exact mechanism by which CD tissue induces epileptogenesis is incompletely understood, but several mechanisms based on molecular observations of the tissue have been proposed.[3] Cytomegalic neurons typify CD tissue and are often found in the most electrophysiologically abnormal regions.[25] These abnormal cells appear to have important interactions with inhibitory γ-aminobutyric acid (GABA) pathways (which appear upregulated) and play a central role in epileptogenesis. Altered membrane properties have also been observed. Differential expression of N-methyl-D-aspartic acid (NMDA) subunit receptors and persistence of undifferentiated neurons are also regularly encountered in histological evaluation of CD and may play an important contributory role in epileptogenesis.[3,25,26] Two different histopathological subtypes have been defined and stratified (IA, IB, and II) that demonstrate clinically important differences such as seizure outcome and neuropsychological deficits.[27] Clinical studies for localization implicate the most active region of epileptogenesis but cannot define the cellular limits of the CD. As a result, all resections in which CD is the predominant pathological finding have an inherent risk for reorganization and surgical failure.

Errors in Localization

Localization of medically intractable epilepsy is based on the principle of concordance of semiology, EEG, and noninvasive functional imaging studies in implicating a particular region of cortex in epileptogenesis. Great advances have been made in each of these techniques such that noninvasive localization is a more accurate process than ever before. EEG advances include use of novel montages and the development of high-density EEG arrays. Functional imaging advances are extensive and include the development and widespread application of techniques in magnetoencephalography (MEG), ictal single photon emission computed tomography (SPECT) with subtraction ictal SPECT scanning coregistered to MRI imaging (SISCOM), and positron emission tomography (PET). Each of these is discussed elsewhere in this book. Despite these considerable advances localization remains a challenging and imperfect process with a real potential for misinterpretation and errors. Errors in localization account for important sources of surgical failure and need for reoperation.

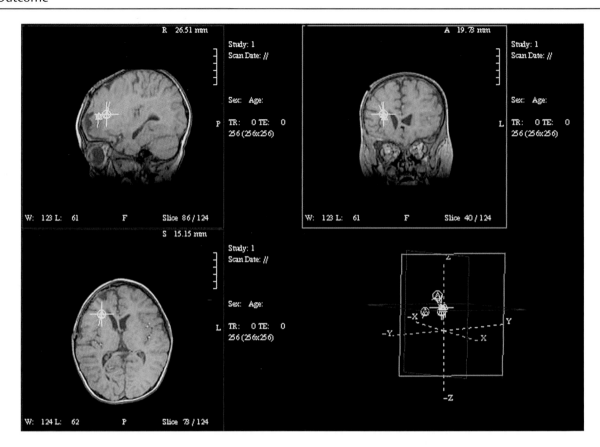

Fig. 36.1 Surgical failure because of reorganization from malformations of cortical development (MCD)-induced epilepsy. This 14-month-old boy initially presented with severe localization-related medically refractile epilepsy and underwent a grid-based resection. He remained seizure free for 7 months postoperatively, and then seizures recurred. This figure illustrates a magnetic source imaging image featuring dipoles showing the recurrence of medically intractable epilepsy at the resection margin of his frontal MCD. Reoperation was performed and localization confirmed with intracranial electrodes. He has been seizure free for more than 5 years.

Patterns in errors of localization can be recognized and organized. The first type of error occurs when an active area of epileptogenesis fails to be recognized. A common example of this error occurs with dual pathology in which a temporal lobe focus of activity is sufficiently active that a simultaneous frontal region of activity is either not detected or ignored. A more common error occurs when an area that is detected by a test is misinterpreted as being less active or less contributory to the overall epilepsy than is the case. This may occur when disease is multifocal or when semiology or other characteristics of the epilepsy appear to implicate other brain regions. Even though concordance is a useful unifying principle of epilepsy localization, it remains a practical reality that information from functional imaging studies often shows significant discordance and that interpretation (which can be very challenging) is always necessary.

Experienced centers usually quickly get a sense for how concordant the localizing information is for a given patient and develop a degree of confidence for the need for intracra-

nial electrodes. A sincere and earnest desire to help a child with severe, progressive, disabling epilepsy can lead to the ill-advised implantation of electrodes despite modest concordance of noninvasive imaging studies. Such "fishing trips" are characterized by a wide and extensive coverage with electrodes and very modest surgical success rates.

Response to Surgical Failure and Consideration for Reoperation

After it has been determined that surgical failure has occurred, consideration for reoperation should be undertaken. Several issues must be addressed to appropriately and accurately make the best recommendation to the patient regarding reoperation. First, it must be determined whether the postoperative seizure pattern is sufficiently severe to warrant the risks of further operative intervention. This involves the comparison of the burden of the epilepsy with

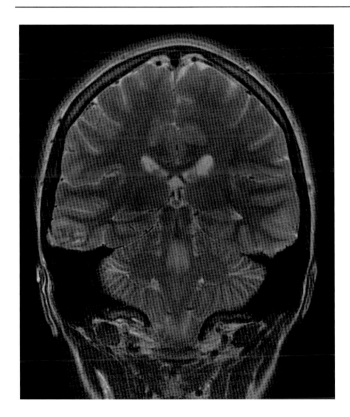

Fig. 36.2 Surgical failure surrounding lesional resection. This 6-year-old girl presented with characteristic partial complex seizures and was found to harbor this temporal lobe mass. Uncomplicated image-guided lesionectomy was performed. Pathology revealed a gangliogloma. Her seizures recurred 3 months postoperatively. A repeat operation was done with invasive recordings, and a grid-based resection was performed. Additional tissue was removed, and she has been seizure free for 3.5 years.

the projected burden of potential neurological morbidity that would occur as a result of extension of the resection. Most focal epilepsy fails at sites adjacent to prior resection margins so it can be roughly estimated that those whose resections were limited by adjacent eloquent cortex would be at significantly higher risk than those in which focal resections were far from eloquent cortex. It is also important to emphasize that not every surgical failure warrants operative intervention or consideration for operative intervention. Some failures are relatively minor; the postoperative seizure pattern is markedly better than that experienced before surgery. In others, the surgical team recognizes that reasonable surgical limits have been reached.

Second the degree to which successful localization can be obtained must be addressed. Occasionally, the original operative intervention improves the capability to monitor and localize, and it becomes immediately evident that ictal onset is diffuse or multifactorial. By contrast, if good localization can be attained then reoperation can be highly successful in achieving long-term seizure control. González-

Martínez and colleagues demonstrated a 52% rate of Engel Class I (seizure free) or Engel Class II (markedly improved) outcomes for reoperation after initial resective epilepsy surgery that proved unsuccessful in imparting long-term control.[28]

■ Reoperation

Reoperation in Grid-Based Resections/ Focal Cortical Resections

Reoperations in Cortical Dysplasia

MCDs are the most common pathological substrate for LRMRE in children.[3] MCDs are inherently difficult to localize noninvasively and require virtually uniform use of invasive electrode recordings for proper localization. Because of the extensive nature of MCDs and the resultant proximity to eloquent regions, invasive recordings also typically serve to define the regions of epileptogenesis and eloquence. Thus, properly localized grids that allow for extensive mapping of the cortex are central to the contemporary operative strategy for nonlesional medically refractile focal epilepsy in childhood (**Fig. 36.2**). Some authors have advocated that more extensive investigation and mapping of the cortex in the child with epilepsy results in better seizure control.[23] Insufficient or improperly placed grids may lead to suboptimal characterization of the region of epileptogenesis and its important relationship to regions of functional eloquence. The resulting uncertainty of localization is an important cause for surgical failure and the need for reoperation.

Reoperation after failed grid localization is inherently difficult because of the scar and fibrosis prompted by the grid. Even when subdural grids are inserted using gentle technique and under a flood of irrigation, an inflammatory reaction ensues over the cortex. Postgrid inflammatory changes are rarely relevant at the time of the initial resection but are highly problematic if the initial resection fails and reoperation is required. Adhesions commonly form between the pia and the dura in areas that have previous interventions for subdural grid placement. This is particularly robust at resection sites, resection margins, and along the edge of the dural closure. Opening the dura alone can become a bloody, time-intensive, and inelegant undertaking. The pial surface is often at least partially disturbed, and the underlying epileptogenic patterns may be affected.

Furthermore, the anatomical structures have often shifted and scarred; gliotic planes infiltrate and distort the margins of resection cavities so as to distort the distinction between normal and abnormal tissue planes. The scarring between pia and dura is particularly problematic in repeat surgery if extensive grid placement is required. Because the scarring often requires direct microsurgical dissection to take it down and allow the placement of subdural electrodes, the placement of grids may be limited only to those regions underlying the craniotomy. Scarring around cortical veins is a particular risk because experience dictates that the scar tissue is often stronger and more robust than the walls of the veins. Thus, ill-advised but well-intended efforts to slide a small electrode into an area of previous scarring where resistance is encountered may result in pronounced hemorrhage.

In spite of the previously mentioned limitations, repeat surgery using invasive electrodes can be undertaken with good outcome. The role for diligence and patience in gentle dissection of the dura from the pia and delicate placement of electrodes into corridors where they can readily and easily be accommodated cannot be overemphasized.

Reoperations after Lobar Resections that Evolve into Hemispherectomy

Several pathologies are distinct in their potential to require repeated lobar resections that evolve ultimately into a need for a hemispherectomy. The most common and most obvious of these is Rasmussen encephalitis, but progression because of reorganization can be seen in LRMRE arising from MCDs or neurocutaneous syndromes such as Sturge-Weber.

Rasmussen encephalitis is an incompletely understood cerebritis thought to be of autoimmune origin. One cerebral hemisphere is selectively involved and gives rise to an epileptic syndrome of progressive and unremitting seizures that typically culminate in a pattern of epilepsia partialis continua (EPC) or unremitting focal partial epilepsy. Seizure patterns and overall clinical course may vary widely, but EPC is highly associated with Rasmussen encephalitis. At early onset, the Rasmussen encephalitis may appear focal and result in focal resection that fails in a short time. The key issues with regard to surgical failure and reoperation focus on the capability to make the correct diagnosis of Rasmussen encephalitis and to make difficult right decisions surrounding timing of hemispherectomy during the long, agonizing clinical demise that typifies Rasmussen encephalitis. It has been a traditional clinical dictum to only surgically intervene when the disease has progressed sufficiently that the hemiparesis has progressed to hemiplegia. However, the awareness of the relentless progressive quality of the disease, the refractile quality of the seizures to antiepileptic drugs, the potential damage imposed to the contralateral hemisphere, and the severe impairment to quality of life associated with EPC have induced controversy over the optimal timing for hemispheric disconnection. Clearly, the clinical presence of EPC in a patient who fails carefully planned and executed lobar resection should prompt an investigation for Rasmussen encephalitis and usher in a careful discussion and consideration of the unique set of issues that surrounds the disease.

Reoperation after Functional Hemispherectomy

Surgical failure in functional hemispherectomy is usually caused by incomplete disconnection. Several different operations have been advocated to remove or disconnect a hemisphere, and each of the procedures has its own area of risk for disconnection.[29] Anatomical hemispherectomies are less frequently performed now because of the inherent advantages conferred by the functional hemispherectomy techniques, such as reduced blood loss, operating times, and incidence of postoperative hydrocephalus and avoiding subpial hemosiderosis.[13,29] As a result, few recent articles discuss technical reasons for failure in anatomical hemispherectomy. Similarly, little is written about technical failures in hemispheric decortication or other procedures designed to accomplish complete disconnection via anatomical subremoval with the exception of peri-insular hemispherotomy (PIH).[30]

PIH has gained wide appeal and use because of the inherently elegant and efficient way in which it takes advantage of the anatomical relationship of the circular sulcus at the margins of the insula, the frontal and temporal "stems" (of subcortically directed white matter), and the underlying cerebral ventricles. However, the last step in PIH involving frontobasal disconnection is often the most frequent cause for failure of complete disconnection in this procedure. This is because of the perception that there is not an anatomical guideline that the surgeon can follow. Binder and Schramm noted that the critical step in frontobasal disconnection is to secure the pericallosal arteries during the callosotomy stage of the operation.[31] They are then followed proximally around the genu of the corpus callosum where they merge with the distal A2 segments of the anterior cerebral artery (ACA). Dissection follows the A2 segments all the way back past the anterior communicating artery (hence becoming A1 segments of the ACA) to the bifurcation with the middle cerebral artery. By using the anatomy of the ACA in this way, absolute frontobasal disconnection is assured without a risk of entering the basal ganglia or hypothalamus.

Regardless of the technique chosen, the critical issue is that the hemisphere is completely disconnected. Meticulous review of postoperative images by the neurosurgical team can ensure that disconnection has been attained or indicate areas in which disconnection may be or is incomplete. As discussed previously, seizure recurrence after hemispherectomy should prompt early MRI that should be carefully inspected to discern any possible areas where disconnection may be incomplete. Indeed, MRI is of greater value than EEG in the immediate postoperative period for the patient demonstrating APOS after hemispherectomy. MRI may demonstrate regions of incomplete disconnection, whereas EEG is notoriously difficult to interpret because EEG cannot distinguish that the diseased hemisphere has been disconnected. Because the tissue remains in place with intact blood supply, the EEG will still indicate a massively diseased hemisphere.

Diffusion tensor imaging (DTI) is a promising recent technique that demonstrates white matter fiber tracks.[52] The capability of DTI to image axonal degeneration after corpus callosotomy and the feasibility of DTI after hemispherectomy were previously demonstrated. These studies attest to the promise of DTI to image tracts that may remain intact after surgery, but it remains to be seen whether these technologies will show great utility or gain widespread clinical utility.[52]

Reoperation in Corpus Callosotomy

Corpus callosotomy involves the surgical disconnection of the two cerebral hemispheres either in part (anterior two-thirds callosotomy) or in its entirety (complete callosotomy). It has been shown in multiple series to be highly effective yet remains underused. Drop seizures and events have been shown most amenable to callosal section, but the procedure is also shown to favorably affect frequency and severity of generalized events when hemispheric bisynchrony appears central in the epilepsy. Operative failure typically either comes from technical failure to attain the intended extent of division of the corpus callosum or from a failure of the two thirds resection to attain the desired clinical endpoint. Postoperative MRI scans, particularly coronal T1 images, can readily identify any regions of the corpus callosum that remain intact after operative intervention. Once postoperative MRI confirms that the desired degree of callosal sectioning has been attained, consideration must be given to determine whether extending the resection to complete callosal section would result in more favorable outcome or whether the benefits of callosal section have been attained and alternative strategies such as implantation of a vagus nerve stimulator should be considered.

Technically, a repeat callosotomy is relatively straightforward if performed in the immediate postoperative period after the initial intervention (as when postoperative MRI indicates a region of incomplete callosal section) and markedly more difficult if the repeat operation is substantially delayed. The most dangerous part of repeat callosotomy involves the removal of the bone flap over the superior sagittal sinus. Scar from the previous operation typically forms between the dura and the underside of the craniotomy flap. This scar can make dissection in the epidural space above the sinus both difficult and very hazardous. Surgical options to deal with this problem include (a) adjusting the trajectory to approach the remaining intact callosum through a nondissected corridor, (b) altering the size or configuration of the bone flap, (c) meticulously trying to dissect the prior bone flap, or (d) considering alternative techniques such as radiosurgery to complete the callosal division. Additional burr holes are often helpful if the choice is to open the prior craniotomy. The formation of scar tissue between the pia

of the involved hemisphere and the overlying dura and the falx cerebri can also account for great difficulty in repeat callosotomy. Because the operation requires exposure of the interhemispheric fissure to gain access to the corpus callosum, the presence of at least some important cortical draining veins can be assured. When scar tissue involves these important vessels, the surgeon must take particular care not to retract on them. Such retraction can result in vessel avulsion right at the point of entry into the superior sagittal sinus. This can result in voluminous bleeding directly from the edge of the sinus, which can prove challenging to control. The logical sequence of control should consist of gentle focal tamponade with Cottonoid patties or cotton balls, incorporation of hemostatic agents such as oxidized cellulose (Surgicel R, Ethicon, Somerville, NJ) or Gelfoam (Pfizer, New York, NY) with further focal tamponade and then judicious use of vascular clips to occlude the open edge of the superior sagittal sinus, as needed.

Once the approach to the corpus callosum (CC) has been accomplished, the region of incomplete section must be addressed. Frameless navigation can be helpful in targeting a region of incomplete section. Consideration must also be given to whether the callosotomy should be extended to incorporate complete callosal section (i.e., conversion of anterior two-thirds callosotomy to complete callosotomy). Characteristically, the tissue in the region of incomplete section is no more difficult to divide than normal tissue, but the exposure to it may be more challenging. The easiest regions to miss are the anterior and superior extent of the genu and the rostrum (for anterior two-thirds CC) and the splenium (for complete CC) of the corpus callosum. Anatomical vascular landmarks are helpful in preventing this. Anteriorly the pericallosal arteries can be followed back, and complete division can be ensured once the anterior communicating artery complex is visualized. Posteriorly, the splenium can be confidently considered divided when the pia-arachnoid planes surrounding the great vein of Galen are encountered. The white matter tissue of the CC is characteristically no more difficult to divide on repeat operation than on the original resection because, by definition, it has not been touched and, as such, is free of scar and fibrosis.

Reoperation after Epileptogenic Lesional Resection

Reoperation for Tumor

Tumors accounted for 19% of all pediatric epilepsy operations, yet 40% of these patients had required prior surgery in the recent survey conducted by The Pediatric Epilepsy Surgery Subcommission of the International League Against Epilepsy.[1] Resection of tumors and vascular lesions results in higher seizure-free outcomes than other pathologies, so the incidence of surgical failure is generally low.[15,28] The most common tumors that characteristically cause refractile seizures in childhood are benign, slow growing, hamartomatous tumors such as gangliogliomas, desmoplastic infantile gangliogliomas (DNTs),[32] and pleomorphic xanthoastrocytomas.[33–36] Each of these tumors is generally benign, with apparently low incidence of anaplastic transformation. A temporal lobe predilection has been observed for those tumors causing seizures. The two related issues surrounding surgical failure and reoperation regarding these tumors are (a) extent of seizure workup that is necessary and appropriate to ensure that the lesion is epileptogenic and (b) whether the resection should be limited to the lesion itself (i.e., a pure lesionectomy) or whether surrounding tissue needs to be taken as well to optimize the likelihood of a seizure-free outcome.[37] Failure to identify and resect the full extent of the epileptogenic region will likely result in postoperative seizures whereas removal of additional tissue potentially will cause increased risks for neurological deficit (**Fig. 36.3**). Experienced centers and surgeons differ on their approaches to lesional epilepsy. Minimalist centers advocate performance of a pure lesionectomy if there is concordance between an imaging abnormality and scalp EEG data. Such an approach streamlines and economizes the preoperative evaluation and is highly effective in a large percentage of cases. However, there are now multiple reports regarding dysplastic cortical areas surrounding the DNT tumors.[38–40] Other studies have demonstrated epileptogenic region in the tissue surrounding the lesion without correlating with abnormal histopathology. Minkin et al reviewed 24 children who underwent resection of DNTs at a single French center between 1986 and 2000.[16] Seizure freedom was realized in 83% of the entire series but 4 of 15 children with temporal lobe DNTs had residual seizures. These authors concluded that lesionectomy was appropriate for extratemporal DNTs but that lesions involving the temporal lobe warranted extensive invasive electrode-based interventions.[16] Zaatreh and colleagues examined a large group of patients undergoing surgery for temporal lobe tumors that caused epilepsy. They found that postoperative seizure freedom was predicted by gross total resection of the tumor and that the extent of tumor resection was largely predictive of outcome.[41] Similarly Khajavi and colleagues found that the extent of temporal tumor resection predicted long-term seizure outcome.[37] Luyken et al reviewed 207 adults and children who underwent resection of a tumor that caused refractile seizures and found that a short duration of seizures, single EEG focus, and absence of additional pathology such as CD or hippocampal sclerosis were predictive of good outcome.[42] Jooma et al[53] studied 30 patients with refractile seizures from temporal lobe lesions and divided them into two groups, depending on whether straightforward lesionectomy or EEG-guided resection was done. They found that the group treated with EEG delineation of the epileptogenic zone achieved a 92% seizure-free rate after surgery, whereas the group undergoing lesionectomy achieved only a 19% rate of seizure freedom. The rate of seizure freedom increased to 63% when the temporal mesial structures were resected at reoperation. This finding prompted this group to conclude that resection of the amygdala and hippocampus concomitant with temporal lesion resection results in the highest rate of seizure freedom.

Reoperation for Vascular Lesions

Although symptomatic medically refractile epilepsy can arise from either cavernous malformations (CCMs) or true arteriovenous malformations (AVMs), it is more common from CCM and it is here that the greatest uncertainty has arisen. CCMs characteristically demonstrate a rim of hemosiderin-stained tissue. The epileptogenic potential of this tissue is uncertain, and the surgical approach to it is controversial.[43] The debate focuses on whether there is a need to remove the hemosiderin-laden tissue or perform invasive epilepsy monitoring or whether simple lesionectomy suffices.[44] Bernotas and colleagues incorporated removal of the hemosiderin-stained tissue into their operative approach for CCMs and reported a 79% incidence of seizure freedom in a group of 87 adult patients who underwent surgical resection of a supratentorial CCM.[45] Benifla and colleagues from Toronto reported an identical incidence of seizure freedom in a group of children who underwent the resection of a temporal CCM as a cause of their medically refractile epilepsy.[15]

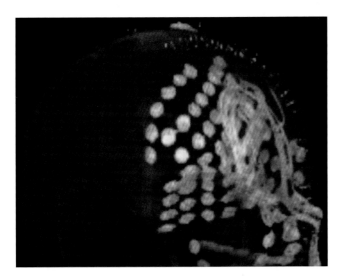

Fig. 36.3 Surgical failure because of difficulty in localization. This 7-year-old girl demonstrated a frontal malformation of cortical development (MCD) as the region of her ictal onset. Even with intracranial recordings, exact localization proved difficult. Interictal activity was highly localized and corresponded to a focal MCD. Ictal activity spread broadly and immediately throughout the whole frontal lobe. A focal resection incorporating the MCD was performed. She acutely recurred with seizures 2 weeks after the resection. A reoperation was performed in which a frontal lobectomy was performed, and she has been seizure free for almost 1 year.

Bauman and colleagues reported on a large adult series from New York in which lesionectomy appeared to suffice.[46] More than two thirds of the patients who underwent surgical resection of a single supratentorial CCM were rendered seizure free in this series. Predictors of good outcome included older age (> 30 years), lack of secondary generalized seizures, small lesions, and localization within the mesial temporal lobe.[46]

CCMs are uncommon lesions in childhood, and the number of reported series in childhood is limited. Perhaps most importantly, the presentation in children appears quite different in that CCMs in children appear to more frequently present with spontaneous intracerebral hemorrhage than medically refractile seizures. Mottolese and colleagues described a series of 35 pediatric patients with intracerebral CCMs and noted the paucity of recurrent seizures and the frequency of spontaneous hemorrhage in presentation.[47] Microsurgical excision was recommended for all symptomatic and enlarging lesions.[47]

True AVMs in children typically warrant aggressive treatment because of their inherent risk of hemorrhage. Typically, surgical removal of the AVM or obliteration via radiosurgery results in marked improvement in seizure control. Both surgical excision and radiosurgery can result in mild, relatively easy-to-control seizures but severe, medically refractile epilepsy has only been rarely reported.[48] Thus, true AVMs are usually treated either by microsurgical excision (with or without embolization) or by radiosurgery, and severe medically refractile epilepsy is rarely either an indication for treatment or a result of treatment.

Reoperation in Temporal Lobectomy in Children

The risk for surgical failure and the need for reoperation is increased if two important differences between pediatric and adult temporal lobe epilepsy are not carefully considered in surgical planning. The first of these differences is that temporal lobe resections in children differ inherently from those in adults because of the pronounced increase in both lesional (40%) and neocortical (CD) temporal lobe epilepsy (30%).[1] Thus, the regions involved are most often lateral and inferior temporal lobe, and pure hippocampal sclerosis is less common in children. Epileptogenic regions within lateral and basal neocortex rapidly spread to and via the mesial limbic pathways to give rise to partial complex seizures that are clinically identical to those emanating from mesial temporal sclerosis commonly seen in adults. Failure to consider the inherent propensity toward neocortical disease in children increases the risk of improper localization and surgical failure.[15,49]

The second important difference in temporal lobe epilepsy in children is the high incidence of dual pathology. This refers to simultaneous regions of epileptogenesis both within the temporal and frontal neocortex that typically arise from parallel regions of CD. There is a predominance of fronto-orbital and inferior frontal localization for the frontal lobe foci. Thus, it is very important to consider the potential for dual pathology in the construction of the operation for pediatric temporal lobe epilepsy. It must be remembered that pure mesial temporal sclerosis is an uncommon finding in pediatric temporal lobe epilepsy. Structural changes in the hippocampus that typify classic adult mesial temporal sclerosis may occur as a result of increased limbic outflow from neocortical seizures in a child. Standard techniques of anterior temporal resection that focus singularly or primarily on the medial structures may have a higher rate of failure. More aggressive monitoring with increased use of invasive electrodes to adequately monitor temporal neocortex and frontal/orbitofrontal neocortex would appear well advised in cases of pediatric temporal epilepsy in which the classic characteristics (clinical, EEG, or imaging) of mesial temporal sclerosis are missing.

If repeat surgery is necessary, many of the same problems are encountered as in other neocortical resections. Typically, the dura is densely adherent to pia. Temporal draining veins may become incorporated and threatened. Gliosis and scar distort normal anatomical planes. These issues are particularly important if prior medial temporal dissection occurred. It is exceptionally important to know whether the pia on the mesial side of the temporal lobe was disturbed at the time of prior resection. The surgeon must assume that it was and that the oculomotor nerve, posterior communicating artery, and cerebral peduncle are not protected.

■ Conclusion

Surgical failure and the need for reoperation are inherent in the surgical treatment of children with medically refractile epilepsy. This is because the primary cause of LRMRE in children is an MCD. Despite considerable technical advances in anatomical and functional imaging studies, the complete extent of CDs remains difficult to discern.[10,50] Great progress has been made, and there is greater cause for hope for the child suffering from LRMRE than at any point in the past.[1,51] However improper localization or insufficient resection may occur, and either is a source of surgical failure. The definition of surgical failure must take into account the realistic preoperative goals for a given intervention for a specific child. Although complete seizure freedom must remain the goal of operative intervention, the traditional definition of any outcome short of complete seizure freedom may be inappropriate in children because of the severity of many of the epilepsy syndromes encountered. Complete resection of the epileptogenic MCD is the most important predictor of good outcome. Consideration for reoperation weighs the burden of the postresection seizure pattern with the potential risks for additional resection. Comprehensive relocalization is essential for cortical resections, but more rapid take backs may be appropriate for disconnection-based procedures (PIH and CC) that show acute postoperative seizures. MRI can indicate regions of incomplete disconnection that can often be re-explored with lower risk than if intervention is delayed until after scar tissue forms.

Reoperation can be highly successful but in general carries somewhat higher risks of failure and complications. Each operation has its own individual considerations if repeat surgery is necessary.

References

1. Harvey AS, Cross JH, Shinnar S, Mathern BW; ILAE Pediatric Epilepsy Surgery Survey Taskforce. Defining the spectrum of international practice in pediatric epilepsy surgery patients. Epilepsia 2008;49(1):146–155

2. Andres M, Andre VM, Nguyen S, et al. Human cortical dysplasia and epilepsy: an ontogenetic hypothesis based on volumetric MRI and NeuN neuronal density and size measurements. Cereb Cortex 2005;15(2):194–210

3. Wang VY, Chang EF, Barbaro NM. Focal cortical dysplasia: a review of pathological features, genetics, and surgical outcome. Neurosurg Focus 2006;20(1):E7

4. Kim DW, Lee SK, Chu K, et al. Predictors of surgical outcome and pathologic considerations in focal cortical dysplasia. Neurology 2009;72(3):211–216

5. Kim SK, Wang KC, Hwang YS, et al. Epilepsy surgery in children: outcomes and complications. J Neurosurg Pediatr 2008;1(4):277–283

6. Wyllie E, Comair YG, Kotagal P, Bulacio J, Bingaman W, Ruggieri P. Seizure outcome after epilepsy surgery in children and adolescents. Ann Neurol 1998;44(5):740–748

7. Awad IA, Nayel MH, Lüders H. Second operation after the failure of previous resection for epilepsy. Neurosurgery 1991;28(4):510–518

8. Schwartz TH, Spencer DD. Strategies for reoperation after comprehensive epilepsy surgery. J Neurosurg 2001;95(4):615–623

9. Hamiwka L, Jayakar P, Resnick T, et al. Surgery for epilepsy due to cortical malformations: ten-year follow-up. Epilepsia 2005;46(4):556–560

10. Knowlton RC, Elgavish RA, Bartolucci A, et al. Functional imaging: II. Prediction of epilepsy surgery outcome. Ann Neurol 2008;64(1):35–41

11. Sinclair DB, Aronyk K, Snyder T, et al. Extratemporal resection for childhood epilepsy. Pediatr Neurol 2004;30(3):177–185

12. Wyllie E. Surgical treatment of epilepsy in children. Pediatr Neurol 1998;19(3):179–188

13. Jonas R, Nguyen S, Hu B, et al. Cerebral hemispherectomy: hospital course, seizure, developmental, language, and motor outcomes. Neurology 2004;62(10):1712–1721

14. Peacock WJ, Wehby-Grant MC, Shields WD, et al. Hemispherectomy for intractable seizures in children: a report of 58 cases. Childs Nerv Syst 1996;12(7):376–384

15. Benifla M, Rutka JT, Otsubo H, et al. Long-term seizure and social outcomes following temporal lobe surgery for intractable epilepsy during childhood. Epilepsy Res 2008;82(2–3):133–138

16. Minkin K, Klein O, Mancini J, Lena G. Surgical strategies and seizure control in pediatric patients with dysembryoplastic neuroepithelial tumors: a single-institution experience. J Neurosurg Pediatr 2008;1(3):206–210

17. Koh S, Nguyen S, Asarnow RF, et al. Five or more acute postoperative seizures predict hospital course and long-term seizure control after hemispherectomy. Epilepsia 2004;45(5):527–533

18. Mani J, Gupta A, Mascha E, et al. Postoperative seizures after extratemporal resections and hemispherectomy in pediatric epilepsy. Neurology 2006;66(7):1038–1043

19. Tigaran S, Cascino GD, McClelland RL, So EL, Richard Marsh W. Acute postoperative seizures after frontal lobe cortical resection for intractable partial epilepsy. Epilepsia 2003;44(6):831–835

20. Ficker DM, So EL, Mosewich RK, Radhakrishnan K, Cascino GD, Sharbrough FW. Improvement and deterioration of seizure control during the postsurgical course of epilepsy surgery patients. Epilepsia 1999;40(1):62–67

21. Park K, Buchhalter J, McClelland R, Raffel C. Frequency and significance of acute postoperative seizures following epilepsy surgery in children and adolescents. Epilepsia 2002;43(8):874–881

22. Cohen-Gadol AA, Wilhelmi BG, Collignon F, et al. Long-term outcome of epilepsy surgery among 399 patients with nonlesional seizure foci including mesial temporal lobe sclerosis. J Neurosurg 2006;104(4):513–524

23. Krsek P, Maton B, Jayakar P, et al. Incomplete resection of focal cortical dysplasia is the main predictor of poor postsurgical outcome. Neurology 2009;72(3):217–223

24. Chamoun RB, Nayar VV, Yoshor D. Neuronavigation applied to epilepsy monitoring with subdural electrodes. Neurosurg Focus 2008;25(3):E21

25. Najm I, Ying Z, Babb T, et al. Mechanisms of epileptogenicity in cortical dysplasias. Neurology 2004; 62(6, suppl 3):S9–S13

26. André VM, Flores-Hernández J, Cepeda C, et al. NMDA receptor alterations in neurons from pediatric cortical dysplasia tissue. Cereb Cortex 2004;14(6):634–646

27. Krsek P, Pieper T, Karlmeier A, et al. Different presurgical characteristics and seizure outcomes in children with focal cortical dysplasia type I or II. Epilepsia 2009;50(1):125–137

28. González-Martínez JA, Srikijvilaikul T, Nair D, Bingaman WE. Long-term seizure outcome in reoperation after failure of epilepsy surgery. Neurosurgery 2007;60(5):873–880, discussion 873–880

29. Cook SW, Nguyen ST, Hu B, et al. Cerebral hemispherectomy in pediatric patients with epilepsy: comparison of three techniques by pathological substrate in 115 patients. J Neurosurg 2004; 100(2, suppl Pediatrics):125–141

30. Cats EA, Kho KH, Van Nieuwenhuizen O, Van Veelen CW, Gosselaar PH, Van Rijen PC. Seizure freedom after functional hemispherectomy and a possible role for the insular cortex: the Dutch experience. J Neurosurg 2007; 107(4, suppl):275–280

31. Binder DK, Schramm J. Transsylvian functional hemispherectomy. Childs Nerv Syst 2006;22(8):960–966

32. Daumas-Duport C, Scheithauer BW, Chodkiewicz JP, Laws ER Jr, Vedrenne C. Dysembryoplastic neuroepithelial tumor: a surgically curable tumor of young patients with intractable partial seizures. Report of thirty-nine cases. Neurosurgery 1988;23(5):545–556

33. Johnson JH Jr, Hariharan S, Berman J, et al. Clinical outcome of pediatric gangliogliomas: ninety-nine cases over 20 years. Pediatr Neurosurg 1997;27(4):203–207

34. Khajavi K, Comair YG, Prayson RA, et al. Childhood ganglioglioma and medically intractable epilepsy. A clinicopathological study of 15 patients and a review of the literature. Pediatr Neurosurg 1995;22(4):181–188

35. Mickle JP. Ganglioglioma in children. A review of 32 cases at the University of Florida. Pediatr Neurosurg 1992;18(5-6):310–314

36. Fried I, Kim JH, Spencer DD. Limbic and neocortical gliomas associated with intractable seizures: a distinct clinicopathological group. Neurosurgery 1994;34(5):815–823, discussion 823–824

37. Khajavi K, Comair YG, Wyllie E, Palmer J, Morris HH, Hahn JF. Surgical management of pediatric tumor-associated epilepsy. J Child Neurol 1999;14(1):15–25

38. Lee J, Lee BL, Joo EY, et al. Dysembryoplastic neuroepithelial tumors in pediatric patients. Brain Dev 2008 [Epub ahead of print]

39. Nishida N, Hayase Y, Mikuni N, et al. A nonspecific form of dysembryoplastic neuroepithelial tumor presenting with intractable epilepsy. Brain Tumor Pathol 2005;22(1):35–40

40. Takahashi A, Hong SC, Seo DW, Hong SB, Lee M, Suh YL. Frequent association of cortical dysplasia in dysembryoplastic neuroepithelial tumor treated by epilepsy surgery. Surg Neurol 2005;64(5):419–427

41. Zaatreh MM, Firlik KS, Spencer DD, Spencer SS. Temporal lobe tumoral epilepsy: characteristics and predictors of surgical outcome. Neurology 2003;61(5):636–641

42. Luyken C, Blümcke I, Fimmers R, et al. The spectrum of long-term epilepsy-associated tumors: long-term seizure and tumor outcome and neurosurgical aspects. Epilepsia 2003;44(6):822–830

43. Hammen T, Romstöck J, Dörfler A, Kerling F, Buchfelder M, Stefan H. Prediction of postoperative outcome with special respect to removal of hemosiderin fringe: a study in patients with cavernous haemangiomas associated with symptomatic epilepsy. Seizure 2007;16(3):248–253

44. Siegel AM, Roberts DW, Harbaugh RE, Williamson PD. Pure lesionectomy versus tailored epilepsy surgery in treatment of cavernous malformations presenting with epilepsy. Neurosurg Rev 2000;23(2):80–83

45. Bernotas G, Rastenyte D, Deltuva V, Matukevicius A, Jaskeviciene V, Tamasauskas A. Cavernous angiomas: an uncontrolled clinical study of 87 surgically treated patients. Medicina (Kaunas) 2009;45(1):21–28

46. Baumann CR, Acciarri N, Bertalanffy H, et al. Seizure outcome after resection of supratentorial cavernous malformations: a study of 168 patients. Epilepsia 2007;48(3):559–563

47. Mottolese C, Hermier M, Stan H, et al. Central nervous system cavernomas in the pediatric age group. Neurosurg Rev 2001;24(2-3):55–71, discussion 72–73

48. Husain AM, Mendez M, Friedman AH. Intractable epilepsy following radiosurgery for arteriovenous malformation. J Neurosurg 2001;95(5):888–892

49. Schramm J. Temporal lobe epilepsy surgery and the quest for optimal extent of resection: a review. Epilepsia 2008;49(8):1296–1307

50. Knowlton RC, Elgavish RA, Limdi N, et al. Functional imaging: I. Relative predictive value of intracranial electroencephalography. Ann Neurol 2008;64(1):25–34

51. Bittar RG, Rosenfeld JV, Klug GL, Hopkins IJ, Simon Harvey A. Resective surgery in infants and young children with intractable epilepsy. J Clin Neurosci 2002;9(2):142–146

52. Wakamoto H, Eluvathingel TJ, Makk M, Juhasz C, Chupani HT. Diffusion tensor imaging of the corticospinal tract following cerebral hemispherectomy. J Child Neurol 2006;21(7):566–571

53. Jooma R, Yeh HS, Privitera MD, Cartner M. Lesionectomy versus electrophysiologically guided resection for temporal lobe tumors manifesting with complex partial seizures. J Neurosurgery 1995;83(2):231–236

37 Postoperative Seizure Control

Seema Adhami and Chellamani Harini

Epilepsy is a common problem in pediatric neurology. In 1975, Davidson and Falconer first showed that surgery could alter the outcome of children with temporal lobe epilepsy (TLE).[1] The last two decades have seen the emergence of surgery as a valuable and viable option in the treatment of refractory focal epilepsy in children. Ten to 20 percent of cases of pediatric epilepsy fall into this category.[2,3] Although much of the early literature on postoperative seizure control refers to adults with epilepsy, the importance of considering surgical treatment in children with intractable epilepsy is well recognized. Issues in pediatric epilepsy surgery differ from those in adults in several respects, including factors that may potentially affect seizure outcome. Children have a higher proportion of neoplastic lesions and malformation of cortical development in the epileptogenic substrate and more frequent extratemporal epileptogenic foci.[2,4–8] Surgery on the developing brain may in itself affect postoperative seizure control in children.

Why is seizure control important as an outcome measure after epilepsy surgery? An obvious answer is that it enables physicians to consider the option of surgical treatment for an individual patient, in addition to providing a prognosis to families presented with the option of surgery for their child with refractory epilepsy. The ultimate aim of any treatment for epilepsy is to improve quality of life. Adult studies have shown that postoperative seizure control is an important predictor of quality of life.[9–11] Seizure frequency has also been related to an increased risk of sudden unexpected death in adults.[12] In children, as opposed to adults, an additional factor is the potentially deleterious effect of recurrent seizures on the developing brain and long-term side effects of antiepileptic drugs on achieving developmental potential.

In this chapter, we address postoperative seizure control in terms of what is known regarding the outcome of epilepsy surgery with respect to subsequent seizure control and factors that may affect postoperative seizure control. This is followed by a discussion of the medical management of epilepsy in children after epilepsy surgery.

■ Outcome with Respect to Seizure Control after Surgery

The most widely accepted classification of postoperative seizure outcome is the scheme proposed by Engel.[13] This scheme stratifies postoperative outcome into four classes, Class I to Class IV. Patients in Class I are free of disabling seizures (excludes early postoperative seizures) and are further subdivided into four categories: (a) completely seizure free since surgery; (b) nondisabling, simple partial seizures or auras only since surgery; (c) some disabling seizures after surgery, but free of disabling seizures for at least 2 years; (d) generalized convulsion with antiepileptic drug withdrawal only. Patients in Class II have rare disabling seizures. This group is divided into four subgroups: (a) initially free of disabling seizures but have rare seizures now; (b) rare disabling seizures since surgery; (c) more than rare disabling seizures after surgery, but rare seizures for the last 2 years; (d) nocturnal seizures only. Class III describes patients with worthwhile improvement and includes patients with worthwhile seizure reduction, or prolonged seizure-free intervals amounting to greater than half the follow-up period, but not less than 2 years. Patients in Class IV have no worthwhile improvement in seizures. Favorable postoperative seizure control is generally considered as an Engel Class I or Class II outcome.

Systematic evaluation of surgical outcome data in children is limited by the heterogeneity of the surgical groups, both in terms of the surgical procedure (e.g., temporal resection, extratemporal resection, hemispherectomy, multiple subpial transection, corpus callosotomy) and the underlying cause of the seizures or epilepsy syndrome. The numbers that fall into a similar category are, therefore, not large. Potential confounders in trying to assess postoperative seizure control may be the different proportion of children in various age groups (between birth and 18 years) in each series, and, more importantly, the duration of postsurgical follow-up. Although a significant body of literature on postoperative seizure control has emerged in the last three decades, there is a lack of prospective, randomized, and controlled studies in children treated surgically for epilepsy.

Postoperative seizure control reported in seven pediatric series[14-20] with reasonable sample size and duration of follow-up is summarized in **Table 37.1**. The average postoperative follow-up in these children ranged from 2.7 years to almost 11 years; 67 to 81% were seizure free after surgery, and a higher proportion, 74 to 86%, had a favorable seizure outcome (Engel Class I or II).

Seizure Control after Surgery for a Structural Lesion

Refractory seizures in children caused by lesions identified on imaging are unlikely to remit with time.[21] The location of the lesion, particularly temporal versus extratemporal, has also been implicated as a factor with potential influence on seizure control after epilepsy surgery.[14,18-20]

Seizure Control after Temporal Lobe Surgery

Evidence from retrospective studies in children treated surgically for intractable epilepsy over the last two and a half decades shows that 58 to 74% of children become seizure free. A larger percentage, 67 to 82%, show favorable seizure control.[3,7,8,20,22,23] Within the last few years, randomized controlled studies have shown the efficacy of surgery compared with medical therapy in TLE in adults.[24,25] Although there are no such randomized controlled trials in children, several pediatric series have documented the effectiveness of temporal resection for seizure control.[16,17,26-28]

In a large series reported by Benifla and colleagues (**Table 37.1**), of the 106 children treated surgically for TLE, 74% were seizure free (Engel Class I) at a mean follow-up period of 67 months. This included 7 who became seizure free after a second procedure. Two additional patients were in Engel Class II, giving a favorable seizure outcome in 75% of patients in this series. Twenty-six patients (25%) had a less favorable outcome (Engel Class III and Class IV). In those who relapsed, the mean time to seizure recurrence was 15 months after surgery.[17] In another cohort of 109 patients who underwent temporal resection and for whom follow-up data for a minimum of 5 years were available, 81.7% became seizure free (Engel Class I), and an additional 4.6% satisfied criteria for Engel Class II, resulting in favorable seizure control in 86% of the 109 patients.[16]

Features associated with an unfavorable outcome after temporal resection are the lack of a structural abnormality on magnetic resonance imaging (MRI), development-associated with disease, widespread disease documented by postoperative electroencephalography (EEG; occult dual disease involving the same temporal lobe, adjacent frontal lobe, or bi-temporal disease), residual tumor or malignant transformation, and the need for emergency temporal

lobectomy secondary to complication of invasive presurgical monitoring.[20]

Seizure Control after Extratemporal Resection

Seizure outcome is usually better after temporal resection than after extratemporal resection (**Table 37.2**) with 72 to 88% seizure-free rates after temporal resection versus 54 to 60% patients becoming seizure free after extratemporal resection.[14,18-20] Nevertheless, in most well-selected patients, surgery for extratemporal lesions provides an improvement in seizure control, with more than 50% of patients achieving a seizure-free status (**Table 37.2**).

Kim and coworkers (**Table 37.2**) found that 88% of the patients who had temporal lobe resection were seizure free, and 90% had favorable seizure outcomes. By comparison, 55% who had extratemporal resection became seizure free, and 64% had a favorable seizure outcome. This finding was despite more invasive presurgical studies in the extratemporal resection group.[20] The mean duration of follow-up was more than 5 years in this study. A smaller series reported by Gilliam and colleagues, with mean follow-up of 2.7 years, showed a 72% seizure-free rate after temporal resection versus 60% seizure free after frontal lobe resection.[14] Another cohort of 113 children from Italy[18] showed that 54% of the patients became seizure free after extratemporal resection. After temporal resection, 91% of the patients were seizure free. The mean duration of follow-up was 55 months.[18]

Factors associated with an unfavorable outcome in those who had extratemporal resection were similar to the factors identified in children who had temporal resection, namely, the lack of a structural abnormality on MRI, development associated disease, more widespread disease than suspected preoperatively, residual tumor, or malignant transformation. Additional factors associated with an unfavorable outcome after extratemporal resection were multilobar resection, limited resection because of the presence of functional cortex, incomplete lesionectomy, or tumor progression.[20]

Seizure Control after Hemispherectomy

Successful postoperative seizure control depends primarily on removing the cortical substrate likely responsible for the seizures. Hemispherectomy has been referred to as the ultimate focal resection and is usually performed in children with diffuse hemispheric pathologies. This includes development related disorders (hemimegalencephaly, diffuse and focal cortical dysplasia [CD], polymicrogyria, microdysgenesis), acquired conditions that may be perinatal or postnatal (infarction/ischemia, infection, trauma, hemiconvulsive–hemiplegic epilepsy), or progressive disorders such as Rasmussen encephalitis and Sturge-Weber syndrome.[29,30] Seizure freedom after hemispherectomy is 70 to 80% in well-selected

Table 37.1 Postoperative Seizure Outcome in Some Pediatric Epilepsy Surgery Studies

Authors	Number of Patients	Age at Surgery, Mean (Range)	Age at Seizure Onset Mean (Range)	Duration of Epilepsy before Surgery	Duration of Follow-up Mean (Range)	Postoperative Seizure Control According to Engel Classification, % (number)			
						Engel I % (No.)	Engel II % (No.)	Engel III % (No.)	Engel IV % (No.)
Gilliam et al[14]	33	7.75 years (8 months–12 years)	2.2 years (6 days–5 years)	—	2.7 years (7 months–6 years)	67% (22)	9% (3)	12% (4)	12% (4)
Bourgeois et al[15]	200	8.3 years (10 months–15 years)	— (6 weeks–12 years)	2.5 years (1 months–12 years)	5.2 years (18 months–17 years)	71.3%	7.2%	2.9%	4.7%
Cossu et al[16]	109	13.2 years (2 months–8.9 years)	5.5 years (birth–17 years)	7.7 years (01.–17.6 years)	10.9 years (5–10.2 years)	81.7%	4.6%	13.8% (15/109)	
Benifla et al[17]	106	13.5 years	5.9 years (1 month–17 years)	5.6 years	67 months (2 years–13 years)	74% (78)	1.8% (2)	5.6% (6)	19% (20)
Massimo et al[18]	113	8.8 years (1–15 years)	3.1 years (0–15 years)	5.7 years (0–14 years)	55.1 months (24–115 months)	68% (77)	9% (10)	10% (11)	13% (15)
Kan et al[19]	58	11.2 years (1.8–21 years)	—	4.8 years (6 months–15 years)	4.7 years (1–8 years)	74% seizure free			
Kim et al[20]	134	8.5 years (8 months–18 years)	4.3 years (birth–14 years)	—	62.3 months (12–168 months)	69% (93)	5% (7)	7% (9)	19% (25)

Source: Gilliam F, Wyllie E, Kashden J, et al. Epilepsy surgery outcome: comprehensive assessment in children. Neurology 1997;48(5):1368–1374; Bourgeois M, Sainte-Rose C, Lellouch-Tubiana A, et al. Surgery of epilepsy associated with focal lesions in childhood. J Neurosurg 1999;90(5):833–842; Mittal S, Montes JL, Farmer JP, et al. Long-term outcome after surgical treatment of temporal lobe epilepsy in children. J Neurosurg 2005; 103(5, suppl):401–412; Benifla M, Otsubo H, Ochi A, et al. Temporal lobe surgery for intractable epilepsy in children: an analysis of outcomes in 126 children. Neurosurgery 2006;59(6):1203–1213, discussion 1213–1214; Cossu M, Lo Russo G, Francione S, et al. Epilepsy surgery in children: results and predictors of outcome on seizures. Epilepsia 2008;49(1):65–72; Kan P, Van Orman C, Kestle JRW. Outcomes after surgery for focal epilepsy in children. Childs Nerv Syst 2008;24(5):587–591; Kim SK, Wang KC, Hwang YS, et al. Epilepsy surgery in children: outcomes and complications. J Neurosurg Pediatr 2008;1(4):277–283

Table 37.2 Seizure Control after Temporal and Extratemporal Resection in Children Treated Surgically for Epilepsy

Author (Number of Patients)	Temporal Resection		Extratemporal Resection	
	n	% Seizure Free	n	% Seizure Free
Gilliam et al[14] (n = 33)	18	72%	15	60%
Massimo et al[18] (n = 113)	43	91%	70	54%
Kan et al[19] (n = 58)	33	85%	25	60%
Kim et al[20] (n = 134[a])	59	88%	56	55%

[a]Nineteen patients who had functional hemispherectomy, corpus callosotomy, or multiple subpial transaction, are not included in table.
Source: Gilliam F, Wyllie E, Kashden J, et al. Epilepsy surgery outcome: comprehensive assessment in children. Neurology 1997;48(5):1368–1374; Sinclair DB, Aronyk KE, Snyder TJ, et al. Pediatric epilepsy surgery at the University of Alberta: 1988-2000. Pediatr Neurol 2003;29(4):302–311; Baker GA, Jacoby A, Buck D, Stalgis C, Monnet D. Quality of life of people with epilepsy: a European study. Epilepsia 1997;38(3):353–362; Kim SK, Wang KC, Hwang YS, et al. Epilepsy surgery in children: outcomes and complications. J Neurosurg Pediatr 2008;1(4):277–283

patients. As most of the hemisphere is removed, pathology may not matter.[20,31,32] In the UCLA series, which included a large percentage of cortical dysplasias and other non-CD destructive lesions, 64% of the 62 patients who had hemi-

spherectomy showed an Engel Class I outcome at 2 years.[33] Seizure-free rates of 54 to 82% have been seen after hemispherectomy for infantile hemiplegia, Rasmussen encephalitis, and Sturge-Weber syndrome.[34–37] **Table 37.3** gives a summary of seizure outcome after hemispherectomy for the treatment of intractable epilepsy in three studies.[29,30,38] In the series reported by Devlin and colleagues,[30] seizure freedom was 82% in those with acquired pathology (11 of 33 cases), 50% in those with progressive disorders (6 of 33 children), and 31% in those with developmental pathology (16 of 33). A worthwhile reduction in seizures was seen across all groups.[30] By contrast, in the series from the Cleveland Clinic Foundation, the etiology of catastrophic epilepsy in 18 children younger than 2 years old who underwent hemispherectomy was not associated with the outcome of seizures after surgery. Incomplete disconnection was the only factor related to seizure outcome in this cohort.[38]

Seizure Outcome in Relation to Pathology of the Epileptogenic Substrate

Low-grade tumors, malformations of cortical development (MCD), mesial temporal sclerosis (MTS), vascular malformations, hypoxic ischemic insults (including in utero ischemic lesions) are all causes of focal epilepsy in children.[14,16–20] **Table 37.4** shows the relative distribution of postoperative pathology reported in six pediatric series and whether pathology is correlated with postoperative seizure control in these patients. Low-grade tumors and MCD, together as well as independently, constitute the most common pathologies identified postoperatively. MTS as an isolated lesion is seen much less often in children (refer to **Table 37.4**). An exception to this is the series reported by Mittal and

Table 37.3 Postoperative Seizure Control after Hemispherectomy

Author (ref)	N	Age at Surgery Mean/Median (Range)	Follow-up Mean/Median (Range)	Seizure Outcome, %			
				Seizure Free	Rare Seizures	Worthwhile Improvement	No Improvement
Vining et al[29]	54	7.1 years (0.2–20.6 years)	6.2 years (0.5–27.3 years)	54%	24%	17%[a]	6%[b]
Devlin et al[30]	33	4.25 years (0.33–17 years)	3.4 years (1–8 years)	52%	9%	30% > 75% seizure reduction	9% < 75% or no seizure reduction
Gonzalez-Martinez et al[38]	18	11.7 months (3–22 months)	34.8 months (12–74 months)	66%		22% > 90% seizure reduction	

[a]Moderate frequency and severity of seizures that interfered to some extent with function.
[b]Frequency and severity of seizures significantly handicapping.
Source: Vining EP, Freeman JM, Pillas DJ, et al. Why would you remove half a brain? The outcome of 58 children after hemispherectomy–the Johns Hopkins experience: 1968 to 1996. Pediatrics 1997;100(2 pt 1):163–171; Devlin AM, Cross JH, Harkness W, et al. Clinical outcomes of hemispherectomy for epilepsy in childhood and adolescence. Brain 2003;126(pt 3):556–566; González-Martínez JA, Gupta A, Kotagal P, et al. Hemispherectomy for catastrophic epilepsy in infants. Epilepsia 2005;46(9):1518–1525.

Table 37.4   Pathology and Postoperative Seizure Control

Author (Number of Patients)	Neoplasm % (Number of Patients)	MCD % (Number of Patients)	MTS % (Number of Patients)	Multiple Findings % (Number of Patients)	Gliosis % (Number of Patients)	Miscellaneous % (Number of Patients)	No Abnormality % (Number of Patients)	Relation of Pathology to Seizure Control after Surgery
Gilliam et al[14] (n = 33)	36.4% (12)	33.3% (11)	3% (1)	3% (1)	6% (2)	12% (4)	6% (2)	Pathology not related to seizure outcome
Mittal et al[16] (n = 109)	35% (38)	35% (38)	45% (49)	25%	—	4.6% (5)	5.5% (6)	Pathology as an independent variable related to seizure outcome
Benifla et al[17] (n = 126)	51% (64)	10% (13)	13% (16)	8% (10)	12% (15)	2% (3)	3% (5)	Better seizure outcome with neoplasm
Massimo et al[18] (n = 113)	38% (43)	83% (94)	10% (11)	24% (27)	—	4% (5)	2% (2)	Better seizure outcome with glial neuronal tumor versus other path
Kan et al[19] (n = 58)	28% (16)	22% (13)	28% (16)	5% (3)	—	17% (10)	—	Seizure outcome best with neoplasm and MTS
Kim et al[20] (n = 124; n for study = 134, no path specimen in 10)	36% (45)	57% (71)	15% (19)	21% (26)	—	—	—	Tumor better outcome than MCD; worse outcome with dual pathology.

Abbreviations: malformations of cortical development, MCD, mesial temporal sclerosis, MTS.
Source: Gilliam F, Wyllie E, Kashden J, et al. Epilepsy surgery outcome: comprehensive assessment in children. Neurology 1997;48(5):1368–1374; Mittal S, Montes JL, Farmer JP, et al. Long-term outcome after surgical treatment of temporal lobe epilepsy in children. J Neurosurg 2005; 103(5, suppl):401–412; Benifla M, Otsubo H, Ochi A, et al. Temporal lobe surgery for intractable epilepsy in children: an analysis of outcomes in 126 children. Neurosurgery 2006;59(6):1203–1213, discussion 1213–1214; Cossu M, Lo Russo G, Francione S, et al. Epilepsy surgery in children: results and predictors of outcome on seizures. Epilepsia 2008;49(1):65–72; Kan P, Van Orman C, Kestle JRW. Outcomes after surgery for focal epilepsy in children. Childs Nerv Syst 2008;24(5):587–591; Kim SK, Wang KC, Hwang YS, et al. Epilepsy surgery in children: outcomes and complications. J Neurosurg Pediatr 2008;1(4):277–283.

colleagues[16]; 45% (49/109) of patients in this series showed MTS and formed the largest single histopathological diagnosis.[16] Among tumors, ganglioglioma, dysembryoplastic neuroepithelial tumor, low-grade astrocytoma, and mixed gliomas are the most frequent, and a smaller number of other tumors, such as pilocytic xanthoastrocytoma, oligodendroglioma, and choroid plexus papilloma, were identified.[14,16–20] In the larger cohorts of children treated for epilepsy by surgical resection, up to 25% of children show more than one pathological finding, that is, dual or multiple pathology.[16,18,20]

As noted in the last column of **Table 37.4**, better postoperative seizure control is achieved when the causative lesion is a low-grade tumor or isolated MTS.[16,17,19] Seizure control is better after resection of glial neuronal tumors compared with other pathologies.[18] Tumors, in general are associated with better postoperative seizure control than MCD. The presence of more than one pathology correlates with a worse seizure outcome.[19,20]

Among children with epilepsy, the most intractable are the youngest patients with cortical dysplasia, tuberous sclerosis, or other structural lesions.[39,40] The structural lesion in these cases is often more extensive than in TLE, which has become the prototypical focal epilepsy syndrome that shows good seizure control after surgery. A study by Mathern and coworkers from UCLA compared seizure outcomes in children with symptomatic seizures from large unilateral CD and non-CD pathologies (e.g., infantile hemiplegia, perinatal stroke, infection, Rasmussen encephalitis, Sturge-Weber syndrome and miscellaneous) with TLE patients who had more focal pathology. Seizure outcomes at 6, 12, and 24 months and 5 years and 10 years after surgery were assessed.[33]

The mean presurgical seizure frequency was significantly greater in the CD and non-CD groups than in the group with

TLE. There was no difference in postoperative seizure frequency among CD, non-CD, and TLE patients at 6, 12, and 24 months and at 10 years. The percentage of seizure-free patients at 2 years after surgery was similar in CD (65% of 64 children), non-CD (56% of 71 children) and TLE (65% of 31 children). At 5 years after surgery, seizure frequency was significantly greater in CD cases compared with TLE. The cause was unclear. The authors believed that most of the recurrent seizures were complex partial seizures and were less debilitating than the original seizures. The number of patients who had follow-up at 5 years and 10 years, however, was small.

There is some evidence to suggest that early and complete surgical resection of CD lesions may contribute to better postoperative seizure control in children with CD than in adults with CD.[41-46]

Seizure Outcome after Reoperation

In children with intractable seizures who do not have a favorable postoperative seizure outcome after initial surgery, it may not be unreasonable to consider a second surgical procedure, particularly in the face of medical intractability. In some of the larger pediatric studies, small numbers of patients underwent reoperation. In one such group, 7 of 134 patients required a second surgery because of poor seizure control after the first surgery. Four of the 7 (57%) patients showed favorable seizure control after reoperation.[20]

■ Seizure Control after Surgical Treatment of Epilepsy in Children without an Obvious Structural Lesion

A structural lesion is not always identified in children with refractory focal epilepsy. MRI may be noncontributory in up to 29% of patients with partial epilepsy.[47] There is no accurate estimate of the prevalence of a normal MRI in children with intractable epilepsy who are potential surgical candidates. In a cohort of 75 children younger than 12 years of age who underwent resective surgery for intractable epilepsy, 35 (47%) had no identifiable focal lesion on MRI.[7]

The identification of a focal epileptogenic lesion on preoperative MRI may affect postoperative seizure control in both adult and pediatric patients, depending on the location of the lesion and the pathology. Postoperative seizure control is less favorable when no MRI lesion is seen.[7,13,23,48-61] In a meta-analysis of 47 studies, an abnormal MRI was found to be a favorable prognostic factor for seizure outcome after surgery.[62] Although postoperative seizure control may be relatively less favorable in children with nonlesional epilepsy compared with those with an identifiable focal le-

sion on MRI, the reduction in seizures is still an important improvement for this patient population, which often has a very high preoperative seizure burden and severe medical intractability.

The literature on postoperative seizure outcome for nonlesional epilepsy is still emerging. Evidence-based data regarding postoperative seizure control in children with intractable nonlesional epilepsy are scarce. There are no controlled studies or standardized guidelines for preoperative evaluation to identify the epileptogenic zone and to assess postoperative seizure outcome, leaving room for selection bias and observer bias. This may account for the variation in the reported success rate of surgery for nonlesional epilepsy with the range of seizure-free outcome being 37 to 51%. Most of these studies consist of adult patients. Conclusions from adult studies cannot necessarily be extrapolated to pediatric or adolescent patients. Multicenter prospective studies are needed to obtain reasonable estimates of seizure outcome in children with nonlesional epilepsy.

Some recent studies (**Table 37.5**) that include predominantly or exclusively children, show relatively better postoperative seizure outcome.[7,63-68] Paolicchi and coworkers,[7] in their cohort of 35 children with nonlesional epilepsy, found that 51% were seizure free. However, 21 of these children were designated as nonlesional based on a 0.5 Tesla MRI. In another pediatric series 36% of 22 patients became seizure free, and 77% had a good outcome.[66] A recently published series of predominately children with nonlesional partial epilepsy[67] gives a better idea of postoperative seizure control up to 10 years after surgery. In this cohort, at 2-year follow-up, 44% were seizure free and 58% had a favorable outcome. After a period of 5 years, the numbers were similar with 44% still seizure free and 59% with a favorable seizure outcome. Ten years after surgery, 38% were seizure free and 68% continued to fall in the favorable outcome category. Even though the number of patients for whom follow-up data were available for 10 years after surgery was approximately 43% of the initial cohort, it is encouraging to see that a favorable reduction in seizures persisted up to 10 years after surgery. These data suggest that surgery, even in nonlesional epilepsy, can improve seizure control and thereby quality of life. Pathology of the resected tissue, for the most part, probably does not influence postoperative seizure control in children treated surgically for epilepsy without a structural lesion on MRI (**Table 37.6**).

■ Factors Affecting Postoperative Seizure Control

Variables potentially affecting seizure outcome after epilepsy surgery can be categorized as presurgical, surgical, and postsurgical. Presurgical factors include age at seizure onset, duration of epilepsy, seizure frequency, age at surgery, and MRI

Table 37.5 Seizure Outcome after Epilepsy Surgery in Patients with Nonlesional Epilepsy

Author	Number of Patients	Age at Onset Mean/Median (range)	Epilepsy Duration	Age at Surgery	Follow-Up Mean (range)	Temporal Resection	Neocortical Temporal/Extratemporal Resection	Seizure Outcome	
								Seizure Free	Favorable[a]
Paolicchi et al[7]	35	2.8 years (0–9.7 years)	Not given	7.7 years (0.5–11.9 years)	5 years (1–10 years)	9	19	51%	74%
Siegel et al[55]	25	12.2 years (0.5–40.3years)	19.2 years (2.9–40.6 years)	31.3 year (16.8–51.8 years)	≥ 2 years	5	19	62%	83%
Blume et al[63]	70	13 years (1–47 year)	17 years (1–41 years)	31 years (6–65 years)	8.1 years (2–12 years)	43	27	37%	50%
Sylaja et al[64]	17	12 years (5.5 – 26 years)	15 years (7–25 years)	27 years (14–44 years)	≥ 1 year	17	NA	29%	41%
Lee et al[65]	89	6.8 ± 6.1 years (2–49 years)	13.5 ± 6.5 years (3–28 years)		At least 2 years (3.54 ± 1.85 years)		NTLE – 31 FLE – 35 PLE – 11 OLE – 11 Multifocal - 1	47.2%	*80%
Ramachandran Nair et al[66]	22	4.3 years (0.5–9 years)	7.4 years (2.5–13 years)	11.7 years (4–18 years)	27 months (9–67 months)	Resection of 2 or more lobes in most		36%	*77%
Jayakar et al[67]	102	3.5 years (0–15.2 years)	Not given	10.7 years (1.5–21 years)	Minimum 2 years	47	54	44%	58%

Abbreviations: Number of patients with nonlesional epilepsy who had surgery, N; temporal lobe epilepsy, TLE; neocortical TLE, NTLE; frontal lobe epilepsy, FLE; parieral lobe epilepsy, PLE; occipital lobe epilepsy, OLE.

[a]Favorable outcome means Engel Class I or II, except *Class I–III.

Source: Paolicchi JM, Jayakar P, Dean P, et al. Predictors of outcome in pediatric epilepsy surgery. Neurology 2000;54(3):642–647; Siegel AM, Jobst BC, Thadani VM, et al. Medically intractable, localization-related epilepsy with normal MRI: presurgical evaluation and surgical outcome in 43 patients. Epilepsia 2001;42(7):883–888; Blume WT, Ganapathy GR, Munoz D, Lee DH. Indices of resective surgery effectiveness for intractable nonlesional focal epilepsy. Epilepsia 2004;45(1):46–53; Sylaja PN, Radhakrishnan K, Kesavadas C, Sarma PS. Seizure outcome after anterior temporal lobectomy and its predictors in patients with apparent temporal lobe epilepsy and normal MRI. Epilepsia 2004;45(7):803–808; Lee SK, Lee SY, Kim KK, Hong KS, Lee DS, Chung CK. Surgical outcome and prognostic factors of cryptogenic neocortical epilepsy. Ann Neurol 2005;58(4):525–532; Ramachandran Nair R, Otsubo H, Shroff MM, et al. MEG predicts outcome following surgery for intractable epilepsy in children with normal or nonfocal MRI findings. Epilepsia 2007;48(1):149–157; Jayakar P, Dunoyer C, Dean P, et al. Epilepsy surgery in patients with normal or nonfocal MRI scans: integrative strategies offer long-term seizure relief. Epilepsia 2008;49(5):758–764.

Table 37.6   Pathology and Outcome in Nonlesional Epilepsy

Author	Number	Normal	Cortical Dysplasia/ Migration Abnormalities	Tumors	Nonspecific Histology[a]	Seizure Outcome
Siegel et al[55]	24	13	1	1	9	Not related to pathology
Blume et al[63]	70 (pathology not available)	19			48	Not related to pathology
Sylaja et al[64]	17	11			6	Hippocampal neuronal loss correlated with excellent outcome
Lee et al[65]	89 (pathology available in 80)		68	1	11	Not related to pathology
Ramachandran Nair et al[66]	22 (pathology available for 21)	4	9	1	7	Not related to pathology

[a]Includes gliosis, heterotopia, chronic inflammation, microinfarct, hippocampal atrophy, hippocampal sclerosis, microdysgenesis, and subpial gliosis.
Source: Siegel AM, Jobst BC, Thadani VM, et al. Medically intractable, localization-related epilepsy with normal MRI: presurgical evaluation and surgical outcome in 43 patients. Epilepsia 2001;42(7):883–888; Blume WT, Ganapathy GR, Munoz D, Lee DH. Indices of resective surgery effectiveness for intractable nonlesional focal epilepsy. Epilepsia 2004;45(1):46–53; Sylaja PN, Radhakrishnan K, Kesavadas C, Sarma PS. Seizure outcome after anterior temporal lobectomy and its predictors in patients with apparent temporal lobe epilepsy and normal MRI. Epilepsia 2004;45(7):803–808; Lee SK, Lee SY, Kim KK, Hong KS, Lee DS, Chung CK. Surgical outcome and prognostic factors of cryptogenic neocortical epilepsy. Ann Neurol 2005;58(4):525–532; Ramachandran Nair R, Otsubo H, Shroff MM, et al. MEG predicts outcome following surgery for intractable epilepsy in children with normal or nonfocal MRI findings. Epilepsia 2007;48(1):149–157.

findings. Surgical variables consist of the site of surgery and extent of resection of the lesion or the identified epileptogenic zone. The main postsurgical variables are histopathology of the resected tissue, acute postoperative seizures, and the duration of follow-up after surgery. On reviewing the literature on this aspect of postoperative seizure control, it becomes apparent that generalizations cannot be made, because reports are often conflicting. The following is a summary of the available data in children undergoing epilepsy surgery.

Presurgical Factors

Age at seizure onset, duration of epilepsy, and age at surgery do not predict seizure outcome in most pediatric epilepsy studies.[7,17] There are, however, reports of lower risk of seizure recurrence with older age of seizure onset.[18] In this context, animal studies on the effect of seizures in the immature brain may be significant.[68,69] The establishment of an epileptogenic network at an early stage of brain maturation may potentially cause an increased susceptibility to seizures than if the first seizure occurs after the main physiological networks have already developed. Most studies do not identify the duration of epilepsy before surgery as a factor predicting outcome. However, at least one pediatric study found that seizures for more than 5 years before surgery correlated with worse seizure control.[16] Other presurgical factors, such as a definite history of febrile seizures (in addition to afebrile seizures), secondary generalization of focal seizures, and multiple seizure types, have been associated with postoperative seizure control. Occurrence of febrile seizures was found to be a favorable predictor of seizure outcome in chil-

dren with TLE,[16,64] whereas secondary generalization was an unfavorable predictor of seizure control,[17] as was the occurrence of multiple seizure types.[55,66]

Patients with a unifocal lesion on MRI have a lower risk of seizure recurrence than those with multifocal lesions on MRI or an unremarkable MRI.[18,20,23] Temporal lobe lesions generally have a better seizure outcome than extratemporal lesions.[14,18–20] Conversely, in a study of 75 children younger than 12 years old who had epilepsy surgery, there was no difference in seizure outcome based on whether the lesion was temporal or extratemporal or whether a lesion was identified on MRI.[7] A good correlation between seizure semiology, neuroradiological findings, and EEG localization is associated with a favorable seizure outcome.[19]

Presurgical localization of the epileptogenic zone is a topic by itself. The prediction of seizure control based on specific and specialized modalities of localization, such as functional imaging, magnetoencephalography (MEG) studies, and invasive EEG monitoring is addressed in the section on preoperative assessment. In general, a high degree of concordance among different methods used to localize the epileptic zone is associated with a favorable seizure outcome.

Surgical Factors

Seizure control is generally better after temporal resection than after extratemporal resection[14,18–20] and after unilobar resection compared with multilobar resection.[14,18,20] As can be expected, partial or incomplete resection of a lesion is associated with a worse seizure outcome.[15,18] A trend toward seizure freedom is seen when resection is complete.[66]

Complete resection may be limited by the presence of eloquent cortex in the epileptogenic zone or poor macroscopic differentiation of the margins of the lesion.

Postsurgical Factors

In children, a low-grade neoplasm is associated with better postoperative seizure control than a nondiagnostic or nonneoplastic histopathology.[17] Histopathological diagnosis of glial neuronal tumor is associated with better seizure outcome.[18] Tumors have a better postoperative seizure outcome than developmental lesions, which are often poorly circumscribed and tend to have a widespread epileptogenic zone that even invasive EEG monitoring may not be able to precisely delineate. Such lesions are not always apparent on MRI, or the visible lesion may be only part of a diffuse structural abnormality.[20] If postoperative EEG shows widespread disease, such as dual disease, bitemporal seizure onset, and multilobar seizures, this is associated with an unfavorable seizure outcome.[20]

Acute postoperative seizures (APOSs) are defined as seizures occurring within the first 7 to 10 days after epilepsy surgery. In a series of patients younger than 18 years of age who underwent surgery for refractory epilepsy, 25% of patients had APOSs. Patients who did not have APOSs had a greater chance of being seizure free compared with those who had APOSs—80% versus 51%.[70] In another pediatric study, in patients undergoing hemispherectomy, the occurrence of more than five APOSs predicted a worse seizure outcome.[71]

It is important to remember that all available data are from retrospective studies and the number of patients with long-term follow-up may not be large. Jarrar and colleagues in a long-term follow-up of temporal lobectomy in children found that at 1 year, 75% were in Engel Class I. At 15 years, only 53% remained in Engel Class I; 86% of the 37 patients in this study had 15 years of follow-up.[26] In a pediatric series of temporal lobe surgery for intractable epilepsy,[17] an overall good seizure outcome occurred in 74% of cases. The mean follow-up in this study was 67 months (range 2–13 years). Of the 20 patients in Engel Class IV in this series, seizures recurred within 4 years in three children but after almost 10 years in another child. This finding supports the notion that seizure outcome may not necessarily remain stable over time. The limitation of the Engel classification is that the class that is assigned to a particular patient is based on postoperative seizure status in the preceding 2 years at the time of last follow-up.[13]

■ Medical Management after Epilepsy Surgery

After surgical treatment of epilepsy, antiepileptic drug (AED) therapy is continued for some time. Discontinuation or a re-

duction in the number of medications is considered after a variable period of time, depending on the postoperative seizure outcome. Most literature on planned discontinuation of AED involves adults with TLE surgery and is retrospective in nature. Approximately one third of patients who have planned discontinuation of AED after a period of being seizure free relapse within 1 to 5 years of withdrawing medication.[72] Most of those who relapse come under control again once medication is restarted. A prospective study examined tapering and discontinuing AED in patients who were seizure free for 1 year. One in three postoperative patients experience a relapse after an attempt to reduce seizure medication.[73] It is suggested but not confirmed that the relapse rate in children after medication withdrawal may be lower. Figures of 10 to 16% have been reported,[74,75] however, a higher relapse rate of 44% has also been reported.[76] Almost two thirds of adults who relapse after a reduction of AED regain remission when medication is restarted. Some, however, never regain a seizure-free state. There is probably a small but definite risk of precipitating uncontrollable epilepsy, including the risk of status epilepticus and death. By some estimates, up to 9% of adult patients[77] and 3% of pediatric patients[74] experience refractory epilepsy associated with AED withdrawal and remain difficult to control after medication is restarted. Overall, however, data suggest that those who relapse in the context of AED reduction are perhaps more likely to regain remission than those who relapse for other reasons.[73]

There are no good evidence-based guidelines on the optimal timing for initiating medication withdrawal or reduction in children and adolescents with a favorable seizure outcome after epilepsy surgery. From some of the reported data, there appears to be little benefit in waiting to attempt AED discontinuation in seizure-free children longer than 1 year after surgery and in seizure-free adults beyond 2 years after epilepsy surgery.[72] Some recent data in children suggest that AED withdrawal may be considered earlier than 1 year after surgery when postoperative seizure control is favorable. Discontinuation of AED less than 6 months after successful epilepsy surgery is associated with higher risk of seizure recurrence than if medication is withdrawn more than 6 months later or not at all, although waiting for more than 1 year after surgery does not appear to be of any additional benefit.[78]

Medication adjustment in the immediate postoperative period and in the first few months after surgery is difficult. It is probably better to simplify the drug regimen preoperatively, particularly in patients on poly therapy. In the immediate postoperative period, fluctuation of AED levels can occur without a change in dose. Careful monitoring of drug levels is suggested. An increase in dose may be needed to prevent breakthrough seizures during this period. Downward dose adjustments can be made once the immediate postoperative effect has disappeared.[79] There is a lack of specific data regarding the pharmacokinetics of the newer AEDs in the immediate postoperative period.

■ Conclusion

Surgery is a useful treatment option in children with refractory epilepsy and should be considered when medical treatment fails to adequately control seizures. Experience over the last two decades suggests that, in well-selected patients, there is a good chance of favorable postoperative seizure control across all etiologies of focal epilepsy and in the youngest and most refractory patients. A large proportion of children who undergo surgery for medically refractory epilepsy are able to discontinue or decrease antiepileptic medication after surgery. In those who relapse, restarting medication usually results in better seizure control than before surgery.

References

1. Davidson S, Falconer MA. Outcome of surgery in 40 children with temporal-lobe epilepsy. Lancet 1975;1(7919):1260–1263
2. Kim SK, Wang KC, Hwang YS, et al. Pediatric intractable epilepsy: the role of presurgical evaluation and seizure outcome. Childs Nerv Syst 2000;16(5):278–285, discussion 286
3. Morrison G, Duchowny M, Resnick T, et al. Epilepsy surgery in childhood. A report of 79 patients. Pediatr Neurosurg 1992;18(5–6):291–297
4. Fish DR, Smith SJ, Quesney LF, Andermann F, Rasmussen T. Surgical treatment of children with medically intractable frontal or temporal lobe epilepsy: results and highlights of 40 years' experience. Epilepsia 1993;34(2):244–247
5. Holmes GL. Intractable epilepsy in children. Epilepsia 1996;37(suppl 3):14–27
6. Leiphart JW, Peacock WJ, Mathern GW. Lobar and multilobar resections for medically intractable pediatric epilepsy. Pediatr Neurosurg 2001;34(6):311–318
7. Paolicchi JM, Jayakar P, Dean P, et al. Predictors of outcome in pediatric epilepsy surgery. Neurology 2000;54(3):642–647
8. Sinclair DB, Aronyk KE, Snyder TJ, et al. Pediatric epilepsy surgery at the University of Alberta: 1988-2000. Pediatr Neurol 2003;29(4):302–311
9. Baker GA, Jacoby A, Buck D, Stalgis C, Monnet D. Quality of life of people with epilepsy: a European study. Epilepsia 1997;38(3):353–362
10. Kellett MW, Smith DF, Baker GA, Chadwick DW. Quality of life after epilepsy surgery. J Neurol Neurosurg Psychiatry 1997;63(1):52–58
11. Vickrey BG, Berg AT, Sperling MR, et al. Relationships between seizure severity and health-related quality of life in refractory localization-related epilepsy. Epilepsia 2000;41(6):760–764
12. Tomson T. Mortality in epilepsy. J Neurol 2000;247(1):15–21
13. Engel J Jr, Van Ness PC, Rasmussen TB, Ojemann LM. Outcome with respect to epileptic seizures. In: Engel J. Jr. Surgical Treatment of the Epilepsies. 2nd ed. New York, NY: Raven Press, Ltd; 1993:609–622
14. Gilliam F, Wyllie E, Kashden J, et al. Epilepsy surgery outcome: comprehensive assessment in children. Neurology 1997;48(5):1368–1374
15. Bourgeois M, Sainte-Rose C, Lellouch-Tubiana A, et al. Surgery of epilepsy associated with focal lesions in childhood. J Neurosurg 1999;90(5):833–842
16. Mittal S, Montes JL, Farmer JP, et al. Long-term outcome after surgical treatment of temporal lobe epilepsy in children. J Neurosurg 2005; 103(5, suppl):401–412
17. Benifla M, Otsubo H, Ochi A, et al. Temporal lobe surgery for intractable epilepsy in children: an analysis of outcomes in 126 children. Neurosurgery 2006;59(6):1203–1213, discussion 1213–1214
18. Cossu M, Lo Russo G, Francione S, et al. Epilepsy surgery in children: results and predictors of outcome on seizures. Epilepsia 2008;49(1):65–72
19. Kan P, Van Orman C, Kestle JRW. Outcomes after surgery for focal epilepsy in children. Childs Nerv Syst 2008;24(5):587–591
20. Kim SK, Wang KC, Hwang YS, et al. Epilepsy surgery in children: outcomes and complications. J Neurosurg Pediatr 2008;1(4):277–283
21. Wyllie E. Surgery for catastrophic localization-related epilepsy in infants. Epilepsia 1996;37(suppl 1):S22–S25
22. Terra-Bustamante VC, Fernandes RM, Inuzuka LM, et al. Surgically amenable epilepsies in children and adolescents: clinical, imaging, electrophysiological, and post-surgical outcome data. Childs Nerv Syst 2005;21(7):546–551
23. Wyllie E, Comair YG, Kotagal P, Bulacio J, Bingaman W, Ruggieri P. Seizure outcome after epilepsy surgery in children and adolescents. Ann Neurol 1998;44(5):740–748
24. Bien CG, Kurthen M, Baron K, et al. Long-term seizure outcome and antiepileptic drug treatment in surgically treated temporal lobe epilepsy patients: a controlled study. Epilepsia 2001;42(11):1416–1421
25. Wiebe S, Blume WT, Girvin JP, Eliasziw M; Effectiveness and Efficiency of Surgery for Temporal Lobe Epilepsy Study Group. A randomized, controlled trial of surgery for temporal-lobe epilepsy. N Engl J Med 2001;345(5):311–318
26. Jarrar RG, Buchhalter JR, Meyer FB, Sharbrough FW, Laws E. Long-term follow-up of temporal lobectomy in children. Neurology 2002;59(10):1635–1637
27. Chen LS, Wang N, Lin MI. Seizure outcome of intractable partial epilepsy in children. Pediatr Neurol 2002;26(4):282–287
28. Sinclair DB, Aronyk K, Snyder T, et al. Pediatric temporal lobectomy for epilepsy. Pediatr Neurosurg 2003;38(4):195–205
29. Vining EP, Freeman JM, Pillas DJ, et al. Why would you remove half a brain? The outcome of 58 children after hemispherectomy–the Johns Hopkins experience: 1968 to 1996. Pediatrics 1997;100(2 pt 1):163–171
30. Devlin AM, Cross JH, Harkness W, et al. Clinical outcomes of hemispherectomy for epilepsy in childhood and adolescence. Brain 2003;126(pt 3):556–566
31. Daniel RT, Joseph TP, Gnanamuthu C, Chandy MJ. Hemispherotomy for paediatric hemispheric epilepsy. Stereotact Funct Neurosurg 2001;77(1–4):219–222
32. Pulsifer MB, Brandt J, Salorio CF, Vining EP, Carson BS, Freeman JM. The cognitive outcome of hemispherectomy in 71 children. Epilepsia 2004;45(3):243–254
33. Mathern GW, Giza CC, Yudovin S, et al. Postoperative seizure control and antiepileptic drug use in pediatric epilepsy surgery patients: the UCLA experience, 1986-1997. Epilepsia 1999;40(12):1740–1749
34. Wilson PJ. Cerebral hemispherectomy for infantile hemiplegia. A report of 50 cases. Brain 1970;93(1):147–180

35. Carson BS, Javedan SP, Freeman JM, et al. Hemispherectomy: a hemidecortication approach and review of 52 cases. J Neurosurg 1996;84(6):903–911

36. Peacock WJ, Wehby-Grant MC, Shields WD, et al. Hemispherectomy for intractable seizures in children: a report of 58 cases. Childs Nerv Syst 1996;12(7):376–384

37. Holthausen H, May TW, Adams CTB, et al. Seizures post hemispherectomy. In: Tuxhorn I, Holthausen H, Boenigk H, eds. Pediatric Epilepsy Syndromes and Their Surgical Treatment. London, UK: John Libbey; 1997:749–773

38. González-Martínez JA, Gupta A, Kotagal P, et al. Hemispherectomy for catastrophic epilepsy in infants. Epilepsia 2005;46(9):1518–1525

39. Sander JWAS, Sillanpaa M. Natural history and prognosis. In: Engel J Jr, Pedley TA, eds. Epilepsy: A Comprehensive Textbook. Philadelphia, PA: Lippincott-Raven; 1997:69–86

40. Tuxhorn I, Holthausen H, Boenigk H. Pediatric Epilepsy Syndromes and Their Surgical Treatment. London, UK: John Libbey; 1997:894

41. Palmini A, Andermann F, Olivier A, et al. Focal neuronal migration disorders and intractable partial epilepsy: a study of 30 patients. Ann Neurol 1991;30(6):741–749

42. Palmini A, Andermann F, Olivier A, Tampieri D, Robitaille Y. Focal neuronal migration disorders and intractable partial epilepsy: results of surgical treatment. Ann Neurol 1991;30(6):750–757

43. Palmini A, Costa Da Costa J, Anderman F, et al. Surgical results in epilepsy patients with localized cortical dysplastic lesions. In Tuxhorn I, Holthausen H, Boenigk H, eds. Pediatric Epilepsy Syndromes and Their Surgical Treatment. London, UK: John Libbey; 1997:216–224

44. Hirabayashi S, Binnie CD, Janota I, Polkey CE. Surgical treatment of epilepsy because of cortical dysplasia: clinical and EEG findings. J Neurol Neurosurg Psychiatry 1993;56(7):765–770

45. Otsubo H, Hwang PA, Jay V, et al. Focal cortical dysplasia in children with localization-related epilepsy: EEG, MRI, and SPECT findings. Pediatr Neurol 1993;9(2):101–107

46. Wyllie E, Baumgartnet C, Prayson R, et al. The clinical spectrum of focal cortical dysplasia and epilepsy. J Epilepsy 1994;7:303–312

47. Semah F, Picot MC, Adam C, et al. Is the underlying cause of epilepsy a major prognostic factor for recurrence? Neurology 1998;51(5):1256–1262

48. Zentner J, Hufnagel A, Ostertun B, et al. Surgical treatment of extratemporal epilepsy: clinical, radiologic, and histopathologic findings in 60 patients. Epilepsia 1996;37(11):1072–1080

49. Zentner J, Hufnagel A, Wolf HK, et al. Surgical treatment of temporal lobe epilepsy: clinical, radiological, and histopathological findings in 178 patients. J Neurol Neurosurg Psychiatry 1995;58(6):666–673

50. Schramm J, Kral T, Grunwald T, Blümcke I. Surgical treatment for neocortical temporal lobe epilepsy: clinical and surgical aspects and seizure outcome. J Neurosurg 2001;94(1):33–42

51. Patel H, Garg BP, Salanova V, Boaz JC, Luerssen TG, Kalsbeck JE. Tumor-related epilepsy in children. J Child Neurol 2001;16(2):141–145

52. Edwards JC, Wyllie E, Ruggeri PM, et al. Seizure outcome after surgery for epilepsy due to malformation of cortical development. Neurology 2000;55(8):1110–1114

53. Kuzniecky R, Ho SS, Martin R, et al. Temporal lobe developmental malformations and hippocampal sclerosis: epilepsy surgical outcome. Neurology 1999;52(3):479–484

54. Mohamed A, Wyllie E, Ruggieri P, et al. Temporal lobe epilepsy due to hippocampal sclerosis in pediatric candidates for epilepsy surgery. Neurology 2001;56(12):1643–1649

55. Siegel AM, Jobst BC, Thadani VM, et al. Medically intractable, localization-related epilepsy with normal MRI: presurgical evaluation and surgical outcome in 43 patients. Epilepsia 2001;42(7):883–888

56. Berkovic SF, McIntosh AM, Kalnins RM, et al. Preoperative MRI predicts outcome of temporal lobectomy: an actuarial analysis. Neurology 1995;45(7):1358–1363

57. Smith JR, Lee MR, King DW, et al. Results of lesional vs. nonlesional frontal lobe epilepsy surgery. Stereotact Funct Neurosurg 1997;69(1–4 pt 2):202–209

58. Cukiert A, Buratini JA, Machado E, et al. Results of surgery in patients with refractory extratemporal epilepsy with normal or nonlocalizing magnetic resonance findings investigated with subdural grids. Epilepsia 2001;42(7):889–894

59. Won HJ, Chang KH, Cheon JE, et al. Comparison of MR imaging with PET and ictal SPECT in 118 patients with intractable epilepsy. AJNR Am J Neuroradiol 1999;20(4):593–599

60. Park SA, Lim SR, Kim GS, et al. Ictal electrocorticographic findings related with surgical outcomes in nonlesional neocortical epilepsy. Epilepsy Res 2002;48(3):199–206

61. Holmes MD, Born DE, Kutsy RL, Wilensky AJ, Ojemann GA, Ojemann LM. Outcome after surgery in patients with refractory temporal lobe epilepsy and normal MRI. Seizure 2000;9(6):407–411

62. Tonini C, Beghi E, Berg AT, et al. Predictors of epilepsy surgery outcome: a meta-analysis. Epilepsy Res 2004;62(1):75–87

63. Blume WT, Ganapathy GR, Munoz D, Lee DH. Indices of resective surgery effectiveness for intractable nonlesional focal epilepsy. Epilepsia 2004;45(1):46–53

64. Sylaja PN, Radhakrishnan K, Kesavadas C, Sarma PS. Seizure outcome after anterior temporal lobectomy and its predictors in patients with apparent temporal lobe epilepsy and normal MRI. Epilepsia 2004;45(7):803–808

65. Lee SK, Lee SY, Kim KK, Hong KS, Lee DS, Chung CK. Surgical outcome and prognostic factors of cryptogenic neocortical epilepsy. Ann Neurol 2005;58(4):525–532

66. Ramachandran Nair R, Otsubo H, Shroff MM, et al. MEG predicts outcome following surgery for intractable epilepsy in children with normal or nonfocal MRI findings. Epilepsia 2007;48(1):149–157

67. Jayakar P, Dunoyer C, Dean P, et al. Epilepsy surgery in patients with normal or nonfocal MRI scans: integrative strategies offer long-term seizure relief. Epilepsia 2008;49(5):758–764

68. Ben-Ari Y, Holmes GL. Effects of seizures on developmental processes in the immature brain. Lancet Neurol 2006;5(12):1055–1063

69. Stafstrom CE. Neurobiological mechanisms of developmental epilepsy: translating experimental findings into clinical application. Semin Pediatr Neurol 2007;14(4):164–172

70. Park K, Buchhalter J, McClelland R, Raffel C. Frequency and significance of acute postoperative seizures following epilepsy surgery in children and adolescents. Epilepsia 2002;43(8):874–881

71. Koh S, Nguyen S, Asarnow RF, et al. Five or more acute postoperative seizures predict hospital course and long-term seizure control after hemispherectomy. Epilepsia 2004;45(5):527–533

72. Schmidt D, Baumgartner C, Löscher W. Seizure recurrence after planned discontinuation of antiepileptic drugs in seizure-free

patients after epilepsy surgery: a review of current clinical experience. Epilepsia 2004;45(2):179–186

73. Berg AT, Vickrey BG, Langfitt JT, et al; Multicenter Study of Epilepsy Surgery. Reduction of AEDs in postsurgical patients who attain remission. Epilepsia 2006;47(1):64–71

74. Hoppe C, Poepel A, Sassen R, Elger CE. Discontinuation of anticonvulsant medication after epilepsy surgery in children. Epilepsia 2006;47(3):580–583

75. Lachhwani D, Wyllie E, Loddenkemper T, Holland K, Kotagal P, Bingaman W. Discontinuation of antiepileptic medications following epilepsy surgery in childhood and adolescence[abstract]. Neurology 2003;60(suppl 1):A259

76. Sinclair DB, Jurasek L, Wheatley M, et al. Discontinuation of antiepileptic drugs after pediatric epilepsy surgery. Pediatr Neurol 2007;37(3):200–202

77. Schiller Y, Cascino GD, So EL, Marsh WR. Discontinuation of antiepileptic drugs after successful epilepsy surgery. Neurology 2000;54(2):346–349

78. Lachhwani DK, Loddenkemper T, Holland KD, et al. Discontinuation of medications after successful epilepsy surgery in children. Pediatr Neurol 2008;38(5):340–344

79. McLachlan RS, Maher J. Management of antiepileptic drugs following epilepsy surgery: a review. Can J Neurol Sci 2000;27(suppl 1): S106–S110, discussion S121–S125

Postoperative Neuropsychological and Psychosocial Outcome

Mary Lou Smith, Irene Elliott, and Suncica Lah

Children with epilepsy are at increased risk for cognitive and behavioral dysfunction, and greater severity of deficits is associated with longer duration of epilepsy disorder and earlier age of onset.[1-4] It has been hoped that improved seizure control from epilepsy surgery in children would lead to improved cognitive and psychosocial functioning. The rationale for such hope has rested on three assumptions[5]: that seizures interfere with brain functioning and their elimination will increase the likelihood of achieving optimal cognitive and psychological attainments; that the cognitive and psychosocial sequelae of epilepsy may not be as entrenched in childhood as they would be later in life, and earlier intervention is a form of prevention; and, that the capacity for plasticity in the young brain would allow for restitution or reorganization to support further development. Therefore, in evaluating the outcome of surgery, the most important question is whether surgery has altered the course of development as it would have unfolded had the child continued to have seizures. In this chapter, we review the neuropsychological and psychosocial outcomes of epilepsy surgery. Emphasis is placed on relatively recent studies, because they are more likely to have used standardized or objective measures than older studies, allowing for a more rigorous evaluation of the impact of surgery.

■ Neuropsychological Outcome

Resection from the Temporal Lobe

An international survey of pediatric epilepsy surgery centers revealed that temporal lobe resections (TLs) make up 23.2% of all resective procedures.[6] Most of the literature on cognitive outcomes has been directed at children undergoing TL. A comprehensive review of the published studies before 2004 that examined children's overall development before and after TL noted that only 3 of 16 studies that examined group outcome found evidence of a significant change (increase) in the IQ after surgery, suggesting that the overall rate of development does not change after surgery.[7] These studies included seizure-free children, as well as children who had some ongoing residual seizures. In turn, it is possible that the rate of development progression after surgery

was underestimated by the inclusion of children who had ongoing seizures. Indeed, two of the reviewed studies found that good seizure outcome was associated with an increase in IQ,[8,9] but two other studies did not.[10,11]

Individual outcomes are examined in only some of the neuropsychological studies. One of the difficulties in reporting the neuropsychological individual outcomes is a lack of consensus on a method to be used to determine whether the change in the score is clinically significant. Some of the previously reviewed studies,[7] however, did examine IQ changes in individual children after TL. Typically, the number of children who showed a significant increase tended to be greater than that of children who had a significant decline after TL. However, studies that have included a comparison group of children with intractable epilepsy in addition to a surgical group have found that the likelihood of change does not differ over time between the two,[11,12] suggesting there is no advantage as a result of surgery.

In adults, TL surgery is associated with a neuropsychological morbidity; patients who undergo language-dominant (in most cases left) TL are at risk of a decline in anterograde verbal memory.[13] In children, the outcome may differ because ongoing maturational changes, difference in etiology, and physiological and functional plasticity may have a significant role in determining the outcome.[14] The review by Lah[7] identified 13 studies that reported on the verbal memory outcome in children who underwent TL, and an additional study has since been published.[10] Interestingly, only four found evidence of a significant decline, six found no evidence of a significant change, and four reported a significant improvement in memory after surgery. As with adults, a decline was more likely to be found after left rather than right TL, except in one study that found that a significant decline was independent of the side of the surgery.[15] Of studies that found evidence of significant improvement, one showed increased verbal memory after right TL,[8] and one found improved verbal memory after left or right TL.[10] Improved visual memory was reported after either right or left TL in one study[16] and after right TL in another.[17]

Of particular interest is a longitudinal study that compared child and adult memory outcome before surgery and at 3 and 12 months after TL.[18] In short-term follow-up, both children and adults showed a significant decline in verbal memory. By the 12-month follow-up, however, children's memory scores were comparable to their preoperative results, but adults' scores were not, suggesting better functional outcome for children compared with adults. Smith, Elliot and Lach,[5] conversely, found no evidence of a significant change in memory scores over time in children who underwent either temporal or extratemporal resection (regression analyses indicated that the site of excision did not have a significant impact on memory outcome). In this study, however, the first follow-up took place at 1 year after surgery, which was the time of the long-term follow-up in Gleissner et al's[18] study, at which point children's results were much improved and comparable to their presurgical scores. Together, these findings suggest that, in children, memory reorganization after TL may occur rapidly.

In their unique longitudinal study, Smith, Elliot, and Lach[5] examined objective and subjective memory in children who underwent temporal or extratemporal excisions and an epilepsy control group at baseline, 1-year follow-up, and 2- to 3-year follow-up. There was no significant change in objective memory scores over time in any of the groups. More importantly, low concordance between objective and subjective memory outcome was noticed. Qualitative analyses of children's narratives indicated difficulty in aspects of everyday memory not measured by the objective memory tests, such as autobiographical and semantic memory. To date, only one case study[19] directly examined autobiographical memory in a boy who was initially seen for a neuropsychological assessment at 9 years of age (some 1½ years after the onset of temporal lobe epilepsy). His scores on memory tests fell in the age-appropriate range, but he had difficulty recalling autobiographical events. He underwent TL at 10 years of age, and follow-up 8 years later showed the same pattern of results. Evidence suggested that his problems in everyday memory may have been caused by impaired memory consolidation.

Clusmann and colleagues[20] compared verbal memory outcome of 25 children who underwent left TLs that included one of the following surgical approaches: lesionectomy plus hippocampectomy (LX+HC), lateral temporal lesionectomy (lat. LX) and amygdalohippocampectomy (AH). Children who underwent left AH had an increased risk of developing more significant memory deficits after surgery compared with children who underwent left LX+HC or lat. LX. The authors warned, however, that this finding might be secondary to factors other than surgical techniques, because the type of procedure used in the surgery was guided by clinical reasons rather than patients being randomized to undergo different surgical procedures.

Outcomes in other cognitive areas, such as attention, language, and visuospatial skills have barely been examined. Improvements in attention have been reported after TL,[18,20] which could be benefits secondary to favorable seizure outcome and reduction of antiepileptic medication. Nevertheless, Clusmann et al[20] found the relationship between attention and seizure outcomes to be nonsignificant, although more than 80% of children were reported to be seizure free.

Adult literature suggests that dominant TL is also associated with a risk of language decline.[21] In children, language-related cognitive decline after TL was first reported by Dlugos et al[22] Nevertheless, Blanchette and Smith[23] questioned the validity of this finding, as they pointed out that Dlugos et al[22] did not use specific language-processing tasks. Instead, they used tasks (such as verbal learning) that involved language but assessed other cognitive skills (i.e., anterograde verbal memory). Blanchette and Smith[23] found that children with left-sided (temporal, $n = 10$; or frontal, $n = 9$) lesions performed worse than children with right-sided lesions irrespective of the seizure site both before and after surgery (on category fluency and language comprehension tasks) but showed no evidence of a significant drop in their language scores after surgery. When changes in individual scores after TL were examined, however, significant changes were observed in several children, with declines most likely to be observed on the phonetic fluency task (5/10 children), irrespective of the side of resection. Subsequently, in a study that used one (combined) language score, Clusmann et al[20] found a significant improvement in language score after right TL and no evidence of a drop after left TL. Gleissner et al,[18] who reported on individual outcomes, found a significant increase (and no significant decline) in language scores in a small number of children after either right or left TL. The number of increases, however, was not significantly greater than could be expected by chance.

Finally, few studies used tasks to examine other specific visuospatial skills. One study found that the number of children who experienced losses in visuospatial skills after right TL was significantly greater than expected at 3 months after surgery.[18] Nevertheless, only a small number of patients still demonstrated losses (relative to preoperative scores) at 12 months after surgery. Interestingly, Clusmann et al[20] found a significant increase in visuospatial skills 1 year after left TL and pointed out that this improvement was in skills typically subserved by the hemisphere contralateral to the previous epilepsy focus.

Resection from the Frontal Lobe

Despite the fact that surgery in the frontal lobe accounts for 17.5% of pediatric resective procedures, which is not greatly different from the proportion of temporal lobe removals,[6] the literature on the neuropsychological outcomes of frontal resections lags considerably behind that for temporal lobectomy, and only two studies were identified.

Twelve children with frontal lobe epilepsy (six left, six right) were compared preoperatively and 1 year after surgery with 12 children (matched for age and side of surgery) who underwent excision from the temporal lobe.[24] The frontal lobe group included six cases of lesionectomy, four cases of lesionectomy plus multiple subpial transactions (MST), and two cases of MST only. The outcomes included attention, executive function, memory, motor coordination, and language. Before surgery, the frontal group had higher IQ but was more impaired in motor coordination than the temporal lobe group. After surgery, there were improvements in attention and memory that were independent of site and side of surgery; the other functions examined did not change. Analysis of individual changes indicated that the majority of patients showed no significant changes over time. Postoperative improvements were not related to complete seizure relief after surgery.

Potential risk to the child's language ability is of concern when undertaking resection in the language-dominant hemisphere. In the series described previously,[24] two patients underwent surgery that involved area 44 in the left hemisphere. One case had bilateral language representation as determined by the intracarotid amobarbital test and had average language function before surgery. Extraoperative cortical stimulation in area 44 did not interfere with her language. Postoperatively, she showed a decrement in verbal fluency and comprehension. The second patient had right hemisphere language dominance, but electrical stimulation caused a speech arrest in a small left frontal region that was spared in surgery. Postoperative, verbal fluency and naming improved.

Verbal fluency, reading, spelling, vocabulary, and comprehension were examined in another study[23] in which all children had left hemisphere language representation. No differences relating to site (frontal versus temporal lobe) were found before or after surgery, and none of these functions was significantly affected after excision from either the frontal or temporal lobes. Children with left hemisphere dysfunction had lower scores on measures of phonemic fluency and comprehension, but laterality, effects were not present for the other tasks.

Resection from the Parietal Lobe

Parietal lobe resections account for fewer than 3% of pediatric cases,[6] and little has been written on either pre- or postoperative function among children who have undergone parietal lobe surgery. In one investigation of 15 children, a relatively high percentage had deficits in intelligence, memory, language, visuospatial processing, attention, executive function, and motor function before surgery.[25] Differences between left- and right-sided cases were not observed; a large proportion had functional deficits discordant with the side of lesion. The most frequent impairment was in the realm of attention. After surgery, change was apparent only in the domain of attention, which was improved. By contrast to these findings, in a small case series of three patients with excisions from the postcentral gyrus, cognitive function was

generally intact and was essentially unchanged in followup.[26] Two of the patients had evaluation of fine motor dexterity on the hands; both showed declines bilaterally after surgery. In these two case series, the patients were quite heterogeneous in terms of the location of the excisions, which may explain the different pattern of findings.

Multilobar Resections

Approximately 13% of pediatric surgery patients have excisions involving two or more lobes.[6] Studies including such patients have often combined them into one group or have not separated them in analyses from patients with TLs or hemispherectomy. With these findings, it is usually not possible to examine any specific effects associated with multilobar resections. In a comparison of children who had excision from one versus multiple lobes, Smith et al[11] found a decrement in the multilobar but not the unilobar group after surgery for skills dependent on perceptual organization but not on other measures of intelligence, memory, academic skills, or attention. IQ has been found not to change after surgery in small combined samples consisting of patients with extratemporal and multilobar resection.[27,28]

Hemispheric Resections

Research on the neuropsychological outcomes of hemispheric resections (HR) is complicated by the marked developmental delays that the majority of the children exhibit before surgery. Their severe impairments and frequent seizures often place limitations on the type and amount of cognitive testing they can undergo. Furthermore, tests may not yield appropriate standardized scores for their chronological age or may not have basal scores low enough to accurately capture the child's level of function. In this section, our review is directed toward studies that have preoperative data as a baseline against which to evaluate outcome and in which direct assessment of neuropsychological status was performed. Single-case studies are not included because they often illustrate exceptional rather than typical outcomes.

The majority of children who undergo HR do not experience a significant change in developmental or cognitive function as a result of surgery.[29–33] Most patients show no or a small change in IQ or developmental quotient (DQ), with more dramatic changes found only in a few. Investigators have attempted to identify variables that may predict which children will improve or decline, but these results are at times contradictory. For example, higher DQ before surgery has been identified as both a factor that predicts both postoperative improvement[30,33] and decline.[32] Some studies identify pathology or seizure type as a predictor of outcome but others do not.[30,32,34,35] Undoubtedly, these varied and sometimes conflicting results may result from small and heterogeneous samples. With few exceptions,[30] the following variables have been shown not to be associated with development before or after hemispherectomy: pre- and postoperative seizure frequency, duration of seizure disorder, postoperative seizure freedom, side of surgery, and change in number of antiepileptic drugs.[29,31,32,34] In the remainder of this section, the results of recent studies with relatively large samples are summarized.

Devlin et al[29] found that 23 of 27 (85%) children remained within the same category of development after surgery. The remaining 4 children showed improvement but remained within the severely or moderately impaired developmental category. None of the patients had a loss in language function after either left- or right-sided HR. Two patients with Rasmussen encephalitis, who had become aphasic before surgery, showed improvement after left HR (one aged 4.2 years, the other 3.8 years at the time of surgery).

In a study of the impact of pathological substrate on outcome after HR in 44 children, the greatest increases after surgery in DQ were found within the cortical dysplasia group, which differed significantly from subgroups with infarct/ischemia or other/miscellaneous pathology but not from the Rasmussen encephalitis group.[30] Close examination of the results showed that even when improvements were found, the children generally remained with significant developmental delays. All patents had DQs below the normal range before and after surgery (and 70.8% were below 50).

The etiology was also investigated in cognitive outcomes in 53 children with Rasmussen encephalitis, cortical dysplasia, or congenital vascular abnormality.[35] IQ scores were available for all patients; several children received measures of other aspects of cognitive function, but the samples sizes by etiology for these tests were quite small and the results for these more specialized tests are reported here only for the Rasmussen group, which had the largest sample. For patients with Rasmussen encephalitis (n = 31), the left hemispherectomy group had lower presurgical IQ, receptive language, and expressive language than the right. At follow-up, changes were found only for expressive language scores, which were lower than they had been preoperatively. For the cortical dysplasia group (n = 15), mean intelligence was very low preoperatively (less than 50), and no effect of side of surgery or time of testing was detected. Among the 7 patients with vascular etiologies, significant changes were not found from the preoperative baseline to the follow-up.

In a study comparing the outcomes of children with symptomatic infantile spasms (IS) and children with symptomatic epilepsy other than IS, the majority of cases underwent either HR or multilobar resections at an early age (mean of 1.8 years for the IS group and mean of 3.3 years in the non-IS group).[34] These children had markedly impaired development of language, cognition, and social interaction before and 2 years after surgery. The social interaction impairments were similar to those associated with autism. Postsurgical development of nonverbal communication was related to

neuropathological and morphometric indexes but not to seizure control or medication. These results emphasize the role of the abnormal brain structure rather than seizures in the developmental deficits in these children.

■ Psychosocial Outcome

Most early studies on postoperative psychosocial functioning in children almost exclusively addressed the effects of temporal lobectomy. These studies consistently identified behavioral, social, and school difficulties before surgery and an association between improved seizure control and better psychosocial outcomes in behavior, mood, self-esteem, and social adaptation. Hermann[36] emphasized the design limitations of these early studies (including variable time to follow-up, a retrospective approach, and nonstandardized measures) and suggested that the findings be considered only as hypotheses for future testing with rigorous, prospective designs. Therefore, the following review emphasizes recent evidence regarding psychosocial outcomes in studies that have avoided some of these methodological weaknesses.

These studies frequently combined temporal lobe, extratemporal, and hemispherectomy cases, and a few include children who have undergone corpus callosotomy. Most studies used standardized instruments that fall into three categories: generic (nonillness specific) measures of psychosocial (emotional, behavioral, social) functioning; health-related quality-of-life (nonillness specific) measures; and epilepsy (illness specific) quality-of-life measures. Few studies included a comparison or control group. The mean follow-up period for prospective studies in this series was still relatively short, at less than 2½ years.

Studies Using Generic Measures

Four prospective studies[11,37–39] have shown that change is not seen on the measures of social function during the first year after surgery. The one study with a longer (2-year) follow-up found that between the first and second year after surgery, significant positive changes emerged on the social subscales for the surgical group, whereas an intractable epilepsy comparison group experienced a decline.[39] Changes in social function likely require time to emerge because parents and children require time to distance themselves from worries surrounding seizures before children begin to engage more fully in social activities and peer interactions.[39]

These same studies have produced mixed results with respect to other aspects of behavior. One found significant improvement on scales of internalizing behavior, thought problems, and aggression 1 year after surgery.[38] In another with a 3-month follow-up, significant improvements were observed on measures of internalizing and externalizing behaviors, thought problems, and attention in the surgery group but not in an intractable epilepsy comparison group.[37] The two other studies included a nonsurgical epilepsy comparison group and found that when changes in behavior were observed at either 1 or 2 years after surgery, they occurred for both the surgical and the nonsurgical.[11,39]

The single retrospective study using generic psychosocial measures examined outcome approximately 2 years after surgery.[40] Parents reported greater social problems in their children compared with the normative sample, and teachers rated children as having significantly more symptoms of anxiety and depression.

Studies Using Health-Related Quality-of-Life Instruments

On measures of health-related quality of life and self-perceived competence,[41] children rated the quality and quantity of their social activities as worse than normative sample before surgery. Six months after surgery, they reported significant improvement in social activities and social competence; at 2 years, children continued to view themselves as more socially accepted and having greater self-worth. Parents also rated significant improvements in the frequency of social activities by 6 months after surgery. Interestingly, parents rated their children as having more positive emotions at 6 months, whereas children did not report improved feelings until 2 years after surgery. The authors concluded that surgery does "set the stage" (p. 258) for improvement in quality of life. Another study of parent (plus some older children) ratings of quality of life before and 1 year after surgery observed a tendency toward improvement in socialization subscale and in overall quality of life in up to 38% of their sample.[42]

Sabaz and colleagues[43] used a parent report epilepsy-specific measure of quality of life and found that children who became seizure free versus those with continuing seizures had greater improvement on overall quality-of-life scores and general health, as well as several subscale scores (cognitive, social, emotional, behavioral, and physical domains of life). Using the same quality-of-life scale but in a retrospective, cross-sectional study comparing Lebanese children 2.4 years after surgery with a group or children who had intractable epilepsy, parents reported that overall quality of life and well-being was better in the surgery group, whereas social and behavioral functioning did not differ between the two groups.[44] Although this study used the same quality-of-life instrument as Sabaz et al,[43] results differed on social and behavioral outcomes, which the authors suggested may be because of the culture in Lebanon, one that emphasizes "strong family ties that tend to be overprotective, encouraging reliance on the family rather than independence" (p. 147). In addition, the authors posited that at school, children were being still viewed as having epilepsy by peers and teachers and suggest, for these reasons,

quality of life after surgery may be different from Western countries.

A retrospective qualitative study,[45] using open-ended interviews to explore several domains that reflect quality of life in a group of adolescents and their mothers 1 to 2½ years after surgery, discovered that outcomes varied by informant. Adolescents reported positive changes in many areas of quality of life, whereas mothers described more negative changes and continuing concerns.

Two studies have addressed psychosocial or quality-of-life outcomes after HR. In a prospective study using parent report questionnaires at baseline and after surgery (mean 5.4 years),[35] no significant behavioral or emotional problems were seen before surgery or at follow-up. Ratings on attention and thought problems subscales improved significantly after surgery. Social interactions and activities were limited before surgery and continued to be so after surgery. A retrospective study[46] compared quality of life in children who underwent HR to that of children who had undergone temporal or frontal lobe surgery and to a nonsurgical epilepsy group. Similar levels of quality of life were found in all groups, indicating that HR is not associated with increased risk over that of other intractable epilepsy groups for poor quality of life.

■ Predictors of Neuropsychological and Psychosocial Outcomes

Research has explored factors that might predict postoperative function or change after surgery including gender, age at epilepsy onset, proportion of life with epilepsy, age at testing or surgery, number of antiepileptic drugs, intellectual ability, site of excision, laterality, and histopathology. Some of these factors have been reviewed in the preceding sections and have been shown to have inconsistent or no predictive power. The two variables that have received most attention are age and seizure status.

There is a strong sentiment that developmental outcomes will be better when surgery is conducted at a very early age. This question is difficult to address experimentally because those children who have surgery very early in life may differ in several important ways (seizure frequency, age of seizure onset, neuropathology) from children who are operated on a later age. When surgery has taken place at school age or later, age has not been predictive of cognitive or psychosocial outcomes.[5,11,39] Recent studies that have examined outcomes after surgery conducted in children at early school age or younger were reviewed for evidence of any advantage associated with timing. Some of these studies included mixed samples of focal resections and HR and did not distinguish outcomes based on type of resection.[32,47]

Freitag and Tuxhorn[47] examined the developmental trajectory of children who had undergone surgery between the ages of 3 and 7 years. The predominant outcome was functioning at follow-up was consistent with the preoperative level. The authors reported that children with shorter intervals between the onset of epilepsy and the surgery had greater developmental gains. However, this result must be considered against the finding that seizure outcome did not predict postoperative cognitive change; cognitive gains were almost exclusively found in seizure-free patients but so were cognitive losses.

In a follow-up (conducted at a median of 6 months after surgery) of 24 children operated on before 3 years of age, younger age at surgery was correlated with improvement in DQ.[32] This effect was limited, however, in that surgery did not influence outcome in children over the age at 12 months at the time of surgery. The effect of age on outcome was further qualified by the finding that only infants with epileptic spasms had significant improvement after surgery. Developmental delays were prominent among the sample, and only two children had DQs in the average range before surgery and three at follow-up. Two other studies of in which all patients had HR before 6 years of age identified few cases of improvement over the low developmental level exhibited at the preoperative stage.[31,33]

The most consistent finding with respect to psychosocial function and quality of life has been that improved seizure control or freedom from seizures predicts improvement in various domains,[24,39,43,46,48] although this effect is not always found.[11] Seizure outcome is not consistently associated with improved cognitive function.[5,11,16,20,24]

Lower (worse) baseline scores were predictive of positive change within some psychosocial or quality-of-life domains in two studies,[11,43] and one study found that younger age at baseline was a significant predictor of improvement on an overall psychosocial measure.[11] A retrospective study of quality of life found that female gender, higher number of antiepileptic drugs, and lower functional independence was associated with worse quality of life.[46]

■ Conclusion and Future Directions

This review demonstrates that there have been mixed findings regarding whether surgery and its impact on seizures results in neuropsychological and psychosocial benefits to the child. Some of the variability in findings is caused by differences in methodology. The field remains characterized by studies with weak methodology and samples that are insufficient to test the influence of the many potentially important variables contributing to outcome. Future studies clearly require prospective designs with a preoperative baseline and an appropriate control group. A recent meta-analysis of long-term outcome in epilepsy surgery showed that noncontrolled studies consistently reported improvements in psychosocial status but that the effect was less clear in controlled studies.[49] Without a comparison group, it is not possible to determine whether change is the result of ongoing maturation or an effect of surgery.

One finding of considerable interest is that parents rate at least certain aspects of their child's quality of life as better after surgery. It is unclear why these findings are not more consistently paralleled in the cognitive, behavioral, and emotional status of the children as captured by other measures. This discrepancy argues for a continuation of research on all aspects of cognitive and psychosocial function that make up aspects of quality of life, their meaning, and their measurement. Finally, the improvements in social function have been documented, but they may take time to emerge. Whether other aspects of the child's cognitive or psychosocial function could improve with time after surgery is an important question.

References

1. Hermann BP, Seidenberg M, Bell B. The neurodevelopmental impact of childhood onset temporal lobe epilepsy on brain structure and function and the risk of progressive cognitive effects. Prog Brain Res 2002;135:429–438
2. Jokeit H, Ebner A. Long term effects of refractory temporal lobe epilepsy on cognitive abilities: a cross sectional study. J Neurol Neurosurg Psychiatry 1999;67(1):44–50
3. Nolan MA, Redoblado MA, Lah S, et al. Intelligence in childhood epilepsy syndromes. Epilepsy Res 2003;53(1–2):139–150
4. Nolan MA, Redoblado MA, Lah S, et al. Memory function in childhood epilepsy syndromes. J Paediatr Child Health 2004;40(1–2):20–27
5. Smith ML, Elliott IM, Lach L. Memory outcome after pediatric epilepsy surgery: objective and subjective perspectives. Child Neuropsychol 2006;12(3):151–164
6. Harvey AS, Cross JH, Shinnar S, Mathern BW; ILAE Pediatric Epilepsy Surgery Survey Taskforce. Defining the spectrum of international practice in pediatric epilepsy surgery patients. Epilepsia 2008;49(1):146–155

7. Lah S. Neuropsychological outcome following focal cortical removal for intractable epilepsy in children. Epilepsy Behav 2004;5(6):804–817
8. Robinson S, Park TS, Blackburn LB, Bourgeois BFD, Arnold ST, Dodson WE. Transparahippocampal selective amygdalohippocampectomy in children and adolescents: efficacy of the procedure and cognitive morbidity in patients. J Neurosurg 2000;93(3):402–409
9. Miranda C, Smith ML. Predictors of intelligence after temporal lobectomy in children with epilepsy. Epilepsy Behav 2001;2(1):13–19
10. Jambaqué I, Dellatolas G, Fohlen M, et al. Memory functions following surgery for temporal lobe epilepsy in children. Neuropsychologia 2007;45(12):2850–2862
11. Smith ML, Elliott IM, Lach L. Cognitive, psychosocial, and family function one year after pediatric epilepsy surgery. Epilepsia 2004;45(6):650–660
12. Bjørnaes H, Stabell KE, Henriksen O, Røste G, Diep LM. Surgical versus medical treatment for severe epilepsy: consequences for intellectual functioning in children and adults. A follow-up study. Seizure 2002;11(8):473–482

13. Davies KG, Bell BD, Bush AJ, Wyler AR. Prediction of verbal memory loss in individuals after anterior temporal lobectomy. Epilepsia 1998;39(8):820–828

14. Smith ML. Presurgical neuropsychological assessment. In Jambaque I, Lassonde M, Dulac O, eds. Neuropsychology of Childhood Epilepsy. New York, NY: Kluwer Academic/Plenum Publishers; 2001:207–214

15. Szabó CA, Wyllie E, Stanford LD, et al. Neuropsychological effect of temporal lobe resection in preadolescent children with epilepsy. Epilepsia 1998;39(8):814–819

16. Mabbott DJ, Smith ML. Memory in children with temporal or extra-temporal excisions. Neuropsychologia 2003;41(8):995–1007

17. Beardsworth ED, Zaidel DW. Memory for faces in epileptic children before and after brain surgery. J Clin Exp Neuropsychol 1994;16(4):589–596

18. Gleissner U, Sassen R, Schramm J, Elger CE, Helmstaedter C. Greater functional recovery after temporal lobe epilepsy surgery in children. Brain 2005;128(pt 12):2822–2829

19. Cronel-Ohayon S, Zesiger P, Davidoff V, Boni A, Roulet E, Deonna T. Deficit in memory consolidation (abnormal forgetting rate) in childhood temporal lobe epilepsy. Pre and postoperative long-term observation. Neuropediatrics 2006;37(6):317–324

20. Clusmann H, Kral T, Gleissner U, et al. Analysis of different types of resection for pediatric patients with temporal lobe epilepsy. Neurosurgery 2004;54(4):847–859, discussion 859–860

21. Davies KG, Bell BD, Bush AJ, Hermann BP, Dohan FC Jr, Jaap AS. Naming decline after left anterior temporal lobectomy correlates with pathological status of resected hippocampus. Epilepsia 1998;39(4):407–419

22. Dlugos DJ, Moss EM, Duhaime A-C, Brooks-Kayal AR. Language-related cognitive declines after left temporal lobectomy in children. Pediatr Neurol 1999;21(1):444–449

23. Blanchette N, Smith ML. Language after temporal or frontal lobe surgery in children with epilepsy. Brain Cogn 2002;48(2–3):280–284

24. Lendt M, Gleissner U, Helmstaedter C, Sassen R, Clusmann H, Elger CE. Neuropsychological outcome in children after frontal lobe epilepsy surgery. Epilepsy Behav 2002;3(1):51–59

25. Gleissner U, Kuczaty S, Clusmann H, Elger CE, Helmstaedter C. Neuropsychological results in pediatric patients with epilepsy surgery in the parietal cortex. Epilepsia 2008;49(4):700–704

26. Lam FW, Weiss SK, Kerr E, Rutka J, Smith ML. Analysis of neuropsychological function in parietal lobe epilepsy surgery patients: Is this surgery well tolerated in children? Epilepsia 2007;48(suppl 6):233

27. Kuehn SM, Keene DL, Richards PMP, Ventureyra ECG. Are there changes in intelligence and memory functioning following surgery for the treatment of refractory epilepsy in childhood? Childs Nerv Syst 2002;18(6–7):306–310

28. Korkman M, Granström M-L, Kantola-Sorsa E, et al. Two-year follow-up of intelligence after pediatric epilepsy surgery. Pediatr Neurol 2005;33(3):173–178

29. Devlin AM, Cross JH, Harkness W, et al. Clinical outcomes of hemispherectomy for epilepsy in childhood and adolescence. Brain 2003;126(pt 3):556–566

30. Jonas R, Nguyen S, Hu B, et al. Cerebral hemispherectomy: hospital course, seizure, developmental, language, and motor outcomes. Neurology 2004;62(10):1712–1721

31. Lettori D, Battaglia D, Sacco A, et al. Early hemispherectomy in catastrophic epilepsy: a neuro-cognitive and epileptic long-term follow-up. Seizure 2008;17(1):49–63

32. Loddenkemper T, Holland KD, Stanford LD, Kotagal P, Bingaman W, Wyllie E. Developmental outcome after epilepsy surgery in infancy. Pediatrics 2007;119(5):930–935

33. Maehara T, Shimizu H, Kawai K, et al. Postoperative development of children after hemispherotomy. Brain Dev 2002;24(3):155–160

34. Caplan R, Siddarth P, Mathern G, et al. Developmental outcome with and without successful intervention. Int Rev Neurobiol 2002;49:269–284

35. Pulsifer MB, Brandt J, Salorio CF, Vining EPG, Carson BS, Freeman JM. The cognitive outcome of hemispherectomy in 71 children. Epilepsia 2004;45(3):243–254

36. Hermann BP. Psychosocial outcome following focal resections in childhood. J Epilepsy 1990;3(suppl):243–252

37. Lendt M, Helmstaedter C, Kuczaty S, Schramm J, Elger CE. Behavioural disorders in children with epilepsy: early improvement after surgery. J Neurol Neurosurg Psychiatry 2000;69(6):739–744

38. Williams J, Griebel ML, Sharp GB, Boop FA. Cognition and behavior after temporal lobectomy in pediatric patients with intractable epilepsy. Pediatr Neurol 1998;19(3):189–194

39. Elliott IM, Lach L, Kadis DS, Smith ML. Psychosocial outcomes in children two years after epilepsy surgery: has anything changed? Epilepsia 2008;49(4):634–641

40. Korneluk YG, Kuehn SM, Keene DL, Ventureyra ECG. Psychosocial functioning following surgical treatment for intractable epilepsy in childhood. Childs Nerv Syst 2003;19(3):179–182

41. van Empelen R, Jennekens-Schinkel A, van Rijen PC, Helders PJ, van Nieuwenhuizen O. Health-related quality of life and self-perceived competence of children assessed before and up to two years after epilepsy surgery. Epilepsia 2005;46(2):258–271

42. Larysz D, Larysz P, Mandera M. Evaluation of quality of life and clinical status of children operated on for intractable epilepsy. Childs Nerv Syst 2007;23(1):91–97

43. Sabaz M, Lawson JA, Cairns DR, et al. The impact of epilepsy surgery on quality of life in children. Neurology 2006;66(4):557–561

44. Mikati MA, Rahi AC, Shamseddine A, Mroueh S, Shoeib H, Comair Y. Marked benefits in physical activity and well-being, but not in functioning domains, 2 years after successful epilepsy surgery in children. Epilepsy Behav 2008;12(1):145–149

45. Elliott IM, Lach L, Smith ML. Adolescent and maternal perspectives of quality of life and neuropsychological status following epilepsy surgery. Epilepsy Behav 2000;1(6):406–417

46. Griffiths SY, Sherman EMS, Slick DJ, Eyrl K, Connolly MB, Steinbok P. Postsurgical health-related quality of life (HRQOL) in children following hemispherectomy for intractable epilepsy. Epilepsia 2007;48(3):564–570

47. Freitag H, Tuxhorn I. Cognitive function in preschool children after epilepsy surgery: rationale for early intervention. Epilepsia 2005;46(4):561–567

48. Keene DL, Higgins MJ, Ventureyra ECG. Outcome and life prospects after surgical management of medically intractable epilepsy in patients under 18 years of age. Childs Nerv Syst 1997;13(10):530–535

49. Téllez-Zenteno JF, Dhar R, Hernandez-Ronquillo L, Wiebe S. Long-term outcomes in epilepsy surgery: antiepileptic drugs, mortality, cognitive and psychosocial aspects. Brain 2007;130(pt 2):334–345

IV Recent Advances

39 New Techniques in Electrophysiological Assessment of Pediatric Epilepsy

Tomoyuki Akiyama, Derrick Chan, and Hiroshi Otsubo

In pediatric epilepsy, neocortical seizures are more common compared with adult epilepsy. Epilepsy monitoring with subdural grid and depth electrodes has been used in pediatric epilepsy surgery to delineate the epileptogenic zone and provide valuable insights into the underlying mechanisms of the epileptogenic network in children with intractable epilepsy.

This chapter presents full-band electroencephalography (EEG), ranging from high-frequency oscillations (HFOs) to infraslow EEG (very slow EEG response or direct current [DC] potential shifts), and including EEG source localization (ESL) and nonlinear analysis techniques of seizure prediction by detecting neural network changes in simplicity or complexity. We discuss their roles in improving our understanding of the complex epileptic networks in children.

Conventional analog EEG consists of five bands between 0.5 Hz and 80 Hz: δ < 4 Hz, θ < 8 Hz, α < 13 Hz, β < 30 to 40 Hz, and γ <80 Hz. Previously limited by EEG data storage capacity, low sampling rate, and low frequency filtration at the amplifier level, the ends of the EEG spectrum comprising HFOs (> 80 Hz) and infraslow EEG (< 0.5 Hz) now lie within current technological capability and are revealing valuable information. Advanced digital EEG has become able to analyze full range of brain activity from scalp to intracranial recordings.

■ Full Band EEG

HFOs

Recent advances in digital EEG technology have enabled us to record HFOs > 80 Hz with high sampling rates of 1 to 10 kHz. HFOs above γ frequency are generally termed *ripples* (80–250 Hz) and *fast ripples* (≥ 250 Hz) based on their frequency ranges.

HFOs in the brain can be physiological or epileptic.[1] Gamma activities and ripples have been noted in the normal and epileptogenic brain; however, fast ripples have been recorded specially in the epileptogenic brain.[2] Examples of physiological HFOs include cognitive γ oscillations of 30 to 70 Hz,[3] 40 to 200 Hz activity in the visual cortex,[4] and 500 to 600 Hz in somatosensory evoked potentials.[5] HFOs can be recorded intracranial EEG at the onset of focal epileptic seizures.[6–10] Power spectral analyses show that the location of HFOs at seizure onset indicate the ictal onset zone.[6–9,11] HFOs are also recorded in interictal EEG in epileptic patients.[2,12–15] Therefore, HFOs have drawn attention in the field of epilepsy surgery.

Recording HFOs

Recording fast ripples up to 500 Hz requires an EEG sampling rate ≥ 1 kHz according to the Nyquist theorem. Monitors to display EEG waveforms need to have high enough resolution to show recorded HFOs properly. Scalp EEG has recorded HFOs up to 120 Hz using a 500 Hz sampling rate for epileptic spasms in children.[16,17] Most studies on HFOs have been done with intracranial macro- and microelectrodes. The electrodes must be placed very close to the area generating HFOs, otherwise HFOs may not be recorded because of focality of the HFOs.

Analysis of HFOs

HFOs analysis encompasses visual and computer evaluation. Visual analysis of HFOs requires high-pass filtering at high frequencies (e.g., 100 Hz) and temporal expansion with high sweep speeds (e.g., 100 mm/s). This filtering and expanding waveform can realize superimposed HFOs in the interictal and ictal discharges.[10,15]

In computer analysis, time–frequency analyses have been widely used. These analyses transform a one-dimensional signal in the time domain into a two-dimensional domain of both time and frequency. Short-time Fourier transform and wavelet transform are common methods. The authors apply multiple band frequency analysis (MBFA) to demonstrate the rapidly changing property of HFOs in time–frequency domains in detail.

Short-time Fourier transform is a well-known method; however, frequency resolution (frequency band width in which the power spectrum is calculated) depends on time resolution (time window width for power spectrum calculation), and there is a trade off between these resolutions.[18,19] To achieve high time resolution to reveal rapid spectral changes of HFOs, frequency resolution has to be sacrificed.

Wavelet transform was developed to capture rapid spectral changes of nonstationary signals.[18,19] In wavelet transform, time resolution is high and frequency resolution is low in analysis of high frequencies. The relationship is reversed at lower frequencies, with low time resolution and high frequency resolution. Wavelet transform is useful in detecting changes in power spectra of HFOs; however it is difficult to investigate changes in frequency in detail, particularly at higher frequencies.

MBFA was developed to analyze rapid spectral changes of evoked potentials over time with high frequency and time resolutions.[20] MBFA decomposes the raw signal into component frequency bands by applying multiple sequential band filters. Application of time windows divides the component frequency bands into chronologically sequential segments for which the power values can be calculated and demonstrated graphically. In MBFA, frequency and time resolutions are fixed for all frequency bands, similar to the short-time Fourier transform.

HFOs in Interictal Periods

Bragin et al[2] used microelectrodes to record ripples at 100 to 200 Hz and fast ripples at 200 to 500 Hz in hippocampus and entorhinal cortex in patients with mesial temporal lobe epilepsy. Staba et al[13] reported interictal HFOs within the bandwidth of 80 to 500 Hz in hippocampus and entorhinal cortex of patients with mesial temporal lobe epilepsy using depth electrodes. The hippocampus and entorhinal cortex ipsilateral to seizure onset showed a higher ratio of the number of fast ripples to ripples compared with the contralateral side. Urrestarazu et al[14,15] also demonstrated interictal 100 to 500 Hz HFOs recorded from depth electrodes in focal epilepsy. Their results indicated that in temporal lobe epilepsy, fast ripples were more restricted than ripples to the electrodes located within the seizure onset zone, especially to the hippocampus.[15]

HFOs in Ictal Periods

Allen et al[6] found 80 to 115 Hz HFOs at the onset of frontal lobe seizures. Fisher et al[7] reported a twofold increase in the 40 to 50 Hz range and up to a fivefold increase in the 80 to 120 Hz portion of power spectrum at seizure onset in patients with various etiologies. Traub et al[8] reported ictal HFOs up to 130 Hz in children with epilepsy secondary to cortical dysplasia. Jirsch et al[10] demonstrated well-localized, segmental, fast ripples at 250 to 500 Hz in mesial temporal lobe seizures. Akiyama et al[21] reported the presence of 60 to 150 Hz HFOs during epileptic spasms of focal origin (**Fig. 39.1**). Ochi et al[22] demonstrated HFOs up to 250 Hz in pediatric focal neocortical seizures.

Propagation of HFOs during Seizures

Ictal HFOs had different patterns and distributions among seizures in pediatric neocortical epilepsy. Ochi et al[22] analyzed spatiotemporal dynamic changes of ictal HFOs by MBFA and compared the distribution and frequency of ictal HFOs with the postsurgical seizure outcome. When HFOs early in the course of a clinical seizure were confined to the ictal onset zone, resection of this zone stopped seizures. However, when the predominant HFO zone extended beyond the resection margins or the area outside resection margins recorded higher frequency HFOs than resection area, seizures continued postoperatively.

Topographic HFO Movie

Visualization of HFOs on the brain surface picture enhances the understanding of the relationship between their topographic distribution and anatomical structures. Akiyama et

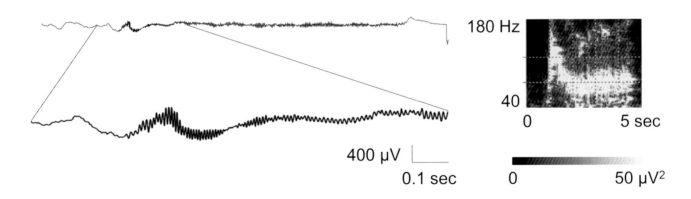

Fig. 39.1 (*Left*) A 5-second EEG section recorded over the epileptogenic zone during epileptic spasms in a 14-year-old patient demonstrates 75 to 145 Hz oscillations lasting 3.5 seconds. Akiyama et al[21] applied multiple band frequency analysis for the same EEG section (*left*) to show power spectrogram (*right*) of 80 to 160 Hz oscillations lasting 0.5 second initially followed by 60 to 100 Hz oscillations for 3 seconds. (From Akiyama T, Otsubo H, Ochi A, et al. Focal cortical high-frequency oscillations trigger epileptic spasms: confirmation by digital video subdural EEG. Clin Neurophysiol 2005;116(12):2819–2825. Adapted with permission.)

al[23] developed a movie mapping technique to demonstrate power changes of ictal HFOs over time during neocortical epileptic seizures. They identified the ictal HFO frequency range and averaged the HFO power values within the frequency bands at each electrode. Topographic maps of HFO power values were superimposed onto a picture of the brain surface. These maps were integrated into a movie file to animate the spatiotemporal changes of ictal HFO power over the grid electrodes correlating with progression of seizures.

HFOs and Muscle Activity

During seizures, intracranial EEG electrodes can record HFOs of extracranial origin caused by ictal muscle movements. Otsubo et al[24] reported confounding of intracranial HFOs during mesial temporal lobe seizures in a patient with recurrent seizures. Power spectral analysis of HFOs using MBFA demonstrated differences in spatial distribution and frequency properties between HFOs originating from the brain and muscles. Muscle HFOs were observed at fixed electrodes close to temporal muscles and were of random scattered frequency bands, whereas ictal epileptic HFOs showed a sustained, high-frequency band in the ictal onset zone and subsequently propagated to other areas through the epileptic network. This phenomenon of extracranial HFOs recorded in intracranial EEG electrodes was termed a *reverse breach rhythm*, compared with a regular *breach rhythm* in which intracerebral discharges appeared at high amplitude through the skull defect.

■ Infraslow EEG

Traditionally dismissed as artifacts and actively filtered out, infraslow EEG activity (often referred to as DC-EEG) has been recognized in association with seizure activity as far back as 1963.[25] DC-EEG implies a frequency of 0 Hz, but in reality infraslow EEG consists of extremely low-frequency signal of < 0.5 Hz.[26]

Interest in this infraslow EEG has waxed and waned[27] because the data collection was hampered by the need of specific equipment. Unlike HFOs, which can be measured by most commercially available EEG recording equipment with a sufficiently high sampling rate and storage capacity, infraslow frequencies require DC-compatible amplifiers with nonpolarizable Ag-AgCl electrodes and stable gel-electrode interfaces. In addition, skin preparation is required to eliminate skin potentials by scraping or puncturing the skin with microneedles.[28]

Visual interpretation of infraslow EEG is complicated by the masking effect of higher frequency activity and difficulty in differentiating between genuine potential changes, artifacts, and surface potential changes related to the blood–brain barrier and cerebral blood flow.[29–31] Applications of infraslow EEG include study of the preterm neonatal brain,[32]

sleep,[33] cognition and motor activity,[34] and seizures. Initial studies on seizures used invasive monitoring in animals and humans and has demonstrated infraslow activity during 3 Hz generalized spike-and-wave discharges,[35,36] temporal lobe seizures in humans and monkeys,[37] and focal epilepsy.[38] Noninvasive recordings of 35 seizures in seven adult patients with temporal lobe epilepsy provided lateralizing information consistent with conventional scalp EEG in all and intracranial EEG in four patients.[39] In both temporal and extratemporal lobe epilepsies, infraslow EEG analysis with source localization gave independent localization data in 6 of 30 patients. Source analysis was done in adult patients who had single epileptic foci and no skull breaches. Surgery was performed in five, all with temporal lobe epilepsy.[40] Further study of the utility of infraslow EEG in neocortical epilepsy and in pediatric subjects is desirable.

■ EEG Source Localization

ESL has been practiced since the advent of the analog EEG. With digital EEG, automated ESL of increasing complexity has become possible. In its broadest sense, ESL can be divided into model-dependent ESL and model-independent ESL. Model-independent ESL constitutes topographical mapping, Laplacian, multivariate statistical, and cortical projection methods.[41]

Model-dependent ESL needs to answer the forward and inverse problems. The accuracy of the forward problem solution is determined by the shape and conductivity of the volume conductor head model. Head models are more critical for ESL than with magnetoencephalography source localization because of heterogeneous conductivities of brain, cerebral spinal fluid, bone, and skin. Therefore one applies one-to-four shell simple models or boundary- or finite-element-method realistic head models. In the inverse problem, an infinite number of source permutations can, in theory, explain a specific potential field recorded at the surface.[42] Modeling the inverse problem is complex. A detailed description is outside the scope of this chapter and is described elsewhere.[41,43,44] Source models can be divided into overdetermined (or dipolar) or underdetermined (distributed source) methods.[43]

Practical concerns in ESL include the number and distribution of electrodes, choice of source and head model, and reference and signal-to-noise ratio.[43] Higher electrode density with interelectrode distances of 2 to 3 cm minimize surface potential distortion.[45–48] Electrode placement can affect results, and incomplete coverage of the head can lead to false localization.[43] Whole head coverage with 64 to 128 electrode array nets or with increased electrode density over the region of interest improved the accurate localization of electrographical source.[49] Accurate estimation of scalp electrode position can be aided by well-applied electrode caps or nets.[50,51] The localization error caused by noise may exceed that caused by slight electrode mispositioning[52–54] or shell versus realistic forward head model.[55]

Correlation of ESL solutions with clinical data has been shown in adult and pediatric epilepsy patients.[56,57] Sperli et al[57] found 90% concordance between ESL and resection margin in a retrospective pediatric epilepsy surgical cohort. Erroneous localizations in dorsal temporal lobes were likely caused by inadequate electrode coverage in these areas. By comparison, positron emission tomography and ictal single photon emission computed tomography data in the same patients localized correctly in 82% and 70%, respectively. Ochi et al[56] reported that the systematic approach of equiva-

lent current dipole analysis using spike detection, clustering analysis for conventional scalp EEG is useful for identifying extratemporal lobe epilepsies in children.

In a prospective unblinded trial, Boon et al[58] were able to analyze 31 of 100 presurgical patients and found ESL influenced operative decision making in 14, usually against invasive monitoring. Comparison of scalp ESL with intracranial depth electrode recordings obtained stable dipole results in only 40%.[59] Pitfalls in ESL are caused by fitting of the simplistic dipole model to real cortical sources with more extensive spatial distribution and complex configuration (**Fig. 39.2**).[60] Comparison of ESL to intracranial recordings with wide cortical coverage including the lateral temporal lobe and depth

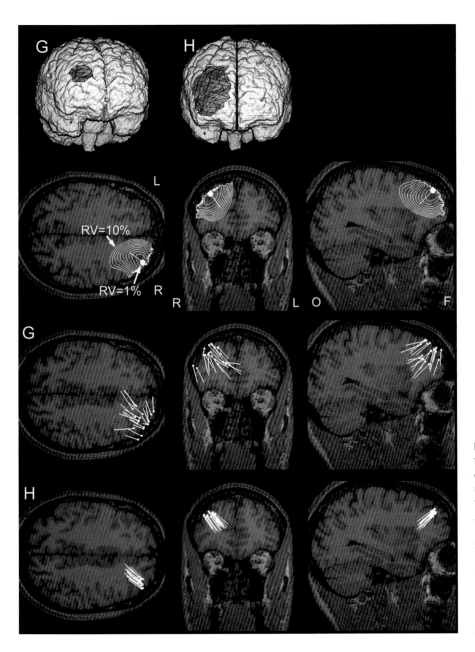

Fig. 39.2 Kobayashi et al,[60] demonstrated the effect of source characteristics on dipole modeling. The top row shows simulated right frontal lobe cortical epileptiform sources covering 6 cm² (source G) and 30 cm² (source H). The second row shows residual variance map after dipole fitting to source G. The third and bottom rows show modeled dipoles corresponding to sources G and H. (From Kobayashi K, Yoshinaga H, Ohtsuka Y, Gotman J. Dipole modeling of epileptic spikes can be accurate or misleading. Epilepsia 2005;46(3):397–408. Adapted with permission.)

sampling to the temporal lobe tip and mesial and inferior structures is desirable[44] to validate ESL.

Seizure Prediction

In most epileptic patients, epileptic seizures occur without any identifiable external precipitating factors. This unpredictability of seizures has a great effect on quality of life and increases the risk of sudden unexpected death or morbidity.[61] A means of advance warning of impending seizures would enable patients equipped with a portable continuous monitoring system to prepare for seizures and their consequences. Furthermore, if the analysis methods could be incorporated into seizure recognition software in, for example, implanted brain stimulators, it might be possible to attenuate or completely prevent impending seizures.

Recent development of the theory of nonlinear analysis, called chaos theory, has enabled analysis of irregular behaviors of complex EEG signals before and around seizure onsets. Nonlinear methods were initially developed to describe the dynamics of complex physical systems with nonlinear components. The nonlinear components imply that their time course does not follow the linearity of the classic deterministic laws but may exhibit nonproportional responses to specific inputs instead.[62] Self-organizing behavior and intermittency are other interesting properties of nonlinear systems that permit transitions between states in the absence of external triggers.

Hughes[63] stated that seizure onset could be predicted several minutes to 4 hours before seizure onset, with a median of 6 to 7 minutes. Martinerie et al[64] studied 11 mesial temporal seizures from 19 patients and demonstrated in most cases (17 out of 19), seizure onset could be anticipated well in advance (between 2 and 6 minutes beforehand) based on decrease in correlation density. In 16 patients with mesial temporal lobe epilepsy recorded by intracranial video-EEG, Elger et al[65] reported that long-lasting and marked reduction of dimensionality, which reflected a continuous increase in the degree of synchronicity, was found, specifically up to 25 minutes before epileptic seizures. This change predicted the occurrence of individual seizures in time. Le Van Quyen et al[66] reported that nonlinear changes in neuronal dynamics allowed a seizure anticipation several minutes in advance in 16 of 17 seizures from nine patients using a new nonlinear similarity analysis. With regard to intracranial EEG of neocortical seizures, Navarro et al[62] applied the nonlinear similarity analysis to 41 seizures from 11 patients with neocortical focal epilepsy and demonstrated that a preictal state was detected in 90% of the patients and 83% of the seizures whatever their location, with a mean anticipation time of 7.5 minutes.

Conclusion

HFO analysis delineates the epileptogenic (part of the interictal) and ictogenic (ictal) zone. When the interictal and ictal HFOs are confined to the possible resection area, the surgical resection of that limited epileptogenic network may stop seizures. Infraslow EEG can show lateralization in temporal lobe epilepsy. Further work will elucidate its utility in neocortical epilepsy and the pediatric population. ESL shows promise in focal epilepsy and comparison with more extensive intracranial data will validate and refine existing models. Nonlinear analysis can demonstrate the behavior of epileptic networks before and around seizure onset. Nonlinear analysis is a promising technique currently for predicting seizure onset, thereby expanding our understanding of epileptogenesis and ictogenesis.

References

1. Le Van Quyen M, Khalilov I, Ben-Ari Y. The dark side of high-frequency oscillations in the developing brain. Trends Neurosci 2006;29(7):419–427
2. Bragin A, Engel J Jr, Wilson CL, Fried I, Mathern GW. Hippocampal and entorhinal cortex high-frequency oscillations (100–500 Hz) in human epileptic brain and in kainic acid–treated rats with chronic seizures. Epilepsia 1999;40(2):127–137
3. Rodriguez E, George N, Lachaux JP, Martinerie J, Renault B, Varela FJ. Perception's shadow: long-distance synchronization of human brain activity. Nature 1999;397(6718):430–433
4. Lachaux JP, George N, Tallon-Baudry C, et al. The many faces of the gamma band response to complex visual stimuli. Neuroimage 2005;25(2):491–501
5. Ozaki I, Suzuki C, Yaegashi Y, Baba M, Matsunaga M, Hashimoto I. High frequency oscillations in early cortical somatosensory evoked potentials. Electroencephalogr Clin Neurophysiol 1998;108(6):536–542
6. Allen PJ, Fish DR, Smith SJ. Very high-frequency rhythmic activity during SEEG suppression in frontal lobe epilepsy. Electroencephalogr Clin Neurophysiol 1992;82(2):155–159
7. Fisher RS, Webber WR, Lesser RP, Arroyo S, Uematsu S. High-frequency EEG activity at the start of seizures. J Clin Neurophysiol 1992;9(3):441–448
8. Traub RD, Whittington MA, Buhl EH, et al. A possible role for gap junctions in generation of very fast EEG oscillations preceding the onset of, and perhaps initiating, seizures. Epilepsia 2001;42(2):153–170
9. Worrell GA, Parish L, Cranstoun SD, Jonas R, Baltuch G, Litt B. High-frequency oscillations and seizure generation in neocortical epilepsy. Brain 2004;127(pt 7):1496–1506
10. Jirsch JD, Urrestarazu E, LeVan P, Olivier A, Dubeau F, Gotman J. High-frequency oscillations during human focal seizures. Brain 2006;129(pt 6):1593–1608

11. Alarcon G, Binnie CD, Elwes RD, Polkey CE. Power spectrum and intracranial EEG patterns at seizure onset in partial epilepsy. Electroencephalogr Clin Neurophysiol 1995;94(5):326–337

12. Bragin A, Wilson CL, Staba RJ, Reddick M, Fried I, Engel J Jr. Interictal high-frequency oscillations (80–500 Hz) in the human epileptic brain: entorhinal cortex. Ann Neurol 2002;52(4):407–415

13. Staba RJ, Wilson CL, Bragin A, Fried I, Engel J Jr. Quantitative analysis of high-frequency oscillations (80-500 Hz) recorded in human epileptic hippocampus and entorhinal cortex. J Neurophysiol 2002;88(4):1743–1752

14. Urrestarazu E, Jirsch JD, LeVan P, et al. High-frequency intracerebral EEG activity (100–500 Hz) following interictal spikes. Epilepsia 2006;47(9):1465–1476

15. Urrestarazu E, Chander R, Dubeau F, Gotman J. Interictal high-frequency oscillations (100-500 Hz) in the intracerebral EEG of epileptic patients. Brain 2007;130(pt 9):2354–2366

16. Kobayashi K, Oka M, Akiyama T, et al. Very fast rhythmic activity on scalp EEG associated with epileptic spasms. Epilepsia 2004;45(5):488–496

17. Inoue T, Kobayashi K, Oka M, Yoshinaga H, Ohtsuka Y. Spectral characteristics of EEG gamma rhythms associated with epileptic spasms. Brain Dev 2008;30(5):321–328

18. Najmi AH, Sadowsky J. The continuous wavelet transform and variable resolution time-frequency analysis. Johns Hopkins APL Tech Dig 1997;18:134–140

19. Muthuswamy J, Thakor NV. Spectral analysis methods for neurological signals. J Neurosci Methods 1998;83(1):1–14

20. Shimoyama I, Kasagi Y, Kaiho T, Shibata T, Nakajima Y, Asano H. Flash-related synchronization and desynchronization revealed by a multiple band frequency analysis. Jpn J Physiol 2000;50(5):553–559

21. Akiyama T, Otsubo H, Ochi A, et al. Focal cortical high-frequency oscillations trigger epileptic spasms: confirmation by digital video subdural EEG. Clin Neurophysiol 2005;116(12):2819–2825

22. Ochi A, Otsubo H, Donner EJ, et al. Dynamic changes of ictal high-frequency oscillations in neocortical epilepsy: using multiple band frequency analysis. Epilepsia 2007;48(2):286–296

23. Akiyama T, Otsubo H, Ochi A, et al. Topographic movie of ictal high-frequency oscillations on the brain surface using subdural EEG in neocortical epilepsy. Epilepsia 2006;47(11):1953–1957

24. Otsubo H, Ochi A, Imai K, et al. High-frequency oscillations of ictal muscle activity and epileptogenic discharges on intracranial EEG in a temporal lobe epilepsy patient. Clin Neurophysiol 2008;119(4):862–868

25. Goldring S. Negative steady potential shifts which lead to seizure discharge. In: Brazier MAB, ed. Brain Function, Cortical Excitability and Steady Potentials. Los Angeles, CA: UCLA Press; 1963:215–236

26. Vanhatalo S, Voipio J, Kaila K. Full-band EEG (FbEEG): an emerging standard in electroencephalography. Clin Neurophysiol 2005;116(1):1–8

27. Gross DW, Gotman J, Quesney LF, Dubeau F, Olivier A. Intracranial EEG with very low frequency activity fails to demonstrate an advantage over conventional recordings. Epilepsia 1999;40(7):891–898

28. Tallgren P, Vanhatalo S, Kaila K, Voipio J. Evaluation of commercially available electrodes and gels for recording of slow EEG potentials. Clin Neurophysiol 2005;116(4):799–806

29. Cornford EM, Oldendorf WH. Epilepsy and the blood-brain barrier. Adv Neurol 1986;44:787–812

30. Duncan JS. Imaging and epilepsy. Brain 1997;120(pt 2):339–377

31. Voipio J, Tallgren P, Heinonen E, Vanhatalo S, Kaila K. Millivolt-scale DC shifts in the human scalp EEG: evidence for a nonneuronal generator. J Neurophysiol 2003;89(4):2208–2214

32. Vanhatalo S, Tallgren P, Andersson S, Sainio K, Voipio J, Kaila K. DC-EEG discloses prominent, very slow activity patterns during sleep in preterm infants. Clin Neurophysiol 2002;113(11):1822–1825

33. Vanhatalo S, Palva JM, Holmes MD, Miller JW, Voipio J, Kaila K. Infraslow oscillations modulate excitability and interictal epileptic activity in the human cortex during sleep. Proc Natl Acad Sci U S A 2004;101(14):5053–5057

34. Birbaumer N, Elbert T, Canavan AG, Rockstroh B. Slow potentials of the cerebral cortex and behavior. Physiol Rev 1990;70(1):1–41

35. Bates JAV. The unidirectional potential changes in petit mal epilepsy. In: Brazier MAB, eds. Brain Function, Cortical Excitability and Steady Potentials. Los Angeles, CA: UCLA Press; 1963:237–279

36. Chatrian GE, Somasundaram M, Tassinari CA. DC changes recorded transcranially during "typical" three per second spike and wave discharges in man. Epilepsia 1968;9(3):185–209

37. Mayanagi Y, Walker AE. DC potentials of temporal lobe seizures in the monkey. J Neurol 1975;209(3):199–215

38. Ikeda A, Terada K, Mikuni N, et al. Subdural recording of ictal DC shifts in neocortical seizures in humans. Epilepsia 1996;37(7):662–674

39. Vanhatalo S, Holmes MD, Tallgren P, Voipio J, Kaila K, Miller JW. Very slow EEG responses lateralize temporal lobe seizures: an evaluation of non-invasive DC-EEG. Neurology 2003;60(7):1098–1104

40. Miller JW, Kim W, Holmes MD, Vanhatalo S. Ictal localization by source analysis of infraslow activity in DC-coupled scalp EEG recordings. Neuroimage 2007;35(2):583–597

41. Lagerlund TD, Worrell GA. EEG source localization (model-dependent and model-independent methods). In: Niedermeyer E, Lopes da Silva F, eds. Electroencephalography, 5th ed. Philadelphia, PA: Lippincott Williams & Wilkins; 2005:829–844

42. Helmholtz H. Über die Methoden, kleinste Zeitteile zu messen, und ihre Anwendung für physiologische Zwecke. Original work translated in: Philos Mag 1853;6:313–325

43. Michel CM, Murray MM, Lantz G, Gonzalez S, Spinelli L, Grave de Peralta R. EEG source imaging. Clin Neurophysiol 2004;115(10):2195–2222

44. Plummer C, Harvey AS, Cook M. EEG source localization in focal epilepsy: where are we now? Epilepsia 2008;49(2):201–218

45. Gevins A, Brickett P, Costales B, Le J, Reutter B. Beyond topographic mapping: towards functional-anatomical imaging with 124-channel EEGs and 3-D MRIs. Brain Topogr 1990;3(1):53–64

46. Spitzer AR, Cohen LG, Fabrikant J, Hallett M. A method for determining optimal interelectrode spacing for cerebral topographic mapping. Electroencephalogr Clin Neurophysiol 1989;72(4):355–361

47. Srinivasan R, Nunez PL, Tucker DM, Silberstein RB, Cadusch PJ. Spatial sampling and filtering of EEG with spline laplacians to estimate cortical potentials. Brain Topogr 1996;8(4):355–366

48. Srinivasan R, Nunez PL, Tucker DM. Estimating the spatial Nyquist of the human EEG. Behav Res Methods Instrum Comput 1998;30:8–19

49. Benar CG, Gotman J. Non-uniform spatial sampling in EEG source analysis. Paper presented at 23rd Conference of IEEE-EMBS; 25–28 October, 2001; Istanbul

50. De Munck JC, Vijn PC, Spekreijse H. A practical method for determining electrode positions on the head. Electroencephalogr Clin Neurophysiol 1991;78(1):85–87

51. Le J, Lu M, Pellouchoud E, Gevins A. A rapid method for determining standard 10/10 electrode positions for high resolution EEG studies. Electroencephalogr Clin Neurophysiol 1998;106(6):554–558

52. Khosla D, Don M, Kwong B. Spatial mislocalization of EEG electrodes—effects on accuracy of dipole estimation. Clin Neurophysiol 1999;110(2):261–271

53. Van Hoey G, De Clercq J, Vanrumste B, et al. EEG dipole source localization using artificial neural networks. Phys Med Biol 2000;45(4):997–1011

54. Wang Y, Gotman J. The influence of electrode location errors on EEG dipole source localization with a realistic head model. Clin Neurophysiol 2001;112(9):1777–1780

55. Vanrumste B, Van Hoey G, Van de Walle R, D'Havé MR, Lemahieu IA, Boon PA. Comparison of performance of spherical and realistic head models in dipole localization from noisy EEG. Med Eng Phys 2002;24(6):403–418

56. Ochi A, Otsubo H, Shirasawa A, et al. Systematic approach to dipole localization of interictal EEG spikes in children with extratemporal lobe epilepsies. Clin Neurophysiol 2000;111(1):161–168

57. Sperli F, Spinelli L, Seeck M, Kurian M, Michel CM, Lantz G. EEG source imaging in pediatric epilepsy surgery: a new perspective in presurgical workup. Epilepsia 2006;47(6):981–990

58. Boon P, D'Havé M, Vanrumste B, et al. Ictal source localization in presurgical patients with refractory epilepsy. J Clin Neurophysiol 2002;19(5):461–468

59. Merlet I, Gotman J. Dipole modeling of scalp electroencephalogram epileptic discharges: correlation with intracerebral fields. Clin Neurophysiol 2001;112(3):414–430

60. Kobayashi K, Yoshinaga H, Ohtsuka Y, Gotman J. Dipole modeling of epileptic spikes can be accurate or misleading. Epilepsia 2005;46(3):397–408

61. Donner EJ, Smith CR, Snead OC III. Sudden unexplained death in children with epilepsy. Neurology 2001;57(3):430–434

62. Navarro V, Martinerie J, Le Van Quyen M, et al. Seizure anticipation in human neocortical partial epilepsy. Brain 2002;125(pt 3): 640–655

63. Hughes JR. Progress in predicting seizure episodes with nonlinear methods. Epilepsy Behav 2008;12(1):128–135

64. Martinerie J, Adam C, Le Van Quyen M, et al. Epileptic seizures can be anticipated by non-linear analysis. Nat Med 1998;4(10):1173–1176

65. Elger CE, Lehnertz K. Seizure prediction by non-linear time series analysis of brain electrical activity. Eur J Neurosci 1998;10(2): 786–789

66. Le Van Quyen M, Adam C, Martinerie J, Baulac M, Clémenceau S, Varela F. Spatio-temporal characterizations of non-linear changes in intracranial activities prior to human temporal lobe seizures. Eur J Neurosci 2000;12(6):2124–2134

40 New Imaging Techniques in Pediatric Epilepsy Surgery

Christoph M. Michel and Margitta Seeck

An essential task in the surgical treatment of epilepsy is the definition of resection margins, which allows the removal of the epileptogenic zone as complete as possible while avoiding neurological deficits. To achieve this goal, the presurgical workup includes precise localization of the epileptogenic cortex and of surrounding functionally eloquent cortical areas. Despite all efforts with conventional neurophysiological and brain-imaging techniques, patients who undergo curative epilepsy surgery may receive incomplete focus resections, leaving them with persistent postoperative seizures. The percentage of patients who are not seizure free postoperatively depends on several clinical aspects. Most studies agree that an extratemporal focus and the absence of magnetic resonance imaging (MRI) lesions carries a less favorable outcome, that is, only 30 to 40% are seizure free after surgical intervention.

Up to now, most of these patients have to undergo invasive preoperative electroencephalography (EEG) monitoring during a period of several days or weeks. This monitoring represents a quite demanding situation for the patient and is related to significant medical risks (e.g., bleeding or infection).[1] Moreover, intracranial electrodes capture neuronal signals only from a small radius of surrounding tissue,[2] which means that the placement of electrodes needs careful elaboration of hypothesis of possible seizure origins. If the intracranial electrodes are not correctly placed, the yield of this exam is reduced. Thus, when patients are supposed to undergo implantation of electrodes for intracranial EEG monitoring, an accurate idea of the cortex to be covered is mandatory.

In addition to the need for exact focus localization, intracranial monitoring may also be required for localization of essential functions, such as motor or language functions, through electrocortical stimulation (ES). ES requires significant time and work-load investment from the medical staff and optimal collaboration from the patient. In addition, the validity of ES alone as a gold standard for functional localization has been questioned, particularly with respect to higher cognitive functions such as language[3,4] and are probably partially replaceable by noninvasive techniques. If this lengthy procedure could be abbreviated, this would be most welcome by the patient and the medical team.

Given the significant impact of proper localization of the focus and adjacent eloquent cortex on the surgical results, considerable research has been devoted to sophisticated imaging methods in epileptic patients. Several techniques are addressed elsewhere in this book. Here we concentrate on electric source imaging (ESI) with high-density EEG, on EEG–functional MRI (fMRI), and on the combination of ESI with fMRI by direct recordings of high density EEG in the MRI scanner and simultaneous analysis of the electric and the hemodynamic activity.

■ Electric Source Imaging

By contrast with fMRI, positron emission tomography (PET) and single photon emission computed tomography (SPECT), ESI directly measures neuronal activity. It is based on the recording of the electric potential field on the scalp using multichannel EEG. The neuronal sources in the brain that produce these scalp potential maps can be estimated using inverse solution algorithms. Despite the nonuniqueness of the inverse problem, sophisticated source and head models now allow a stable and reliable identification of the active neuronal populations in the brain that produces the scalp measurements.[5–8] The high temporal resolution (milliseconds) allows tracing the flow of neuronal activity in the whole brain in real time. This high temporal resolution is of fundamental importance in the application to focus localization, where fast propagation of interictal and ictal activity is the rule rather than the exception.[9,10] This fast propagation is the reason why ESI and the related technique magnetic source imaging [based on the magnetoencephalogram (MEG)] have particularly attracted epileptologists. MEG is discussed in detail elsewhere in this book, and a recent literature review on its use in presurgical epilepsy is provided in Lau et al.[11] MEG relies on the same electrophysiological phenomena (temporally synchronized and spatially aligned postsynaptic potentials) and on the same mathematical underpinnings as ESI. The difference between EEG and MEG has been discussed and debated repeatedly,[12–16] but in principle, EEG (when recorded with a sufficient number of electrodes) has higher sensitivity than MEG in the sense that it records neuronal activity independent of the dipole orientation and that it is more susceptive for deeper sources.[17] In clinical routine, the practical advantages of the EEG are obvious, particularly in pediatric and ictal recordings. A very comprehensive review on the yield of ESI in epilepsy can be found in Plummer et al.[18] Here we only summarize the basic features and results of ESI.

Number and Positioning of the Electrodes for ESI

The question of the number of electrodes that is needed for proper ESI refers to the question of spatial sampling of the potential field on the scalp and the spatial frequency of this field. Undersampling the field bears the risk of not properly capturing the field extrema and field inversions and thus misinterpreting the sources of this field.[6] It has been estimated that electrode spacing of approximately 1 cm is needed to properly measure the potential field.[19] Because the electrodes should also cover the low basal temporal and occipital scalp regions, more than 100 electrodes are needed for correct spatial sampling.[20] A systematic evaluation of the question of number of electrodes in epileptic patients was performed with a 123-channel ESI recording. The interictal spikes in 14 patients were subsampled to 63 and to 32 channels, and the results were compared with the original 123-channel ESI.[21] Localization of the estimated epileptic zone with these three electrode arrays was evaluated with respect to the distance of the resected structure that rendered all patients seizure free. This study showed that localization precision increased significantly with increasing number of electrodes.

However, this study, like many others, used conductivity values of the skull that are probably not adequate. Several recent studies have shown that the skull resistivity is considerably lower than previously assumed[22-24] and, therefore, the spatial frequency of the scalp potential field is considerably higher. This lower resistivity is particularly true in newborns and young children, because the resistivity depends on the skull thickness.[25,26] Consequently, 256 or more electrodes would be needed in children to minimize spatial sampling errors. Fortunately, this requirement is met by several recent systems, which are commercially available and allow recordings of 256 electrodes or more.[27] Fast application of electrode caps with a large number of electrodes is now readily possible, making high-density EEG feasible in clinical routine.[28,29]

Source Model

EEG source imaging in epilepsy often uses distributed source localization procedures instead of the initially proposed equivalent dipole fitting procedures (see Plummer[18] for a review). Distributed source models have the advantages that there is no need for a priori assumption of the number of sources and that they allow an estimation of the extent of the active sources. Distributed source models also better localize propagated activity that often includes multiple simul-

taneous active sources. Distributed source models estimate the "best" current density distribution in the whole three-dimensional brain space that produced a given recorded scalp potential field.[6] The source space is restricted to the gray matter of the cortex obtained from MRI segmentation. Because the problem is highly underdetermined (there are much more solution points than electrodes), additional constraints are needed. Such constraints can be purely mathematical or can incorporate biophysical or physiological knowledge or even incorporate findings from other structural or functional imaging modalities.[30] Many advances in source models have been made in recent years. The use of realistic head models and the coregistration of the solutions with the individual three-dimensional brain MRI has ultimately converted the EEG to a functional imaging procedure as capable as other imaging techniques, in keeping with the advantage of directly recording neuronal activity in real time. Examples are shown in **Fig. 40.1**.

Clinical Applications of ESI

Most of the clinical ESI studies analyzed interictal spike activity. Ray and colleagues[31] convincingly showed in simultaneous intracranial and scalp recordings that the analysis of scalp spikes provides more reliable localizing information about the epileptogenic zone than the analysis of ictal activity because of limited propagation of spikes. This good localizing information is, however, only true if the beginning phase of the spike is analyzed and not the peak of the spike, which already reflects propagated activity. Lantz and colleagues[10] systematically studied spike propagation in 16 patients with symptomatic focal epilepsy who were all seizure free after surgery. The source analysis of the 128-channel recordings revealed that the best localization was obtained when analyzing the EEG at 50% of the rising phase of the spike. In all cases, the active brain area laid within the resected structure. However, at the spike peak, the source maximum was outside the epileptogenic zone in 5 of the 16 patients.

We evaluated the clinical yield and localization precision in a group of 32 patients with different types of focal epilepsy, all recorded with 128 electrodes.[28] A correct localization on a lobar level was found in 93.7% of the cases. In the 24 patients who were operated, the maximal ESI source laid within the resected area in 79%.

Even better accuracy was obtained when using statistical parametric mapping (SPM) or nonparametric mapping applied to the distributed source analysis. The earliest significantly active voxels before the spike peak (compared with a prespike period) highly accurately identified the epileptogenic focus in several studies.[32-34] In a pediatric epilepsy surgical cohort, SPM was used to study the yield of ESI from standard clinical EEG (i.e., 19–29 scalp electrodes).[34] Interictal recordings of 30 children (13 temporal, 17 extratemporal)

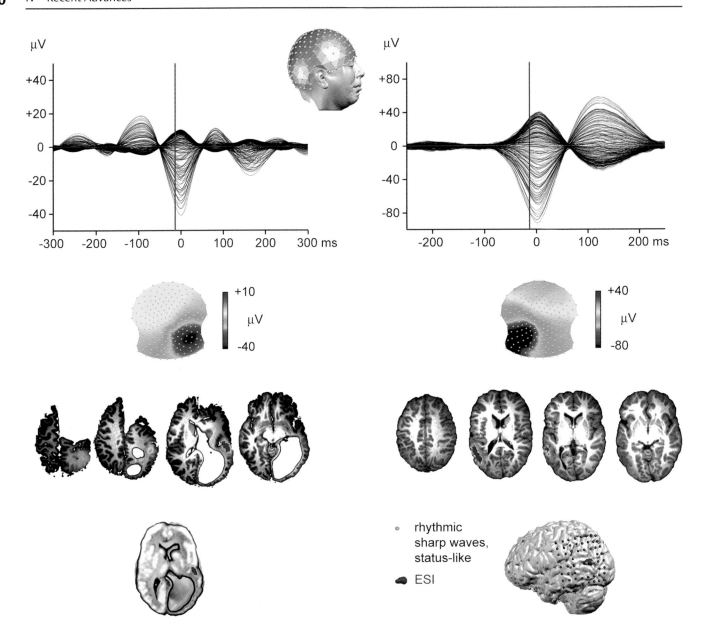

Fig. 40.1 Electric source imaging (ESI) in two patients and correspondences with other noninvasive or invasive investigations. Left: 17-year-old boy with chronic focal epilepsy and complex cerebral malformation of the right hemisphere. Right: 15-year-old girl with tuberous sclerosis with numerous tuber in both hemispheres, including a large tuber in the left posterior temporal lobe. The top row shows the overlapped waveforms of the averaged spikes recorded from 204 electrodes. The inset illustrates the location of the 204 electrodes on a template head. The second row shows the scalp potential map at the rising phase of the spike. The third row gives the result of the linear distributed inverse solution (LAURA) applied to this map, coregistered with the individual brain. The fourth row shows other exams in these patients with highly corresponding results. Left: interictal positron emission tomography, coregistered with the magnetic resonance imaging (MRI) and the ESI solution. A hypometabolism is seen concordant with the ESI maximum. Right: Subdural grid recording coregistered with the MRI and the ESI solution, showing the correspondence of the ESI of the sharp waves with their subdural electrode recordings. The ESI result of the patient on the left shows that even large liquid-filled brain lesions permit correct source localization, despite eventually altered conductivity values. (From Brodbeck V, Lascano AM, Spinelli L, Michel CM. Accuracy of EEG source imaging of epileptic spikes in patients with large brain lesions. Clin Neurophysiol 2009; 120:679–685.)

were analyzed, and their results were compared with ictal SPECT and interictal PET. Localization of the epileptogenic region agreed with the PET in 82% and with the SPECT in 70%, whereas ESI correctly identified the focus in 90% of the patients. However, the study also showed the limitation of the low number of electrodes, particularly with respect to basal mesial temporal sources, where ESI localized incorrectly in the insula or basal frontal regions in a few patients.

Localization of Eloquent Cortex with ESI

Today, fMRI is the most established tool of noninvasive imaging and is discussed elsewhere in this book. Several investigations showed a good correlation between the distance of the resection margin and the motor area identified by fMRI as determined by the presence or absence of the neurological deficit postoperatively.[35] However, despite relatively reliable identification of sensorimotor areas with the fMRI (see **Figs. 40.2** and **40.3**), there are drawbacks that affect its clinical acceptance. Sunaert[36] discussed the different reasons: besides a relatively high drop-out rate for technical reasons (e.g., movement artifacts, distortions, system instabilities), the most important problem in patients with brain lesions is the possibility of altered vasoactivity that can lead to neurovascular uncoupling and incorrect lack of the BOLD (blood oxygen dependent) activation. Consequently, absence of an fMRI activity in a given area does not necessarily indicate that this region is not implied in the function.

MEG and EEG source imaging can be an alternative to localize functional cortex in the presurgical planning. High-resolution MEG systems have been on the market somewhat longer and have, therefore, been used for this purpose in several studies, particularly for localization of sensory and motor cortex. These studies showed good correlation between sensory and motor evoked fields and ES.[37,38] Similar good localization has been achieved with ESI applied to somatosensory evoked potentials.[39] A recent comparative study of the yield of EEG and MEG for localizing somatosensory activity in children with focal epilepsies indicated comparable good localization precision in all subjects with structurally normal cortex.[40] Interestingly, this study showed that EEG source localization was superior to MEG in patients with central structural lesions, because of more radial orientation of the dipoles in theses cases that were not seen by MEG. The authors concluded that "these findings strongly contradict the view that the EEG is in general less exact or less helpful in mapping cortical activity under clinical condition"[40, p 1733]. This conclusion was based on a study with 122-channel MEG and only 33-channel EEG (i.e., a setting rather unfavorable for EEG). It may be speculated that ESI is even more precise if more EEG channels are used.[41] Because this is now easily obtained in clinical routine,[28] high-resolution ESI of somatosensory evoked activity should be considered for noninva-

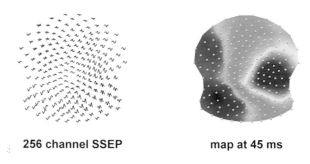

256 channel SSEP   **map at 45 ms**

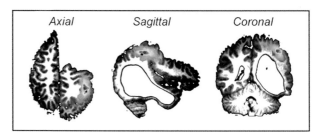

Axial   *Sagittal*   *Coronal*

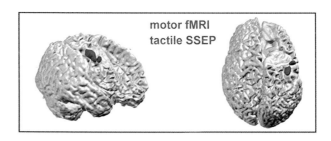

motor fMRI
tactile SSEP

Fig. 40.2 Mapping of the sensorimotor cortex with functional magnetic resonance imaging fMRI and electric source imaging (ESI) in the same patient as in **Fig. 40.1** (*left*) with the complex right hemispheric malformation. *Top:* Somatosensory evoked potentials (SSEP) by tactile stimulation of the left thumb and the scalp potential map at 45 milliseconds. *Middle:* Localization of the sources for the 45-millisecond map estimated by a linear distributed inverse solution (LAURA) constraint to the gray matter of the patient's own MRI, showing a focal activation of the right somatosensory cortex. *Bottom:* coregistration of the tactile SSEP sources and the significant BOLD response of a left hand movement in the individual MRI of the patient. Despite extremely complex lesions, the sensory–motor cortex is correctly identified by the combination of these two techniques.

sive presurgical functional localization of the somatosensory cortex, particularly in patients with cortical malformations (**Fig. 40.2**).

The use of MEG or ESI for localization of language cortex is rather sparse. However, there is some evidence that the posterior language cortex is better retrieved with MEG, a region that is inconsistently identified with fMRI.[42] More studies are needed to judge the yield of magnetic or electric source imaging in localization of language areas in the individual patient.

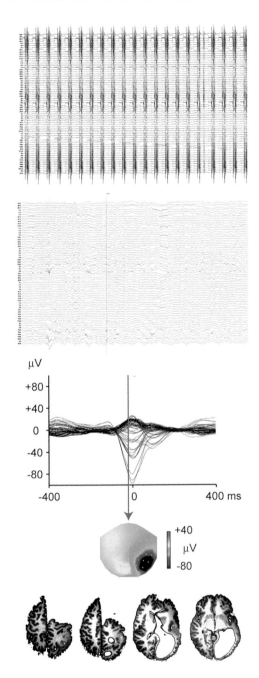

Fig. 40.3 Sixty-four-channel electroencephalography (EEG) recording of the same patient as in Figs. 40.1 and 40.2 within the 3T magnetic resonance imaging (MRI) scanner during continuous ESI sequences. *1st row:* Uncorrected EEG, showing the gradient artifacts. *2nd row:* EEG after correction for the imaging and the pulse artifact. *3rd row:* Overlapped waveforms (64 channel) of the averaged spikes identified in the EEG within the scanner. These spikes were also used for the correlation with the BOLD response (see also **Fig. 40.4**). The scalp potential maps at the rising phase of the spike are shown and the result of the distributed linear inverse solution applied to this map. The same head model and solution space as for the 204-channel recording in Fig. 40.1 was used. Note the highly similar map and source localization of the spike recorded inside and outside the scanner.

■ EEG–fMRI

The combination of EEG and fMRI has become possible thanks to MRI-compatible EEG systems.[43] In the last few years, powerful artifact removal algorithms for the EEG signals have been developed that allow us to recover the EEG during scans, despite the large gradient artifact they produce.[44,45] **Fig. 40.4** shows a corrected 64-channel EEG recording during fMRI acquisition in a 3T scanner.

The EEG–fMRI combination has become of particular interest for the localization of epileptogenic foci. Several groups have repeatedly shown the possibility to detect spike-related activity in the fMRI when the BOLD response is correlated with the epileptic discharges recorded in the simultaneous EEG. In particular, in chronic focal epilepsy, EEG-fMRI appeared as a promising localizing tool with high spatial resolution.[46–50] Recent studies also demonstrated interesting results in patients with idiopathic generalized epilepsy using EEG–fMRI combination,[51–53] demonstrating patterns of thalamic activations and frontal and parietal lobe deactivations. The reasons for negative BOLD response related to interictal activity are not yet clear and could be related to steal phenomenon secondary to the increased blood flow, to abnormal coupling between neuronal activity and blood flow in the pathological area, or to decreased or inhibited synaptic activity (for a discussion see Gotman[54]).

The overall clinical yield of the EEG–fMRI combination is relatively low. A recent detailed study of 63 consecutively recruited patients with focal epilepsy revealed significant BOLD changes that were concordant with electroclinical results in only 17 patients (27%).[55] A similar low number was reported by our group.[56] This low yield is partially because of the impossibility to detect interictal epileptic discharges in the scanner, especially with small amplitudes. In the study of Salek-Haddadi and colleagues,[55] no spikes were detected in 25 patients (40%). Whether this is because of distorted EEG, despite effective artifact corrections or because of other electromagnetic or physiological factors (e.g., patient is awake and tense, which may reduce epileptic discharges) is unclear. Another important problem is movements that make proper fMRI acquisition analysis impossible, in particular in small children and retarded subjects. In the study of Salek-Haddadi and collaborators,[55] 4 patients had to be discarded because of artifacts. From the remaining 34 patients with spikes, 11 patients showed no significant BOLD changes. That means that even if spikes were detected, they did not correlate with any significant BOLD responses in 32%. From the 23 patients with significant BOLD changes, either positive or negative, 6 showed areas of BOLD response that were not concordant with the clinical data. Finally, from the 17 cases (27%) with concordant responses, only 7 patients showed unambiguous fMRI signals (i.e., only activated areas that corresponded with the electroclinical data). The remaining 10 patients

Tactile SSEP

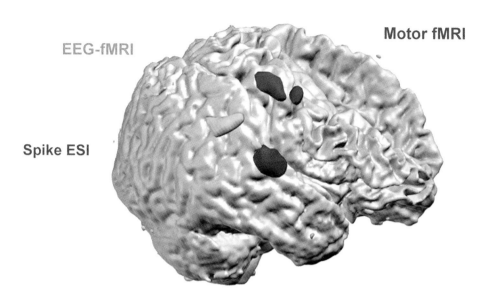

EEG-fMRI

Motor fMRI

Spike ESI

Fig. 40.4 Results of the multimodal imaging in the same patient as in the previous figures. All results are coregistered with the magnetic resonance imaging of the patient. Concerning the location of the epileptic focus, electroencephalography–functional magnetic resonance imaging (fMRI) overlaps with electric source imaging (ESI) in the right superior posterior temporal gyrus. The second BOLD response in the parietal lobe had no correspondence in the ESI and might be caused by propagation. Concerning the sensory–motor cortex, the motor area of the left-hand side was identified in the right frontal lobe with the fMRI, and the somatosensory hand area with the 204-channel tactile somatosensory cuoked potentials (SSEP) just posterior to it, allowing a precise localization of the central sulcus in this patient.

showed activations related to the real focus as well as additional noncorresponding areas, providing ambiguous results of which BOLD response is truly significant with respect to primary focus localization difficult.

An important limitation of the EEG–fMRI for the localization of epileptic discharges is the low temporal resolution of the fMRI. As already discussed, interictal epileptic discharges propagate within a few milliseconds to remote brain areas. These secondary activations can be as active as the primary focus and therefore consume as much as oxygen. The temporal blurring of the BOLD response over seconds makes it virtually impossible to separate discharges from the primary focus and those from propagated areas. It is, therefore, rather the rule than the exception to find multiple areas of BOLD changes, and additional tools are needed to determine their functional–anatomical relationship.

■ Combination of ESI and EEG-fMRI

Although the high spatial resolution of the fMRI makes the EEG–fMRI an interesting technique to precisely localize the epileptogenic focus, the inherent low temporal resolution does not allow us to tease apart primary from secondary foci. Because this temporal resolution is exactly the strength

of ESI, the most rational approach is to combine these two techniques. This combination was already demonstrated in a case report by Seeck and colleagues[46]: ESI analysis at different time points during the spike-wave complex identified the generators of epileptogenic discharges (left lateral frontal) and differentiated them from areas activated by propagation (mesial frontal bilaterally and right frontal). Surgical resection of the initial left frontal area with subsequent seizure freedom confirmed the correctness of this localization. A more recent study by Boor and colleagues[57] compared multiple dipole analysis obtained by 23-channel EEG with EEG–fMRI in 11 patients with benign childhood epilepsy with centrotemporal (rolandic) spikes. In all patients, multiple dipole analysis located underlying spike sources (several 100 spikes were averaged in each patient) in the rolandic face or hand region, as expected. In 10 of the 11 patients, a second (or even a third) dipole was found in remote areas with delays of approximately 20 milliseconds, most likely representing propagation. The fMRI analysis provided results only in 4 of the 11 patients (36%). In these 4 patients, the expected rolandic areas showed increased BOLD response, but additional areas in the central cortex, the sylvian fissure, and the insula also showed response. Most of these areas (but not all) corresponded to the propagated dipoles as identified by the ESI.

However, the previously discussed studies[46,57] and similar other studies[58-60] used the EEG recorded outside the scanner to compare with the BOLD response, assuming that the spatiotemporal behavior of the spikes are the same inside and outside the magnet. It is well known in clinical practice that the propagation behavior of single spikes is quite variable, even in patients known for stable unifocal epilepsy. Very powerful correction algorithms are currently available, so that artifact-reduced, high-density EEG (more than 64 channels) can be retrieved inside the magnet.[45] Therefore, ESI analysis can now be performed on the same spikes that are associated to BOLD response, as shown in **Fig. 40.4**. This allows us to directly combine the high spatial resolution of the fMRI with the high temporal resolution of the ESI.

■ Conclusion

The complete resection of the epileptic focus while preventing new neurological or cognitive deficits after brain surgery depends on the precise mapping of all vital functions and the dysfunctional zone in the individual patient. Despite the advancement of noninvasive functional brain mapping, preoperative mapping of functional and dysfunctional cortex still relies largely on invasive procedures with recording from and stimulation of intracranial electrodes. This costly and lengthy procedure is associated to a certain risk of morbidity and mortality. A better integration of the noninvasive techniques is, therefore, highly warranted.

High density ESI is noninvasive, easily applied in less cooperative patients, and relatively inexpensive compared with other imaging tools. ESI with its temporal resolution in the millisec-ond range is ideal to provide information regarding the distinction between the primary focus and propagated areas. ESI can also be used to map eloquent cortex with good precision, using high-density evoked potentials, as shown by some studies.

fMRI is a powerful tool to localize cortical functions with high spatial precision, especially the sensorimotor cortex, if the vasoactivity is not altered by the pathology. fMRI can also be used to localize the epileptic focus by measuring the EEG inside the scanner and determining BOLD responses related to spike activity. However, for multiple reasons, the yield appears relatively poor, although the exact reasons for the multitude—or lack—of activations are still unclear.

Because none of the available imaging techniques is ideal in all circumstances, a multimodal imaging approach is best applied. **Fig. 40.4** illustrates this integration of multimodal noninvasive imaging techniques for the localization of pathological (epileptic) and eloquent cortex in an individual patient. It illustrates that the combination is most powerful to delineate pathological and functionally relevant brain areas.

In the future, we may be able to obtain simultaneously fMRI, EEG–fMRI, and ESI. However, many issues remain to be resolved for the time being related rather to an incomplete understanding of fMRI response pattern in epileptic subjects and proper EEG acquisition inside the scanner.

Acknowledgments

The authors are supported by the Swiss National Science Foundation (grants #32-111783 and 32-113766) and by the Biomedical Imaging Center (CIBM) Geneva-Lausanne. We thank Laurent Spinelli for the image fusioning and Verena Brodbeck and Agustina Lascano for data acquisition and analysis.

References

1. Hamer HM, Morris HH, Mascha EJ, et al. Complications of invasive video-EEG monitoring with subdural grid electrodes. Neurology 2002;58(1):97–103

2. Seeck M, Spinelli L. Intracranial monitoring. Suppl Clin Neurophysiol 2004;57:485–493

3. Schäffler L, Lüders HO, Beck GJ. Quantitative comparison of language deficits produced by extraoperative electrical stimulation of Broca's, Wernicke's, and basal temporal language areas. Epilepsia 1996;37(5):463–475

4. Seeck M, Pegna AJ, Ortigue S, et al. Speech arrest with stimulation may not reliably predict language deficit after epilepsy surgery. Neurology 2006;66(4):592–594

5. Baillet S, Mosher JC, Leahy RM. Electromagnetic brain mapping. IEEE Signal Process Mag 2001;18:14–30

6. Michel CM, Murray MM, Lantz G, Gonzalez S, Spinelli L, Grave de Peralta R. EEG source imaging. Clin Neurophysiol 2004;115(10):2195–2222

7. He B, Lian J. High-resolution spatio-temporal functional neuroimaging of brain activity. Crit Rev Biomed Eng 2002;30(4–6):283–306

8. Liu Z, Ding L, He B. Integration of EEG/MEG with MRI and fMRI. IEEE Eng Med Biol Mag 2006;25(4):46–53

9. Alarcon G, Guy CN, Binnie CD, Walker SR, Elwes RD, Polkey CE. Intracerebral propagation of interictal activity in partial epilepsy: implications for source localisation. J Neurol Neurosurg Psychiatry 1994;57(4):435–449

10. Lantz G, Spinelli L, Seeck M, de Peralta Menendez RG, Sottas CC, Michel CM. Propagation of interictal epileptiform activity can lead to erroneous source localizations: a 128-channel EEG mapping study. J Clin Neurophysiol 2003;20(5):311–319

11. Lau M, Yam D, Burneo JG. A systematic review on MEG and its use in the presurgical evaluation of localization-related epilepsy. Epilepsy Res 2008;79(2–3):97–104

12. Barkley GL, Baumgartner C. MEG and EEG in epilepsy. J Clin Neurophysiol 2003;20(3):163–178

13. Baumgartner C, Pataraia E. Revisiting the role of magnetoencephalography in epilepsy. Curr Opin Neurol 2006;19(2):181–186

14. Malmivuo J, Suihko V, Eskola H. Sensitivity distributions of EEG and MEG measurements. IEEE Trans Biomed Eng 1997;44(3):196–208

15. Liu AK, Dale AM, Belliveau JW. Monte Carlo simulation studies of EEG and MEG localization accuracy. Hum Brain Mapp 2002;16(1):47–62

16. Malmivuo JA, Suihko VE. Effect of skull resistivity on the spatial resolutions of EEG and MEG. IEEE Trans Biomed Eng 2004;51(7):1276–1280

17. Baumgartner C. Controversies in clinical neurophysiology. MEG is superior to EEG in the localization of interictal epileptiform activity: Con. Clin Neurophysiol 2004;115(5):1010–1020

18. Plummer C, Harvey AS, Cook M. EEG source localization in focal epilepsy: where are we now? Epilepsia 2008;49(2):201–218

19. Freeman WJ, Holmes MD, Burke BC, Vanhatalo S. Spatial spectra of scalp EEG and EMG from awake humans. Clin Neurophysiol 2003;114(6):1053–1068

20. Srinivasan R, Tucker DM, Murias M. Estimating the spatial Nyquist of the human EEG. Behav Res Methods Instrum Comput 1998;30:8–19

21. Lantz G, Grave de Peralta R, Spinelli L, Seeck M, Michel CM. Epileptic source localization with high density EEG: how many electrodes are needed? Clin Neurophysiol 2003;114(1):63–69

22. Oostendorp TF, Delbeke J, Stegeman DF. The conductivity of the human skull: results of in vivo and in vitro measurements. IEEE Trans Biomed Eng 2000;47(11):1487–1492

23. Lai Y, van Drongelen W, Ding L, et al. Estimation of in vivo human brain-to-skull conductivity ratio from simultaneous extra- and intra-cranial electrical potential recordings. Clin Neurophysiol 2005;116(2):456–465

24. Ryynanen OR, Hyttinen JA, Malmivuo JA. Effect of measurement noise and electrode density on the spatial resolution of cortical potential distribution with different resistivity values for the skull. IEEE Trans Biomed Eng 2006;53(9):1851–1858

25. Fifer WP, Grieve PG, Grose-Fifer J, Isler JR, Byrd D. High-density electroencephalogram monitoring in the neonate. Clin Perinatol 2006;33(3):679–691, vii

26. Grieve PG, Emerson RG, Isler JR, Stark RI. Quantitative analysis of spatial sampling error in the infant and adult electroencephalogram. Neuroimage 2004;21(4):1260–1274

27. Holmes MD, Brown M, Tucker DM. Are "generalized" seizures truly generalized? Evidence of localized mesial frontal and frontopolar discharges in absence. Epilepsia 2004;45(12):1568–1579

28. Michel CM, Lantz G, Spinelli L, De Peralta RG, Landis T, Seeck M. 128-channel EEG source imaging in epilepsy: clinical yield and localization precision. J Clin Neurophysiol 2004;21(2):71–83

29. Holmes MD. Dense array EEG: methodology and new hypothesis on epilepsy syndromes. Epilepsia 2008;49(suppl 3):3–14

30. He B, Lian J. Electrophysiological Neuroimaging: solving the EEG inverse problem. In: He B, ed. Neuroal Engineering. Berlin: Springer 2005:221–261

31. Ray A, Tao JX, Hawes-Ebersole SM, Ebersole JS. Localizing value of scalp EEG spikes: a simultaneous scalp and intracranial study. Clin Neurophysiol 2007;118(1):69–79

32. Zumsteg D, Friedman A, Wennberg RA, Wieser HG. Source localization of mesial temporal interictal epileptiform discharges: correlation with intracranial foramen ovale electrode recordings. Clin Neurophysiol 2005;116(12):2810–2818

33. Zumsteg D, Andrade DM, Wennberg RA. Source localization of small sharp spikes: low resolution electromagnetic tomography (LORETA) reveals two distinct cortical sources. Clin Neurophysiol 2006;117(6):1380–1387

34. Sperli F, Spinelli L, Seeck M, Kurian M, Michel CM, Lantz G. EEG source imaging in pediatric epilepsy surgery: a new perspective in presurgical workup. Epilepsia 2006;47(6):981–990

35. Håberg A, Kvistad KA, Unsgård G, Haraldseth O. Preoperative blood oxygen level-dependent functional magnetic resonance imaging in patients with primary brain tumors: clinical application and outcome. Neurosurgery 2004;54(4):902–914, discussion 914–915

36. Sunaert S. Presurgical planning for tumor resectioning. J Magn Reson Imaging 2006;23(6):887–905

37. Ganslandt O, Fahlbusch R, Nimsky C, et al. Functional neuronavigation with magnetoencephalography: outcome in 50 patients with lesions around the motor cortex. J Neurosurg 1999;91(1):73–79

38. Cheyne D, Bostan AC, Gaetz W, Pang EW. Event-related beamforming: a robust method for presurgical functional mapping using MEG. Clin Neurophysiol 2007;118(8):1691–1704

39. Gross DW, Merlet I, Boling W, Gotman J. Relationships between the epileptic focus and hand area in central epilepsy: combining dipole models and anatomical landmarks. J Neurosurg 2000;92(5):785–792

40. Bast T, Wright T, Boor R, et al. Combined EEG and MEG analysis of early somatosensory evoked activity in children and adolescents with focal epilepsies. Clin Neurophysiol 2007;118(8):1721–1735

41. Lantz G, Grave de Peralta Menendez R, Gonzalez Andino S, Michel CM. Noninvasive localization of electromagnetic epileptic activity. II. Demonstration of sublobar accuracy in patients with simultaneous surface and depth recordings. Brain Topogr 2001;14(2):139–147

42. Salmelin R. Clinical neurophysiology of language: the MEG approach. Clin Neurophysiol 2007;118(2):237–254

43. Ives JR, Warach S, Schmitt F, Edelman RR, Schomer DL. Monitoring the patient's EEG during echo planar MRI. Electroencephalogr Clin Neurophysiol 1993;87(6):417–420

44. Allen PJ, Josephs O, Turner R. A method for removing imaging artifact from continuous EEG recorded during functional MRI. Neuroimage 2000;12(2):230–239

45. Grouiller F, Vercueil L, Krainik A, Segebarth C, Kahane P, David O. A comparative study of different artefact removal algorithms for EEG signals acquired during functional MRI. Neuroimage 2007;38(1):124–137

46. Seeck M, Lazeyras F, Michel CM, et al. Non-invasive epileptic focus localization using EEG-triggered functional MRI and electromagnetic tomography. Electroencephalogr Clin Neurophysiol 1998;106(6):508–512

47. Krakow K, Woermann FG, Symms MR, et al. EEG-triggered functional MRI of interictal epileptiform activity in patients with partial seizures. Brain 1999;122(pt 9):1679–1688

48. Lazeyras F, Blanke O, Perrig S, et al. EEG-triggered functional MRI in patients with pharmacoresistant epilepsy. J Magn Reson Imaging 2000;12(1):177–185

49. Lemieux L. Electroencephalography-correlated functional MR imaging studies of epileptic activity. Neuroimaging Clin N Am 2004;14(3):487–506

50. Al-Asmi A, Bénar CG, Gross DW, et al. fMRI activation in continuous and spike-triggered EEG-fMRI studies of epileptic spikes. Epilepsia 2003;44(10):1328–1339

51. Gotman J, Grova C, Bagshaw A, Kobayashi E, Aghakhani Y, Dubeau F. Generalized epileptic discharges show thalamocortical activation and suspension of the default state of the brain. Proc Natl Acad Sci U S A 2005;102(42):15236–15240

52. Aghakhani Y, Bagshaw AP, Bénar CG, et al. fMRI activation during spike and wave discharges in idiopathic generalized epilepsy. Brain 2004;127(pt 5):1127–1144

53. Laufs H, Lengler U, Hamandi K, Kleinschmidt A, Krakow K. Linking generalized spike-and-wave discharges and resting state brain activity by using EEG/fMRI in a patient with absence seizures. Epilepsia 2006;47(2):444–448

54. Gotman J. Epileptic networks studied with EEG-fMRI. Epilepsia 2008;49(suppl 3):42–51

55. Salek-Haddadi A, Diehl B, Hamandi K, et al. Hemodynamic correlates of epileptiform discharges: an EEG-fMRI study of 63 patients with focal epilepsy. Brain Res 2006;1088(1):148–166

56. Lantz G, Spinelli L, Menendez RG, Seeck M, Michel CM. Localization of distributed sources and comparison with functional MRI. Epileptic Disord 2001;special issue:45–58

57. Boor R, Jacobs J, Hinzmann A, et al. Combined spike-related functional MRI and multiple source analysis in the non-invasive spike localization of benign rolandic epilepsy. Clin Neurophysiol 2007; 118(4):901–909

58. Lemieux L, Krakow K, Fish DR. Comparison of spike-triggered functional MRI BOLD activation and EEG dipole model localization. Neuroimage 2001;14(5):1097–1104

59. Bagshaw AP, Kobayashi E, Dubeau F, Pike GB, Gotman J. Correspondence between EEG-fMRI and EEG dipole localisation of interictal discharges in focal epilepsy. Neuroimage 2006;30(2):417–425

60. Grova C, Daunizeau J, Kobayashi E, et al. Concordance between distributed EEG source localization and simultaneous EEG-fMRI studies of epileptic spikes. Neuroimage 2008;39(2):755–774

61. Brodbech V, Lascano AM, Spinelli L, Michel CM. Accuracy of EEG source imaging of epileptic spikes in patients with large brain lesions. Clin Neurophysiol 2009; 120:679–685

41 Optical Imaging Techniques in Neocortical Epilepsy

Daryl W. Hochman and Michael M. Haglund

Changes in the level of neuronal activity can alter the way in which visible light is absorbed and scattered by brain tissue.[1,2] Increases in action potential firing within organized networks of cortical neurons elicit transient optical changes that are localized in the tissue to the areas undergoing increased activity. Because these optical changes arise from the tissue itself and do not involve the application of dyes or contrast-enhancing agents, they are often referred to as intrinsic optical signals (IOSs). IOS imaging involves attaching a sensitive digital camera to an operating microscope, illuminating the cortical surface with light at appropriate wavelengths, and acquiring series of images that can then be processed and analyzed using digital imaging techniques and statistical modeling. This relatively straightforward technique makes it possible to acquire movies showing dynamic patterns of the IOS resulting from action potential firing. IOS-imaging has been used as an experimental technique in the laboratory since the 1980s to study the functional organization of sensory cortex in nonhuman primates.[3] It has been most often applied in the laboratory for studying the visual cortex, where it is possible to map functional units such as ocular dominance and orientation selectivity columns.[4] In recent years, IOS imaging has been adapted to the operating room where it has been shown to be capable of mapping language, motor, and sensory cortex, as well as the spread of epileptic activity in human subjects.[1,5–10]

High-resolution IOS imaging has several important limitations. These include its restriction to mapping activity on the exposed cortical surface and its temporal and spatial relationships to neuronal activity, which are still not completely understood. In spite of these limitations, IOS imaging has several major advantages, giving it the potential to be a widely useful tool in the operating room for online mapping of functional and epileptic tissue. Its main advantages are its ability to safely map patterns of cortical activity with micron-level resolution and its relative low cost. Because IOS imaging uses nonionizing light and does not require the use of potentially phototoxic optical dyes, it can safely map the cortex without any possibility of causing tissue damage. In addition, an IOS imaging system is a fraction of the cost and far simpler and more portable than other imaging technologies, such as functional magnetic resonance imaging (fMRI) and positron emission tomography.

A more complete understanding and interpretation of the activity-evoked optical changes in the cortex is required to allow IOS imaging to become a practical and useful clinical tool. An important issue that needs to be better understood is how accurately optical changes at various wavelengths localize normal and epileptic neuronal activity. Resolving this issue requires better elucidating the hemodynamic changes responsible for generating the activity-evoked optical changes in the neocortex. The remainder of this chapter focuses on this issue.

■ Relationships between the Optical Signal, Cerebral Hemodynamics, and Cortical Activity

Changes in the intrinsic optical properties of cortical tissue are thought to arise from activity-evoked changes in blood volume and blood oxygenation.[2] Action potential firing by cortical neurons is known to elicit a transient redistribution of blood within the active tissue, resulting in significant localized increases in blood flow and blood volume.[11] Signaling molecules, such as adenosine and nitric oxide, are released by neurons during action potential firing and diffused through the extracellular space to cause nearby pial arterioles to dilate.[12] It is known that the smallest pial arterioles with diameters less than 100 μm are the major mediators of this activity-evoked redistribution of blood within the neocortex.[13] Poiseuille's equation predicts that blood flow is related to the fourth-power of vessel diameter,[14] and hence small changes in neuronal activity are transformed into large increases in blood flow and volume through dilation of the pial arterioles, whose diameters can increase by 30% above their resting baseline size. The dramatic increase in flow velocity means that the transit time of hemoglobin molecules within the vicinity of the active tissue is significantly reduced, resulting in an increase in the amount of oxygenated hemoglobin in that portion of the venous network receiving the blood from the active tissue.[11] Blood oxygen dependent (BOLD)-fMRI, for example, relies on the detection of this activity-evoked increase in oxyhemoglobin (OxyHb).

IOS imaging takes advantage of the fact that OxyHb and deoxyhemoglobin (Hb) absorb light throughout the visible spectrum differently from each other (**Fig. 41.1A**). Their absorption

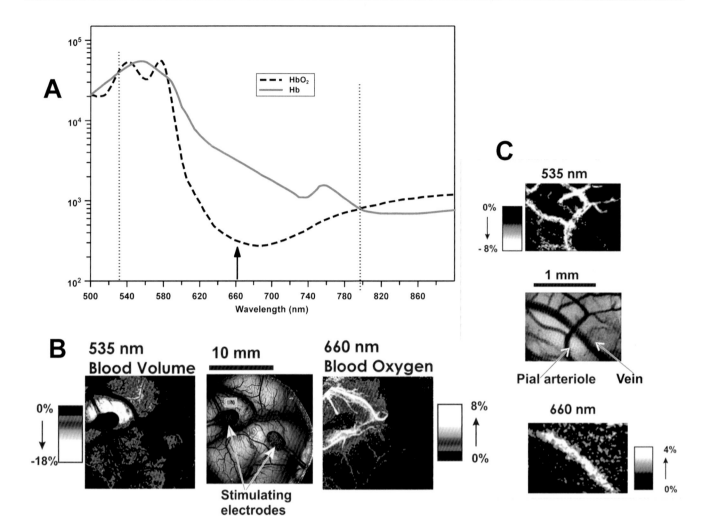

Fig. 41.1 **(A)** Plots of the optical absorption spectra for oxyhemoglobin (HbO$_2$) and deoxyhemoglobin (Hb). Plots are shown of the amount of light absorbed by HbO$_2$ (*dashed black line*) and Hb (*solid gray line*) across the optical spectrum, plotted on a logarithmic scale in units of Molar extinction coefficient (M^{-1}cm^{-1}) on the *y* axis versus wavelength (nm) on the *x* axis. HbO$_2$ and Hb both absorb exactly the same amount of light at certain wavelengths, such as 535 nm and 800 nm (*vertical dotted lines*). These wavelengths of equal optical absorption for both light-absorbing species are known as isosbestic points. Imaging at isosbestic points is useful for mapping changes in blood volume independent of changes in blood oxygenation. At 660 nm (*vertical arrow*), the difference between HbO$_2$ and Hb is maximal, and hence imaging at this wavelength is maximally sensitive to changes on blood oxygenation. **(B)** Low-magnification optical imaging of electrical stimulation-evoked activity in monkey cortex. The center image shows the position of the bipolar stimulating electrode on the cortical surface. The cortex was stimulated for 4 seconds with a current (6 mA; 60Hz biphasic) that was just below the after-discharge threshold. The leftmost image shows a map of the blood volume changes acquired with 535 nm light. As is typical, the largest changes occurs predominantly around one of the two stimulating electrodes. The largest optical changes at this wavelength appear to occur diffusely throughout the tissue surround the electrode and are absent in the larger blood vessels. The rightmost image shows the blood oxygenation map acquired with 660 nm light. At this wavelength, the largest changes occur in the larger veins nearest the stimulating electrodes. **(C)** High-magnification optical imaging of electrical stimulation-evoked cortical activity. These images show highly magnified changes occurring within the small square region drawn above the left electrode in the middle figure of **(B)**. The middle figure shows the microvascular network within the field of view, where the pial arteriole is approximately 30 μm in diameter. During stimulation, the pial arterial dilated approximately 30% above its resting diameter, mediating the blood volume change within that region of tissue. The top image shows that blood volume changes that were acquired with 535 nm light, demonstrating that the optical changes were restricted to the dilating pial arteriole. The bottom image shows that the blood oxygenation images acquired with 660 nm light were restricted to the small veins. The graphs in **(A)** were generated from publicly available data on the Internet compiled by Scott Prahl, Oregon Medical Laser Center at http://omlc.ogi.edu/spectra/hemoglobin/summary.html, tabulated from data by W. B. Gratzer, Medical Research Council Laboratories, Holly Hill, London, UK, and N. Kollias, Wellman Laboratories, Harvard Medical School, Boston, MA, USA. (The pictures in Figs. 41.1B, C were modified from Haglund MM. Hochman DW. Imaging of intrinsic optical signals in primate cortex during epileptiform activity. Epilepsia 2007;48 (suppl 4):65–74. Reprinted and modified by permission from Wiley-Blackwell.)

spectra show that at certain wavelengths, such as 535 nm (green light) and 800 nm (near-infrared light), OxyHb and Hb both absorb exactly the same amount of light, and hence optical imaging at these wavelengths would be insensitive to changes in the oxygen content of blood. By contrast, optical imaging at 660 nm (red light) would be expected to be highly sensitive to changes on blood oxygenation because OxyHb and Hb are maximally distinguishable at this wavelength. Several predictions follow from the facts described in the preceding section. First, it would

be expected that during activation, the cortex would absorb more light when illuminated with 535 nm light (i.e., become darker). This follows from the fact that dilating microscopic pial arterioles result in an increase in the number of light-absorbing hemoglobin molecules within a volume of tissue, and so more light would be expected to be absorbed at 535 nm, a wavelength that is insensitive to changes in blood oxygenation. By contrast, it would be expected that the veins receiving blood from active tissue would absorb less light or become brighter

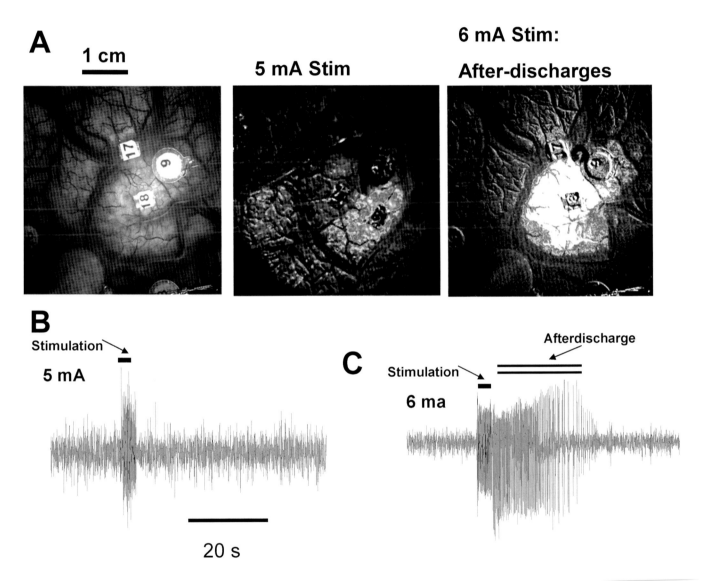

Fig. 41.2 Optical imaging of electrical stimulation-evoked after-discharge (ictal) activity in the human cortex. This figure shows a comparison of the blood volume changes elicited by a stimulation current that was just below the after-discharge threshold (5 mA) to those elicited by a current at the after-discharge threshold (6 mA) that elicited approximately 30 seconds of discharge activity. The left-most image in **(A)** shows the position of the bipolar electrodes on the cortical surface that are labeled "17" and "18," and the surface electroencephalography (EEG) recording electrode labeled "9." The

middle image shows the blood volume changes imaged at 535 nm resulting from 4 seconds of stimulation in which no after-discharge activity was elicited. The rightmost image in **(A)** shows the pattern of blood volume changes occurring during the after-discharge activity after 4 seconds of stimulation with 6 mA current. Note the increase in spread and magnitude of the optical changes. **(B)** and **(C)** show the simultaneously acquired EEG recordings at 5 mA and 6 mA, respectively. The after-discharge activity in **(C)** is indicated by the double horizontal lines above the EEG recording.

under illumination 660 nm light. This follows from the facts that there would be an increase in HbO_2 in the venous network, and HbO_2 absorbs less than Hb at this wavelength (**Fig. 41.1A**). These hypotheses have recently been tested and validated in the monkey cortex[2] (**Fig. 41.1B** and **41.1C**). IOS imaging was performed in those studies at sufficiently high magnification to reveal the optical changes occurring within the microscopic pial arterioles and surrounding venous network during electrical stimulation of the cortical surface. It can be seen that the optical changes at 535 nm are restricted to the dilating pial arterioles that absorb more light after cortical activation. At 660 nm, the optical changes are restricted to the nearby veins that become brighter at the same time (**Fig. 41.1C**). These experiments suggest optical changes at 535 nm are restricted to the dilating pial arterioles nearest to the neurons that fire action potential; hence, IOS imaging at this wavelength would be expected to generate maps that reliably localize cortical areas of increased activity. Optical changes at 660 nm are localized to the venous network, which receives blood from active cortical areas that is more highly oxygenated during increased neuronal activity. Because the more oxygenated blood may flow into vessels that may be located at various distances from the site of activation, it would be expected that IOS imaging at 660 nm would be less reliable for localizing active cortical areas. In summary, these recent studies suggest that IOS-imaging at 535 nm, which reflects activity-evoked changes in blood volume, may be an accurate and reliable method for intraoperative cortical mapping.

Intraoperative IOS imaging studies on human subjects further support the notion that IOS imaging of blood volume changes at 535 nm can be used to reliably map functional and epileptic activity.[1] We have recently performed a more extensive series of careful studies on the use of 535 nm IOS imaging for localizing cortical activity. One experimental method for investigating that ability of IOS imaging for mapping epileptic activity involves electrical stimulation of the cortex at various currents that are either below or at the threshold for eliciting after-discharge activity, which is electrophysiologically similar to ictal discharges (**Fig. 41.2**). Through stimulation of the cortex for 4-second durations with an Ojemann Stimulator (Integra Lifesciences Corporation, New Jersey, USA; 60 Hz, biphasic), it is typical to find stimulation currents that are just sufficient to reliably and repeatedly elicit after-discharges. Stimulation at a

current that is just 1 mA below this after-discharge threshold will fail to elicit any after-discharges. **Fig. 41.2A** shows data from one such experiment in which 6 mA was found to be the after-discharge threshold. In these experiments, it is found that after-discharge activity generates optical changes at 535 nm that are of significantly greater magnitude and of longer duration than optical changes elicited by neuronal activity below the after-discharge threshold. Further, the optical changes are observed to spread into cortical areas that are more distant from the stimulating electrodes during the after-discharge activity. These observations suggest that epileptic activity may have a distinctly different optical signature from nonepileptic activity. Intraoperative IOS imaging in combination with electrical stimulation may thus provide a reliable means to map epileptogenic cortical tissue.

■ Making IOS Imaging a Practical Clinical Tool

IOS imaging is currently an experimental technique that will require further development before it can become a practical method for intraoperative cortical mapping. Necessary steps include (a) further elucidation of the accuracy and reliability for localizing epileptic and functional activity and (b) further development of data processing and analysis techniques to provide a meaningful representation of optical imaging data to the neurosurgeon. This first step will require further human and animal studies aimed at carefully correlating optical changes to normal and epileptic electrophysiological activities. The second step is necessary because intraoperatively acquired optical data are extremely noisy—contaminated with artifacts from heartbeat, respiration, and random movements in the case of awake subjects. Data analysis methods need to be developed that remove the noise from the optical data while preserving the underlying activity-evoked signal. Ideally, these techniques will allow for a statistical analysis, so that, for example, optical maps can be generated that represent areas of optical changes with a well-defined statistical confidence level. Preliminary work in this area shows that statistical modeling of optical imaging data with dynamic linear models may be a promising approach to addressing this issue.[15]

References

1. Haglund MM, Hochman DW. Optical imaging of epileptiform activity in human neocortex. Epilepsia 2004;45(suppl 4):43–47
2. Haglund MM, Hochman DW. Imaging of intrinsic optical signals in primate cortex during epileptiform activity. Epilepsia 2007;48(suppl 4):65–74
3. Grinvald A, Frostig RD, Lieke E, Hildesheim R. Optical imaging of neuronal activity. Physiol Rev 1988;68(4):1285–1366
4. Xiao Y, Casti A, Xiao J, Kaplan E. Hue maps in primate striate cortex. Neuroimage 2007;35(2):771–786
5. Haglund MM, Ojemann GA, Hochman DW. Optical imaging of epileptiform and functional activity in human cerebral cortex. Nature 1992;358(6388):668–671
6. Cannestra AF, Pouratian N, Bookheimer SY, Martin NA, Beckerand DP, Toga AW. Temporal spatial differences observed by functional

MRI and human intraoperative optical imaging. Cereb Cortex 2001;11(8):773–782

7. Sato K, Nariai T, Sasaki S, et al. Intraoperative intrinsic optical imaging of neuronal activity from subdivisions of the human primary somatosensory cortex. Cereb Cortex 2002;12(3):269–280

8. Schwartz TH, Chen LM, Friedman RM, Spencer DD, Roe AW. Intraoperative optical imaging of human face cortical topography: a case study. Neuroreport 2004;15(9):1527–1531

9. Sato K, Nariai T, Tanaka Y, et al. Functional representation of the finger and face in the human somatosensory cortex: intraoperative intrinsic optical imaging. Neuroimage 2005;25(4):1292–1301

10. Zhao M, Suh M, Ma H, Perry C, Geneslaw A, Schwartz TH. Focal increases in perfusion and decreases in hemoglobin oxygenation precede seizure onset in spontaneous human epilepsy. Epilepsia 2007;48(11):2059–2067

11. Roland PE. Brain Activation. New York, NY: Wiley-Liss; 1997

12. Iadecola C. Neurovascular regulation in the normal brain and in Alzheimer's disease. Nat Rev Neurosci 2004;5(5):347–360

13. Mchedlishvili G. Arterial Behavior and Blood Circulation in the Brain. New York, NY: Plenum Press, 1987

14. Fung YC. Biomechanics: Circulation. New York, NY: Springer; 1997

15. Hochman DW, Lavine M, Haglund MM. Dynamic linear modeling of optical brain data. Paper presented at: Statistical Analysis of Neuronal Data Meeting. Pittsburgh, PA, 2006; May 29–31

Index

Note: Page numbers followed by *f* and *t* indicate figures and tables, respectively.